Dementia

A Clinical Approach

Second Edition

Dementia
A Clinical Approach
Second Edition

JEFFREY L. CUMMINGS, M.D.

Director, UCLA Alzheimer's Disease Center and Associate Professor of Neurology and Psychiatry UCLA School of Medicine; Chief, Behavioral Neuroscience Section, West Los Angeles Veterans Affairs Medical Center, Los Angeles, California

D. FRANK BENSON, M.D.

The Augustus S. Rose Professor of Neurology, Department of Neurology and Reed Neurological Research Center, UCLA School of Medicine, Los Angeles, California

BUTTERWORTH–HEINEMANN
Boston London Oxford Singapore Sydney Toronto Wellington

Every effort has been made to ensure that the drug dosage schedules within this text are accurate and conform to standards accepted at time of publication. However, as treatment recommendations vary in the light of continuing research and clinical experience, the reader is advised to verify drug dosage schedules herein with information found on product information sheets. This is especially true in cases of new or infrequently used drugs.

 Recognizing the importance of preserving what has been written, it is the policy of Butterworth–Heinemann to have the books it publishes printed on acid-free paper, and we exert our best efforts to that end.

Library of Congress Cataloging-in-Publication Data

Cummings, Jeffrey L., 1948–
  Dementia : a clinical approach / Jeffrey L. Cummings, D. Frank Benson.—2nd ed.
    p. cm.
  Includes bibliographical references.
  Includes index.
  ISBN 0-7506-9065-8 (casebound : alk. paper)
  1. Dementia. I. Benson, D. Frank (David Frank), 1928–
II. Title.
  [DNLM: 1. Dementia. WM 220 C971d]
  RC521.C86 1991
  616.8′3—dc20
  DNLM/DLC
  for Library of Congress   91-8289
                                                                   CIP

British Library Cataloguing in Publication Data
Cummings, Jeffrey L.
  Dementia : a clinical approach.—2nd. ed.
  1. Dementia
  I. Title II. Benson, D. Frank (David Frank) 1928–
  616.8983

  ISBN 0-7506-9065-8

Butterworth–Heinemann
313 Washington Street
Newton, MA 02158–1626

10 9 8 7 6 5 4 3
Printed in the United States of America

Contents

Preface to the Second Edition ix
Preface to the First Edition xiii
Acknowledgments xvii

1. Dementia: Definition, Prevalence, Classification, and
    Approach to Diagnosis 1
    Definition of Dementia 1
    Epidemiology 3
    Classification of Dementia and Systematic Approach to
    Diagnosis 9
    Differential Diagnosis of the Dementia Syndrome 13

2. Mental Status Examination 19
    Clinical Mental Status Examination 20
    Screening for Mental Status Dysfunction 38
    Psychological Testing 40

3. Cortical Dementias: Alzheimer's Disease and Other Cortical
    Degenerations 45
    Dementia of the Alzheimer Type (DAT) 46
    Pick's Disease 75
    Differentiating DAT from Pick's Disease and Other
    Disorders 87
    Focal Cortical Atrophies 90

4. Subcortical Dementias in the Extrapyramidal Disorders 95
    Huntington's Disease 95
    Progressive Supranuclear Palsy (PSP) 108
    Parkinson's Disease 113
    Wilson's Disease 128
    Hallervorden-Spatz Syndrome 136

Amyotrophic Lateral Sclerosis (ALS)–Parkinsonism–
    Dementia Complex   139
Spinocerebellar Degenerations   142
Idiopathic Calcification of the Basal Ganglia (ICBG)   150

5. Vascular Dementias   153
    Characteristics of Vascular Dementia   154
    Types of Vascular Dementia   156
    Etiologies of Vascular Dementia   169
    Cerebral Hypoperfusion as a Cause of Dementia   174
    Evaluation of Vascular Dementia   174
    Treatment of Vascular Dementia   175

6. HIV Encephalopathy, Jakob-Creutzfeldt Disease, and Other
    Infectious Dementias   177
    Viral and Prion Dementias   178
    Jakob-Creutzfeldt Disease   189
    Other Infectious Dementias   198

7. Dementia in Metabolic Disturbances and Toxic Conditions   217
    Metabolic Disturbances   219
    Toxic Dementias   249
    Dementia and Peripheral Neuropathy   264

8. Hydrocephalic Dementia   267
    Pathophysiology of Hydrocephalus   269
    Pathologic States Producing Hydrocephalic Dementia   273
    Symptomatology of Hydrocephalic Dementia   279
    Diagnostic Techniques   282
    Pathology   286
    Treatment   288
    Prognosis   290

9. Dementia Syndromes Associated with Psychiatric Disorders:
    The "Pseudodementias"   293
    Mood Disorders   294
    Schizophrenia   302
    Hysterical Dementia   304
    Ganser's Syndrome   305
    Miscellaneous Pseudodementias   306

10. Dementias Associated with Trauma, Neoplasms, Enzyme
    Deficiencies, Multiple Sclerosis, and Other Acquired
    and Inherited Disorders   307

Acquired Dementias 307
Inherited Disorders with Dementia 322
Miscellaneous Inherited Dementing Disorders 330

11. Aging and Senility 335
Clinical Alterations in Senility 336
Laboratory Changes in Senility 340
Postulated Causes of Senility 341
Differential Problems 343
Treatment of Senility 343

12. Laboratory Aids in the Diagnosis of Dementia 345
Clinical Laboratory and Pathologic Studies 346
Radiologic Examinations 351
Electrophysiologic Studies 357
Nuclear Medicine Investigations 361

13. Treatment, Long-Term Management, and Working with
Caregivers 365
Medical Issues in Long-Term Care 366
Behavioral Management in Long-Term Care 368
Community Resources 373
Nursing Home Care 377
Caregivers 379
Legal Counseling 380
Ethical Issues 381

14. Conclusions and Directions 383
Generalizations Concerning the Dementias 383
Changing Concepts of DAT 386
Future Trends 387

References 391
Index 531

Preface to the Second Edition

The first edition of this volume appeared in 1983 coincident with an emerging awareness of the importance of dementia as a major public health problem. Since that time, dementia of the Alzheimer type (DAT) by itself has become the fourth leading cause of death in the United States and other industrialized/computerized nations, and one family in every three is said to have a member with a dementia syndrome. *Dementia: A Clinical Approach* proved to be a valuable guide to understanding and evaluating dementia patients, and we were encouraged to update the volume with a second edition. We hope that this new version of the text will serve as a useful source of information and guidance to those who consult it.

There have been many changes in the field of dementia research and care since the first edition of *Dementia* appeared, and we have tried to incorporate those relevant to diagnosis and management in this revised volume. In the clinical arena, major strides have been made in diagnostic procedures, particularly neuroimaging. Magnetic resonance imaging (MRI) has come into widespread use and, where it is available, has virtually replaced X-ray computerized tomography (CT) as the technology of choice for the evaluation of the dementia patient. Its usefulness stems primarily from its sensitivity to ischemic and demyelinating lesions of the brain. Positron emission tomography (PET) scanning has become more widely available although it is still largely confined to a few centers and its application to the study of dementia remains in its infancy. Glucose metabolism studies with PET reveal distinctive patterns of cerebral activity in different disease states including DAT, Pick's disease, progressive supranuclear palsy, and others. Single photon emission computed tomography (SPECT) is also becoming more accessible, and its resolution is improving. This method for measuring cerebral perfusion requires less complex technical support than does PET and is likely to become the principal functional image useful in the evaluation of dementia syndromes. Characteristic patterns of decreased bilateral parietal lobe perfusion in DAT and diminished frontal lobe perfusion in frontal lobe degenerations such as Pick's disease have been identified. With the introduction and increased application of functional brain imaging such as PET and SPECT, diagnostic approaches to degenerative disorders are being altered, and the negative evaluation of the 1980s and before is being replaced by identification of distinctive clinical and laboratory findings in the major diseases. Wherever possible, information regarding these new imaging techniques have been incorporated with the description of the laboratory evaluation of each disease state.

Clinical diagnosis and research has also benefited from the evolution of standard nomenclatures. The latest revision of the *Diagnostic and Statistical Manual of Mental Disorders* as well as the Alzheimer's Disease Work Group of the Department of Health and Human Services have provided useful definitions of DAT and other dementias that provide a common basis for communication. We have either used these definitions or provided cogent reasons for not doing so in this edition of *Dementia*.

Geriatrics has also grown as a discipline since we initiated the first volume and has convincingly demonstrated that dementia in the elderly must be approached with full cognizance of the special circumstances of aging. Multiple illnesses, cohort effects, altered pharmacokinetics, tissue aging, and many other aspects of aging impact on dementia. We have tried to reflect this perspective here.

Another major area of growth in dementia research and care concerns long-term management, the continuum of care, and working with families. Most dementia patients will progress through a series of increasingly dependent states, and many will spend the last few years of their lives in nursing homes. Providing a continuum of resources such as day care, respite care, and institutional residence is becoming increasingly important; but few medical schools or training programs provide any experience in the problems that arise in the course of extended care. It is evident that families provide most of the care of dementia patients and that effective care of the dementia patient entails developing a successful working alliance with family caregivers. Spouses are required to put aside the expectations of their senior years to care for a partner who dies gradually over a 10-year period. Caregivers need education about diseases, interventions, and prognosis as well as the aid available through support groups, individual counseling, and other community resources (day care, and so forth). They require legal, medical, and social support. Those involved in the care of dementia patients must be knowledgeable in these areas, and we have added an entirely new chapter (13) to the book to discuss these concerns.

Acquired immune deficiency syndrome (AIDS) and its attendant dementia syndrome were barely known when the first edition of *Dementia* was published. This tragic illness has since become the most common infectious cause of dementia as well as the most common nontraumatic dementia in young adults. No discussion of dementia could be complete without careful consideration of HIV encephalopathy, and we have added this information to the second edition (Chapter 6).

Enormous effort has been expended in the investigation of the neurobiological basis of dementing disorders in the past few years. The focus of this book is clinical; it is not an in-depth review of the available scientific literature. In many instances, however, laboratory observations illuminate aspects of the clinical phenomenology, and we have tried to provide this clinically relevant information. In addition, updated references to much of this material are included and the reader may use these to further explore the basic science issues.

It is our hope that this new edition of *Dementia* will serve the practitioner as a useful guide to these complex and challenging illnesses.

J. L. C.
D. F. B.

Preface to the First Edition

This book is the result of the authors' collaboration in the evaluation of demented patients for almost a decade, spanning a period when ideas concerning dementia have been in a state of flux and our concepts about acquired intellectual impairment have evolved and changed. Most recent investigative work has focused on the basic science aspects of dementia, particularly the physical and chemical alterations occurring in Alzheimer disease. The results of this research have been valuable and exciting, but a considerable gap has opened between the new information and its application in the clinical management of demented patients. Our aim is to clarify for the practitioner the clinical use of this recently acquired knowledge.

Central to present understanding of the dementing disorders is the concept of cortical versus subcortical patterns of dementia. This differentiation, which can be made on clinical grounds, permits distinction between the irreversible dementias such as Alzheimer disease and those dementing illnesses caused by a potentially treatable underlying process. Alzheimer disease has often been a diagnosis made by exclusion; the systematic approach to evaluation presented here seeks to guide the practitioner in diagnosing dementing illnesses based on positive clinical findings.

Written for neurologists, psychiatrists, geriatricians, internists, and other professionals confronted with the ever-increasing number of demented individuals and the difficult problems they raise, *Dementia: A Clinical Approach* is intended as a compendium of useful information, as a reference and guide to the literature, and as a tool for use in the investigation of patients suffering from dementia. We have not attempted to present an update of all the new research findings in Alzheimer disease and other dementias; that material has been well reviewed in several recent publications. Ours is a clinical approach.

A working definition, classification, and systematic diagnostic approach to dementia are presented in Chapter 1, and individual sections of the following chapters are devoted to Alzheimer disease, Pick disease, vascular and infectious dementias, dementias in extrapyramidal syndromes, hydrocephalic dementias, toxic and metabolic disturbances of mental function, and intellectual compromise in traumatic, neoplastic, and demyelinating disorders. The mental status alterations accompanying normal aging are described and contrasted with those of dementia. The characteristics of dementias associated with cerebral cortical dysfunction are distinguished from those produced by disruption of subcortical function, and the usefulness of subcortical features for the identification of potentially treatable disorders is emphasized. Separate chapters are devoted to the mental status examination in dementia and to laboratory evaluation of the demented patient. New information concerning laboratory studies, including the use of positron emission tomography and x-ray computed tomography, is presented.

Many of the ideas set forth in this book are not entirely own own; we have been inspired and our thinking has been modified by colleagues in many institutions. In particular, the work on which this volume is based has depended on input of friends and collaborators in the West Los Angeles Veterans Administration Medical Center, the UCLA Department of Neurology, the Boston Veterans Administration Medical Center, the Boston University Department of Neurology, the National Hospital for Nervous Diseases, Queen Square, London, and the Institute of Psychiatry, Maudsley Hospital, London. In addition, the authors have been privileged to attend several national and international meetings devoted to the study of aging and dementia; this volume reflects many of the new ideas proposed at those meetings.

Numerous individuals have contributed directly or indirectly to the material that appears in this book; space permits mention of only a few. Professor Leo Duchen, Director of the Department of Neuropathology, Institute of Neurology and National Hospital for Nervous Diseases, Queen Square, London, generously shared his time and expertise and contributed most of the photographs of pathologic specimens shown in Chapters 3 and 5. Dr. David Kuhl and Dr. Michael Phelps of the Divisions of Biophysics and Nuclear Medicine, Department of Radiological Sciences, Laboratory of Biomedical and Environmental Sciences, UCLA School of Medicine, have collaborated with us and encouraged study of demented patients with the positron emission tomographic techniques they have developed. Funds from the Augustus Rose Chair in Neurology contributed important support toward completion of this work. Our secretaries, Norene Hiekel and Bonita Porch, spent many hours preparing the manuscript, proofreading, checking refer- ences, and the like, and have earned our enduring gratitude. Finally, com- pletion of this book would have been impossible without the constant support and encouragement we received from our wives, Inese Verzemnieks and Donna Benson.

J. L. C.
D. F. B.

Acknowledgments

We would like to thank all of our readers who found the first edition of *Dementia* useful and encouraged us to update and revise it. Many of our friends spotted errors in the first edition or provided valuable suggestions for material to be developed in the second edition. Acknowledgment is also due our colleagues and the Fellows in the UCLA Neurobehavior Program who challenge and motivate us to better understand the dementing illnesses. We must also thank our patients and their families: they are our greatest teachers, and without their guidance, we would never have found our way through the labyrinth to our current point of view. Bonita Porch provided faithful support for the development of the manuscript, and Norene Hiekel also provided devoted secretarial support. Our wives, Inese and Donna, have endured the sacrifices required for this volume without complaint; their love and understanding made this project possible.

1
Dementia: Definition, Prevalence, Classification, and Approach to Diagnosis

Dementia is an acquired syndrome of intellectual impairment produced by brain dysfunction. Its prevalence is rapidly increasing, and adequate care of the burgeoning population of demented individuals requires a knowledgeable approach to diagnosis and management. The purpose of this volume is to provide clinicians involved in the evaluation, diagnosis, and treatment of demented patients with a useful guide to identification and management of the dementia syndrome. This chapter reviews the definition, prevalence, and differential diagnosis of dementia. A systematic approach to evaluation of demented patients is introduced and the division of dementias into cortical and subcortical types is presented. The remaining chapters discuss use of the mental status examination in the clinical evaluation of demented patients, the many illnesses that can produce a dementia syndrome, and laboratory studies available to aid in differential diagnosis. A clinical approach is stressed throughout; distinctions between dementia and normal aging are drawn; and appropriate management and family care is described.

DEFINITION OF DEMENTIA

Operationally, dementia can be defined as an acquired persistent impairment of intellectual function with compromise in at least three of the following spheres of mental activity: language, memory, visuospatial skills, emotion

1

or personality, and cognition (abstraction, calculation, judgment, executive function, and so forth) (Cummings et al., 1980a). This definition is based on evaluation of disturbances that are readily testable at the bedside or may be quantitated using neuropsychological testing. The stipulation that the intellectual impairment must be acquired distinguishes dementia from the congenital mental retardation syndromes. The examiner must be certain that the failed material was previously within the intellectual grasp of the patient before considering the diagnosis of dementia. Persistence is included as a criterion to exclude confusional states frequently noted in acute traumatic, metabolic, and toxic disorders. Conditions lasting hours to days are more appropriately regarded as acute confusional states or delirium, whereas those lasting weeks to months are properly considered dementias. The definition excludes patients with relatively isolated neuropsychological disturbances such as aphasia or amnesia that occur with focal brain lesions. On the other hand, few if any dementias are truly global. Throughout this book we emphasize that it is the retention of specific intellectual functions contrasting with the deterioration of others that gives rise to identifiable neuropsychological patterns within the dementia syndrome. These patterns are both anatomically and etiologically revealing. Except for a few metabolic, toxic, and infectious conditions that advance rapidly to coma and death, dementing processes do not affect all intellectual abilities to similar degrees.

The identification of a dementia syndrome does not imply any specific cause, and the definition is equally applicable to reversible and irreversible changes in mental status. Structural, metabolic, toxic, and psychiatric etiologies are included. Thus recognition of a dementia syndrome is not a cause for nihilistic despair; rather, it is a diagnostic challenge that demands thorough evaluation of the patient for potentially treatable processes that may be producing or exacerbating the intellectual impairment.

Historically, the term *dementia* has been used in a variety of ways. It was introduced into American neuropsychiatric terminology by Benjamin Rush in 1812 (Slaby and Wyatt, 1974). He borrowed the term from Pinel, the great French psychiatrist, who had used it to refer to patients with intellectual deterioration and idiocy (Alexander and Selesnick, 1966). Since its introduction, the term has been defined and redefined, each new meaning reflecting the progressive evolution of knowledge concerning the types of disorders that produce intellectual deterioration as well as changing conceptions about criteria for identifying and diagnosing dementia.

Currently, dementia is often used synonymously with organic brain syndrome. The latter is too broad to be used meaningfully since it includes focal syndromes such as aphasia and amnesia as well as the dementias. The modifiers "acute" and "chronic" have been appended with the implication that acute organic brain syndromes are short-lived, reversible forms of intellectual impairment secondary to metabolic or toxic disturbances whereas chronic organic brain syndrome indicates a chronic condition based on irreversible structural changes in the central nervous system (CNS). Well founded as these ideas may have been, they are now obsolete. Dementia such as that associated with normal-pressure hydrocephalus may begin abruptly after head trauma or subarachnoid hemorrhage, is produced by structural alterations in the nervous system and yet may reverse completely with appropriate surgical intervention. On the other hand, metabolic disturbances such as hypothyroidism or vitamin B_{12} deficiency can exist undetected for years and produce insidiously progressive and sometimes permanent intellectual impairment. Thus hydrocephalic dementias are based on structural changes but may be reversible, whereas some metabolic and toxic disorders may be chronic and irreversible. These inconsistencies indicate the need for abandoning organic brain syndrome in favor of the more adequate term *dementia.*

A widely used definition of dementia is that of the revised third edition of the *Diagnostic and Statistical Manual of Mental Disorders* (DSMIIIR) (American Psychiatric Association, 1987). This definition requires that the patient have impairment of short- and long-term memory in addition to abnormalities in at least one of the areas of mental function: abstract thinking, judgment, language, praxis, visual recognition, constructional abilities, or personality. These disturbances must be sufficiently severe to interfere with work, social activities, or relationships with others. The abnormalities must not occur exclusively during the course of delirium, and there must be evidence of an organic etiology or evidence that the disorder cannot be attributed to a "nonorganic" mental disorder such as depression. This definition has several limitations. First, by requiring that all demented patients have a memory impairment, it excludes disorders such as Pick's disease that have preserved memory in the early and middle phases of the illness (Chapter 3). Second, the requirement of social or occupational disability renders the definition imprecise and unquantifiable—patients with minimally demanding circumstances would not be considered demented with the same disability that would warrant that diagnosis in a more exacting situation. Third, by excluding psychiatric disorders including depression as potential causes of dementia, the definition prohibits consideration of the dementia syndrome of dementia, an increasingly recognized clinical condition (Chapter 9). The definition used throughout this volume has the advantage of flexibility and quantifiability. In common disorders such as Alzheimer's disease, both definitions apply equally well and identify the same patient population as demented; it is the less common conditions that the DSMIIIR definition may fail to recognize.

EPIDEMIOLOGY

Prevalence of Dementia

The rapidly increasing incidence of dementia has been called an approaching epidemic (Plum, 1979) and a deluge (Wells, 1981). These alarmist terms appear justified when it is realized that most dementias are found in people over the age of 65 years and that the elderly population is increasing rapidly in both absolute numbers and percentage of the population. In 1950, 8 percent of the population of the United States was over 65 years, accounting for 12.3 million people. By 1978, the proportion had risen to 11 percent and amounted to 22 million individuals. It is estimated that by the year 2030 those over age 65 will constitute between 17 and 20 percent of the population, about 51 million persons (Plum, 1979; Schoenberg, 1986). The cost of caring for demented patients soared from its 1978 level of $12 billion per annum to its current $30 billion annual economic toll (Hay and Ernst, 1987).

The actual prevalence of dementia, including mild as well as severe cases and patients remaining at home as well as those in hospitals, institutions, and nursing homes, has been difficult to determine, and the true prevalence of dementia is unknown. All studies concur, however, in suggesting that dementia is a major problem among the elderly and will be an even larger public health concern as the size of the aged population increases. In a recent review of 20 published studies of the prevalence of dementia in various countries of the world, Ineichen (1987) found prevalence rates ranging from 2.5 to 24.6 percent of those over age 65. The variability among studies reflected different definitions of dementia, use of instruments of different sensitivity, different sampling techniques, and different approaches to extrapolating results to a larger population. No systematic differences emerged suggesting an increased risk in any particular world population. In a similar meta-analysis, Henderson (1986) reported that the observed prevalence of mild dementia varied from 1.5 to 21.9 percent; of moderate dementia, from 1.1 to 13 percent; and of severe dementia, from 0.6 to 12.1 percent. In a study of a racially balanced population in Copiah County, Mississippi, based on a house to house survey that incorporated 97 percent of all inhabited dwellings in the county, Schoenberg et al (1985) found that the prevalence of *severe* dementia among individuals over age 40 was 1 percent. The figure rose to 7 percent for individuals 80 years old or older. There were no marked differences between men and women or between blacks and whites. Average figures for the prevalence of dementia would suggest that approximately 6 percent of those over age 65 manifest severe dementia, and an additional 10 to 15 percent have mild to moderate intellectual impairment (Gunner-Svensson and Jensen, 1976; Kay et al, 1970; Mortimer et al, 1981; Nielsen, 1962). The prevalence of dementia doubles approximately every five years after age 65 (Jorm et al, 1987). Kokmen and coworkers (1989) found the following age-specific prevalence rates for moderate to severe dementia in the region of Rochester, Minnesota: age 60–64, 0.2 percent; age 65–69, 0.9 percent; age 70–74, 2 percent; age 75–79, 4 percent; age 80–84, 9 percent; and age 85 and older, 16 percent. A similar marked age-related increase in dementia was noted when the incidence (new cases/100,000/year) was studied in this same population. Schoenberg and colleagues (1987) found the incidence rate to be 0.004 percent for 30- to 59-year-olds, 0.09 percent for 60- to 69-year-olds, 0.5 percent for 70- to 79-year olds, and 1.4 percent for those 80 years old and older. The high frequency of dementia among the elderly leads to a heavy use of health care resources. Dementia accounts for more admissions and hospital in-patient days than does any other psychiatric condition in the geriatric-age group (Christie, 1982; Kay et al, 1970).

The severity and prevalence of dementia are also highly correlated with the type of health care facility studied. The prevalence of severe dementia is 54 percent among the elderly in state hospitals; 30 percent, in nursing homes; and 15 percent in retirement communities; it is reportedly 94 percent, 87 percent, and 80 percent respectively for dementia of at least mild degree in these facilities (Goldfarb, 1962). There is a definite tendency for the more severe dementias to be concentrated in hospitals and publicly supported facilities.

Prevalence of Types of Dementia

The information quoted above did not establish the prevalence of different types of dementia, and the relative frequency of dementia of different etiologies has proved remarkably difficult to ascertain. Most studies surveying the various causes of the dementia syndrome have been hospital-based. As already noted, this is a selected population; patients hospitalized for dementia have more severe intellectual impairment and progressive disorders such as Alzheimer's disease and multi-infarct dementia are likely to be over-represented, whereas the milder dementias that accompany chronic systemic illnesses, trauma, and depression will be underrepresented.

Table 1–1 presents nine studies of groups of demented patients, representing 1363 individuals admitted for evaluation of progressive intellectual deterioration. Most of the studies are based on patients admitted to neurologic or psychiatric units and include relatively few cases of dementia associated with chronic medical problems such as uremia, hepatic failure, pulmonary and cardiac disease, or endocrinopathies (most of these patients would be admitted to medical units for management). The relative absence of movement disorders (16 patients with Huntington's disease and 6 patients with Parkinson's disease) suggests that the dementias accompanying these conditions and other specific neurologic syndromes are also underrepresented in these studies. Similarly, fewer toxic causes of intellectual impairment are listed than would be expected. Only 8 cases of intoxication were recorded among the 1363 evaluations, whereas Learoyd (1972) found that at least 16 percent of all psychiatric admissions of geriatric-age individuals were directly attributable to the effects of psychoactive drugs. Most such patients are probably recognized and managed as outpatients, but many may

TABLE 1-1.   Relative prevalence of different types of dementia among patients referred for evaluation of progressive intellectual deterioration.

Final diagnosis	Marsden and Harrison (1972)	Freemon (1976)	Victoratos et al (1977)	Smith and Kiloh (1981)	Hutton (1981b)	Maletta et al (1982)	Benson et al (1982)	Erkinjuntti et al (1987)	Thal et al (1988)
	No. (%)	No. (%)	No. (%)	No. (%)	No. (%)	No. (%)	No. (%)	No. (%)	No. (%)
Alzheimer's disease	48 (45)	26 (43)	30 (57)	84 (42)	22 (22)	43 (43)	22 (24)	73 (26)	264 (70)
Alcoholic dementia	6 (6)	4 (7)	1 (2)	30 (15)	12 (12)	7 (7)		5 (2)	3 (1)
Multi-infarct dementia	8 (8)	5 (8)	5 (10)	22 (11)	12 (12)	10 (10)	31 (34)	70 (25)	18 (4.8)
Infections	4 (4)		2 (4)	1 (1)	2 (2)			2 (1)	
Metabolic conditions				2 (1)	9 (9)	3 (3)	15 (17)	5 (2)	5 (1)
Neoplasms	8 (8)	2 (3)	4 (8)	3 (2)	4 (4)	1 (1)	2 (2)	4 (2)	3 (1)
Hydrocephalus	5 (5)	7 (12)	1 (2)	8 (4)	1 (1)	1 (1)	4 (4)	5 (2)	2 (1)
Toxic conditions		5 (8)			2 (2)	1 (1)			
Posttrauma	1 (1)		1 (2)	5 (3)	2 (2)			3 (1)	3 (1)
Postanoxia			1 (2)	1 (1)					
Subdural hematoma			1 (2)					2 (1)	
Huntington's disease	3 (3)	4 (7)		5 (3)		2 (2)		2 (1)	
Parkinson's disease			1 (2)					5 (2)	
Miscellaneous	8 (8)	6 (10)	3 (6)	19 (10)	8 (18)	3 (3)	8 (9)	22 (8)	50 (16)
Dementia associated with a psychiatric disorder	15 (15)	1 (2)		20 (10)	18 (18)	28 (28)	6 (7)	46 (16)	11 (3)
Not demented	----	----	2 (4)	----	8 (8)	1 (1)	2 (2)	36 (13)	16 (4)
Totals	106	60	52	200	100	100	90	280	375

go unrecognized with their cognitive deterioration attributed to idiopathic dementia.

The dementia syndrome of depression is another category underrepresented in Table 1–1. None of the studies shown were subjected to follow-up verification, and existing studies of the stability of neuropsychiatric diagnosis over time suggest that the final diagnosis might be changed in a sizeable number of cases. Studies of patients diagnosed as having presenile dementia (probable Alzheimer's disease) and reexamined 5 to 15 years later show that from 25 to 57 percent failed to deteriorate in the expected manner and were subsequently rediagnosed (Kendell, 1974; Nott and Fleminger, 1975; Ron et al, 1979). In these surveys, depression was the principal disorder that went unrecognized as the cause of intellectual deterioration. Current, more stringent criteria for the diagnosis of Alzheimer's disease (Chapter 3) have improved diagnostic accuracy, but distinguishing among disorders that lack specific biologic markers is still fraught with error.

Alzheimer's disease represents 45 percent of the total cumulative dementias shown in Table 1–1 and was diagnosed in 22 to 70 percent of patients in the individual studies. This wide variation in the apparent prevalence of Alzheimer's disease reflects variations in referral patterns and diagnostic approaches. Sampling and diagnostic biases increase both the actual and the apparent number of patients with Alzheimer's disease in most reported studies. The selection of the more severe and progressive dementias for in-hospital evaluation and management, exclusion of the many metabolic and systemic causes of dementia, failure to include most dementing disorders associated with specific neurologic disorders, and underrecognition of depression and drug intoxication as sources of intellectual impairment combine to produce an overrepresentation of Alzheimer's disease in the reported series. This trend is further complicated by the tendency to regard Alzheimer's disease as a diagnosis of exclusion based on the absence of other identifiable causes of dementia. Such a category is bound to include all unrecognized causes of dementia in addition to true cases of Alzheimer's disease. Thus, the 22 to 70 percent of cases of dementia (Table 1–1) diagnosed as Alzheimer's disease almost certainly overestimates the actual occurrence of Alzheimer's disease as a cause of intellectual impairment in the general population. This is not to de-emphasize the importance of that disease as a cause of dementia or to disparage the efforts currently being directed at understanding and treating it. Rather, this is an attempt to show the true magnitude of the problem of dementia when all sources and causes are considered. Even though its relative occurrence has probably been exaggerated, Alzheimer's disease is a common disorder and, because of its untreatable and relentless course, one of the most important causes of dementia.

The accuracy of diagnosis of Alzheimer's disease has been improved by the introduction of the diagnostic criteria developed by the National

Institute of Neurologic and Communicative Disorders and Stroke and the Alzheimer's Disease and Related Disorders Association Work Group (McKhann et al, 1984)(Chapter 3). With these guidelines, the accuracy of diagnosis has been reported to be as high as 88 percent (Tierney et al, 1988), although some studies report clinicopathologic concordance as low as 63 percent even with these improved standards (Boller et al, 1989).

Progress in the clinical care of patients with Alzheimer's disease and more successful research into dementia of the Alzheimer type depend on reliable clinical identification of the disease. A systematic approach to diagnosis is outlined later in this chapter, and positive criteria for the identification of Alzheimer's disease are presented in Chapter 3. These criteria allow the diagnosis to be based as much as possible on identifiable clinical features rather than approaching Alzheimer's disease as diagnosis of exclusion or a post-mortem diagnosis.

Multi-infarct dementia is the second most common cause of dementia in the cumulative totals of Table 1–1 and was identified in as few as 8 percent and as many as 34 percent in the individual series. Again referral patterns and diagnostic rigor no doubt play a role in the readiness with which clinicians consider the diagnosis of vascular dementia. In general, heightened awareness of the potential role of vascular disease in intellectual impairment and improved techniques for detecting ischemic brain injury (particularly magnetic resonance imaging) are leading to an increased recognition of vascular dementia.

The few available autopsy series of demented patients are subject to even greater collection biases than are the clinical studies. Most subjects have been of advanced age with severe dementia and have died in chronic care institutions from complications of their dementing process. Fifty percent of such patients have Alzheimer's disease, approximately 20 percent have multi-infarct dementia, and 15 to 20 percent have a combination of the two conditions (Jellinger, 1976; Tomlinson et al, 1970). While this is valuable information, the selection process makes it impossible to extrapolate to the causes of dementia in a general population. In addition, the increased occurrence of Alzheimer-type neuropathologic changes in the brains of elderly individuals—whether demented or not—makes interpretation of autopsy material difficult without careful quantitative studies of the changes.

Thus available studies provide limited insight into the relative importance of the different etiologies of dementia. Table 1–1 can be used only as a general guide to the prevalence of different causes of intellectual deterioration among patients referred for evaluation of dementia.

CLASSIFICATION OF DEMENTIA AND SYSTEMATIC APPROACH TO DIAGNOSIS

Differential involvement of CNS structures by dementing processes produces identifiable patterns of neuropsychological deficits. Although dementia has often been considered a global disorder, there is no dementing illness that involves all areas of the brain equally or affects all neuropsychological activities to the same degree. Rather, each type of dementia involves some structures more and others less or not at all; the specific topography of involvement is manifested clinically by differing patterns of mental status alteration.

Two basic patterns of neuropsychological impairment have been distinguished within the dementia syndrome and have been labeled according to the major associated neuroanatomic involvement. The first pattern includes *cortical* dementias such as Alzheimer's disease and Pick's disease that affect primarily the cerebral cortex. The second major category has been termed *subcortical* dementia and includes the extrapyramidal disorders, hydrocephalus, white matter diseases, and subcortical vascular diseases that produce maximal dysfunction in the basal ganglia, thalamus, and brainstem. A *mixed* category also exists, including conditions such as some forms of multi-infarct dementia, toxic-metabolic conditions, and slow virus infections that involve both cortical and subcortical structures. Controversy has arisen with regard to the use of the term *subcortical* since some of the dementias included in that group involve either the frontal cortex or frontal-subcortical connections (Mayeux et al, 1983). Anatomically and physiologically, the basal ganglia, selected nuclei of the thalamus, and the prefrontal cortex form a unified frontal-subcortical system, and involvement of any portion will disrupt functions of the entire circuit. Similar deficits will result regardless of the area affected (Alexander et al, 1986; Nauta, 1971, 1979; Rosvold, 1972). The term *subcortical* has been retained for these disorders because the major impact of most of the conditions (extrapyramidal disorders, hydrocephalus, and toxic-metabolic disorders) is on the subcortical components of the system. A classification of the different etiologies of dementia based on whether they affect primarily cortical or subcortical structures is presented in Table 1–2.

The clinical characteristics of the cortical and subcortical types of dementia are shown in Table 1–3 (Cummings, 1986, 1990; Cummings and Benson, 1984). The mental status changes of patients with cortical dementias are fully explained in Chapter 3 and are summarized here. These deficits resemble those in focal processes involving the cerebral cortex and include aphasia with naming difficulties and impaired comprehension, memory disturbances (including deficits in both new learning and remote recall), agnosia, and apraxia. Visuospatial and constructional disturbances may be prominent, calculating ability is disrupted, and judgment is poor. Dressing

TABLE 1–2.   Classification of the major causes of dementia based on the occurrence of features of cortical or subcortical dysfunction.

Cortical dementias	Dementias with combined cortical and
Alzheimer's disease	subcortical dysfunction
Frontal lobe degeneration	Multi-infarct dementias
Subcortical dementias	Infectious dementias
Extrapyramidal syndromes	Slow virus dementias
Parkinson's disease	General paresis
Huntington's disease	Toxic and metabolic
Progressive supranuclear palsy	encephalopathies
Wilson's disease	Systemic illnesses
Spinocerebellar degenerations	Endocrinopathies
Idiopathic basal ganglia	Deficiency states
calcification	Drug intoxications
Hydrocephalus	Heavy metal exposure
Dementia syndrome of depression	Industrial dementias
White matter diseases	Miscellaneous dementia syndromes
Multiple sclerosis	Posttraumatic
Human immunodeficiency	Postanoxic
virus (HIV) encephalopathy	Neoplastic
Vascular dementias	Etc.
Lacunar state	
Binswanger's disease	

disturbances and environmental disorientation are frequently evident. Personality may be relatively preserved, but disinterest and/or disinhibition may appear (Cummings, 1982; Cummings and Benson, 1986). In contrast to the abnormal mental state, the basic neurologic examination remains remarkably normal in patients with cortical dementias until the late phases of disease. Gait, posture, tone, and reflexes are preserved. In contrast to the abnormal language, speech retains normal volume and articulation.

The clinical characteristics of the subcortical dementias contrast sharply with those of the cortical dementing processes. The cardinal features of the mental status of patients with subcortical dementias are a slowing and dilapidation of cognition, forgetfulness, and alterations in affect (Albert et al, 1974; Cummings and Benson, 1984; McHugh and Folstein, 1975). Along with the typical bradykinesia evident in motor function, there is a slowing of speech, cognition, and comprehension. Memory disturbances include forgetfulness characterized by difficulty in spontaneously retrieving information. The patients are aided by clues and structure, and can often be shown to have learned much that they cannot recall without prompting. Patients with subcortical dementias also have an impairment of cognition that is difficult to characterize accurately and has been termed *dilapidation* (McHugh and Folstein, 1975). Thus they may correctly perform individual

TABLE 1–3.   Clinical characteristics of cortical and subcortical dementias.

Characteristic	Cortical dementia	Subcortical dementia
Verbal output		
Language	Aphasic	Normal
Speech	Normal	Abnormal (hypophonic, dysarthric, mute)
Mental status		
Memory	Amnesia (learning deficit)	Forgetful (retrieval deficit)
Cognition	Abnormal (acalculia, poor judgment, impaired abstraction)	Abnormal (slowed, dilapidated)
Visuospatial	Abnormal	Abnormal
Affect	Abnormal (unconcerned or disinhibited)	Abnormal (apathetic or depressed)
Motor system		
Posture	Normal*	Abnormal (stooped, extended)
Tone	Normal*	Usually increased
Movements	Normal*	Abnormal (tremor, chorea, asterixis, dystonia)
Gait	Normal*	Abnormal

*Motor system impairment with increased tone and a tendency to assume flexed postures becomes evident in the final stages of the cortical dementias.

steps of a complex problem but fail to synthesize the elements properly to achieve the correct answer; producing strategies and manipulating the necessary sequential steps is impossible. The final feature of the subcortical dementias is a disturbance of mood. Depression is the most commonly described disorder, and mania and apathy have also been observed. Decreased motivation is apparent in most cases.

Motor activity is often markedly altered in disorders manifesting subcortical dementia. Posture may be stooped as in Parkinson's disease or hyperextended, as in progressive supranuclear palsy; movements are slow, and choreoathetosis, tremor, dystonia, or asterixis may be present; tone is usually increased and speech output is dysarthric.

Recognition of these two basic clinical patterns of dementia, reflecting primarily cortical or subcortical involvement of the nervous system, is a major initial step toward establishment of an etiologic diagnosis and appropriate management.

Figure 1–1 presents a systematic approach to the diagnosis of specific causes of the dementia syndrome. The first step is to distinguish dementias with features of cortical involvement from those with subcortical characteristics or mixed cortical and subcortical attributes. Alzheimer's and Pick's

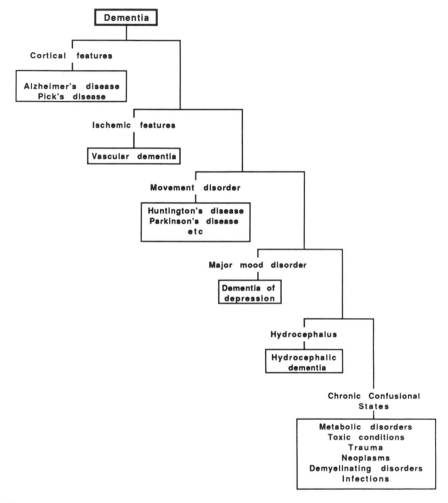

FIGURE 1–1.   Systematic approach to diagnosis of the etiologies of the dementia syndrome.

disease are thus identified as cortical dementias. Next, those dementias occurring in individuals with evidence of extensive intracranial vascular disease—abrupt onset, stepwise deterioration, and focal neurologic symptoms and signs—are identified as vascular dementias. Then dementias associated with extrapyramidal syndromes such as Huntington's disease or Parkinson's disease are distinguished. The dementia syndrome of depression is next considered in patients with signs of a major mood disorder, and hydrocephalus is diagnosed by radiologic evaluation. The remaining category, designated chronic confusional states, is a heterogeneous class including chronic toxic and metabolic encephalopathies as well as dementias associated with trauma, neoplasms, subdural hematomas, demyelinating disorders, CNS infections, and so forth. Laboratory studies, EEGs, and neuroradiologic procedures are necessary to help identify individual diseases within each group. The approach outlined in Figure 1–1 will lead to identification of most causes of dementia in the individual presenting progressive intellectual deterioration.

DIFFERENTIAL DIAGNOSIS OF THE DEMENTIA SYNDROME

Dementia must be differentiated from several focal syndromes and from delirium. Aphasia, amnesia, and the acute confusional states in particular require management and intervention strategies different from those of dementia and must be distinguished from dementia syndromes.

Aphasia

Fluent aphasia with normal or increased verbal output, naming difficulties, and impaired comprehension may be seen as part of a dementing illness affecting the cerebral cortex but may also occur as a result of a focal lesion affecting the posterior aspect of the language-dominant hemisphere. The presence of a language disturbance interferes with testing many aspects of the mental status including calculations, recent and remote memory, and abstraction. If the comprehension defect is severe, most components of the mental state are untestable. The general behavior of the two groups of patients, however, is different. In contrast to demented patients, those with focal aphasic syndromes usually show active engagement in conversation and a desire to communicate; they recognize what is happening around them, and they participate in ward and home activities; they are usually topographically oriented; and they remember people, places, and routines even though they cannot express this memory in words. Nonverbal memory tests and tests of abstraction not dependent on language may demonstrate intact extralinguistic intellect. These features help distinguish patients with a focal lesion from those with cortical dementias (Chapters 3 and 5 give additional details).

Amnesia

Amnesia, like aphasia, may masquerade as dementia, although it is usually easily distinguished if the definition of dementia is adhered to. The diagnosis of dementia depends on the presence of compromise in multiple areas of neuropsychological activity, whereas amnesia implies a deficit primarily involving recent memory (Benson, 1978). Memory is impaired in nearly all types of dementia: in subcortical dementias forgetfulness is apparent, and in cortical dementias learning new information and recollection of remote material are disturbed. Specific amnesic disorders usually result from bilateral lesions involving the medial limbic structures and/or diencephalon, including the hippocampus, fornix, mamillary bodies, and mediodorsal nuclei of the thalamus. Amnesia may result from posterior cerebral artery occlusion, anoxia, hypoglycemia, herpes simplex encephalitis, trauma, temporal lobe surgery, electroconvulsive therapy, and thiamine deficiency states (Benson, 1978; Symonds, 1966). In amnesia the focal nature of the damage spares other intellectual activities, and careful testing distinguishes the amnesia syndrome from dementia.

Acute Confusional States

The most characteristic feature of delirium or acute confusional states is reduction or impairment of attention (Strub, 1982). Other cardinal features are abrupt onset, short duration, impaired memory, incoherence of thought and conversation, hallucinations, delusions, disturbances of the sleep-wakefulness cycle, abnormal EEG, and evidence of systemic illness (Beresin, 1988; Chedru and Geschwind, 1972; Engel and Romano, 1959; Lipowski, 1980a, b, 1987; Wolff and Curran, 1935).

Table 1–4 compares the typical features of acute confusional states with those of cortical dementias. The onset of an acute confusional state is usually sudden, coinciding with the appearance of a systemic illness or toxic exposure. Most episodes are of brief duration. Postural or action tremors, myoclonus, asterixis, and slurred speech may be prominent in delirium. Similarly, speech tends to be slurred in the acute confusional states and normal in the cortical dementias. Motor activity and speech articulation are spared in cortical dementias. In addition to the attentional disturbances of delirium, hallucinations, delusions, fear, and anxiety may be florid manifestations and are much more prominent than is common in cortical dementia. In contrast, language may be normal in confusional states, or a subtle naming deficit and a propensity to misname objects may be the only language problems (Cummings et al., 1980b; Weinstein and Kahn, 1952), whereas language abnormalities are common in cortical dementias. Chedru and Geschwind (1972) noted that in delirium writing is disturbed out of proportion to many other functions. Omission and substitution of letters and words, errors in consonants and grammatic words, and a tendency to perseverate on the final letters of words occur frequently. The EEGs obtained during delirious episodes are nearly always markedly abnormal, with diffuse slowing in the delta range (Cadilhac and Ribstein, 1961; Pro and Wells, 1977;

TABLE 1–4.   Clinical characteristics of acute confusional states and cortical dementias.

Characteristic	Cortical dementia	Acute confusional state
History		
Onset	Insidious	Sudden
Duration	Months to years	Hours to days
Course	Constant	Fluctuating
Motor signs	None (until late)	Postural tremor, myoclonus, asterixis
Speech	Normal	Slurred
Mental stutus		
Attention	Normal, distractable (late)	Inattention, fluctuating arousal, variably alert
Memory	Amnesia	Impaired by poor attention
Language	Aphasia	Normal or mild anomia; misnaming may be prominent; dysgraphia often prominent
Perception	Hallucinations not prominent	Visual, auditory, and/or tactile hallucinations may be florid
Mood/affect	Disinterested and/or disinhibited	Fear and suspiciousness may often be prominent
Review of systems	Involvement of extraneural organ systems usually absent	History of systemic illness or toxic exposure
EEG	Normal or mildly slow	Pronounced diffuse slowing

Romano and Engel, 1944). The EEG abnormalities are usually more profound than are those seen in all but the most advanced dementias. The fatality rate is greater for delirium than it is for dementia (Rabins and Folstein, 1982); 15 to 30 percent of patients admitted in a delirium die within one month of admission (Beresin, 1988; Lipowski, 1983).

Delirium is an etiologically nonspecific syndrome with a wide differential diagnosis. The causative factors may be divided into four general categories: (1) primary cerebral disease including infection, tumors, trauma, epilepsy, and stroke; (2) systemic illnesses that affect brain function such as metabolic disorders, infections, cardiopulmonary dysfunction, and collagen diseases; (3) intoxication with exogenous substances including medical drugs, intoxicants, and industrial agents; and (4) withdrawal from substances after dependency has developed including abstinence from alcohol or sedative-hypnotic agents (Lipowski, 1987). Elderly patients are particularly vulnerable to delirium because of the high frequency of systemic disorders in the aged and the high rate of administration of drugs for medical management. Drug administration is further complicated by changes in pharmacodynamics and increased end-organ sensitivity in older individuals (see Chapter 7 for more details). In one study, patients admitted for management of an acute confusional state manifested the following toxic and metabolic conditions: drug intoxication, 39 percent of cases; fluid and electrolyte disturbances and alcohol withdrawal, 11 percent each; infection, 5 percent; and endocrine abnormalities, 2 percent (Purdie et al, 1981). General surgery in the elderly is followed by delirium in 10 to 14 percent of patients, and hip surgery may produce delirium in as many as 50 percent of elderly patients (Lipowski, 1987).

There is an intimate relationship between chronic dementia syndromes and acute confusional states; almost half of patients admitted in a delirium will be found to have an underlying dementia (Purdie et al, 1981). In these patients, infections account for most of the acute changes (23 percent) with fluid and electrolyte imbalance and iatrogenic intoxications responsible for many of the remaining cases (14 percent each)(Purdie et al, 1981). Congestive heart failure, pulmonary dysfunction, anemia, and other chronic disorders have also been found to complicate dementing illnesses and contribute to the underlying intellectual impairment (Larson et al, 1984). Radiologic studies of medically ill patients with and without delirium indicate that structural brain changes predispose patients to the development of acute confusional states (Koponen et al, 1987). Thus delirium must be sought in dementia patients manifesting acute changes in intellectual function, and an underlying dementia should be considered in patients presenting with delirium.

Differentiation of acute confusional states from dementia associated with chronic metabolic encephalopathies is not simple, and the nosologic status of the chronic toxic and metabolic dementias is controversial. The onset of the mental status impairments associated with chronic metabolic disturbances is often insidious and may persist for months or years (for example, with chronic obstructive pulmonary disease or uremia). In some cases, a systemic disturbance may not be readily apparent, particularly in some of the dementias associated with chronic exposure to toxins. Insidious onset and inapparent etiology are characteristics shared with degenerative, vascular, neoplastic, and hydrocephalic dementias. On the other hand, as in the acute confusional states, patients with chronic toxic and metabolic disorders may manifest fluctuations of arousal, impaired attention, hallucinations, and agitation. Using the syndromic approach to dementia emphasized above, we have grouped the chronic toxic and metabolic disorders with the dementias rather than with the acute confusional states.

The chronic confusional states have many features in common with disorders that affect primarily subcortical structures. Motor abnormalities, speech disturbances, impaired attentional mechanisms, and relative integrity of language function occur in both groups. The major impact of metabolic and toxic disturbances appears to be on the reticular system and frontal-subcortical circuit functions. Thus the chronic confusional states have features of subcortical dementia. Naming and memory may also be compromised, however, and thus a mixed cortical-subcortical pattern of mental status impairment may be exhibited.

2

Mental Status Examination

While the definition of dementia as an acquired impairment of intellectual capacity appears simple and straightforward, the key term *intellectual capacity* defies precise definition. The clinician need not worry about an exact meaning of intellectual capacity, but an ability to demonstrate alterations in mental functions is crucial to the recognition of dementia. This chapter offers suggestions to aid in this admittedly difficult task. Probing the mental state is the essential beginning for evaluation of any demented patient.

An impression of a patient's mental status can generally be discerned from the history and description of the patient's activities by family members. This is abetted by results of general physical, neurologic, psychiatric, and selected laboratory examinations. A formal mental assessment is necessary to establish the severity and to characterize the dementia. While a detailed evaluation is not necessary in all patients, some assessment of intellectual competence is valuable. Screening tests for mental status can be performed rapidly and can direct attention toward mental abnormalities. An example is presented at the end of this chapter. A longer and more complete examination is usually needed, however; the examination taught and used in the Neurobehavioral Training Program, UCLA School of Medicine and West Los Angeles Veterans Administration Medical Center will be outlined. For greater depth or alternative approaches, books covering this topic by Denny-Brown (1957) and Strub and Black (1977) can be reviewed, and most textbooks of neurology and psychiatry offer outlines for mental status evaluation. Formal neuropsychological testing augments the mental status examination and in most instances provides better quantification of intellectual deficits. The information obtained from neuropsychological testing is rarely etiologically specific. It is, however, worthwhile for establishing the degree of mental impairment and particularly valuable for determining progression (or static state) through serial evaluation.

CLINICAL MENTAL STATUS EXAMINATION

For convenience, the full mental status evaluation is discussed under 10 separate headings. These are somewhat artificial, and not all aspects of each heading are useful for all patients. The clinician's task is to use those tests that offer information of value for a particular patient. While a short, rigid series of tests will provide a decent overview, the examiner should be prepared to evaluate pertinent areas in greater depth. The best information for clinical diagnosis of dementia will come from this type of probing.

State of Awareness

A mandatory first step is a careful determination of the patient's level of awareness at the time of testing.

Abnormal awareness is demonstrated by inability to maintain a coherent line of thought and can be separated into two basic types: 1) depressed or fluctuating arousal, associated with impairment in the level of awakeness, and 2) distractability, a fully awake state but with inability to maintain attention. While most subjects with a depressed state of awareness have some mixture of the two, differentiation is of considerable clinical significance.

Is the patient alert or dull, wide awake or drowsy? If the patient is somnolent, can he or she be aroused to full awareness or will arousal produce only partial awakening? If the patient is aroused, can attention be sustained or does the patient drift back into sleep? Can the patient keep his or her eyes open, or do they remain shut; are the eyes fixed or do they follow movements?

Both the state and any fluctuation in the level of conscious awareness during testing must be recorded. The nursing staff and/or relatives should be questioned about changes in the level of awareness occurring during the day or night. Special inquiries should be made about diurnal variations. The examiner should be aware that fluctuations in the level of awareness may interfere with ongoing experiences to such an extent that the patient does not present a full, coherent, and correct history.

If the patient is less than totally alert and awake, the alterations should be documented and measured as accurately as possible. This is best accomplished by recording the nature of the stimulus necessary to evoke a response and the character of that response. Thus if the patient will awaken to loud calling of his or her name but eventually drifts off, necessitating restimulation, this pattern should be recorded. If a painful pinch of the Achilles tendon or firm rubbing of the sternum is needed to evoke a response, both the stimulus and the degree of response should be recorded. While terms such as delirium, stupor, coma, lethargy, drowsiness, and so on are frequently used, they are inexact at best. Description of both stimulus and response represents a far better gauge of an abnormal level of awakeness and provides useful data for later comparison.

Disturbed states of awakeness are common and are extremely important for the clinician. Depressed awakeness suggests a disturbance involving the reticular activating system, usually indicating malfunction at the brainstem level. While this may be on the basis of mass lesion or traumatic insult, more commonly it is associated with metabolic and toxic abnormalities such as drug overdose, hypoxia, alcohol abuse, and the like. It is usually easy to identify disturbances of the level of awakeness, and if the stimulus/response approach noted above is used, the disturbances are relatively easy to quantitate. Serial documentation of the level of arousal is a valuable clinical test for determining whether therapeutic intervention is succeeding.

Considerably more difficult to demonstrate and understand is a patient's inability to maintain a coherent line of thought in the state of full awakeness. The condition has been called the acute confusional state (Strub, 1982). Unfortunately, this state is easily overlooked, a situation that leads to misinterpretation of other items of the mental status evaluation. While the confused patient can attend for short periods, this ability is rapidly lost and attention wanders or, more exactly, is captured by other stimuli that appear (stimulus-bound). It is important to separate this condition from dementia; most confusional states are acute in onset and have a specific, remediable cause. Misdiagnosis as dementia may ignore a fully reversible acute medical problem. While not so readily localized when the confusional state results from focal pathology, the problem is usually located somewhat higher in the neuraxis than are disorders causing decreased alertness, usually involving the medial posterior frontal (septal) area or frontal-subcortical connections. Again, toxic and metabolic disturbances are the most common causes of the awake-confused state.

While observation is usually adequate to define the abnormality of awakeness, formal testing is needed to quantify the awake-confused state. Most frequently used is the digit span; at a rate of about one per second, the examiner recites a few numbers and immediately asks the patient to repeat them. When it is successful, a series with one additional number is offered and so on until the patient makes an error. The "magic number seven plus or minus two" (Miller, 1956) is considered normal. A patient failing at five or fewer digits has a significant attention problem. Another easy bedside evaluation of attention is the "A test," a simplified continuous-performance task. The examiner slowly recites random letters of the alphabet with the patient instructed to indicate each time "A" is presented. More than a single omission in 60 seconds suggests an attention disturbance. Purely clinical observations monitoring the patient's conversation and behavior during the interview can prove useful. Patients with disturbed attention tend to ramble, lose the train of their conversation and fail to maintain coherence in thought. Verbal incoherence may provide a solid indication of disrupted attention. Throughout this volume, the word *confusion* is used only when referring to an attentional deficit. Unfortunately, many practitioners (and teachers) interchange confusion with disorientation (actually a memory function) or use the term to refer to vague uncharacterized mental status changes. This unrestricted use of the word is misleading and usually indicates more about the mental state of the examiner than about that of the patient.

While they are clearly separate from dementia, disorders of awakeness and attention are often superimposed on a more general intellectual disturbance. Various combinations of awakeness/attention disorder have been called delirium (Lipowski, 1980a, b), mental concomitants of physical disease (Bleuler, 1975), toxic or metabolic encephalopathy (Adams and Victor, 1977, 1989), acute organic reaction (Lishman, 1987), and acute confusional state (Strub, 1982; Cummings, 1985). The disorders are clinically significant. Lipowski (1980a) states that over a quarter of elderly patients suffering delirium in hospitals will die even though most causes are amenable to therapy (Strub, 1982). Recognition of the problem and differentiation from the more chronic dementing disorders may be life saving. Lesser degrees of attention disorder are frequent in dementia, and their impact on determination of the mental state deserves consideration.

General Appearance and Behavior

This portion of the mental status test evaluates the patient's general behavior and demeanor. Many observations of significance can be made. For instance, how does the patient spend the day? What are the patterns of eating and sleeping? Is the patient clean or messy? Is the patient concerned about self-care, including keeping hair combed and clothes neat, using cosmetics properly, and so on? What is the patient's behavior toward other patients, doctors, nursing staff, relatives, and others? What is the patient's general motor and mental attitude? Is the patient relaxed, or is there an appearance of tension and restlessness? Is the patient alert and kinetic or slow and hesitant? Is there a great deal of apparently purposeless movement? Does the patient respond normally to external events? Gestures, grimaces, and evidence of bodily motor expression should be observed. The amount of activity and variations in activity patterns through the day should be noted.

Is there resistance or negativity, or is the patient the opposite, in a passive state? Finally is the patient continent or incontinent?

Many of these observations are difficult to make in the period of a single evaluation. Family members or nursing staff can often be helpful. In particular, the examiner must be aware of incontinence and cannot rely on immediate observations. The nursing staff strives to keep patients free of their own excrement. In fact, the patient who looks abnormally neat and clean and is in bright, fresh pajamas or sheets while others appear less neat is to be suspected of recent soiling. A question to the nursing staff concerning the presence of incontinence always receives a definite response. Family members often provide valuable, detailed accounts of the patient's ongoing activity level, sleep patterns, and social competence.

Mood and Affect

Emotion is a difficult term to define as it includes a number of rather disparate states and activities. Two components, however, mood and affect, are relatively easy to explain although often difficult to distinguish accurately in a patient. Mood is used to indicate the inner feeling tone and subjective feelings of the patient while affect can be considered the outward expression of emotion. Emotion is a combination of these complicated by a third aspect, personality, which refers to total behavior over time. Personality can influence the patient's immediate emotional state but is determined by genetic background, premorbid learning, and underlying brain disease.

Mood and affect can be dissociated, and when they are being evaluated in the mental status examination, the examiner should consider them separately. Mood is probed by asking the patient specific questions concerning feelings, for example, "how do you feel inside?," "what are you feeling now?," or "do you feel blue?" Some will respond to a question about their "spirits" and more intelligent patients may provide considerable insight following inquiry into their present mood. The examiner should ask about depression, including current or past suicidal thoughts. An important question concerns the patient's attitudes toward the future, both to seek depressive mood and as a probe of the patient's ability to anticipate needs and formulate plans. Variations of mood are difficult to express in words. While happiness or sadness is fairly easily stated, fear, apprehension, suspicion, perplexity, and anxiety are often composites of feelings and are difficult to put into words. One must be cautious not to overinterpret the patient's explanation of mood.

Affect is behavior that is judged primarily by observation and, as such, is more readily recorded. One should look for evidence of flatness or hypokinesia. Lability of affective responses is also of considerable pertinence. Negativity and denial suggest that the patient is concealing, or is unaware of, true feelings. While these observations are pertinent, the examiner must again be cautioned not to overinterpret apparent abnormalities of affect.

Mood and affect, even when they are clearly demonstrated, are not necessarily congruent; in organically disturbed patients the affect may not reflect underlying mood. A common error in mental status evaluations is to misinterpret psychomotor retardation as depression. For instance, the patient with parkinsonism often shows evidence of both motor and mental retardation. This patient may also have a depressed mood, but this is not constant and must be specifically sought, not inferred from the apathetic, retarded appearance. The euphoria present in some brain-damaged individuals, most notably in those with advanced multiple sclerosis, may be a facade overlying a seriously depressed mood. Another glaring discrepancy between mood and affect occurs in pseudobulbar palsy where excessive, uninhibited responses (affect) may not reflect the underlying mood or may grossly exaggerate actual feelings.

Changes in personality are frequently among the earliest features heralding the onset of a dementing process, and dementia should be in the differential diagnosis of all patients manifesting a sudden alteration in personality and emotional behavior.

It is a good rule for the clinician to accept that any complaint (by patient or family) of an altered personality is due to organic brain dysfunction. Dementia is often a concomitant finding.

Speech and Language

Speech represents the mechanical act of expression, the neuromuscular alterations needed to produce communication. Although phonated expression is most often considered, this definition also refers to the mechanical aspects of writing and to the motor aspects of gesture. *Language* refers to symbolic communication; a specific language system is the set of communication symbols used by persons of the same cultural background. The ability to comprehend (decode) and to express (encode) a common body of symbols falls within this definition. Language can be subdivided into four distinct elements: 1) gesture; 2) prosody, the passage of information by tone or inflection; 3) semantics, the corpus of words that symbolize objects, places, and so on; and 4) syntax, the relationship of language items.

Aphasia is the loss or impairment of language caused by brain damage. *Alexia* is the loss or impairment of the ability to comprehend printed language. *Agraphia* is the loss or impairment of the ability to communicate in written language. *Dysarthria* refers to disordered phonated speech and covers many different speech disorders; *hypophonia* is a notable decrease in vocal volume. *Mutism* refers to an inability to phonate.

Motor Aspects of Verbal Speech

A fairly thorough evaluation of the mechanics of vocal output can be performed rather simply. First, the patient's spontaneous speech is monitored (preferably not during history taking as the examiner's attention must be focused elsewhere). Next the patient is asked to read from a text; this is followed by a request that the patient maintain an "aah" sound for as long as possible. Finally, the patient is asked to say three syllables, "puh," "tuh," and "kuh," separately and then to say all three syllables as a single word "putukuh." These simple acts will demonstrate most motor speech disorders. With these three tests one can judge the quality of the patient's respiration, phonation, resonance, and articulation. Various combinations of disturbance of these qualities indicate anatomically specific varieties of dysarthria (Metter, 1985). Almost without exception, abnormality of motor speech output indicates subcortical dysfunction.

Language Functions

Although it is difficult, language can be evaluated in the clinic and in fact clinical testing may be more useful than are formal language batteries for diagnostic purposes. Six language functions can be monitored in the clinic: 1) spontaneous verbal output, 2) comprehension of spoken language, 3) repetition of spoken language, 4) naming, 5) reading, and 6) writing.

Spontaneous verbal output should be monitored for evidence of fluency of output. Flow alone, however, is not a sufficient criterion. Table 2–1 presents seven characteristics that distinguish fluent from nonfluent aphasic outputs. Non-fluent aphasia output suggests abnormality that involves the anterior or frontal language area of the left hemisphere; conversely, a fluent verbal output, particularly when accompanied with paraphasia, reflects posterior left hemisphere abnormality (Benson, 1967).

Comprehension of spoken language is difficult to assess. Three simple tests are considered standard: 1) request to perform an act (for example, "Clap your hands") or a sequence of acts (for example, "Take a sheet of paper, fold it in half, and give it to the examiner"), 2) yes/no questions (for example, "Are you standing up now?" or "Is your name Jones?"), and 3) requests to point to objects (for example, "Point to your nose, your shoe, the entrance to this room"). Unfortunately each of these approaches can be altered by nonlanguage problems leading to misinterpretation. For instance, motor apraxia can prevent a patient from performing commands that are understood. Similarly some aphasics cannot produce accurate yes or no responses either by voice or by gesture although they may understand the question. Even the simplest task of pointing to an object must be learned and then can be failed because of perseveration. Careful testing can provide a gauge of the ability to comprehend in most patients. An additional test,

TABLE 2–1.   Characteristics of aphasic verbal output.

Characteristic	Nonfluent	Fluent
Rate	Slow (<50 wpm)	Normal (100–200 wpm)
Effort	Increased, struggling	Normal
Articulation	Abnormal, dysarthric	Normal
Phrase length	Short (one to two words)	Normal (five to eight words)
Prosody (melody, rhythm, inflection, timbre)	Abnormal	Normal
Content	Relative decrease in relational (syntactic) words	Relative decrease in meaningful (semantic) words
Paraphasia	Relatively infrequent Literal	Relatively frequent Literal, semantic, neologistic

Modified from DF Benson. Fluency in aphasia: Correlation with radioactive scan localization. Cortex 1967;3:373–394.

the handling of sequences of material (for example, "Point to your nose, your shoulder, and your foot in that order") challenges two levels of comprehension. The first is the ability to point successfully to the individual items; the second demands maintenance of the serial order; success at the first level but failure at the second most often indicates frontal disorder.

Repetition of spoken language is relatively simple to test and provides crucial information. The examiner asks the patient to repeat digits, words, and multisyllabic words, phrases, and sentences. If the patient succeeds, sentences with many functor words (for example, "no ifs, ands, or buts" or "if he comes soon we will all go away with him") can be offered. Failure to repeat may be through omission, substitution, altered order, mispronunciation, or limitation of the span level and if it is present in an aphasic patient usually indicates left hemisphere perisylvian dysfunction (Benson, 1979a).

Naming is a sensitive language function that is often abnormal. Three modes of testing are suggested: 1) ability to name on confrontation (the examiner points to objects, body parts, colors, or actions and asks that their names be given), 2) monitoring of verbal output (in particular, the examiner should note any decreased use of the specific, meaningful words needed for a sentence to make clear sense), and 3) production of names in a specific category (for example, names of animals, cities, articles of clothing, or words beginning with a specific letter of the alphabet—each timed for about 60 seconds). The latter test, category naming, may be abnormal in patients whose language otherwise appears intact, and if that is so, it also indicates frontal dysfunction or psychomotor slowing.

Reading is tested in two manners: 1) out loud and 2) for comprehension. It is best to request that the patient read out loud first but particular attention should be given to demonstration of whether the material has been understood. This can be tested by writing single words that are names of objects in the room then by asking the patient to read them aloud and point to the object. If this is successful, sentences describing objects in a moderately abstract way can be used (for example, "Point to the source of illumination in this room"). It is not unusual in demented individuals to find that one reading task is performed successfully (for example, reading aloud) while the other (for example, reading comprehension) is failed.

Writing is the most vulnerable language skill and is disturbed almost any time there is a language disorder. Writing a sentence to command (for example, "Describe today's weather") offers good screening data on the mental state. *Agraphia* may be purely mechanical based on paralysis, chorea, and the like or a truly aphasic verbal output. Combinations of mechanical and aphasic agraphia are common. In testing writing ability it is usually well to start by asking the patient to sign his or her name. It must be remembered, however, that ability to produce a signature is not a sufficient test of writing ability. The patient should be asked to write words or sentences to dictation and if this is successful to produce a spontaneous sentence on a topic designated by the examiner.

Visuospatial Functions

As a corollary to language testing, nonverbal brain functions should be tested. The classic examples are tests of visuospatial competence such as copying and drawing. Visuospatial tests are excellent screening devices, as damage to many portions of the brain not probed by routine neurologic testing (the so-called silent areas) can cause abnormal responses on visuospatial tasks. The most basic test of nonverbal function is the ability to copy drawings (drawing to command is more complex as it probes visual memory as well as visuospatial competence). Both two- and three-dimensional drawings should be used. Figure 3–1 (p. 51) presents examples of drawings that can be used. With few exceptions, healthy individuals and most individuals with serious psychogenic disorders will produce adequate copies. In contrast, individuals with structural brain damage that involves the frontal, parietal, or occipital lobe of either hemisphere usually fail to copy the drawings accurately. Damage to the temporal lobe, however, does not appear to produce alterations in drawing skill (Nahor and Benson, 1970). Inability to copy can stem from lesions in many different areas in the brain, so that these tests are good for screening but are poor anatomic markers.

Many other tests can be used to assess nonverbal mental functioning. The patient can be asked to connect a series of numbers (trails test) or to draw on command a complex figure such as a house, a clock face, or the like. The ability to localize principal cities on a rough outline map of the United States, to reproduce figures made by the examiner out of matches, and to reproduce designs with specially colored blocks (if available) test a patient's visuospatial discrimination. Abnormal performance on any of these tests indicates an organic disturbance. Disturbed visuospatial discrimination is an early finding in Alzheimer's disease and is present in many other types of dementia.

Additional Cortical Functions

Praxis

Apraxia is a word that is used broadly and inconsistently, but one aspect, an inability to carry out purposeful movements on oral verbal command, is often of value. Failure, exclusive of motor or comprehension defects, has been called *motor apraxia* (Geschwind, 1975; Heilman and Gonzalez Rothi, 1985). The patient should be requested to perform buccal-lingual activities such as whistling, coughing, or puffing out the cheeks; limb activities such as folding the arms, waving goodbye, beckoning, saluting, and kicking; and finally whole-body activities such as standing up, turning around, bowing, or boxing. Complex acts demanding a series of coordinated activities can be requested: for example, asking the patient to take a piece of paper, fold it in three, place it in an envelope, seal the envelope, and give the envelope to the examiner tests for "ideational apraxia" as well as comprehension disturbance. Interpretation of praxis disturbances, particularly their neuroanatomic localization, is a complicated and somewhat controversial task beyond the scope of this chapter, but the presence of motor apraxia, the inability to carry out on command a motor act that is easily performed spontaneously, is an important observation (Benson and Geschwind, 1976), and apraxia is present in some types of dementia.

Topographic Disorientation

A patient's ability to find his or her way in familiar parts of his or her own neighborhood or home or to find his or her own bed in the hospital can be impaired in the course of a dementing illness. The ability to localize cities, oceans, and so on on a map is also of consequence. The two acts are not the same; personal topographic competence may be intact in a patient who cannot localize cities on a map, and conversely a person with no problems in map orientation who gets lost in familiar surroundings (Landis et al, 1986) is significant. Inability to find one's own way in familiar areas (environmental disorientation) is usually associated with right medial posterior lesions (Cummings et al, 1983a), whereas disturbed map localization capability indicates right posterior convexity lesion. Both variations occur in demented individuals.

Right-Left Disorientation

Testing a patient's ability to point to or to move individual body parts on the right or left side of their own or the examiner's body on oral command probes the ability to discern right and left. Complex instructions such as "touch your right ear with your left hand" can be given. Some patients fail these tests in a random manner, suggesting inability to discern right from left while others always point to a single side, indicating neglect of the opposite side or perseveration. Still others may fail to handle the sequence of commands correctly and some fail to comprehend the words. Right-left orientation can be disrupted by diverse lesions, but in conjunction with acalculia, finger agnosia, and dysgraphia (the features of the Gerstmann syndrome), it reliably indicates dysfunction of the posterior left hemisphere.

Finger Agnosia

The patient is asked to name each of the fingers. If this test is failed, the patient is asked to show the finger named by the examiner. If the patient still fails, the examiner can stimulate one finger of the patient's hand held out of sight and ask that the same finger of the opposite hand be moved. The last test can be failed because of deafferentation and the first two because of aphasia, but careful testing and correlation with other information allow demonstration of an unusual disturbance.

Identification of Other Body Parts

The patient is asked to point to individual parts of the body (neck, ankle, ear, and so forth) and to name parts of the body. Disturbance (autotopagnosia) is indicative of significant brain disturbance and may have neuroanatomic localizing significance (parietal lobe) if coupled with other appropriate findings.

Unawareness or Neglect

The examiner should note if the patient tends to ignore or neglect one portion of the body (particularly one side) or even verbally denies defect or ownership of the neglected portion (anosognosia). Lesser degrees of neglect

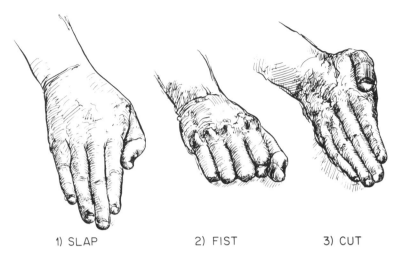

1) SLAP   2) FIST   3) CUT

FIGURE 2–1.   Positions for the Luria three-hand test of sequencing. The steps can be identified verbally as "slap," "fist," and "cut." Many demented patients have difficulty learning the sequence and are less aided than are normal subjects by the verbal reinforcement. (Reprinted by permission of the publisher from DF Benson and DT Stuss, "Motor abilities after frontal leukotomy," Neurology [Ny] 1982;32:1353–1357.)

can be demonstrated in the neurologic examination by tests of double simultaneous stimulation using visual, somesthetic, or auditory stimuli to show unilateral extinction.

Dressing Difficulties

It is important to note whether the patient tends to dress and groom one side of the body while ignoring the other (unilateral neglect); or gets muddled in attempting to put on a garment, inserting a limb into the wrong area and orienting the garment incorrectly (body-garment disorientation); or has sequential problems (undergarments worn over street clothes). Dressing problems should be correlated with other data; body-garment (visual-spatial) dressing disturbances most often indicate right parietal lobe dysfunction whereas the unilateral neglect disturbance indicates contralateral disorder.

Motor Sequences

Sequential hand movements monitor motor sequencing competency (Fig. 2–1). Tests include imitating simple rhythms; performing go/no-go testing (when the examiner taps once the patient taps twice, but when the examiner taps twice the patient does not tap); producing a series of multiple loops (Fig. 2–2) or copying a sequence of script such as m n m n m n. While

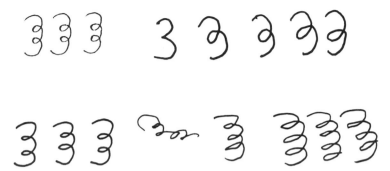

FIGURE 2–2.   Multiple-loop test: model (left) and pathologic responses by demented patients (right).

often considered tests of frontal lobe function, failure may also reflect subcortical pathology (frontal system dysfunction) (Stuss and Benson, 1986).

With the exception of some of the language dysfunctions, cortical function tests are not specific for cerebral localization; as a rule, they do indicate organic mental problems, often focal, and cerebral localizing information may be obtained by demonstrating a pattern of such deficits. There is a tendency for the more visually oriented tests, particularly topographic disorientation and disturbances in visuospatial discrimination, to indicate right hemisphere disorder, just as right-left disorientation and apraxia are more often seen with left hemisphere disturbance. Unilateral neglect is a powerful indicator of opposite hemisphere dysfunction. Great emphasis should not be put on localization based on an individual test, however; it is more important that its presence should alert the clinician to the probability of an underlying organic disorder.

Memory

To test memory, three psychologically distinct activities should be noted: (1) the ability to attend to information offered, (2) the ability to learn (retain) new information, and (3) the ability to retrieve information learned in the past. In addition, the examiner should seek evidence of confabulation and excessive forgetfulness. Each function is tested separately; each represents a different aspect of memory; but, in practice, several components of memory processing may be abnormal simultaneously.

Immediate Recall

The ability to retain a small amount of information with complete accuracy for a short period of time has been called *immediate recall*. Characteristically, this function is evaluated by determining the digit span, the test described earlier in the section entitled "State of Awareness." Letter and word spans are variations. Some authorities suggest that span tests do not test memory, as material handled in immediate recall is not necessarily retained permanently (memorized). Disturbance of this function, however, greatly impairs ability to learn and is often associated with poor memory and disorientation. Immediate recall is an essential initial step in the process of learning.

Ability to Learn New Material

The ability to learn new material is often called *recent memory* (also *short-term memory, secondary memory,* or *consolidation*). The major activity of this step is learning. Many different tests can probe the ability to learn: (1) Orientation for time and place must be learned on an ongoing basis; significant abnormality in either indicates disturbed learning capability. (2) The examiner can give his or her name and minutes later ask the patient to recall the name. (3) Three or four unrelated words can be offered with the patient repeating them several times and then, following a delay of 5 to 10 minutes in which other testing is performed, the patient is asked to recall the words. All words should be recalled; in the face of learning disability there will be failure. (4) A variation of this procedure is the so-called Babcock sentence ("The one thing a nation needs in order to be rich and strong is a large, secure supply of wood"), a supraspan sentence that is offered repeatedly until it is "learned." Most normal subjects will repeat it accurately by the third trial; individuals with significant learning defects may never master the entire sentence. (5) A supraspan word list (8 or 10 unrelated words) can be recited three or four times with the patient repeating as many as possible until the entire list is learned or failure to learn is proved (learning curve). Nonverbal learning can be assessed by pointing to three objects in the room and asking the patient to recall them after three minutes or asking the patient to reproduce (from memory) the drawings copied earlier during visuospatial testing.

Ability to Retrieve Old Learned Information

Often called *remote* or *long-term memory,* this function is difficult to test because the examiner does not know what the patient has known in the past. General questions concerning politics, personal history, the names of the presidents, or personal questions on such topics as military career or family life can be asked. Unfortunately, the examiner rarely knows whether the patient has ever known this information or, in cases of personal information, whether the answers offered are correct. If the patient was given a supraspan word list to test learning, a request to reproduce the list after a 10-minute delay probes retrieval competency. If none or only a portion of the list is recalled, prompting, first by category clues and, failing this, by selection from multiple choice, can be offered. Failure to recall spontaneously but good success after prompting indicates a retrieval problem. In amnesia, learning new information will be seriously disturbed whereas recall of remote material may be relatively preserved (Benson, 1978). In most dementias, elements of both recent and remote memory are compromised.

Confabulation

The presentation by a patient of bizarre or incorrect information to general questioning has been called confabulation (Berlyne, 1972). Often this is merely a wrong answer such as presenting an incorrect day or date, the wrong place on questions of orientation, or a recital of recent personal activities that did not occur. At times, however, confabulations can be bizarre, the spontaneous presentation of unreal or impossible activities. Confabulation is often associated with disturbances in the ability to learn although this is not an absolute correlation and is better correlated with a patient's inability to monitor his or her own responses and be self-corrective (Mercer et al, 1977). Confabulation suggests a frontal malfunction occurring in conjunction with disturbances of learning new material.

Forgetfulness

Forgetting to remember should be noted. Everyone tends to forget, and this tendency increases with normal aging; with only slight prompting, most of this information can be remembered. Forgetting represents a problem in initiating retrieval, not in learning new information. Forgetfulness may become a serious problem in many types of dementia and is a significant finding (Chapters 1 and 4). There is no single test for demonstrating forgetfulness; it may be suspected from the examination, but can be tested only in a crude manner. When standard learning tests are failed, the examiner can provide cues to see if the patient can then remember most of the information taught. Differentiating inability to learn (amnesia) from forgetfulness may be crucial for distinguishing varieties of dementia. In general, amnesia has been correlated with cortical dementia, particularly with Alzheimer's disease, and forgetfulness with subcortical disorders.

Cognitive Functions

Having assessed the level of verbal and nonverbal skills, the ability to learn new information, and to some extent the ability to retrieve information from the fund of knowledge, the next step in the mental status examination is determination of the patient's ability to use these functions, a group of skills that can be called *cognition*. For present purposes, cognition will be defined as the ability to manipulate knowledge. The fund of information, evaluated as a memory retrieval function, represents material already learned; the ability to use bits of this in conjunction with other information to arrive at a new answer can be considered a process of manipulation. Testing of this function, at least to some degree, offers an estimate of the patient's current intellectual competence. Bedside tests of cognition are crude, but even sophisticated psychometric tests offer at best only rough estimations of this function. Significant loss or, conversely, maintenance of the ability to manipulate knowledge is a crucial finding in the diagnosis of dementia. Several ways of gauging cognition are suggested, all somewhat tangential to "intelligence" but useful for diagnostic purposes.

Calculating Ability

Calculation demands a manipulation of already-learned number functions. For success, both number language and number concept must be intact before learned arithmetic processes can be performed. Can the patient correctly read or write numbers of one, two, or more digits? Can he or she accurately count objects and guess, without counting, the approximate number of objects displayed? Can the patient handle simple rote arithmetic such as $4 + 3$ or 6×5? Failure indicates either a lack of education or a significant disturbance in retrieval of old learned material.

If these functions are intact, the ability to compute, actually to handle and manipulate numbers, can be tested. Problems of addition, subtraction, multiplication, and division are presented (addition and multiplication are the easiest to interpret). Results must be correlated with the educational background and occupational status of the patient. Individuals of limited educational background may fail formal mathematical tasks but demonstrate competence when asked to handle money. One commonly used test of calculation is the ability serially to subtract 7 beginning with 100; it must be recognized, however, that this test demands, in addition to cognitive function, good memory, good sequencing ability, and intact attention. With these facts in mind, serial 7s can be considered a good general test of cognition. Simple calculations ($47 + 18 = $ ——; $82 - 16 = $ ——, etc.) are easier to interpret, however.

Interpretation of Proverbs

For many years, proverb interpretation has been used to probe cognitive function but it has always proved difficult to analyze. In general terms, proverb interpretation challenges the ability to abstract. Actually, it challenges the patient's ability to use linguistic metaphors. A concrete (mere repetition or rephrasing of the statement given by the examiner) or bizarre response is considered pathologic. Educational level and prior familiarity with proverbs as well as cognitive competency are important in the patient's response. Some proverbs are considerably easier to interpret than are others;

the examiner should start with simple idioms and progress to proverbs that are sufficiently hard to challenge the patient. Examples are:

(Easy)   He is wearing a loud necktie.
                  He gave me a cold shoulder.
                  Two men see eye to eye.
(Medium)   Rome wasn't built in a day.
                  Don't cry over spilled milk.
                  Don't change horses in the middle of the stream.
(Hard)   A new broom sweeps clean.
                  Still waters run deep.
                  People who live in glass houses shouldn't throw stones.

It is generally said that the mentally impaired patient will give concrete responses while the mentally ill will produce more bizarre responses. This is not always true, and proverb interpretation must be correlated with other findings.

Similarities and Differences

These are also classic tests of a patient's ability to analyze and manipulate knowledge. The shortcomings and limitations noted for proverb interpretations also influence the responses to similarities and differences. The basic integrity of cognitive function can be judged from both the quality and the correctness of the response. Some examples of similarities and differences that can be used include:

How are a coat and a shirt alike?
How are an apple and a banana alike?
How are a bee and a flower alike?
What is the difference between a dog and a wolf?
What is the difference between a river and a canal?
What is the difference between a lie and a mistake?

Although crude and not designed for careful gradation, clinical tests of cognition can provide the examiner with an estimate of the patient's competence in manipulating knowledge and offer a useful characterization of mental function.

Thought Content

Several aspects of the content of the patient's thinking deserve consideration as part of any mental status evaluation. While abnormal content is usually considered most pertinent in the primary psychiatric disorders, its presence in dementia should be noted.

Obsessional Thoughts and Preoccupation

The examiner should seek evidence of anxiety or preoccupation concerning the present life situation as well as similar responses to either the past or the future. Often, only direct questioning concerning such activities can elicit pertinent evidence. Patients often deny morbid preoccupations, but careful questioning particularly following establishment of good rapport, can elicit evidence of serious problems.

1. Does the patient have a morbid concern about his or her personal safety or about that of others?
2. Do such worries interfere with the patient's ability to concentrate? To sleep? To work?
3. Does the patient describe phobias, obsessional ruminations, compulsive actions, or rituals?
4. Is there suggestion of suicidal ideation?

Abnormal Beliefs and Interpretations

Delusions may be present in either psychogenic or organic brain problems and can be important for understanding a dementing condition. The onset of delusion in the older, previously well patient suggests an organic factor (Miller et al, 1986b). Again, only careful questioning, specifically probing for these possibilities, can lead to pertinent information. One should look for:

1. Misinterpretation in relation to the environment. Does the patient have ideas of reference or influence, of beliefs of persecution, of being treated in a special way, or of being the subject of an experiment? Is there other evidence of organized misinterpretation or delusions?
2. Are there misinterpretations concerning the body? Does the patient complain of bodily changes, unpleasant body odor, malformation, or ugliness that is not truly present?
3. Does the patient have abnormal interpretations concerning self? Are there delusions of extreme incompetence or the opposite, major degrees of influence; are there intrusions into the patient's line of thought, reading, and so on?

Abnormal Perception of the Environment, Body, or Self

Hallucinations and illusions are frequently present in both primary psychiatric and organically produced brain abnormalities and should always be sought as part of the mental status evaluation. This problem can be divided into three portions:

1. Misperception of the environment. Does the patient tell of auditory, visual, olfactory, gustatory, or tactile hallucinations or illusions? Does the patient have feelings of familiarity or unfamiliarity of events? Is there depersonalization or derealization? Does the patient describe feelings of déjà vu? These findings can occur in many different disorders, with epileptic seizures and drug abuse the most common. Primary psychiatric disorders such as schizophrenia and severe depression also produce hallucinations. The presence of hallucinatory activity does not rule out a dementing process, and the demented patient may hallucinate following ingestion of therapeutic doses of regularly prescribed medications.
2. Misperceptions of the body. Does the patient tell of feelings of deadness, alterations of body sensations, or pain? Does the patient complain of somatic hallucinations, misperception of body size, shape, or appearance? Again, these misperceptions are most commonly described in psychiatric disorders but may be present in dementia.
3. Misperceptions of self. Depersonalization, an awareness of being able to look at one's own body and react to it in a dismembered manner, and the presence of serious blocking of thought processes or bizarre ideas can be present in either organic mental disturbances or psychiatric disorders.

The physician should record the content of any abnormal thought processes. The time of occurrence, whether episodic or paroxysmal, and the presence of precipitating factors should all be noted. While more often associated with the acute mental alterations of a psychiatric or acute confusional nature, morbid thoughts, delusions, and hallucinations can and do occur in dementia (Cummings and Victoroff, 1990).

Insight and Judgment

Disordered judgment is often one of the early indicators of impending dementia but has always proved difficult to demonstrate. The classic judgment questions (for example, what should you do if you find a stamped, addressed envelope on the street?) probe old, overlearned platitudes, not current judgment competency; the responses can be misleading and are never to be trusted. Judgment can be evaluated best through monitoring the patient's ability to cope with everyday problems (for example, maintaining a checking account or essential correspondence and competency in business or home decisions). Most often this information is not readily available to the examiner, but the patient or a family member will often volunteer incidents that indicate judgment deficiency. In some instances, objective evidence or at least suggestion of deficit can be discerned by probing the patient's insight into his or her current mental/physical status. In particular, after completion of a full examination, a simple question to the patient—"And what do you think is your trouble?"—may demonstrate a lack of realization or a serious misinterpretation of the problem.

Patient/Examiner Relationship

Unlike formal psychological testing, results of much of the mental status examination are directly or indirectly dependent on judgment evaluations by the examiner. Some effort must be made to include the quality of the relationship between patient and examiner in the interpretation of these results. Several suggestions can be offered.

Rapport

At the end of the examination the examiner should evaluate how friendly and open the relationship with the patient was, whether the patient was frank and honest or guarded, evasive, and negative. Would the examiner regard the interview as warm and trusting or as cold and formal? Was there any suggestion that the patient was exaggerating or giving dishonest answers? The patient's responses to both the examination and the examiner are important factors in the overall quality of the mental status examination.

Examiner's Reaction

The examiner should rate his or her own reaction to the patient. Everyone has likes and dislikes among different personalities and these feelings may influence interpretation of the test results. Did the patient produce feelings of sympathy, concern, sadness, anxiety, frustration, impatience, or anger? Did the examiner ever have difficulty controlling responses toward the patient? In the end, the examiner must honestly consider whether some aspect of the attitude toward the patient could have modified the interpretation of performance on the mental status examination.

SCREENING FOR MENTAL STATUS DYSFUNCTION

For most bedside or office evaluations, the clinician must quickly probe wide areas of the patient's mentation. Table 2–2 presents four steps selected because of their sensitivity and usefulness in screening for mental state abnormality in dementia. When an abnormality is identified, additional,

TABLE 2–2.   Steps in the minimum screening mental status examination.

Awareness	Degree of awakeness
	Degree of attention
Language	Naming to confrontation
	Category word list
	Writing to command
Learning	Orientation for time and place
Visual-spatial	Ability to copy three-dimensional shapes

more specific testing is necessary. If a rapid but more quantitative assessment of mental function is desired, the clinician may perform one of a variety of short standardized mental status examinations such as those of Blessed et al (1968), Folstein et al (1975), Jacobs et al (1977), and Mattis (1976).

Step 1: In any mental status evaluation, determination of the level of awareness is imperative. This should be accomplished first because all remaining evaluations depend on the level of awareness. Two major disturbances are sought: First, any lessening of the normal level of awakeness such as lethargy, drowsiness, sleepiness, stupor, coma, and so on are recorded and levels quantitated as described above. Second, the patient's ability to maintain attention should also be noted.

Step 2: At least a cursory evaluation of language function is needed. Most mental function tests depend on verbal responses to questions, and abnormal language (aphasia) can modify verbal interrogation. Two subtests—naming ability and writing to command—are particularly sensitive and therefore act as good screening tests; abnormality of either demands additional directed analysis of language function. A third test—the ability to present a list of words in a specified category—is sensitive to both language and frontal sequencing disorders.

Step 3: Information concerning the patient's ability to learn (memorize) new material is essential. One easy test of this function in the clinical setting is orientation to time and place, information that must be learned on an ongoing basis. Incorrect responses demand careful probing for an acquired inability to learn new material.

Step 4: Evaluation of the ability to copy three-dimensional drawings is a sensitive index of cerebral dysfunction. This act demands competent function by a number of otherwise silent areas of the cerebral hemispheres, areas that can harbor serious abnormalities without demonstrable abnormality on more basic neurologic or mental status tests.

Indication of abnormality in any portion of the screening examination warrants a considerably more thorough evaluation of the mental state. While this can be performed through formal psychometric examinations, excellent information can be gathered from the physician's clinical evaluation, and in many instances, this provides information unavailable from any laboratory study. Appropriate differentiation of varieties of dementia is often dependent on clinical assessment.

Performing the mental status examination is a complex, somewhat obscure, and decidedly difficult task. Nonetheless it is a key in any evaluation of dementia. In general, mental status testing is more important in the diagnosis and management of dementia than any individual laboratory tests.

PSYCHOLOGICAL TESTING

The first procedure that many clinicians request in evaluating an individual with dementia is a psychological examination, both to confirm the presence of dementia and to offer diagnostic clues as to etiology. Psychological tests are useful for the first goal but at present provide limited help for the second.

A number of reasons can be cited why psychological testing is currently of limited value in differential diagnosis. One important factor is that most currently used psychological techniques are derived from abnormal psychology, the study of functional psychiatric disorders. The original tests were designed to demonstrate psychiatric abnormality; they separated organic from psychogenic disorders but were not designed to differentiate the causes of organic mental problems (Shapiro et al, 1957).

Most clinical psychologists are not experienced in the use of neuropsychological tests for etiologic diagnosis of dementia. Relatively few well-trained neuropsychologists are working in this field and, even in their hands, the approach has remained limited. Great strides are being made in devising psychological tests for the evaluation of organic problems, but the tools remain nonspecific and the resultant data must be reviewed with care.

Despite these shortcomings, psychological testing can be an important adjunct in the evaluation of dementia and can be expected to become consistently more effective in the future. A broad variety of tests are available. Some approaches use extensive batteries demanding trained neuropsychologists skilled in the evaluation of brain-damaged patients (Fuld, 1978; Gainotti et al, 1980; Boller et al, 1980). Others are elementary scales for use at the bedside or office, designed to provide an overview of the presence and/or severity of a mental impairment (Blessed et al, 1968; Folstein et al, 1975) or some specific disturbance such as depression or vascular abnormality (Beck, 1963; Hachinski et al, 1975). Psychological testing based on scaled tests with dependable replicability provides an excellent means to determine progression of mental impairment and, when appropriately used, gives valuable information concerning altered mental functions in a demented patient.

One limiting factor for physicians is the wide variety of tests used. Most psychologists are familiar with a limited range of instruments, usually a battery of tests. Currently, four distinctly different, often noninterchangeable neuropsychologic assessment approaches are popular in the United States: the Wechsler tests of intelligence and memory abetted by an assortment of associated tests, the Halstead-Reitan battery, the Luria tests, and the "process" approach. The first group centers on the Wechsler intelligence test (1955) and the Wechsler memory test (1945) augmented by a number of related tests. While probably the most widely used, most heterogeneous, and potentially the most complete, variability in the ancillary tests limits this group as a standardized battery.

The second group, originally devised by Halstead (1940) with documentation and improvements by Reitan (1955 and 1964), is frequently used in the United States. The Halstead-Reitan battery is best standardized and offers considerable experience with results in organic mental problems (Reitan and Davison, 1974). Experienced users claim that it can provide accurate localization of disease within the central nervous system (Reitan, 1964). The battery was devised almost 50 years ago, however, and has undergone few alterations in several decades. Thus many innovations in both psychological thinking and testing are omitted. Of even greater concern is the fact that the diagnostic data relate to older disease classifications, making interpretation difficult. Some portions of this battery have proved so useful, however, that most psychologists who employ the Wechsler tests include one or more Halstead-Reitan subtests.

A third group of neuropsychological tests has become popular more recently and is advocated by a small but ardent group of psychologists. This series was originally devised and perfected by the Russian neuropsychologist Luria (1964 and 1966). It has been translated into English and revised for contemporary use by several investigators (Christensen, 1975; Golden, 1981). The Luria test is relatively short (at least in comparison to the others), is relatively easy to administer, and provides useful information on a broad variety of organic mental problems. In the hands of a seasoned clinician such as Professor Luria, it offered a maximum of information for a minimum investment of time and effort. Unfortunately as it is used by less accomplished neuropsychologists, this short test is open to errors of omission, misinterpretation, and misdiagnosis. Nonetheless the Luria test is gaining use and exerts an influence on current thinking in neuropsychology.

Finally, the process approach to neuropsychology emphasizes analysis of the strategies used by the patient to achieve results in the testing situation in addition to the absolute test results (Kaplan, 1990). Many types of neuropsychological instruments may be used including those mentioned above, and different sets of instruments may be chosen for a particular patient depending on the nature of the referring question, the deficits exhibited by the patient, and the intended application of the test results (for example, documentation of deficit, monitoring of recovery, assessing an intervention, localization of lesion, and development of a rehabilitation program). Even more than with the other batteries, it is the skill and experience of the psychologist that is the key to success with the process approach.

To complement the four major approaches, an array of highly specialized tests exists, many designed to probe single functions. Tests of attention, memory, language (aphasia examinations), musical ability, calculating ability, visuospatial discrimination, and so on are available in a wide and confusing array. Lezak (1976, 1983) has attempted to list and describe the major tests of neuropsychology; her book outlines hundreds of individual tests with descriptions and commentary. No book can be complete and current with the newest developments, however, and tests are being added regularly as psychologists devise new means to investigate specific questions. The best of these are used by other psychologists and eventually become part of the standard armamentarium. Selected combinations of old and new tests can provide relevant diagnostic information and innovations further improve neuropsychological testing for dementia. Unfortunately many psychologists are unaware of, or cannot perform, the best tests for a given problem. The situation is in flux but in a healthy and progressive flux.

In addition to these general neuropsychologic techniques, attempts have been made to produce dementia batteries, combinations of neuropsychological evaluations selected to provide specific information for the diagnosis of dementia. Most techniques such as the batteries of Fuld (1978), Gainotti and co-workers (1980), and Rosen (1980), are aggregates of standardized and validated tests selected because of proven value in the diagnosis of dementia. These batteries successfully identify the major problems of Alzheimer's disease. While a diagnosis of dementia may be confirmed by such batteries, the etiology is likely to remain an unknown quantity. Different profiles of neuropsychological dysfunction occur in cortical and subcortical dementia syndromes (see Chapters 1, 3, and 4 for further discussions of this distinction). Cortical disorders such as Alzheimer's disease produce deficits in instrumental functions such as language, memory, and praxis whereas subcortical disorders adversely affect fundamental functions such as motivation, rate of information processing, attention, and mood (Albert, 1978; Cummings, 1986; Cummings and Benson, 1984). Dementia assessment batteries must be sensitive to deficits in both major domains to be maximally useful to the clinician. Tests of naming, language comprehension, list learning and recall, and constructions are required for the detection of cortical dysfunction; tasks assessing executive and organizational function and speed of processing are necessary to detect defects in subcortical function. Better techniques for the differentiation of dementia through neuropsychological testing are needed; early efforts demonstrate that improvem. anticipated with refinements in, and increased experience w. administration.

Short Mental Status Tests

One serious drawback to the use of a dementia battery is the duration of testing. Testing can take from two to six hours to complete and include complex and demanding material, often well beyond the competence or patience of a demented patient. Many dements cannot respond to the test items, producing information of little value. To avoid this problem, investigators have devised simple tests, often requiring just a few minutes and using material of such simplicity that only the most severely degenerated patient will be unable to produce some scorable responses. Called dementia scales, several have been validated with age and education controls (Blessed et al, 1968; Folstein et al, 1975; Jacobs et al, 1977). These scales can provide valuable information concerning the severity of dementia but offer little information for determination of etiology.

An early example is the dementia scale that Blessed and colleagues (1968) used in their correlation study of Alzheimer's type neuropathologic changes. The Blessed Dementia Scale has two sections—first a series of questions probing cognitive function and second, a questionnaire outlining the patient's self-care capabilities and activities of daily living. Numerical values were set for both scales and a combined number, a dementia score, was obtained. The test was easy to administer, provided replicable results, and clearly demonstrated the progression of dementia.

The most widely used short test is the Mini-Mental State Examination of Folstein, Folstein, and McHugh (1975), a short series of problems that challenge a variety of mental functions and provide a single numerical score. A similar test (Jacobs et al, 1977) demonstrates significant mental impairment in the elderly. The Mini-Mental State Examination and the self-care section of the Blessed scale have been combined in many Alzheimer's disease centers. No short scale can be a discriminating diagnostic tool, but each is useful for screening purposes and can gauge the severity of mental impairment even in advanced dementia.

A different short scale of value for the clinician is the Hachinski Ischemia Scale (Hachinski et al, 1975) (see Chapter 5), a set of observations from the history and examination that suggests the presence of cerebrovascular disease of sufficient severity to be the source of the dementia. There are 13 topics with weighted scores; the potential score ranges from 0 (no suggestion of cerebrovascular disease) to 18 (serious problems). A score above 7 suggests the presence of vascular disease whereas scores below 4 imply that the mental impairment is not on a vascular basis. The Hachinski

Ischemia Scale has been correlated with cerebral blood flow studies (Hachinski et al, 1975) and autopsy findings (Rosen et al, 1980) and is considered a reliable indicator of cerebrovascular disease. Rosen and colleagues demonstrated that some of the items were not discriminatory and suggested that a shorter set of items could provide diagnostically significant information. A high score on the Hachinski scale may have causes other than vascular disease, but in the appropriate clinical context, the test is of definite value.

Other useful tools include the depression scales (Hamilton, 1967; Beck, 1963; Zung, 1965; Folstein and Luria, 1973), questionnaires to be filled out by the patient, members of the family, or the clinician that probe for significant affective disorder. While of proven value, both false positive and false negative results occur in the demented population and the scales should not be interpreted too literally.

Used as an adjunct to clinical impressions, psychological tests and rating scales can be of immense value to the clinician. As independent, uncorrelated entities, however, these tools may be misleading and incorrect. Their value correlates directly with the degree of their integration into the overall clinical picture. Used with intelligence, neuropsychological tests are effective in dementia studies and will become increasingly important as sophistication in their use becomes more widespread.

3

Cortical Dementias: Alzheimer's Disease and Other Cortical Degenerations

A few degenerative diseases affect primarily the cortical mantle and produce disorders of intellectual function. Dementia of the Alzheimer's type (DAT) and frontal lobe degenerations such as Pick's disease are the two principal cortical dementias. DAT is the most well known of all dementing disorders and probably accounts for more cases of dementia than any other single disease entity, between 35 and 60 percent of progressive dementias evaluated in hospital-based settings (Chapter 1). Pick's disease is much more rare, 10 to 15 times less common than DAT. The two disorders share many features and have often been considered clinically indistinguishable. DAT, however, has pathologic changes concentrated in the associative areas of the parietal, temporal, and frontal lobes and the hippocampus. Pick's disease preferentially affects the anterior temporal and frontal areas. These contrasting patterns of topographic involvement produce different behavioral manifestations that often allow clinical identification of the underlying process (Cummings, 1982).

DAT and Pick's disease are not diffuse or global disorders. Areas of cortex subserving primary motor, somatosensory, and visual functions are relatively spared and subcortical structures do not become involved until late in the clinical course, well after the dementia is firmly established. Other dementia-producing conditions (vascular, infectious, traumatic, or neoplastic) may involve the cerebral cortex, but they are less selective, and subcortical structures are also routinely affected to produce clinical syndromes with mixed cortical and subcortical features (Chapters 5, 6, and 10). In this chapter, the cortical dementias are discussed individually and their distinguishing characteristics are emphasized.

DEMENTIA OF THE ALZHEIMER TYPE (DAT)

In 1907 Alois Alzheimer described the disease that came to bear his name (Wilkins and Brody, 1969). In the insane asylum in Frankfurt-am-Main, he observed a 51-year-old woman who manifested persecutory delusions, had impaired memory, and could not find her way about her own apartment. Her language abnormalities included a naming disturbance, paraphasic substitutions, and impaired comprehension. In contrast, her gait, coordination, and reflexes were unaffected. She gradually deteriorated and died after four and a half years of hospitalization. At the autopsy, the brain appeared grossly atrophic. Microscopic study revealed cortical cell loss, neurofibrillary degenerative changes involving many of the neurons, and numerous miliary foci (neuritic plaques) throughout the cortex. The clinical and pathologic features reported by Alzheimer are now considered classic characteristics of the disease.

A perfect epidemiologic study of the prevalence of DAT has not been accomplished, and the exact frequency of the disease in the United States or the world is unknown. The results of existing studies vary substantially, reflecting differing sampling strategies (house-to-house, random, or purposive sampling), differing sensitivity of screening instruments (highly sensitive tests will have a higher false positive rate, less sensitive tests will have a higher false negative rate), and differing criteria for diagnosis of DAT. Most screening instruments have low specificity and tend to exaggerate the number of dementia patients diagnosed as DAT. In a house-to-house survey of patients with severe dementia in a racially balanced county in Mississippi, Schoenberg and colleagues (1985) found an overall prevalence of DAT of 0.45 percent among all individuals above age 40 and a 4 percent prevalence among those age 80 and older. In contrast, Pfeffer and colleagues (1987), using highly sensitive tests for intellectual impairment, studied the prevalence of DAT in a southern California retirement community and found that 15.3 percent among those over age 65 and 36 percent of those over age 80 met criteria for the disease. Most studies have identified prevalence rates of approximately 6 percent among individuals over age 65 (Broe et al, 1973; Gruenberg, 1978; Roth, 1978). Using this mean figure, Rocca and colleagues (1986) estimated that there were 1,414,000 cases of DAT in the United States in 1980 and that there will be 2,008,000 cases by the year 2000.

The most striking correlate of the prevalence of DAT is the age of the victim. In the study by Broe and colleagues (1973), the prevalence rose from

2.4 percent among those under age 75 to 10.9 percent among those over age 75. Similarly, in the Mini-Finland survey, Sulkava and colleagues (1985) identified DAT in 2 percent of 65- to 74-year-olds, 6 percent of those 75 to 84, and 14.8 percent in those 85 and older. Although studies vary in conclusions regarding the exact prevalence of DAT, they concur in observing a steady rise in the disease from age 60 to at least age 80.

The incidence as well as the prevalence of DAT is highly correlated with the age of the population studied. Schoenberg and colleagues (1987) noted that the incidence rose from 4.4/100,000 in those 30 to 59 years old, to 95.8/100,000 in those 60 to 69 years old, to 530.7/100,000 in the 70 to 79 year old group, and finally to 1,431.7/100,000 in those over age 80 years.

Although DAT typically begins after age 50 years, onset as early as the fourth decade of life has been reported (Ferraro and Jervis, 1941; Jervis and Soltz, 1936; Lowenberg and Waggoner, 1934). Gender has little influence on the prevalence or incidence of DAT. Several studies have found a slightly increased occurrence among females (Jorm et al, 1987; Rocca et al, 1986; Sulkava et al, 1985), but the markedly increased prevalence among women reported in carly studies probably reflected the relative longevity of women and a disproportionate number of females surviving into the period of greatest risk for the disease.

The prevalence of DAT is determined by a combination of its incidence and the survival of the patients after onset. The survival of DAT patients is increasing over time probably as a result of both earlier diagnosis and more aggressive medical management of the late medical complications such as aspiration pneumonia and urinary tract infections. Currently the average length of survival after diagnosis is approximately 8 years (Barclay et al, 1985; Treves et al, 1986). An occasional patient may have a rapidly progressive course leading to death in less than a year (Ehle and Johnson, 1977; Watson, 1979), and rare patients may survive 20 or more years after onset of the disease.

Until recently, the diagnosis of DAT was reserved for those patients whose illness began before the age of 65 years whereas those with intellectual deterioration beginning later were considered to have senile dementia. The division into senile and presenile forms at age 65 is arbitrary: Identical pathologic changes are found in both age groups, and the clinical features are similar in the two populations. Growing recognition of the many causes of dementia in the so-called senile period makes the former nomenclature untenable. In this volume, DAT is regarded as a specific entity with characteristic clinical and pathologic changes irrespective of age at onset. It has been suggested but not yet conclusively established that the age of the patient may modify the manifestations of the illness, and some elderly patients may have a more benign course, exhibit less severe language alterations, and have less marked pathologic changes.

A substantial number of families in which DAT is inherited as a mendelian dominant trait have been described (Cook et al, 1979; Essen-Moller, 1946; Feldman et al, 1963a; Landy and Bain, 1970; Lowenberg and Waggoner, 1934; McMenemy et al, 1939; Wheelan, 1959).

Families with clearcut autosomal dominant inheritance and 50 percent risk profile for siblings and offspring comprise approximately 20 percent of reported cases of DAT. In these families, the disease tends to appear in the sixth or seventh decade of life, and some studies suggest that the familial cases are more likely to exhibit such features as aphasia, apraxia, more rapidly progressive course, more prominent myoclonus, and increased platelet membrane fluidity (Breitner and Folstein, 1984; Pratt, 1970; Zubenko et al, 1988). Several recent genetic investigations, however, suggest that the hereditary contribution to the occurrence of DAT has previously been underestimated. These studies indicate that a much larger number of cases of DAT may be familial and that older onset as well as younger onset cases predict an increased risk among family members (Breitner et al, 1988; Farrer et al, 1989; Huff et al, 1988; Martin et al, 1988; Mohs et al, 1987). Not all cases appear to be familial, however, and sporadic as well as hereditary forms of the disease may exist (Fitch et al, 1988).

Twin studies have failed to elucidate the inheritance pattern, since identical twins concordant (Cook et al, 1981) and discordant (Davidson and Robertson, 1955; Hunter et al, 1972; Nee et al, 1987) for DAT have been reported. In addition to an increased incidence of the disease in the families of probands with DAT, there is an increased number of family members with Down's syndrome, lymphoproliferative disorders, and an abnormal number of chromosomes (Cook et al, 1979; Heston and Mastri, 1977; Heston et al, 1981; Jarvik, 1978). Correspondingly, nearly all elderly patients with Down's syndrome develop DAT (Olson and Shaw, 1969) or die of hematologic malignancies. The possible significance of these observations is discussed below.

Clinical Characteristics

Clinically, patients with DAT undergo steadily progressive intellectual deterioration. Remissions do not occur and plateau periods of arrested progression are extremely rare. The rate of intellectual decline is relatively regular although variations in individuals over the course of the illness are not uncommon (Katzman et al, 1988). The sequence in which higher cognitive functions are lost and the temporal order in which behavioral and neurologic disabilities occur are important clues for establishing the clinical diagnosis. The clinical course of the disease can be divided conveniently into three stages (Table 3–1) (Berg et al, 1982; Coblentz et al, 1973; Henderson and MacLachlan, 1930; Lishman, 1978; Sim, 1965; Sjøgren, 1950; Sjøgren et al, 1952). Memory disturbance is nearly always the feature that heralds

TABLE 3–1.   Principal clinical findings in each stage of DAT.

Stage I (duration of disease 1 to 3 years)
    Memory—new learning defective, remote recall mildly impaired
    Visuospatial skills—topographic disorientation, poor complex constructions
    Language—poor wordlist generation, anomia
    Personality—indifference, occasional irritability
    Psychiatric features—sadness or delusions in some
    Motor system—normal
    EEG—normal
    CT/MRI—normal
    PET/SPECT—bilateral posterior parietal hypometabolism/hyperfusion
Stage II (duration of disease 2 to 10 years)
    Memory—recent and remote recall more severely impaired
    Visuospatial skills—poor constructions, spatial disorientation
    Language—fluent aphasia
    Calculation—acalculia
    Praxis—ideomotor apraxia
    Personality—indifference or irritability
    Psychiatric features—delusions in some
    Motor system—restlessness, pacing
    EEG—slowing of background rhythm
    CT/MRI—normal or ventricular dilatation and sulcal enlargement
    PET/SPECT—bilateral parietal and frontal hypometabolism/hypoperfusion
Stage III (duration of disease 8 to 12 years)
    Intellectual functions—severely deteriorated
    Motor—limb rigidity and flexion posture
    Sphincter control—urinary and fecal incontinence
    EEG—diffusely slow
    CT/MRI—ventricular dilatation and sulcal enlargement
    PET/SPECT—bilateral parietal and frontal hypometabolism/hypoperfusion

onset of the disease. Poor judgment is evident and the patient is unable to reason through problems. Carelessness in work habits and household chores and spatial and temporal disorientation also occur early. The patient becomes lost in familiar surroundings and, while still able to follow well-established routines, any new challenge reveals the deficits. Indifference, irritability, or suspiciousness may contribute to the initial symptomatology. In the second stage of illness, aphasia and apraxia appear along with other cognitive deficits. The initial indifference characteristically worsens and restlessness with frequent pacing appears; occasional incontinence may occur. Terminally there is impairment of virtually all intellectual capacities, motor disabilities become evident, and both urinary and fecal incontinence are present.

    The initial memory disturbance in DAT is characterized by impaired ability to learn new material and mild difficulty recalling remote information.

Poor learning appears regularly in the initial stages of the disease and is nearly always the first intellectual deficit noted by the patient's family or workmates (Lishman, 1978; Sjøgren, 1950; Sjøgren et al, 1952; Stengel, 1943). In rare patients, word-finding difficulties and naming disturbances antedate the memory changes (Goodman, 1953), but the diagnosis of DAT should be regarded skeptically if recent memory loss is not among the earliest features observed.

Neuropsychological investigation of the memory defect indicates that these patients have difficulty encoding information. Information is rapidly lost from short-term memory and storage for eventual recall is compromised (Miller, 1971, 1972). Automatic as well as effortful types of mnemonic abilities are compromised in DAT: Priming of the stimulus material, category cueing, categorical organization of the stimuli, associating the stimulus with its superordinant category at the time of presentation, enriching the encoding environment, providing multiple choice alternatives for recognition of stimuli, and self-generation do little to facilitate later recall (Butters et al, 1983; Davis and Mumford, 1984; Dick et al, 1989 a,b; Grober et al, 1988; Kramer et al, 1988; Salmon et al, 1988; Weingartner et al, 1981). Deficits are evident in tests of both verbal and nonverbal memory (Sahakian et al, 1988). Remote memory is also rendered abnormal in DAT, but a temporal gradient of recall with less involvement of remote than of recent information is demonstrable (Beatty et al, 1988b; Moskovitch et al, 1981; Sagar et al, 1988a). Not all aspects of memory are disturbed in DAT. Procedural memory, the learning of motor tasks, undergoes little decrement until the late stages of the illness (Eslinger and Damasio, 1986). Confabulation occurs in DAT, but it is usually not marked and commonly appears several years after onset of the illness (Polatin et al, 1948; Sourander and Sjøgren, 1970; Uyematsu, 1923).

Like memory, visuospatial skills are impaired early in the course of DAT (Adams and Victor, 1977; Sim and Sussman, 1962; Sim et al, 1966; Sjøgren et al, 1952). The patients get lost in familiar surroundings, lose their way while driving, and may eventually become disorientated in their own homes. Simple drawing tests reveal that they are unable to copy three-dimensional representations accurately and often fail to reproduce more elementary figures (Fig. 3–1)(Henderson et al, 1989; Moore and Wyke, 1984; Pan et al, 1989). Neuropsychological testing confirms the visuospatial compromise (Gainotti et al, 1980), and on the Wechsler Adult Intelligence Scale, patients obtain their lowest scores on performance subtests that depend on visuospatial ability (that is, block design) (Perez et al, 1975). Preliminary investigations suggest that DAT patients may exhibit more profound involvement on tests of constructional performance than they do on tests of egocentric space such as map reading (Brouwers et al, 1984). Dressing disturbance, another manifestation of impaired spatial comprehension, is common in the middle phases of the disease (Boyd, 1936–1937;

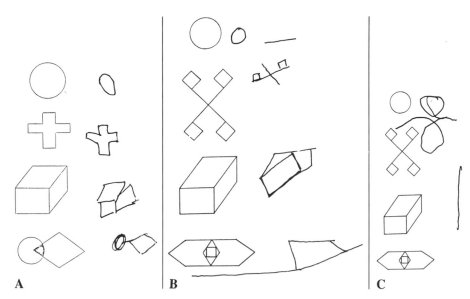

FIGURE 3–1.   Progression of constructional disturbances in Alzheimer's disease: (A) one year after onset, (B) three years after onset, and (C) eight years after onset.

Henderson and MacLachlan, 1930; Jervis, 1937; Rothschild, 1934; Wheelan, 1959).

Language changes are a sensitive indicator of cortical dysfunction, and the specific pattern of linguistic disturbance aids in the diagnosis of DAT. The first abnormalities to become apparent in spontaneous speech are impaired word finding and circumlocution imparting an empty quality to the verbalizations (Goodman, 1953; Hier et al, 1985; Henderson and Maclachlan, 1930; Rothschild, 1934; Whitworth and Larson, 1989). Testing at this time usually reveals that object naming is preserved, but the ability to generate lists of words in a given category is impaired (Benson, 1979a, b; Isaacs and Kennie, 1973). Early in the course of the dementia, patients do better when they are asked to construct a list of animal names than when they are asked to give lists of words beginning with a specific letter. Performance on both types of list construction is soon seriously compromised (Miller and Hague, 1975; Rosen, 1980). As the disease progresses, spontaneous speech becomes increasingly empty and a frank anomia becomes apparent (Bayles and Tomoeda, 1983; Flicker et al, 1987; Fuller, 1912; Gustafson et al, 1978; Malamud and Lowenberg, 1929; Rothschild and Kasanin, 1936). On tests of confrontation naming, naming of low-frequency items fails first followed by difficulty in naming more common objects (Barker and Lawson, 1968; Lawson and Barker, 1968). Paraphasia becomes evident along with the anomia. Verbal paraphasias are the first to occur;

literal paraphasias and neologisms tend to be confined to the later stages of the disease (Bayles and Tomoeda, 1983; de Ajuriaguerra and Tissot, 1975). The verbal paraphasias become progressively less related to the target word as the disease advances (Schwartz et al, 1979).

Comprehension of spoken language is also progressively impaired (Faber-Longendoen et al, 1988; Sjøgren et al, 1952), and repetition of phrases or sentences may be disturbed but is usually relatively spared until late in the course. The spontaneous speech of some patients with DAT closely resembles the fluent paraphasic output of transcortical sensory aphasia (Albert, 1980; Appell et al, 1982; Cummings et al, 1985; Goodman, 1953; Lowenberg and Waggoner, 1934; Rothschild, 1934). Some patients manifest a markedly reduced verbal output (Heston et al, 1966; Sjøgren et al, 1952; Wheelan, 1959) but the sparse output has the same fluent paraphasic characteristics of more talkative patients. Nonfluent agrammatic verbal output of the Broca's or transcortical motor type does not occur in DAT. The syntactic and phonologic aspects of language are relatively preserved until the late stages whereas the semantic aspects undergo progressive deterioration (Kempler et al, 1987; Schwartz et al, 1979; Cummings et al, 1985). Social and practical aspects of language are also progressively disturbed as the dementia advances. The patient's ability to converse is impaired; the listener is frequently unable to follow a coherent line of thought in the verbal output, and the patient is not engaged with the listener (Albert, 1980, 1981). This is one of the principal differences between the language of patients with DAT and those with fluent aphasias secondary to focal vascular insults (Benson et al, 1982). Inappropriate intrusion of words and themes from earlier conversations and earlier testing is also characteristic of the spontaneous speech of patients with DAT (Fuld et al., 1982). Reading comprehension is impaired in patients with DAT although reading aloud may be relatively preserved until fairly late in the course (Cummings et al, 1986). Aphasic agraphia is evident coincident with the disturbances in spontaneous speech, and orthography deteriorates as the disease advances (Folstein and Breitner, 1981; Horner et al, 1988; Rapcsak et al, 1989a).

In the middle and later phases of the illness, a variety of reiterative speech disturbances may become evident. Echolalia, the tendency to repeat words and phrases addressed to the patient, occurs in some (Kasanin and Crank, 1933; Neumann and Cohn, 1953; Sjøgren, 1950). Palilalia, the tendency to repeat words and phrases initiated by the patient, and logoclonia, repetition of the final syllable of a word, may appear as language deteriorates further (Bayles et al, 1985; Fuller, 1912; Hannah, 1936; Rothschild, 1934; Sjøgren, 1950; Wheelan, 1959). Terminally vocalization is reduced to the production of repetitive sounds unrecognizable as language (Jervis, 1937; Stern and Reed, 1945), and complete mutism may eventually occur.

The pattern of linguistic changes occurring during the course of DAT demonstrates that the loss of language is not a global deterioration and does

TABLE 3–2.   Progressive changes in verbal output in DAT.

Stage I
    Empty, circumlocutory spontaneous speech
    Poor word-list generation
    Mild anomia
Stage II
    Anomia
    Paraphasia
    Comprehension impaired
    Difficult to engage in conversation
Stage III
    Paraphasias less related to target word
    Echolalia, palilalia, logoclonia
    Dysarthria
    Terminal mutism

not affect all aspects simultaneously (Table 3–2). With few exceptions, progressive changes occur in a predictable sequence, and the language characteristics of the patient depend on the stage of disease. The earliest abnormalities are emptiness of spontaneous speech and poor word-list generation; next, anomia, paraphasia, and impaired comprehension evolve; fluent aphasia of a transcortical sensory type but with poor engagement in the conversation then appears; and finally reiterative speech disturbances such as palilalia and logoclonia become manifest. Terminally the patient makes only unintelligible sounds or is mute. Throughout the process the semantic and pragmatic aspects of language are progressively impaired, whereas the syntactic and phonologic components are relatively spared. There are many similarities between fluent aphasias secondary to focal left posterior cerebral insults and the aphasic disturbances of DAT. The progressive linguistic deterioration, the increasingly distant relationship between the target word and the verbal paraphasia, and the loss of engagement of the patient in conversation characterize DAT and distinguish the two conditions. (See Chapter 5 for a discussion of the special problems involved in distinguishing the angular gyrus syndrome from dementia of the Alzheimer type.)

Speech, the mechanical aspect of language production, remains normal throughout most of the course of DAT (Cummings et al, 1985). Articulation and voice volume are spared along with other elementary motor functions. As the disease progresses into later stages, stuttering (Barrett, 1913; Essen-Moller, 1946; Gustafson et al, 1978) and/or a slurring dysarthria may occur (Boyd, 1936–1937; English, 1942; Gustafson et al, 1978; Heston et al, 1966; Miller and Hague, 1975; Sjøgren et al, 1952).

Apraxias and agnosias are difficult to study in DAT. Investigators reporting these disorders have used a variety of definitions of praxis and gnosis, and when one is examining patients, it is difficult to distinguish agnosia and apraxia from disabilities related to aphasia, visuospatial disturbance, and amnesia. Some reliable information has been collected, however. Polatin and associates (1948) considered agnosias to be characteristic of DAT, and approximately one-third of the patients studied by Sjøgren and co-workers (1952) had visual agnosia. Rochford (1971) showed that, in some demented patients, poor confrontation naming was due to impaired visual recognition rather than aphasic anomia. Performance on tests naming body parts (where substantial nonvisual cues are available) was superior to performance on object-naming tests of equal difficulty. Agnosia has been less intensively studied in the course of DAT. Patients retain the ability to recognize objects and to use them appropriately beyond the time that they can name them accurately. In the verbal domain, Cummings and colleagues (1986) demonstrated that patients with advanced dementia were able to correctly read words aloud. This indicates that their perception of the stimulus was largely intact even though they were unable to comprehend the meaning of the word, findings consistent with an associative verbal agnosia. Prosopagnosia, the failure to recognize familiar faces, appears together with other forms of agnosia (English, 1942; Essen-Moller, 1946; Goodman, 1953; Henderson and MacLachlan, 1930; Uyematsu, 1923). Impaired self-recognition may be involved in the production of "mirror sign" where patients address their own images when they encounter a mirror (Henderson and MacLachlan, 1930; Sjøgren et al, 1952; Stengel, 1943).

Two types of apraxia occur in DAT: ideational apraxia, the failure correctly to pantomime the sequence of events of a complex motor act such as filling and lighting a pipe, and ideomotor apraxia, the inability to do on command an act that can be performed spontaneously. The obligatory use of a body part as a substitute for an object (such as using the index finger to brush the teeth rather than pretending to hold a toothbrush) is a particularly common manifestation of ideomotor apraxia in DAT (Rapcsak et al, 1989b). The apraxias are rarely an early component of the illness; they are found in about one-third of stage I patients and in 70 to 80 percent of patients in the second stage of the disease (Della Sala et al, 1987; Sjøgren, 1950; Sjøgren et al, 1952). On rare occasions, apraxia antedates other features of the illness.

In addition to the cardinal cortical disturbances of aphasia, amnesia, apraxia, and agnosia, a variety of other intellectual deficits becomes manifest as the disease advances. Disturbances of calculation are evident by the second stage of the disease and may be due to visuospatial or aphasic impairments or to primary acalculia (Adams and Victor, 1981; Lishman, 1978). Poor judgment, loss of abstraction capabilities, distractibility, right-left confusion, and poor concentration may begin early and become more apparent as the disease advances. Motivation, problem-solving abilities, interpersonal skills, logic, and reasoning are all progressively impaired. The intellectual deficits combine to devastate cognition, and terminally there is no evidence of ongoing higher intellectual function.

Personality and social behavior are not markedly changed during the early phases of DAT despite insidious intellectual deterioration (Sim et al, 1966). These preserved behaviors allow patients to continue functioning socially and often lead others to underestimate or excuse the patient's disabilities. Thus it is not uncommon to discover that individuals with severe memory impairment, empty speech, and impaired abstraction and calculation abilities are continuing to go to work, and the extent of their dementia becomes evident only when some novel or demanding situation arises. Indifference is a common early manifestation, and patients frequently have a bewildered facial expression. As the disease becomes established, indifference, disengagement, and loss of investment in activities and relationships are evident; with progression to the later stages of the illness, disinhibited, agitated, and self-centered behaviors become more apparent (Petry et al, 1988, in press; Rubin et al, 1987 a,b). Disruptive, aggressive behavior is not uncommon in the later stages of DAT (Swearer et al, 1988). Witzelsucht, or inappropriate jocularity and frequent laughing, occurs in a few patients. Larson and colleagues (1963) found that 69 percent of their 377 patients with DAT had simple dementia without personality or character alterations, 18 percent became paranoid, and 10 percent had affective disturbances. The Klüver-Bucy syndrome, a complex behavioral condition including sensory agnosia, dietary changes, hypermetamorphosis (mandatory exploration of environmental stimuli as soon as they are noted), altered sexuality, and hyperoral behavior may emerge in the final stages of DAT (Lilly et al, 1982; Lishman, 1978; Sourander and Sjøgren, 1970).

The occurrence of depression in DAT is controversial, with reported frequencies ranging from 0 to 87 percent (Cummings and Victoroff, 1990; Wragg and Jeste, 1989). The evaluation of mood changes in DAT is complicated by the overlapping symptoms that can occur in both disorders such as agitation, loss of interest, loss of insight, and sleep and appetite changes. Depressive statements may be made in the early phases of DAT and mild to moderate symptoms of depression may occur at nearly any point in the disease course, but major depressive episodes appear to be rare (Cummings et al, 1987).

Psychosis and delusions are common in DAT. Approximately 50 percent of patients exhibit delusions in the course of the disease and in some cases they are the presenting manifestation (Cummings et al, 1987; Wragg and Jeste, 1989). Delusional beliefs are usually of a persecutory nature involving fears of personal harm, theft of property, or infidelity of the spouse. Capgras syndrome, the false belief that someone (usually the patient's spouse) has been replaced by an identical-appearing imposter, has also been reported (Merriam et al, 1988; Rubin et al, 1988).

Disturbances of sleep, appetite, and sexual behavior also occur in DAT. Patients exhibit frequent nocturnal awakenings, and studies of sleep architecture reveal diminished slow wave sleep (Stage 3 and Stage 4), decreased rapid-eye-movement sleep, increased latency to onset of rapid-eye-movement sleep, and sleep fragmentation (Lowenstein et al, 1982; Merriam et al, 1988; Prinz et al, 1982; Swearer et al, 1988). Appetite may either increase or decrease in the course of DAT; weight loss is common in the later stages of the illness. Sexual activity is usually diminished in the DAT although a few patients may exhibit a transient period of increased sexual interest (Kumar et al, 1988; Merriam et al, 1988). Sexual aggressiveness is rare (Kumar et al, 1988; Rabins et al, 1982).

A variety of endocrinologic abnormalities have been identified in DAT. The most extensively studied is the dexamethasone suppression test (DST). In normal individuals, administration of exogenous dexamethasone results in a reduction of the serum cortical level when assayed several hours later. A substantial number of depressed patients as well as a few patients with other conditions have been shown to fail to suppress serum cortisol in response to the dexamethasone. Abnormal DSTs can be demonstrated in approximately half of all DAT patients. Abnormal DST results do not correlate with the mood state of the patient but are more common in more severely demented individuals (Davous et al, 1988; Greenwald et al, 1986; Jenike and Albert, 1984; Pomara et al, 1984; Raskind et al, 1982). Other endocrinologic abnormalities reported in DAT include a reduced response of the pineal gland to 5-methoxypsoralen (low melatonin level), poor response of vasopressin to osmotic stimulation and metoclopramide, muted thyroid-stimulating hormone response to thyroid-releasing hormone, blunted-growth hormone response to edrophonium, and reduced prolactin response to thyrotropin-releasing hormone (Lampe et al, 1988; Newhouse et al, 1986; Norbiato et al, 1988; Souetre et al, 1989; Thienhaus et al, 1987). These abnormalities are not sufficiently consistent or unique to have diagnostic significance but suggest that suprahypothalamic or hypothalamic control of endocrinologic function is frequently impaired in DAT.

An initial loss of spontaneity is frequently followed by a prolonged period of restless hyperactivity with purposeless pacing and carphologia (purposeless handling and picking). (Cummings and Victoroth, 1990; Hughes, 1970; Lishman, 1978; Rothschild, 1934; Sjøgren, 1950). No elementary motor abnormalities appear until late stages; in the final few years, the patient gradually develops extrapyramidal rigidity, gegenhalten, or spasticity (Jervis and Soltz, 1936; Sim and Sussman, 1962; Sim et al, 1966). The terminal position, if the patient survives sufficiently long, is one of quadraplegia in flexion (Adams and Victor, 1977; Sjøgren et al, 1952; Yakovlev, 1954).

Ophthalmoplegia does not occur in DAT, but eye movement abnormalities can be identified when studied with electro-oculography. There are errors in tracking visual targets, and saccades are hypometric. Gaze impersistence is also common (Fletcher and Sharpe, 1986, 1988; Hutton et al, 1984).

Seizures, although uncommon in DAT, may occur in the later stages of illness and occasionally are seen early (Hauser et al, 1986; Hughes, 1970; Jervis and Soltz, 1936; Lishman, 1978; Polatin et al, 1948; Sim and Sussman, 1962; Sim et al., 1966). Myoclonic jerks—sudden, unsustained muscular contractions—are not uncommon in later stages (Faden and Townsend, 1976; Gimenez-Roldan et al, 1971; Hauser et al, 1986; Jacob, 1970; Mayeux et al, 1981a). Failure to recognize this fact has led to confusion of the diagnosis of DAT with Jakob-Creutzfeldt disease. In the latter, myoclonus is usually evident within six months of onset whereas in DAT it commonly appears after the patient has had the illness for several years. Jacob (1970) observed that myoclonus is more common among familial cases of DAT.

Terminally urinary and fecal incontinence occur and primitive reflexes including grasp and suck responses become evident (Adams and Victor, 1981; Lishman, 1978; Paulson, 1977; Tweedy et al, 1982). The patients eventually die of aspiration pneumonia, urinary tract infection, or infection of decubitus ulcers.

The clinical phenomenology of DAT goes through a characteristic evolution with the early appearance of mild language, constructional, and memory disturbances followed by a stage of aphasia and progressive intellectual decline. Indifference and disengagement characterize the patients' demeanor, and motor abnormalities do not appear until the final stages of disease. This progression is outlined in Tables 3–1 and 3–2. These features are sufficiently characteristic of disease progression that they may be regarded as guidelines for the positive identification of DAT. Major deviations from the clinical picture should raise serious questions about the diagnosis, and the patient should be reevaluated for remediable causes of dementia. This approach avoids the pitfalls of diagnosis by exclusion discussed in Chapter 1.

Variations in the presentation and course of DAT that depart from the model described above have been documented. Aphasia, amnesia, or visuospatial deficits may dominate the early clinical presentation (Foster et al, 1983). The occurrence of psychosis, myoclonus, or evidence of nondrug-induced extrapyramidal dysfunction may occasionally be the predominant early manifestations and may portend a poor prognosis with more rapid clinical decline (Chui et al, 1985; Mayeux et al, 1985). Several studies have suggested a relationship between early onset, more profound language disorder, and a positive family history of DAT (Breitner and Folstein, 1984; Chui et al, 1985; Filley et al, 1986; Seltzer and Sherwin, 1983) whereas others have failed to confirm such relationships.

The ability to accurately diagnose DAT on the basis of clinical signs and symptoms has improved dramatically. In early follow-up studies, the accuracy of clinical diagnosis was found to be between 50 and 60 percent (Nott and Fleminger, 1975; Ron et al, 1979). With the construction of more rigorous diagnostic criteria, the rate of correct identification has risen to between 85 and 95 percent (Molsa et al, 1985; Sulkava et al, 1983; Tierney et al, 1988; Wade et al, 1987). These are two principal approaches to criterion-based diagnosis of DAT: the diagnostic guidelines of the revised third edition of the *Diagnostic and Statistical Manual of Mental Disorders* (DSMIIIR) (American Psychiatric Association, 1987) and the criteria of the National Institute of Neurological and Communicative Disorders and Stroke and the Alzheimer's Disease and Related Disorders Association (NINCDS–ADRDA)(McKhann et al, 1984). *DSMIIIR* criteria require that the patient have a dementia syndrome with memory impairment that is gradually progressive and that all alternate causes of dementia have been excluded. NINCDS-ADRDA criteria are more explicit and adopt a stratified approach providing for *definite, probable,* and *possible* diagnoses of DAT (Table 3–3). *Definite DAT* is the diagnosis when the patient meets clinical criteria for *probable DAT* and has histopathological evidence of DAT obtained by autopsy or biopsy. *Probable DAT* is identified when the presence of dementia syndrome has been established by a structured clinical questionnaire (such as the Mini-Mental State Examination [Folstein et al, 1975]) and confirmed by neuropsychological testing; there are deficits in two or more areas of cognition; there is progressive worsening of memory and other cognitive functions; there is no disturbance of consciousness; the disorder began after age 40 and before age 90; and there is no systemic or other brain disease present that could account for the progressive deficits in memory and cognition. *Possible DAT* is applied when a dementia syndrome is present and has no non-DAT explanation but the onset, presentation, or course are atypical; a second systemic or brain disorder is present but is not thought to be the cause of the dementia; or there is gradual progression of a single cognitive deficit in the absence of an alternate cause.

Identification of the classic DAT syndrome is aided by the DAT Inventory presented by Cummings and Benson (1986). This is a numerical approach awarding maximum points (2) for each of 10 features of DAT-impaired memory, aphasia, constructional disturbances, poor abstraction/calculation, disengaged/indifferent personality, intact articulation, normal gait and posture, absence of a movement abnormality (parkinsonism, tremor, and the like), and preserved psychomotor speed. Scores of 1 or 0 are awarded for moderate or marked deviations from these standard features. Using a cutoff score of 14, the inventory proved to have high accuracy in distinguishing between DAT and non-DAT dementias.

Laboratory Investigation

The diagnosis of DAT is based on recognition of the characteristic clinical features and is supported by demonstration of the typical cortical changes

TABLE 3–3. NINCDS-ADRDA criteria for definite, probable, and possible DAT.

Definite DAT
   Clinical criteria for Probable DAT
   Histopathologic evidence of DAT (autopsy or biopsy)
Probable DAT
   Dementia established by clinical examination and documented by mental status
      questionnaire
   Dementia confirmed by neuropsychological testing
   Deficits in two or more areas of cognition
   Progressive worsening of memory and other cognitive functions
   No disturbance of consciousness
   Onset between ages 40 and 90
   Absence of systemic or other brain diseases capable of producing a dementia
      syndrome
Possible DAT
   Atypical onset, presentation, or progression of a dementia syndrome without a
      known etiology
   A systemic or other brain disease capable of producing dementia but not
      thought to be the cause of the dementia is present
   There is a gradually progressive decline in a single intellectual function in the
      absence of any other identifiable cause
Unlikely DAT
   Sudden onset
   Focal neurological signs
   Seizures or gait disturbance early in the course of the illness

G McKahnn et al, "Clinical diagnosis of Alzheimer's disease: Report of the NINCDS-ADRDA Work Group, Department of Health and Human Services Task Force on Alzheimer's Disease," Neurol 1984;34:939–944.

postmortem. There are no pathognomonic laboratory results; rather, laboratory studies aid in the diagnosis by excluding conditions that may resemble DAT. A few tests such as F^{18}-flourodeoxyglucose position emission tomography (FDG PET) and single photon emission computed tomography (SPECT) have characteristic changes in DAT, but these fall short of being pathognomonic of the illness. Results of routine blood, serum, and urine studies are normal, and the cerebrospinal fluid (CSF) is normal or shows only a slight elevation of protein content. Research investigations have identified a number of abnormalities in serum and blood components of these patients, but their exact significance is uncertain. Cellular immunity involving T-cell lymphocytes is impaired (Behan and Behan, 1979); serum levels of antibodies against brain tissue are elevated (Nandy, 1978); and there are abnormalities of serum haptoglobin types (Stam and Op den velde, 1978), serum protein electrophoresis (Behan and Feldman, 1970), and serum immunoglobulin levels (Eisdorfer et al, 1978). Aneuploidy, an abnormal number of chromosomes, is found in the lymphocytes of some patients with DAT (Cook et al, 1979; Jarvik, 1978).

Numerous investigations of CSF in DAT have sought a diagnostically useful biological marker of the disorder. Although abnormalities have been identified, none has proved unique to DAT, and no currently available CSF test can be regarded as diagnostic. Among elements shown to be reduced in CSF compared to age-matched control subjects are corticotropin-releasing hormone, corticotropin, somatostatin, biopterin, glycine, glutamine, alpha-melanocyte-stimulating hormone, angiotensin-converting enzyme, and vasopressin (Jolkkonen et al, 1987; Kay et al, 1986; May et al, 1987; Mazurek et al, 1986a,b; Rainero et al, 1988; Raskind et al, 1986; Reinikainen et al, 1987; Smith et al, 1985; Sunderland et al, 1987; Zubenko et al, 1986). Results of studies of CSF catecholamines and serotonin are less consistent, but most investigators report that homovanillic acid, a dopamine metabolite, is diminished (Bareggi et al, 1982; Palmer et al, 1984; Thal, 1985). Controversy also surrounds studies of CSF cholinesterase and beta-endorphin; several investigators have reported diminished levels in DAT while others have failed to confirm these observations (Atack et al, 1988; Kaiya et al, 1983; Raskind et al, 1986; Thal, 1985; Tune et al, 1985; Zubenko et al, 1986).

The electroencephalogram (EEG) and computerized tomographic (CT) scan have been widely used in the differential diagnosis of DAT. Harner (1975) emphasized that most treatable causes of dementia are associated with prominent EEG abnormalities whereas the degenerative cortical dementias show few abnormalities in the early stages of development. There is a reduction of EEG amplitude and a slight slowing of alpha activity at the onset of DAT. As the disease advances, the background consists of low- to medium-amplitude, irregular theta activity. Frontally predominant delta activity is gradually superimposed, and fast activity is lost. Asymmetry of the slow-wave activity is not uncommon, but focal features are rare (Gordon, 1968; Gordon and Sim, 1967; Harner, 1975; Kiloh et al, 1972; Liddell, 1958; Swain, 1959; Weiner and Schuster, 1950). The EEG records obtained during barbiturate-induced sleep reveal poorly developed sleep spindles, scanty fast activity, and few K-complexes (Letemendia and Pampiglione, 1958). There is modest correlation between the EEG slowing and the severity of the mental status compromise (Gordon and Sim, 1967; Kaszniak et al, 1979; Weiner and Schuster, 1950), and the EEG is superior to the CT scan as a predictor of dementia (Kazniak et al, 1978). There is a tendency for the degree of EEG slowing to be less profound than is the severity of the accompanying dementia until the terminal stages, and the EEG may not change during substantial periods of the disease. Computerized EEG (CEEG) and brain mapping studies have been pursued in DAT. Preliminary results demonstrate that DAT patients can be distinguished from normal controls; in most studies, the maximal abnormalities are found in the posterior tem-

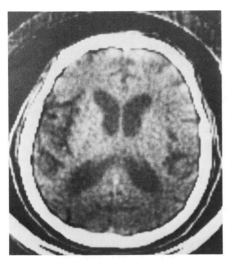 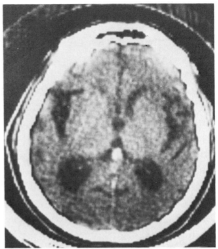

FIGURE 3-2.   CT scan shows enlarged sulci and dilated ventricles indicative of cerebral atrophy in a case of advanced DAT.

poral regions of the brain (Brenner et al, 1986; Duffy et al, 1984; Leuchter et al, 1987; Pentilla et al, 1985). The sensitivity of these techniques to early alterations and the occurrence of changes specific to DAT remain to be demonstrated.

Auditory and visual evoked responses may be useful in the evaluation of patients with DAT. Long-latency event-related components of the auditory evoked potential reflecting attention and decision-making processes are abnormal in many patients. The P300 wave often has a significantly longer duration and smaller amplitude than is present in matched controls whereas the N100 and P200 waves associated with stimulus-related aspects of sensation are usually normal (Goodin et al, 1978; Syndulko et al, 1982). Both short- and long-latency visual evoked responses have been found to be delayed, and the response amplitudes are abnormal (Visser et al, 1976). Prolonged P300 latencies are not unique to DAT and do not aid in distinguishing DAT from other dementing disorders (Neshige et al, 1988).

CT is an important tool in the evaluation of the demented patient. It reliably detects subdural hematomas, hydrocephalus, brain tumors, abscesses, and large cerebral infarctions that may produce dementia and simulate DAT. Patients with clinically diagnosed DAT usually have enlarged ventricles and widened cortical sulci demonstrable by CT scanning (Fig. 3-2). Patients with more advanced disease tend to have the greatest amount of atrophy (Donaldson, 1979), and serial scanning reveals that cerebral atrophy occurs more rapidly than expected in normal-aged individuals (Brinkman and Largen, 1984). Visualization of enlarged sulci and/or ventricles, however, is not a reliable predictor of dementia (Kazniak et al, 1978; Wu et al, 1981), and demented patients without atrophy and atrophy in patients without dementia have been described (Fox et al, 1975; Huckman et al, 1975). Sulcal enlargement and ventricular dilatation occur with normal aging, and most studies have failed to demonstrate reliable differences between patients with DAT and age-matched controls (Kazniak et al, 1978). Attempts to correlate dementia with diminished brain density have been inconsistent, and the diagnostic specificity of these changes has not been determined (Bondareff et al, 1981; Colgan et al, 1986; Naeser et al, 1980, 1982; Wilson et al, 1982). In any individual patient, dementia cannot be diagnosed on the basis of CT findings, and DAT remains a clinical, not a radiologic, diagnosis (Wells and Duncan, 1977).

Magnetic resonance imaging (MRI) has proven to be a superior tool to CT in the evaluation of the demented patient. MRI demonstrates the structural pathology recognized by CT and is much more sensitive to the existence of ischemic brain injury, routinely revealing abnormalities not visualized by CT (Erkinjuntti et al, 1987; Johnson et al, 1987a). There are no pathognomonic MRI findings in DAT, and MRI studies in DAT and normal aging may be indistinguishable.

Studies of cerebral blood flow demonstrate dynamic metabolic alterations occurring in the brain of the demented patient. Cerebral blood flow is consistently reduced in patients with DAT and the reductions correlate with the severity of the dementia (Grubb et al, 1977; Obrist et al, 1970; Yamaguchi et al, 1980). Decreases in blood flow are usually most pronounced in the posterior temporal and parieto-occipital regions (Barclay et al, 1984; Deutsch and Tweedy, 1987; Gustafson and Risberg, 1974; Hagberg and Ingvar, 1976; Prohovnik et al, 1988). It appears that the fluent aphasia seen in early and intermediate stages of DAT correlates with diminished posterior hemispheric flow, whereas the reduced spontaneous speech, echolalia, and mutism of the late stages correlate with more pronounced reduction in frontal lobe flow (Gustafson et al, 1978). Mental effort fails to activate these areas of reduced flow in demented patients (Ingvar et al, 1975; Yamaguchi et al, 1980).

SPECT has become a valuable tool offering information supportive of the diagnosis of DAT. SPECT uses a photon emitting radiotracer in conjunction with computerized reconstruction to provide images indicative of regional cerebral perfusion. Two tracers are currently in common usage: N-isopropyl iodine-123 iodoamphetamine (IMP) and technetium-99m-hexamethylpropyleneamine oxime (HM-PAO). Most studies reveal globally decreased cerebral perfusion with the most marked reductions in the posterior parietal cortex (Costa et al, 1988; Jagust et al, 1987; Johnson et al, 1987b, 1988; Neary et al, 1987). The pattern of posterior temporal-parietal perfusion is characteristic of DAT, correlates with the severity of intellectual compromise, and is unlike the perfusion patterns observed in most other dementing

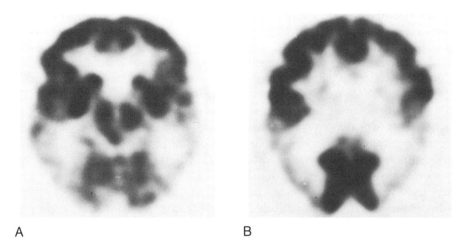

A   B

FIGURE 3–3.   A PET of a patient with DAT reveals decreased metabolic activity in the posterior temporal and parietal association cortices and sparing of subcortical metabolism.

illnesses (Costa et al, 1988; Jagust et al, 1987; Neary et al, 1987). Not all DAT patients, however, exhibit the characteristic pattern (Smith et al, 1988a), and imitation of the pattern by alternative disorders may occur.

Emission-computed tomography using fluorine 18-labeled deoxyglucose or oxygen 15 demonstrates a decrease in cerebral metabolic activity in DAT (Benson, 1982a; Benson et al, 1981b; Frackowiak et al, 1981). The posterotemporal, parietal, and frontal association cortices have markedly reduced metabolism (Fig. 3–3). Metabolic activity of the primary motor, somatosensory, and visual cortices as well as most of subcortical structures is normal or only slightly diminished. In the early phases of the illness, parietal hypometabolism is most marked; as the disease progresses, premotor metabolic reductions also become severe (Haxby et al, 1988). Neocortical metabolic abnormalities correlate with language and visuospatial deficits but may precede their occurence by one to three years (Cutler et al, 1985; Grady et al, 1988; Haxby et al, 1986). Patients with more marked language deficits exhibit more severe metabolic changes in the left hemisphere; those with disproportionate visuospatial impairment have more hypometabolism of the right hemisphere; patients with memory abnormalities as their most apparent clinical feature manifest no metabolic asymmetries (Foster et al, 1983; Haxby et al, 1985).

Neuropsychological assessment of demented patients aids in the identification and quantification of cognitive and memory deficits, but it does little to aid in the diagnosis of the etiologic condition. Perez and colleagues (1975) found that patients with DAT and those with multi-infarct dementia performed similarly on the Wechsler Adult Intelligence Scale, although the former consistently performed more poorly. Tierney and associates (1987) also found that a battery of neuropsychological tests distinguished DAT patients from normal controls but did not differentiate DAT from vascular dementia. Gainotti and co-workers (1980) compared the performance of patients with DAT with individuals suffering from depression or subcortical dementia on a battery of neuropsychological tests. The former group did significantly worse on tests of constructional abilities and tasks requiring verbal or visuospatial memory. Studies comparing the neuropsychological performance of DAT patients with victims of Parkinson's disease, Huntington's disease, progressive supranuclear palsy, and multiple sclerosis reveal that DAT patients have greater language and memory impairment while a subcortical pattern of dementia is observed in the other conditions (Brandt et al, 1988; Filley et al, 1989; Huber et al, 1986; Pillon et al, 1986). Psychometric testing is sometimes able to detect early changes and predict which members of families with dominantly inherited DAT will develop the illness (Feldman et al, 1963a; Folstein and Breitner, 1981).

Neuropathology

The clinical manifestations of DAT reflect the topography and progression of the cerebral cortical neuronal degeneration. The neuropathologic material available from autopsied patients necessarily represents only the most advanced stage of disease, and the course of the disorder must be hypothetically reconstructed on the basis of the pathologic changes found at death.

Grossly, the brains are atrophic, often weighing less than 1000 gm (Corsellis, 1976; Tomlinson, 1977). The atrophy is most pronounced in the temporoparietal and anterior frontal regions. Sparing of the occipital cortex and the primary motor and somatosensory cortices may be apparent (Jervis, 1937; McMenemy, 1940).

On histologic examination, the neurons of the cerebral cortex in DAT show striking changes. The neuronal alterations include neurofibrillary tangles, neuritic plaques, and granulovacuolar degeneration. Identical changes occur in the aging brain unaccompanied by dementia, although the changes are less abundant than they are in the brains of demented patients (Tomlinson, 1977). Amyloid angiopathy is present in a majority of cases (Esiri and Wilcock, 1986). The diagnosis of DAT thus depends on an identifiable clinical pattern combined with characteristic neuropathologic findings.

Neurofibrillary tangles consist of neurofibrils that are contorted, thickened, and conglutinated into bizarre triangle and loop shapes in the neuronal cytoplasm (Fig. 3–4) (Jervis, 1971a). The tangles occur preferentially in the pyramidal neurons of the neocortex, the hippocampus, and the amygdala. They also occur in the raphe nuclei of the brainstem and the neurons of the

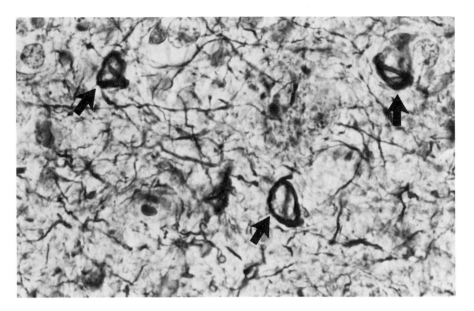

FIGURE 3-4.   Most of the cortical neurons have dark-staining neurofibrillary tangles (arrows) in the cell cytoplasm (Glees. X600).

locus ceruleus (Bondareff et al, 1982; Hirano and Zimmerman, 1962; Ishii, 1966). The tangles are shown to best advantage by silver stains.

Electron microscopic examination of the tangles reveals that they are composed of paired helical filaments. Each neurofilament is 100 Å wide and the helix has a twist every 800 Å (Kidd, 1964; Terry, 1978). Attempts to characterize the protein structure of the filaments in neurofibrillary tangles are evolving (Iqbal et al, 1975; Selkoe, 1980; Selkoe et al, 1981). Studies using monoclonal antibodies have identified atypically phosphorylated tau proteins (45–62 kDa) as a component of the paired helical filaments contributing to both neurofibrillary tangles and neuritic plaques (Grundke-Iqbal et al, 1986). Alz 50, another monoclonal antibody, recognizes a 68 kDa protein possibly related to tau in cells with neurofibrillary tangles and in cells forming abnormal filaments (Tabaton et al, 1988).

Neurofibrillary tangles are not unique to DAT. Table 3–4 lists the principal conditions in which they have been found. Their occurrence in normal aging and in elderly patients with Down's syndrome has been mentioned. A number of extrapyramidal syndromes have neurofibrillary tangles in neurons of rostral brainstem nuclear structures. Postencephalitic Parkinson's disease characteristically has neurons with tangles in the substantia nigra and locus ceruleus, brainstem reticular formation, and hippocampus (Hirano and Zimmerman, 1962). Patients with progressive supranuclear palsy have neurofibrillary tangles distributed in the rostral brainstem and

TABLE 3–4.   Conditions with neurofibrillary tangles as a characteristic neuropathologic finding.

Clinical	Experimental
DAT	Aluminum encephalopathy
Normal aging	Lead encephalopathy
Elderly Down's syndrome	Spindle-inhibitor encephalo-
DAT-Pick's disease complex	myelopathy
Postencephalitic Parkinson's disease	Iminodipropionitrile encephalo-
Progressive supranuclear palsy	myelopathy
Guamanian ALS-parkinsonism-dementia	Vitamin E deficiency
complex	Copper deficiency
Subacute sclerosing panencephalitis	Retrograde and wallerian de-
Hereditary cerebellar ataxia	generation
Infantile neuroaxonal dystrophy	
Vincristine and vinblastine	
encephalomyelopathy	
Dementia pugilistica	

subthalamic areas (Steele et al, 1964). Electron microscopic studies have shown that, unlike the twisted tangles of DAT, the neurofilamentous tangles of progressive supranuclear palsy are straight (Powell et al, 1974; Roy et al, 1974; Tellez-Nagel and Wisniewski, 1973; Tomonaga, 1977). Tangles resembling those of DAT have been found in patients with the amyotrophic lateral sclerosis–parkinsonism–dementia complex of Guam (Chen, 1981; Hirano and Zimmerman, 1962), subacute sclerosing panencephalitis (Mandybur et al, 1977; Wisniewski et al, 1979), infantile neuroaxonal dystrophy, vincristine, and vinblastine encephalomyelopathies (Shelanski and Wisniewski, 1969; Wisniewski et al, 1970), lead encephalopathy, tuberous sclerosis, Hallervorden-Spatz disease, lipofuscinosis (Wisniewski et al, 1979), and dementia pugilistica (Corsellis et al, 1973). Rarely, neuropathologic investigation of demented patients has revealed the coexistence of abundant neurofibrillary tangles with changes typical of Pick's disease (Berlin, 1949; Kosaka et al, 1976), findings of Huntington's disease (McIntosh et al, 1978), or extensive formation of Lewy bodies (Forno et al, 1978; Rosenblum and Ghatak, 1979). Experimentally, neurofibrillary tangles have been induced by lead or aluminum intoxication (Klatzo et al, 1965; Nicklowitz, 1975; Wisniewski et al, 1970, 1980); spindle inhibitors such as vincristine, vinblastine, colchicine, and podophyllotoxin; lathyrogenic agents such as iminodipropionitrile (IDPN); copper or vitamin E deficiency; and retrograde and wallerian degeneration (Wisniewski et al, 1970). The occurrence of neurofibrillary tangles in such a diverse array of conditions suggests that they may represent a nonspecific neuronal response to injury. In the healthy cell, neurofilaments facilitate transport of intracellular elements in the axon

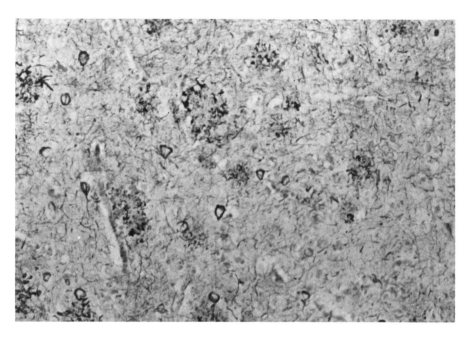

FIGURE 3–5.   Neuritic plaques in the cortex contain a central core of amyloid surrounded by degenerating neuronal processes (Glees. X600).

(Peters et al, 1976), and this mechanism is disrupted when neurofibrillary tangles are present.

Neuritic plaques are minute areas of tissue degeneration consisting of granular deposits and remnants of neuronal processes. The plaques are roughly spherical, measuring 5 to 150 μ in diameter, and they stain deeply with silver impregnation (Fig. 3–5). The plaques are concentrated in the cerebral cortex and hippocampus but also occur in the corpus striatum, amygdala, and thalamus (Corsellis, 1976; Jervis, 1971a). Amyloid plaques similar to classical senile plaques have been found in the cerebellum in some cases of familial DAT (Pro et al, 1980). Typical plaques have a three-tiered structure with an outer zone of degenerating neuritic processes, a middle zone of swollen axons and dendrites, and a central amyloid core (Kidd, 1964). When examined by electron microscopy the plaques appear to be composed of thickened axis cylinders, abnormal dendritic processes, abnormal boutons terminaux, and neuronal processes packed with thickened neurofibrils and dense lamellar bodies surrounding a central area of amyloid fibers (Kidd, 1964; Luse and Smith, 1964; Terry et al, 1964). Synapses are markedly reduced throughout the plaque (Krigman et al, 1965). Astrocytic hypertrophy occurs near the plaque rim and microglia are visible within the plaque (Friede and Magee, 1962; Jervis, 1971a). Histochemically, there is an early increase in oxidative enzyme activity in the area of the plaque followed by a late decrease in enzymatic activity and mitochondrial content (Friede and Magee, 1962). The oxidative activity is localized to the dense lamellated bodies of the plaques (Suzuki and Terry, 1967). Silicon has been found to be increased in the rim and core of senile plaques (Nikaido et al, 1972). The altered synaptic connectivity and function within the plaque impairs intercellular communication and disrupts the essential role of the synapse in learning, memory, and cognition (Gonatas et al, 1967). In addition to DAT, neuritic plaques are found in patients with Down's syndrome, lead encephalopathy, Jakob-Creutzfeldt disease, and kuru (Mandybur, 1979).

The third characteristic histologic finding involving the neurons in DAT is granulovacuolar degeneration. The change consists of clusters of intracytoplasmic vacuoles up to 5 μ in diameter, containing a granule 0.5 to 1.5 μ in size. The central particles are well stained with routine hematoxylin and eosin methods. In DAT, granulovacuolar degeneration is highly selective for the pyramidal neurons of the hippocampus (Corsellis, 1976). Increased frequency and severity of granulovacuolar degeneration is also present in the hippocampi of nondemented persons beyond the age of 60 years, but few people without dementia have severe changes (Tomlinson and Kitchner, 1972; Woodard, 1962).

The fourth major histologic hallmark of DAT is the presence of an amyloid angiopathy. Once thought to represent an unusual variant of DAT, it has now been conclusively demonstrated that amyloid deposits are present in nearly all cases (Esiri and Wilcock, 1986). The amyloid changes have been demonstrated in cerebral biopsies early in the disease course. The cerebrovascular amyloid is identical in structure to the amyloid comprising the core of neuritic plaques (Arai et al, 1987; Roberts et al, 1988). The beta-amyloid (also known as the amyloid A4 protein) of DAT is not elevated in serum but has been detected in extracerebral vessels in skin, subcutaneous tissue, and intestine (Rumble et al, 1989).

In addition to the neurofibrillary tangles, neuritic plaques, granulovacuolar degeneration, and amyloid angiopathy, the affected cortical areas in DAT have loss of neurons, accumulation of neuronal lipofuscin, and astrocytic hyperplasia within the cortex (Corsellis, 1976; Dowson, 1982; Esiri and Wilcock, 1986; Jervis, 1971a; Terry et al, 1981). Golgi studies reveal progressive disintegration of the dendritic domain of involved neurons. The horizontal dendritic branches are affected first followed by changes in the apical shaft and the cell body (Scheibel, 1978). Nuclear and nucleolar volume, RNA content of neurons, and neuronal protein synthesis are reduced (Crapper et al, 1979; Mann et al, 1981), and progressive loss of neurons is reflected in decreased ganglioside content of cerebral tissue. Mild gliosis of the white matter is evident and there is a corresponding decrease in white matter cerebrosides (Suzuki et al, 1965).

The histologic diagnosis of DAT depends on the abundance as well as

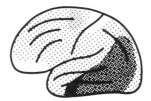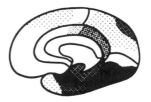

FIGURE 3–6.   Distribution of pathologic changes in the cerebral cortex in DAT. Lightly stippled areas indicate mild to moderate involvement; darkly stippled areas are maximally affected. (Reprinted by permission of the publisher from Brun and Gustafson, 1978).

on the presence of typical histologic changes. A number of sets of histologic criteria for the diagnosis of DAT, based on the abundance of the pathological alterations, have been developed and a consensus for the histopathologic diagnosis of DAT has not been achieved (Ball et al, 1988). National Institute of Aging criteria indicate that, in any patient less than age 50, neurofibrillary tangles or neuritic plaques exceeding 2 to 5 per field (200 × magnification) are abnormal; between 50 and 65 years of age, there may be some tangles in individuals without dementia, and the number of plaques must exceed 8 per field to be of diagnostic significance; for patients age 66 to 75 years, the number of plaques must exceed 10 per field to be considered abnormal; and for those over age 75, there must be more than 15 plaques per field (Khachaturian, 1985).

DAT is not a diffuse process, and the histologic changes occur in specific topographic patterns (Fig. 3–6). Granulovacuolar degeneration occurs almost exclusively in the hippocampus, and the neurofibrillary tangles and senile plaques also involve the cortex selectively. The changes are most severe in the temporoparieto-occipital junction area with prominent involvement of the temporolimbic regions and the posterior cingulate gyrus (Brun and Gustafson, 1978). The anterior cingulate gyrus, the primary motor cortex, the primary somatosensory cortex, and the occipital area are largely spared. In limbic cortex, the hippocampus, entorhinal areas, and the amygdala are affected. Within the hippocampus, layers II and IV of the subiculum are preferentially affected (Hyman et al, 1984). The pattern of amygdaloid involvement is selective with preferential involvement of the corticomedial nuclear groups and sparing of the ventrolateral nuclei (Corsellis, 1970; Herzog and Kemper, 1980; Hooper and Vogel, 1976). Cell loss, granulovacuolar degeneration, and neurons with neurofibrillary tangles also occur in the nucleus basalis (Whitehouse et al, 1981, 1982b). The nucleus basalis has a diffuse cholinergic projection to the cerebral cortex, and its involvement accounts for the marked cholinergic deficit in DAT. Nucleus basalis is also involved in Pick's disease, parkinsonism-dementia complex of Guam, Parkinson's disease, and several other neurologic disorders (Cummings and

Benson, 1987, Hilt et al, 1982; Nakano and Hirano, 1983; Whitehouse et al., 1982a). Cell density and activity are also diminished in the locus ceruleus and in the vagal nuclei of the brainstem (Mann et al, 1982).

Studies of neurotransmitters in DAT reveal transmitter-specific alterations as well as regional selectivity of the changes. Chemical assays demonstrate a preferential involvement of enzymes involved in the cholinergic system. Acetylcholine, choline acetyltransferase, and acetylcholine esterase have all been shown to be preferentially decreased in DAT (Bowen et al, 1976, 1978; Davies, 1979; Davies and Maloney, 1976; Perry et al, 1977; Richter et al, 1980; White et al, 1977). Postsynaptic acetylcholine receptors are normal or only moderately decreased in DAT (Davies and Verth, 1978), suggesting that the disease predominantly affects presynaptic cholinergic neurons. The distribution of the chemical changes closely parallels the topography of the histologic alterations. Choline acetyltransferase, an enzyme involved in acetylcholine synthesis, is significantly reduced in hippocampus, midtemporal gyrus, and parietal and frontal cortices. Normal levels are found in the brainstem, cerebellum, precentral and postcentral gyri, and the occipital cortex (Davies, 1978; Zubenko et al, 1988b).

In addition to the marked and consistent reductions in the cortical cholinergic system, a variety of other transmitters and modulators are also affected in DAT. Among neurotransmitters, levels of gamma-aminobutyric acid, serotonin, and norepinephrine are diminished whereas dopaminergic neurons are unaffected (D'Amato et al, 1987; Ellison et al, 1986; Palmer et al, 1987). Neuropeptides that are reduced in DAT include somatostatin, substance P, corticotropin releasing factor, and vasopressin; neuropeptide Y, cholecystokinin, and vasoactive intestinal peptide are normal or variably reduced; neurotensin levels have been normal, and oxytocin levels are slightly increased (Beal et al 1986, 1987; Davies et al, 1982; Ferrier et al, 1983; Mazurek et al, 1986 a,b; Rossor et al, 1982; Winblad et al, 1982). Receptor changes have also been assessed in DAT. Not all studies are consistent, but most investigations suggest modest reductions in muscarinic and nicotinic cholinergic receptors, moderately reduced S1 and S2 serotoninergic receptors, mildly decreased subcortical dopaminergic receptors (D1 and D2), anatomically selective loss of alpha-1 and alpha-2 adrenergic receptors, moderately decreased gamma-aminobutyric acid receptors, and mild to marked reductions in corticotropin-releasing factor receptors (Katzman and Thal, 1989). Most studies suggest that the neurochemical changes are more marked in early-onset than late-onset DAT patients (Bondareff et al, 1987).

Correlation studies have shown a relationship between the intensity of the neuropathologic changes and enzyme deficits and the severity of the associated dementia. Originally, this correlation was doubted because of the frequency with which the characteristic histologic changes of DAT are found in nondemented elderly people. Quantitative studies were required to demonstrate the relation of the dementia to the neuropathologic alterations. Mean plaque count correlates with a dementia score indicating the degree of debility and with psychological test performance (Blessed et al, 1968; Roth et al, 1966). The plaque count also correlates closely with the diminished level of choline acetyltransferase activity (Perry et al, 1978).

In summary, the pathologic changes of DAT include neurofibrillary tangles, neuritic plaques, granulovacuolar degeneration, neuron loss, and astrocytic gliosis. Involved neurons have a progressive degeneration of the dendritic arbor, decrease in protein synthetic activity, and impaired neuroaxonal transport. Neuronal function, cellular connectivity, and synaptic relations are disrupted. Presynaptic cholinergic neurons are preferentially affected, and the involved neurons are concentrated in the posterotemporal, parietal, and frontal association cortices and the hippocampus. There is correlation between the severity and pattern of intellectual compromise and the abundance and topography of neuronal changes, but there are no completely pathognomonic pathological features of DAT; definite diagnosis depends on identification of a characteristic clinical syndrome with pathologic confirmation of supportive histopathological alterations.

Two related conditions need consideration when discussing the pathology of DAT: familial amyloid angiopathy and the occurrence of Alzheimer-type changes in the brains of patients with Down's syndrome. Amyloid angiopathy is a consistent feature of DAT. It rarely, however, leads to vascular occlusion and infarction. In some families, however, intracerebral hemorrhage with amyloid angiopathy is common and in others a spastic paralysis secondary to spinal cord involvement occurs along with the progressive dementia (Worster-Drought et al, 1940, 1944).

Alzheimer-type changes are found in the cerebral cortex of virtually all patients with Down's syndrome who survive beyond age 40 (Ellis et al, 1974; Olson and Shaw, 1969; Ropper and Williams, 1980; Solitare and Lamarche, 1966). Neuritic plaques are present in small numbers by the second decade and are abundant by the third. Neurofibrillary tangles and granulovacuolar degeneration appear with advancing age (Burger and Vogel, 1973). Neurofibrillary changes are particularly abundant in the hippocampus (Ball and Nuttall, 1980). Several reports have found evidence of progressive mental deterioration in elderly patients with Down's syndrome corresponding to the Alzheimer-type pathology (Blumbergs et al, 1981; Crapper et al, 1975; Jervis, 1948; Lai and Williams, 1989; Owens et al, 1971; Wisniewski et al, 1985).

Etiology

The etiology of DAT is unknown. Several alternative etiologic hypotheses have been offered, including aluminum intoxication, disordered immune function, viral infection, deficits in the formation of cellular filaments, and hereditary predisposition. Aluminum intoxication as a possible causative agent gained attention when it was discovered that rabbits exposed to toxic amounts of aluminum developed neurofibrillary tangles (Klatzo et al, 1965). Initial investigations (Crapper et al, 1976) suggested a minimal elevation in brain aluminum content in DAT, but the importance of slight increases was undetermined and further studies have failed to confirm an elevation (McDermott et al, 1977, 1979). Analyses of cerebrospinal fluid (CSF) and serum aluminum levels were normal in DAT (Delaney, 1979; Shore et al, 1980), and intraneuronal aluminum content was also normal (Markesbery et al, 1981). Furthermore, in dialysis dementia, a disease known to be associated with significantly elevated levels of brain aluminum, neurofibrillary tangles are not found (Dunea et al, 1978; Lederman and Henry, 1978; Rozas et al, 1978). The neurofibrillary tangles induced experimentally by aluminum administration differ from those of DAT in that they are straight rather than twisted and are distributed in the brainstem and spinal cord instead of in the cortex (Yates, 1979). Aluminum accumulation has been demonstrated in the nuclear region of neurons with neurofibrillary tangles (Perl and Brody, 1980); at present, the role of this metal in the etiology or pathogenesis of DAT is uncertain.

Several observations indicate that immune function is disturbed in DAT. Behan and Feldman (1970) found serum protein abnormalities in 66 percent of patients. The abnormalities included decreases in albumin and increases in alpha-$_1$-antitrypsin, alpha-$_2$-macroglobulin, and haptoglobin fractions. Immunoglobulin levels in the CSF are normal (Jonker et al, 1982). Elevated levels of anti-brain antibody have also been demonstrated in DAT (Nandy, 1978), and some of these patients have been shown to have impaired cellular immune responses (Behan and Behan, 1979) and impaired immunoregulation (Miller et al, 1981). Amyloid is also a product of cells involved in the immune system, and altered immune function could explain its presence in neuritic plaques and its occurrence in cerebral vessels (Glenner, 1978). At present it is unknown whether these immunologic abnormalities are primary and thus of possible etiologic significance or secondary to some more basic process. Markers for a genetic susceptibility to DAT have been sought among victims of the illness, but to date no peculiarities of histocompatibility antigens have been found (Henschke et al, 1978; Sulkava et al, 1980; Whalley et al, 1980).

A viral etiology has been proposed, but thus far it has not been possible reliably to transmit DAT by inoculating experimental animals with tissue from the brains of affected patients. Animals injected with brain material from two familial cases of DAT developed a spongiform encephalopathy similar to Jakob-Creutzfeldt disease, but other animals inoculated with the same tissue showed no neurologic deterioration, and the possibility of contamination has not been excluded. Inocula from many other patients with

DAT have produced no neurologic disease (Goudsmit et al, 1980). Neurofibrillary tangles have reportedly been induced in cultured fetal neurons exposed to an extract prepared from the brain of a patient (De Boni and Crapper, 1978), but the observation has not been confirmed by other investigators. Nuclear bodies, sometimes associated with viral encephalitides, have been observed in astrocytes in DAT (Grunnet, 1975), but these bodies are present in many illnesses inciting an astrocytic reaction and may bear no specific relation to DAT. A viral etiology is far from proved but remains an unconfirmed possibility. Patients with DAT should be excluded from blood donation (Cook and Austin, 1978), and caution should be exercised in handling their tissues at autopsy.

A growing body of evidence implicates a basic defect in microtubular function in the etiology or pathogenesis of DAT. Down's syndrome, lymphoproliferative disorders, and chromosomal aneuploidy all occur more frequently than expected in the families of DAT patients (Cook et al, 1979; Heston, 1976; Heston and Mastri, 1977; Heston et al., 1981). Furthermore, chromosomal aneuploidy is more common among aged women than it is among elderly men, an epidemiologic characteristic shared with DAT (Jarvik, 1978). Patients with Down's syndrome have an increased incidence of both hematologic malignancies and DAT. Microtubular dysfunction contributes to the neurofibrillary pathology of DAT and the abnormal mitosis of Down's syndrome and may play a role in the myeloproliferative disorders (Heston, 1976; Yunis et al, 1981). Jarvik and co-workers (1982) found that polymorphonuclear leukocytes derived from DAT patients migrate toward a warmer area more slowly than do normal leukocytes or leukocytes derived from patients with other types of dementia. Microtubules are necessary for directed migration, and if they are confirmed, these findings would further implicate a basic microtubular deficit.

The most convincing evidence for a specific etiology of DAT has been garnered from genetic investigations. Several studies have revealed a 50-percent prevalence of DAT among the first degree relatives of unselected DAT patients, suggesting that autosomal dominant heredity may account for a majority of cases (Breitner et al, 1988; Farrer et al, 1989; Huff et al, 1988; Martin et al, 1988; Mohs et al, 1987). The risk period for expression of the genetic burden extends to age 90.

Treatment

There is no curative therapy for DAT; treatment remains symptomatic. The demonstration of selectively decreased levels of cholinergic enzymes in the brains of patients gave rise to the hope that administration of acetylcholine precursors or facilitators of cholinergic synaptic transmission would reverse or improve cognitive and memory impairments (Smith and Swash, 1978).

Unfortunately the results of these studies have been disappointing. Oral administration of choline, lecithin, and deanol, all of which have been shown to act as central acetylcholine precursors, failed to produce any reliable change in cognition or memory although in some studies there was a tendency for mildly affected patients to show limited improvement (Boyd et al, 1977; Christie et al, 1979; Corser et al, 1979; Etienne et al, 1978, 1979, 1981; Kaye et al, 1982; Renvoize and Jerram, 1979; Smith et al, 1978). More promising results have been obtained from experiments using intravenous administration of anticholinesterase agents or combinations of physostigmine plus an acetylcholine precursor (Christie et al, 1981; Davis et al, 1979; Peters and Levin, 1979; Summers et al, 1981). Likewise, short-term studies of oral physostigmine reveal mild improvement on neuropsychological tests in 30 to 40 percent of treated patients; long-term administration has shown the response to be sustained (Mohs et al, 1985; Stern and Mayeux, 1987, 1988). Tetrahydroaminoacridine (THA), another cholinesterase inhibitor, has been reported to produce mild to marked improvement in DAT, but the high rate of liver toxicity (approximately 30 percent of treated patients exhibit elevated liver enzymes) mandates caution in its use (Gauthier et al, 1988; Nyback et al, 1988; Summers et al, 1986). Intraventricular infusion of a cholinergic receptor agonist, bethanechol, has also been explored in DAT; some patients may evidence a mild improvement in cognition and behavior (Harbaugh, 1988; Penn et al, 1988), but the high morbidity of the procedure (from insertion of the intraventricular cannula and intra-abdominal pump) makes its widespread use impractical. Vasopressin has also been administered in an attempt to improve memory but without success (Durso et al, 1982). Interpretation of many pharmacologic studies is hampered by failure to adequately define the experimental population. A practical, reliable, and successful treatment of the cholinergic defect in DAT is not available, but better diagnostic evaluation, closer attention to disease stage, and development of more effective cholinergic agents may lead to improved results.

A variety of other agents has been used to treat DAT. Cerebral vasodilators, central nervous system stimulants, anabolic agents, anticoagulants, vitamins, chelating agents, hyperbaric oxygen, and precursor amino acids have been administered with little reproducible benefit (Funkenstein et al, 1981; Hier and Caplan, 1980; Meyer et al, 1977; Waters, 1988).

In daily management, minor tranquilizers should be avoided as they often increase confusion and further impair cognition. Combativeness, aggressiveness, and delusions are best controlled with small doses of major tranquilizers such as the phenothiazines or butyrophenones (Gottlieb and Piotrowski, 1990). If depression is significant, an antidepressant agent with few anticholinergic side effects (for example, desipramine) may afford some relief (Gierz et al, 1989). Drugs with pronounced anticholinergic activity may lead to frank psychosis and should not be used. Attention must be directed to correcting even minor degrees of dehydration, limiting any unnecessary drug administration, and avoiding sensory deprivation and social isolation (Snyder and Harris, 1976). Behavioral and psychological therapies with goals of maintaining and maximizing remaining capacities, increasing reality orientation, and reducing the patient's and his or her family's sense of helplessness may also be beneficial (Eisdorfer et al, 1981). Legal and financial as well as psychological counseling for the family are important, and forewarning family members about the expected alterations and deterioration in behavior may help maintain the integrity of family support for the DAT victim. Strategies for the long-term management of DAT and other dementia patients are discussed more comprehensively in Chapter 13.

PICK'S DISEASE

In 1892, Arnold Pick first described the clinical and gross pathologic features of a unique dementing illness. The patient Pick observed was a 71-year-old man with a three-year history of progressive dementia. On examination, the patient had a prominent aphasia with many verbal paraphasic errors plus difficulty recognizing objects. The patient died several months later, and an autopsy performed by Chiari revealed prominent atrophy in a lobar distribution involving the frontal and temporal lobes (Pick, 1977). The histologic characteristics of the disease were first described by Alzheimer in 1911, and in 1926, Onari and Spatz began use of the eponym Pick's disease (Neumann, 1949).

Pick's disease usually has its onset between the ages of 40 and 60 years (Haase, 1977; Slaby and Wyatt, 1974), but cases beginning as early as age 21 (Lowenberg et al, 1939) and as late as age 80 (Binns and Robertson, 1962) are reported. Death occurs within 2 to 15 years of onset with most patients surviving 6 to 12 years (Slaby and Wyatt, 1974). Men may be at greater risk for the disease than may women (Heston et al, 1987). Pick's disease is a relatively rare disorder; DAT is at least 10 to 15 times more common (Jervis, 1971b). Although the cumulative risk for DAT is greater when cases with a presenile onset are considered, the numerical disparity is less profound (Heston and Mastri, 1982; Heston et al, 1987). Eighty percent of cases of Pick's disease occur sporadically while 20 percent are familial (Ferraro and Jervis, 1936). In the familial cases, autosomal dominant transmission is the pattern of inheritance (Groen and Endtz, 1982; Malamud and Waggoner, 1943; Sanders et al, 1939; Schenk, 1958–1959).

Clinical Characteristics

Like DAT, the clinical course of Pick's disease can be divided into three stages (Table 3–5) (Cummings, 1982; Nichols and Weigner, 1938; Robertson

TABLE 3–5.   Clinical characteristics of the three stages of Pick's disease.

Stage I (duration of disease 1 to 3 years)
    Personality—loss of tact and concern
    Judgment—impaired
    Executive function—loss of planning and abstraction
    Memory—relatively preserved
    Visuospatial orientation—intact
    Language—normal or semantic anomia, circumlocutory
    Calculation—relatively preserved
    Klüver-Bucy syndrome—elements may be evident
    Motor system—normal
    EEG—normal
Stage II (duration of disease 3 to 6 years)
    Language—verbal stereotypes; impaired comprehension; aphasia
    Memory—relatively spared
    Visuospatial orientation—relatively spared
    Judgment—deteriorated
    Executive function—deteriorated
    Motor system—relatively normal
    EEG—slowing of background rhythm
    CT/MRI—focal frontal and/or temporal atrophy
    PET/SPECT—bilateral frontal lobe hypometabolism or hypoperfusion
Stage III (duration of disease 6 to 12 years)
    Language—mute or incomprehensible
    Memory—deteriorated
    Visuospatial skills—deteriorated
    Cognition—severe deficits
    Motor system—extrapyramidal syndrome or mixed pyramidal and extrapyramidal
        signs
    EEG—diffusely slow or focal frontal and temporal slowing
    CT/MRI—focal frontal and/or temporal atrophy
    PET/SPECT—bilateral frontal lobe hypometabolism or hypoperfusion

---

et al, 1958; Sjøgren et al, 1952). The initial stage is characterized by prominent personality changes and emotional alterations. Judgment is impaired early and insight is compromised. Social behavior deteriorates and a psychiatric diagnosis is often entertained. Language abnormalities are among the earliest intellectual alterations to occur. In the second stage of disease, deterioration of mental status becomes evident and aphasia is more prominent. Cognitive changes are more pronounced, but memory and mathematical and visuospatial skills may remain relatively unimpaired during this phase. In the third and final stage of the disease, a progressive extrapyramidal syndrome usually appears, intellectual deterioration affects all areas of intellectual function, and the patient becomes mute and incontinent.

Death results from a terminal pulmonary, urinary tract, or decubitus ulcer infection.

A wide variety of personality changes can occur in the initial stages of Pick's disease. Apathy, irritability, depression, jocularity, and euphoria have been described (Brun and Gustafson, 1978; Cummings and Duchen, 1981; Ferraro and Jervis, 1936; Kahn and Thompson, 1933–1934; Robertson et al, 1958). Judgment is poor and personality deterioration frequently includes socially inappropriate activity, sexual indiscretions, loss of personal propriety, and other behavioral disinhibition. Stereotyped behavioral routines and rigid rituals may be observed. Personality alterations often precede the appearance of intellectual deterioration in Pick's disease and may aid in differentiating it from other dementing illnesses. Lishman (1978) observed that it is chiefly by its mode of onset that Pick's disease can be identified clinically. Disturbances indicative of frontal lobe dysfunction may be evident on neuropsychological assessment early in the disease course (Knopman et al, 1989). Maze tests, trail-making tests, and card-sorting tasks reveal deficits in planning and abstraction.

Among the more striking neurobehavioral alterations heralding the onset of Pick's disease is the Klüver-Bucy syndrome (Aronson and Aronson, 1973; Balajthy, 1964; Cummings and Duchen, 1981; Gustafson et al, 1978; Lilly et al, 1982; Pilleri, 1966). This syndrome was first produced in monkeys by surgically ablating both temporal lobes including the amygdalae and hippocampi (Bucy and Klüver, 1955; Klüver and Bucy, 1939). The lesioned monkeys developed a striking behavioral syndrome consisting of emotional blunting with loss of both fear and affective responses, altered dietary preferences, hypermetamorphosis (mandatory exploration of environmental stimuli as soon as they are noticed), prominent oral exploratory behavior, sensory agnosia-like behavior involving vision and hearing, and altered sexual activity in some cases. In Pick's disease, the entire syndrome may not develop, but a sufficient number of elements may be present to permit clinical recognition. Patients with Pick's disease have exhibited various combinations of affective disturbances, hypersexuality, gluttony, hyperorality, hypermetamorphosis, and visual or auditory agnosia (Akelaitis, 1944; Aronson and Aronson, 1973; Balajthy, 1964; Davison, 1938; Gustafson et al, 1978; Pilleri, 1966; Sanders et al, 1939; Swain, 1959). Affective changes and increased eating with weight gain are particularly common (Cummings and Duchen, 1981). Visual object agnosia, prosopagnosia, and/or auditory agnosia indicate a defect in sensory recognition (Cummings and Duchen, 1981; Ferraro and Jervis, 1936; Kahn and Thompson, 1933–1934; Malamud and Boyd, 1940; Malamud and Waggoner, 1943; Rewcastle and Ball, 1968; Schochet et al, 1968).

Emotional and affective changes characterize the early stages of Pick's disease, but cognitive compromise becomes evident as the disease progresses, and aphasia tends to appear early and dominate the middle stage. Rarely, aphasia has been the earliest abnormality noted (Wechsler, 1977; Wechsler et al, 1982). Empty speech, word-finding difficulties, circumlocution, and impaired confrontation naming are the first manifestations of the evolving language impairment (Balajthy, 1964; Binns and Robertson, 1962; Cummings and Duchen, 1981; Davison, 1938; Lowenberg et al, 1939; Sanders et al, 1939; Wechsler et al, 1982). Semantic anomia in which the sound of the word loses all meaning (Benson, 1979b) is an early finding in some patients. Verbal paraphasia occurs, but a fluent paraphasic logorrhea of the transcortical sensory type such as is often seen in DAT is uncommon. Robertson and associates (1958) noted that patients with Pick's disease may use generic terms such as "thing" and rely on particular words to convey several meanings, substituting from their restricted vocabularies an available word for other unrecalled terms. As the disease progresses, impaired comprehension of language also becomes evident. Pure word deafness or auditory agnosia may contribute to the comprehension deficit (Cummings and Duchen, 1981; Holland et al, 1985). Echolalia and a tendency to use verbal stereotypes and to repeat the same stories over and over become prominent as the disease advances (Binns and Robertson, 1962; Cummings and Duchen, 1981; Ferraro and Jervis, 1936; Hassin and Levitin, 1941; Neumann, 1949; Stengel, 1943; Thorpe, 1932). Mayer-Gross and co-workers (1937–1938) labeled the tendency of Pick's disease patients monotonously to retell the same anecdote the "gramophone syndrome." With progression into the final phases of illness, many patients become completely mute (Cummings and Duchen, 1981; Gustafson et al, 1978; Lowenberg, 1936; Lowenberg et al, 1939; Neumann, 1949; Schochet and Earle, 1970; Stengel, 1943). Written language has rarely been studied in Pick's disease. Akelaitis (1944) examined a letter written by one of his patients and noted omissions of articles and conjunctions and improper use of verb tense and mood. Holland et al (1985) described in detail a patient with Pick's disease whose ability to read and write persisted for several years after auditory comprehension declined and mutism became evident.

Memory is often preserved into the middle or late stages of Pick's disease. It may be difficult to test because of profound aphasia or agnosia, but the general behavior of the patient demonstrates at least partial preservation of memory skills (Brun and Gustafson, 1978; Cummings and Duchen, 1981, Knopman et al, 1989; Lishman, 1978; Stengel, 1943).

Visuospatial abilities are also relatively preserved until the later stages of the disease. Patients may be able to copy figures and learn their way around hospitals long after language and emotional behavior are severely compromised (Brun and Gustafson, 1978; Cummings and Duchen, 1981; Robertson et al, 1958; Sjøgren et al, 1952). Similarly, mathematical skills have been noted to be spared in the early phases of the disorder in contrast to DAT (Wechsler et al, 1982).

Generalized hyperalgesia suggesting a bilateral thalamic syndrome was observed in several patients with Pick's disease by Robertson and co-workers (1958), but other investigators have failed to substantiate this finding.

With progression into the final phases of the illness, impairment of memory, visuospatial skills, and other intellectual capacities is apparent, and the patients become profoundly demented. Abnormalities of motor and sensory systems are conspicuously absent during most of the course of the disease, but as it advances, a parkinsonian type of extrapyramidal syndrome may become evident and pyramidal system abnormalities may appear (Akelaitis, 1944; Cummings and Duchen, 1981; Lowenberg et al, 1939; Malamud and Waggoner, 1943; Pilleri, 1966; Sanders et al, 1939). Myoclonus sometimes occurs in late stages (Aronson and Aronson, 1973; Malamud and Waggoner, 1943; Sanders et al, 1939), but seizures are uncommon in Pick's disease. Terminally, the patients are mute and immobile with urinary and fecal incontinence.

Laboratory Evaluation

There are no laboratory findings pathognomonic of Pick's disease, but studies may be helpful by demonstrating other disorders that may mimic the clinical picture. Routine investigations of blood, serum, urine, and cerebrospinal fluid (CSF) yield unremarkable results. In some preliminary studies, Constantinidis (1979) and colleagues (1981) found increased levels of urinary zinc in these patients, but this finding has not been confirmed. EEGs tend to remain normal until late in the course of the illness (Gordon and Sim, 1967; Swain, 1959). When EEG abnormalities appear, diffuse slowing is the usual pattern although focal frontal or temporal slow-wave activity is noted occasionally (Cummings and Duchen, 1981). CT may provide supportive evidence for the diagnosis. The X-ray CT scan in Figure 3–7 shows temporal lobe atrophy in one patient with Pick's disease, and similar scans with lobar atrophy of the temporal and/or frontal lobes have been reported in others (Cummings and Duchen, 1981; Groen and Endtz, 1982; McGeachie et al, 1979; Wechsler et al, 1982). Magnetic resonance imaging likewise frequently reveals lobar atrophy involving the frontal lobes, temporal lobes, or both (Figure 3–8). Positron emission CT reveals diminished cortical glucose metabolism in the association cortices of the frontal and temporal lobes (Kamo et al, 1987) and SPECT studies demonstrate profound hypoperfusion of the frontal regions.

Brain biopsy has occasionally been attempted to facilitate premorbid diagnosis of Pick's disease, but the results have been disappointing. Surgical trauma may induce neuronal swelling that resembles the inflated cells of Pick's disease (Smith et al, 1966) leading to false positive diagnoses, and the prominent spongiform changes that occur in the cortex in advanced cases may lead to confusion with Jakob-Creutzfeldt disease. Neurons with char-

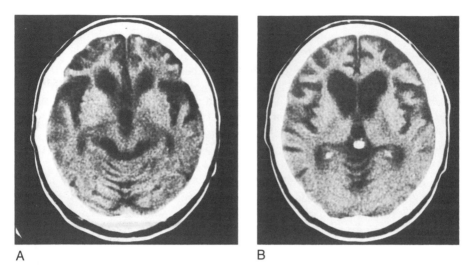

A   B

FIGURE 3–7.   CT scan demonstrates frontal lobe atrophy in a patient with Pick's disease.

acteristic Pick's bodies diagnostic of the disease are most abundant in the medial temporal areas where they are not readily accessible to biopsy. In the absence of specific treatment, the use of biopsy for diagnostic purposes is to be discouraged (except in centers where research on the pathologic material is available).

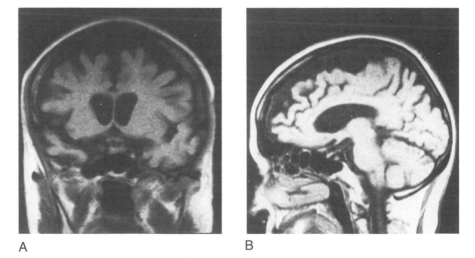

A   B

FIGURE 3–8.   MRI scan reveals atrophy of the temporal and frontal lobes in a patient with Pick's disease: (A) coronal, (B) sagittal.

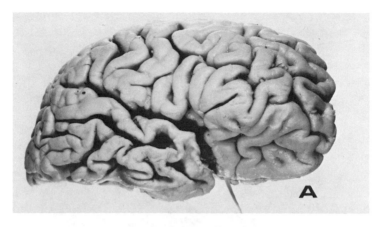

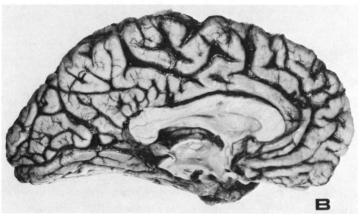

FIGURE 3–9.   View of the lateral aspect (A) of the brain in Pick's disease shows temporal lobe atrophy. The medial aspect of the brain of a Pick's disease patient (B) shows temporal and frontal atrophy.

Neuropathology

At autopsy, the brains of Pick's disease patients are reduced in size, often weighing less than 1000 gm (Neumann, 1949). In most cases the atrophy has a lobar distribution involving the temporal and/or frontal lobes (Fig. 3–9), and this pattern may be helpful diagnostically when histologic changes are equivocal. Approximately 25 percent show primarily temporal lobe atrophy; 25 percent show primarily frontal lobe involvement; 40 to 50 percent have combined frontal and temporal lobar atrophy; and a small number have atrophic changes in the posterior hemispheric regions (Corsellis, 1976; Ferraro and Jervis, 1936; Sjøgren et al, 1952). The atrophy is bilaterally symmetric in approximately 30 percent of cases, has a left-sided predomi-

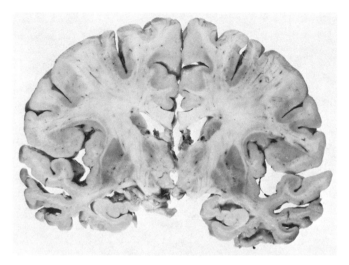

FIGURE 3–10.   Coronal sections of the brain in Pick's disease reveal inferior and lateral temporal atrophy and dilatation of the temporal portion of the ventricular system. Note the widened sulci and knife-edged gyri.

nance in 50 percent, and involves primarily the right side in 20 percent. An abrupt transition is sometimes evident between involved and uninvolved cortical regions, and there is a tendency for selective sparing of the precentral gyrus and the posterior one-third of the superior temporal gyrus (Corsellis, 1976; Sanders et al, 1939; Schochet et al, 1968). The anterior and medial temporal areas and the orbitofrontal cortex show the most severe atrophic changes (Corsellis, 1976; Cummings and Duchen, 1981; Sanders et al, 1939; Schenk and van Mansvelt, 1955). Coronal sections (Fig. 3–10) reveal deep sulci and knife-edged gyri in the atrophic areas. The temporal horns are more dilated than are other parts of the ventricular system.

The histopathologic alterations in Pick's disease are highly distinctive. The two characteristic findings are intracytoplasmic Pick bodies and "inflated" neurons. Pick bodies are dense intracellular structures occurring in the neuronal cytoplasm (Fig. 3–11). They are approximately the same size as the nucleus, stain deeply in silver preparations, and tend to occur singly (Corsellis, 1976; Jervis, 1971b; Scharenberg, 1958; Schochet and Earle, 1970). The cells containing the Pick bodies are mildly enlarged and the nucleus is displaced to the edge of the cell. Small neurons tend to be more involved than are large ones and superficial cortical layers show more changes than do the deep strata (Corsellis, 1976; Jervis, 1971b; Lowenberg, 1936). Pick bodies do not occur in normal aging and are unusual in diseases other than Pick's disease, but they have occasionally been seen in small numbers in inherited diseases of the white matter, general paresis, encephalitis, Binswanger's disease, lead poisoning, gliomas, metastases, and tub-

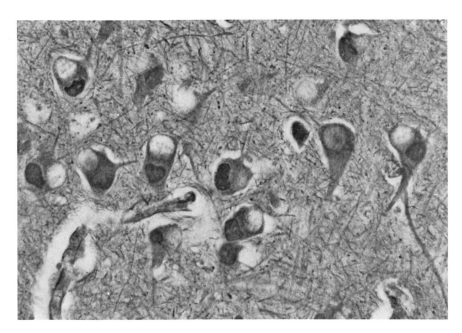

FIGURE 3–11.   Most of the medial temporal lobe neurons have highly argyrophilic Pick bodies in the cytoplasm. The nuclei are unstained (von Braunmuhl: original magnification X500).

erous sclerosis (Hirano et al, 1968; Williams, 1935). The other clinical and pathologic features of these conditions readily differentiate them from Pick's disease. Electron microscopic studies of the Pick bodies reveal that they are composed of 100-Å neurofilaments and 240-Å neurotubules irregularly conglutinated into an intracytoplasmic mass (Corsellis, 1976; Rewcastle and Ball, 1968; Schochet et al, 1968; Towfighi, 1972; Wisniewski et al, 1972). Pick bodies react with monoclonal antibodies directed against neurofilament proteins and antitubulin antisera (Munoz-Garcia and Ludwin, 1984). Antibodies against phosphorylated tau protein intensely stain Pick bodies and monoclonal and polyclonal anti-ubiquitin antibodies stain Pick bodies and the parikarya of inflated cells (Murayama et al, 1990). Both straight and twisted filaments have been observed. Free ribosomes, vesicles and short cisternae of the endoplasmic reticulum, lipochrome granules, and lamellar aggregates of lipid material also participate in the formation of Pick bodies. The bodies are not membrane-bound and bear no particular resemblance to viral inclusions. They are not inclusions in the usual sense of particles originating from extraneuronal sources.

Another characteristic neuronal change in Pick's disease is the inflated cell. These are enlarged neurons with silver-staining cytoplasm and displaced nuclei. No discrete body is evident within the cytoplasm. Electron microscopy demonstrates that the cytoplasm is filled with haphazardly distributed neurofilaments and neurotubules identical to those found in the Pick bodies (Wisniewski et al, 1972). In some cases, neurons identical to inflated cells but not greatly enlarged have been observed (Bouton, 1940; Cummings and Duchen, 1981). These smaller argyrophilic neurons may represent transitional cells in evolution or disappearance of more classic inflated neurons.

Not all patients with frontal or temporal lobar atrophy have inflated cells or neurons with Pick bodies, and this has given rise to controversy regarding the grounds for pathologic diagnosis of the disorder. Pick's bodies are found in 20 to 30 percent and inflated cells in approximately 60 percent of cases that in all other respects are typical of Pick's disease (Constantinidis et al, 1974; Jervis, 1971b). Neumann (1949) proposed that Pick's disease be divided into type I and type II varieties, indicating the presence or absence respectively of the characteristic neuronal alterations. Later, she and Cohn (1967) suggested that the two types might represent different disease entities. They emphasized the extensive gliosis of white matter and proposed the name progressive subcortical gliosis for the variety without Pick bodies or inflated neurons. Several disorders with disproportionate frontal lobe atrophy are now recognized; they are discussed below and are summarized in Table 3–6.

Golgi studies of the neuronal arborization demonstrate an almost complete lack of dendritic spines on the cortical pyramidal cell dendrites. The overall size of the dendritic domain is little affected, but the individual neuritic processes are denuded and the cell bodies are often surrounded by halos of astrocytes (Wechsler et al, 1982).

In addition to these distinctive alterations, a variety of other pathologic changes occur in Pick's disease. Neuron loss, astrocytic hyperplasia, and microglial cell proliferation are evident in the affected cortical regions. In areas of profound cortical involvement, spongiform changes occur (Corsellis, 1976; Cummings and Duchen, 1981; Lowenberg et al, 1939; Malamud and Waggoner, 1943). When Pick cells are lacking, the spongy changes may cause confusion with Jakob-Creutzfeldt disease. White matter in the atrophic areas is also severely involved. Extensive astrocytic gliosis is present and loss of myelin occurs where gliosis is severe (Fig. 3–12) (Corsellis, 1976; Cummings and Duchen, 1981; Jervis, 1971b; Neumann, 1949).

Topographically, Pick's disease involves predominately the anterior hemispheric regions (Fig. 3–13). Within that distribution, anterior limbic areas including the inferior and medial temporal regions and the orbitofrontal cortex are most affected (Brun and Gustafson, 1978). Parahippocampal and adjacent hippocampal areas and the entire amygdaloid complex contain the greatest abundance of Pick cells (Ball, 1979; Cummings and Duchen, 1981). Neuron loss and astrocytic gliosis occur to a variable extent in the basal ganglia and in the thalamus, subthalamic nucleus, and nucleus basalis; Pick

TABLE 3-6.   Features that distinguish DAT and Pick's disease.

DAT	Pick's Disease
Clinical features	
Amnesia early	Amnesia late
Visuospatial disturbances early	Visuospatial disturbances late
Acalculia prominent early	Calculations relatively spared early
Personality changes late	Personality changes early
Klüver-Bucy syndrome late	Klüver-Bucy syndrome early
Speech-language disturbances	Speech-language disturbances
Palilalia	Stereotyped speech
Logoclonia	Terminal mutism
Seizures more common	Seizures less common
Computed tomography	
Widespread atrophy	Temporal and/or lobar atrophy
Gross pathology	
Posterior hemispheric atrophy	Anterior hemispheric atrophy
Amygdala involvement	
Central and medial nuclear groups affected	All nuclear groups affected
Histopathology	
Neurofibrillary tangles	Pick bodies
Senile plaques	Inflated cells
Granulovacuolar degeneration	White matter gliosis
Dendritic domain shrunken	Loss of dendritic spines
Chemopathology	
Cholinergic neurons preferentially involved	No selective transmitter involvement

cells are most abundant in the cortex and rare in the subcortical structures in most cases (Akelaitis, 1944; Corsellis, 1976; Cummings and Duchen, 1981; Hilt et al, 1982; Jervis, 1971b; Munoz-Garcia and Ludwin, 1984; Uhl et al, 1983; Winkleman and Book, 1949).

Neurochemical investigations reveal that cortical cholinergic systems and somatostatin are unaffected in Pick's disease (Hansen et al, 1988; Wood et al, 1983). In the basal ganglia, concentrations of cholinergic system enzymes are variably diminished, and levels of gamma-aminobutyric acid, substance P, and dopamine are reduced (Kanazawa et al, 1988). Trace element analysis in cortex demonstrates significantly increased levels of chlorine, iron, manganese, sodium, and phosphorus; levels of chromium, cesium, rubidium, and selenium are reduced. Zinc levels are normal (Ehmann et al, 1984). Diminished concentrations of galactolipids (Scicutella and Davies, 1987) and increased levels of intracellular and extracellular gangliosides (Kamp et al, 1986) have been described in Pick's disease.

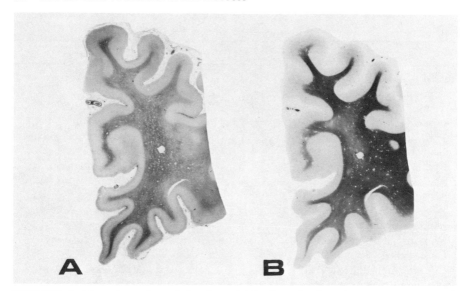

FIGURE 3–12.   A section of the frontal lobe is stained to demonstrate astrocytic gliosis (A) and myelin (B). There is marked subcortical gliosis, and where glial staining is most intense, there is pallor or myelin staining. (A) Holzer technique, (B) luxol-fast blue/cresyl violet.

Etiology

The etiology and pathogenesis of Pick's disease are unknown. Most investigators consider the disease an idiopathic degenerative process affecting the neuronal cell body (Critchley, 1931; Lowenberg et al, 1939; Sanders et al, 1939; Winkleman and Book, 1949). Others note the similarity between the neuronal changes of Pick's disease and those following axonal injury, and suggest that the disease is an axonal disorder with secondary changes in the cell soma (Williams, 1935; Wisniewski et al, 1972).

Based on the observation of increased urinary zinc excretion in a group of patients with Pick's disease, Constantinidis (1979) and colleagues (1981) proposed that a defect in zinc transport by plasma protein leads to elevated intracortical zinc levels and selective disruption of glutamate function in hippocampal and adjacent areas. Recent studies, however, have demonstrated normal levels of zinc in the cortex (Ehmann et al, 1984) offering little support for the zinc hypothesis. At present there is insufficient evidence concerning any of the etiologic possibilities to allow a comprehensive explanation of the neurobiologic mechanisms of Pick's disease.

Treatment

The treatment of Pick's disease is symptomatic. Aggression and combativeness are managed with small doses of the major tranquilizers. Reality

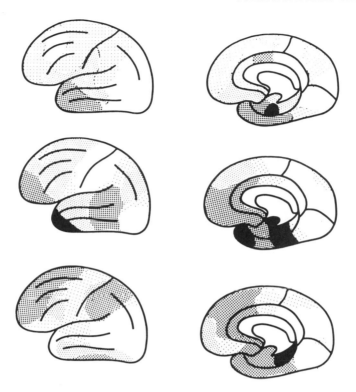

FIGURE 3–13.   Distribution of pathologic changes in the cerebral cortex in Pick's disease (cases with temporal, frontal, and combined involvement are depicted). Light stippling indicates mild to moderate involvement; darkly stippled areas are maximally affected. (Reprinted by permission of the publisher from A Brun and L Gustafson, "Limbic lobe involvement in presenile dementia," Arch Psychiat Nervenkr 1978; 226:79–93.

orientation, adherence to standard routines, and supportive guidance will allow the patient to stay in the home as long as possible. When the Klüver-Bucy syndrome is present, dietary restrictions may be necessary to prevent excessive weight gain. As immobility occurs, preventive measures are instituted to avoid urinary tract infections, aspiration pneumonia, and decubitus ulcers.

DIFFERENTIATING DAT FROM PICK'S DISEASE AND OTHER DISORDERS

The differentiation of DAT from Pick's disease is clinically challenging and may sometimes be impossible. The distinction is important, however, because behavioral expectations and management strategies differ for the two diseases. The two diseases share many features: both are idiopathic cortical dementing diseases that begin in late middle or old age and progress to death in 6 to 12 years. Language disturbances are prominent in both diseases, and motor abnormalities do not appear until late in the clinical course. The EEGs are normal in the early phases of both diseases and show progressive slowing as they evolve. Despite these similarities, there are enough differences in the clinical phenomenology of the two to allow at least tentative separation of most cases.

Table 3–6 summarizes the principal features that distinguish DAT and Pick's disease. The differential value of the clinical characteristics depends on when they appear in the temporal course of the illness, and the diseases are most readily separated on the basis of early behavioral changes (Lishman, 1978). The clinical finding that most consistently distinguishes them is the early appearance of amnesia in DAT, contrasting with the relative preservation of memory in the early stages in Pick's disease (Brun and Gustafson, 1978; Cummings and Duchen, 1981; Lishman, 1978; Nichols and Weigner, 1938; Sim et al, 1966; Stengel, 1943). Like memory, spatial orientation is compromised early in DAT and preserved in the early stages of Pick's disease (Cummings and Duchen, 1981; Haase, 1977). Mathematical skills may also be preserved in the initial stages of Pick's disease compared with early appearance of acalculia in dementia of the Alzheimer type. The early loss of intellectual abilities combined with the relative preservation of social skills and personal propriety in DAT contrasts with the personality changes and behavioral disturbances with sparing of specific intellectual skills that characterize the initial stages of Pick's disease (Brun and Gustafson, 1978; Gordon and Sim, 1967; Lishman, 1978; Polatin et al, 1948).

Among the early behavioral changes occurring in Pick's disease is the Klüver-Bucy syndrome (Cummings and Duchen, 1981). This syndrome has been observed in DAT, but only in its final phases (Sourander and Sjøgren, 1970). The Klüver-Bucy syndrome can occur as a consequence of any process affecting both temporal lobes and has been observed in adrenoleukodystrophy (Powers et al, 1980), after herpes encephalitis (Lilly et al, 1982; Marlowe et al, 1974), after temporal lobe surgery (Sawa et al, 1954; Terzian and Dalle Ore, 1955), with bilateral seizure foci in posttraumatic epilepsy (Liddell and Northfield, 1954), in amyotrophic lateral sclerosis (ALS) dementia (Dickson et al, 1986), and in arteriosclerotic cerebrovascular disease, hypoglycemic cerebral damage, and toxoplasmic encephalitis (Poeck, 1969).

Language disturbances occur in both conditions. Empty speech and poor word-list generation occur early in DAT; semantic anomia and circumlocution are evident early in Pick's disease. As the diseases progress, different patterns of linguistic deterioration occur. Patients with DAT develop fluent aphasias of the transcortical sensory type (Albert, 1981; Cummings, 1982; Goodman, 1953) and with further progression, palilalia and logoclonia become prominent. The typical linguistic changes of Pick's include anomia, auditory agnosia, excessive use of verbal stereotypes, and echolalia (Cummings, 1982; Cummings and Duchen, 1981; Ferraro and Jervis, 1936; Holland et al, 1985; Kahn and Thompson, 1933–1934; Wechsler et al, 1982). Mutism is more common in the later stages of Pick's disease than in DAT.

Seizures are not common in either of the cortical dementias but occur more often in the late stages of DAT (Ferraro and Jervis, 1936; Haase, 1977; Nichols and Weigner, 1928; Polatin et al, 1948; Stengel, 1943).

CT or MRI may provide information that aids in distinguishing the two conditions. If atrophy is present on the scans of patients with DAT, it tends to be widespread whereas temporal and/or frontal lobar atrophy may be demonstrable on the scans of those with Pick's disease (Cummings and Duchen, 1981; McGeachie et al, 1979; Wechsler et al, 1982). Lobar atrophy cannot be considered pathognomonic of Pick's disease, however, since atrophy affecting primarily the frontal and temporal lobes has been reported in occasional DAT patients (Tariska, 1970).

Clinical differences between the conditions reflect the differences in regional distribution of the underlying cellular and neurochemical changes. The relative preservation of personality, early loss of spatial orientation, and tendency to develop fluent aphasia in DAT correlate with the propensity of the disease to involve posterior hemispheric regions (Brun and Gustafson, 1978; Mayer-Gross et al, 1937–1938). In Pick's disease the early deterioration of personality and behavior and relative preservation of visuospatial skills reflect degeneration of the anterior hemispheric areas and limbic system (Brun and Gustafson, 1978; Cummings and Duchen, 1981). The early appearance of Klüver-Bucy syndrome in Pick's disease correlates with severe anterior temporal and diffuse amygdaloid changes (Cummings and Duchen, 1981), contrasting with limited amygdaloid involvement and late appearance of Klüver-Bucy syndrome in DAT (Corsellis, 1970; Herzog and Kemper, 1980; Hooper and Vogel, 1976; Sourander and Sjøgren, 1970).

DAT must also be distinguished from focal lesions involving the posterior aspect of the left hemisphere. Depending on its location and extent, such a lesion will produce a Wernicke, anomic, or transcortical sensory type of aphasia (Benson, 1979a). In addition, angular gyrus involvement produces the Gerstmann syndrome and the syndrome of alexia with agraphia. Gerstmann syndrome includes agraphia, acalculia, finger agnosia, and right-left disorientation and is frequently accompanied by constructional disturbances. Thus a relatively discrete lesion in the posterior portion of the left hemisphere results in disturbances of language, visuospatial skills, and diverse cognitive functions. No motor, sensory, or visual field deficit may occur. These patients are easily misdiagnosed as having DAT (Benson et al, 1982). The clinical features that distinguish this syndrome from DAT are a history of hypertension or other cardiovascular disease, relatively abrupt onset, behavioral evidence of preserved memory even when language disturbances prevent rigorous memory testing, and preservation of the pragmatic aspects of language so that the patient continues to attempt interpersonal discourse despite the aphasic disturbance. Minimal right-sided abnormalities such as hyperreflexia of the muscle stretch reflexes, loss of associated movements of the right arm while walking, or diminished optokinetic nystagmus when the target is moving toward the patient's left hemisphere provide supportive evidence for a focal left-sided lesion. Left-sided EEG abnormalities or neuroimaging findings will further substantiate the diagnosis. Recognition of this syndrome is particularly important because the prognosis and management of the two conditions are considerably different. (Chapter 5 contains a more extensive discussion of this differential diagnostic problem.)

Other syndromes such as multi-infarct dementia, general paresis, and Jakob-Creutzfeldt disease may involve the cerebral cortex, but subcortical involvement is present also. These diseases are discussed in chapters devoted to dementias with mixed subcortical and cortical features.

FOCAL CORTICAL ATROPHIES

Pick's disease is not the only disorder that can produce geographically restricted atrophic changes in the cerebral cortex; several other conditions associated with focal cortical atrophy have been described (Table 3–7). Predominance of parietal atrophy is seen in DAT and in corticobasal degeneration (also known as corticodentatonigral degeneration)(Gibb et al, 1989; Rebeiz et al, 1968). DAT has been extensively described above. Corticobasal degeneration is a rare syndrome that combines cortical and subcortical features. Patients often have an extrapyramidal syndrome and supranuclear gaze palsy resembling progressive supranuclear palsy, but they also have prominent evidence of parietal lobe dysfunction including constructional disturbances and "alien hand" sign, along with dementia and aphasia (Gibb et al, 1989; Rebeiz et al, 1968). At autopsy, neuronal loss, gliosis, and Pick cells are seen in the frontal lobe, basal ganglia, rostral brainstem, and thalamus. The distribution of pathological changes differs from that of classical Pick's disease.

Frontal Lobe Degenerations

Among diseases producing frontal or frontal and temporal lobe atrophy are Pick's disease, frontal lobe degeneration of the non-Alzheimer type, progressive subcortical gliosis, amyotrophic lateral sclerosis (ALS)-dementia syndrome, adult-onset neuronal intranuclear hyaline inclusion disease, and hereditary dysphasic dementia. There have been no demographic studies addressing the prevalence of these disorders; but among 26 cases diagnosed clinically as suffering from dementia syndromes with a predominance of frontal lobe features, Brun (1987) found that 16 had frontal lobe degener-

TABLE 3-7.   Disorders associated with focal cortical atrophy.

Disease	Lobar predominance	Principal histopathology
DAT	Parietal	Neurofibrillary tangles, neuritic plaques, amyloid angiopathy, granulovacuolar degeneration, neuronal loss, cortical gliosis
Corticobasal degeneration	Parietal	Pick cells, neuronal loss, cortical gliosis
Pick's disease	Frontal/temporal	Pick bodies
Frontal lobe dementia	Frontal/temporal	Nonspecific neuronal degeneration
Progressive subcortical gliosis	Frontal/temporal	White matter gliosis
ALS dementia	Frontal	Nonspecific neuronal degeneration
Neuronal intranuclear hyaline inclusion disease	Frontal	Hyalin inclusion bodies in neurons and glial cells
Hereditary dysphasic dementia	Frontal	Argyrophilic intracellular material
Primary progressive aphasia	Left hemisphere	Spongiform changes or Alzheimer-type changes
Posterior cerebral atrophy	Posterior hemispheric regions	Subcortical gliosis or Alzheimer-type changes

ation of the non-Alzheimer type, 4 had Pick's disease, 2 had DAT, 3 had Jakob-Creutzfeldt disease, and 1 had bilateral thalamic infarctions. *Frontal-lobe degeneration of the non-Alzheimer type* refers to a clinicopathological syndrome characterized behaviorally by features indicative of frontal lobe dysfunction (similar to Pick's disease) and pathologically by "simple" neuronal degeneration without Alzheimer or Pick type of histologic changes. The pathological alterations are concentrated in the temporal and frontal lobes (Brun, 1987; Englund and Brun, 1987; Gustafson, 1987; Knopman et al, 1990; Neary et al, 1988; Risberg, 1987). *Progressive subcortical gliosis* is a syndrome with frontal lobe features and marked gliosis of subcortical structures including the frontal lobe and temporal lobe white matter, thalamus, and inferior olivary nuclei (Neumann and Cohn, 1967; Verity and Wechsler, 1987). A frontal or temporal lobe type dementia may rarely precede or accompany the onset of ALS. At autopsy, the patients exhibit nonspecific neuronal degeneration and gliosis especially of the upper cortical layers. There may be sponginess of the neuropil. The changes are most severe in the frontal and medial temporal regions (Dickson et al, 1986; Finlayson et al, 1973; Horoupian et al, 1984). *Adult-onset neuronal intranuclear hyaline inclusion disease* is a frontal-lobe type dementia with prominent irritability, aphasia, and memory impairment. Extrapyramidal features may be present. At autopsy, there is neuronal loss and gliosis, and cells in the involved regions contain intranuclear hyaline inclusion bodies. Pathological alterations may occur in the cerebral cortex, caudate nucleus, and cerebellum (Munoz-Garcia and Ludwin, 1986). *Hereditary dysphasic dementia* is a rare autosomal dominant disease with prominent language abnormalities. Post mortem examination reveals frontal/temporal lobe atrophy, neuronal loss, conspicuous spongiform changes in the outer layers of the cortex, intracellular argyrophilic cytoplasmic fibrillary material, and subcortical Lewy body formation. Classic Alzheimer-type or Pick's type pathology is lacking (Morris et al, 1984).

Primary Progressive Aphasia

Other brain regions may also be subjected to focal atrophy, notably the left hemisphere in primary progressive aphasia and posterior hemispheric regions in posterior cortical atrophy. Primary progressive aphasia, as the name suggests, is a syndrome of progressive aphasia without dementia until the final phases of the illness (Mesulam, 1982). In most cases, the aphasic output has been of a nonfluent type with comprehension deficits. Anomia and shortened phrase length are characteristic. The disorder may be manifest as aphasia without dementia for five to eight years before deficits in other neuropsychological spheres become evident. Fluorodeoxyglucose positron emission tomography reveals marked left hemisphere hypometabolism with preservation of right hemispheric metabolic activity (Chowluk et al, 1986). The syndrome is etiologically heterogeneous: some cases have had topographically restricted spongiform changes without distinctive intracellular changes while others have had Alzheimer-type changes or Pick's disease at post mortem (Green et al, 1990; Kirshner et al, 1987; Mesulam, 1982; Poeck and Luzzatti, 1988; Snowden et al, 1989).

Posterior Cortical Atrophy

Posterior cortical atrophy may also be produced by several diseases. The clinical syndrome is dominated by elements of Balint's syndrome (optic ataxia, "sticky" fixation, simultanagnosia), alexia, agraphia, fluent aphasia, visual agnosia, and components of Gerstmann's syndrome (agraphia, acalculia, right-left disorientation, finger agnosia)(Benson et al, 1988). A variety of underlying diseases have been found in cases with this clinical presentation and studied at autopsy including progressive subcortical gliosis, Alzheimer-type changes, and Jakob-Creutzfeldt disease (Benson and Zaias, in press).

4

Subcortical Dementias in the Extrapyramidal Disorders

Many extrapyramidal disorders manifest a dementia syndrome with features that distinguish it from the cortical dementias discussed in Chapter 3. The clinical characteristics include mental slowness, inertia and lack of initiative, forgetfulness, dilapidation of cognition, and mood disturbances (Chapter 1). Diseases associated with subcortical dementia affect the basal ganglia, thalamus, and rostral brainstem structures or the associated frontal lobe projection regions of these nuclei. The patients typically exhibit a prominent movement disorder—bradykinesia, tremor, rigidity, chorea, myoclonus, dystonia—as part of their clinical symptomatology in addition to the intellectual deterioration. Huntington's disease, progressive supranuclear palsy, Parkinson's disease, Wilson's disease, Hallervorden-Spatz disease, idiopathic basal ganglia calcification, and the spinocerebellar degenerations are the principal movement disorders with dementias.

HUNTINGTON'S DISEASE

Huntington's disease is an idiopathic degenerative disorder of the nervous system with a characteristic triad of clinical features consisting of chorea, dementia, and a history of familial occurrence. The disease is inherited as an autosomal dominant trait with complete penetrance, affecting half the offspring of an afflicted individual. The gene for the disease is located on the short arm of chromosome 4 (Gusella et al, 1983). Males and females are equally likely to have the disease. The average course from onset to death is 14 years, and the average age of onset is 35 to 40 years. Approximately 5 percent of cases begin before age 20; 30 percent have their onset between 40 and 49 years of age; 17 percent begin between 50 and 59; and 5 percent begin after age 60 (Hayden, 1981). Considerable variation in age of onset may occur within families (Sax et al, 1989). Prevalence is 40 to 70 per 1,000,000 population (Hogg et al, 1979; Myrianthopoulos, 1966).

Dementia

In his original paper describing the disease that bears his name, George Huntington (1872) noted that "as the disease progresses the mind becomes more or less impaired, in many amounting to insanity, while in others mind and body gradually fail until death relieves them of their sufferings." He also noted that the form of insanity suffered by the patients often leads to suicide. Huntington's observations have been amply confirmed. Dementia is a constant feature of the disease and depression is exceedingly common. Suicide accounts for the deaths of 7.8 percent of males and 6.4 percent of females suffering from Huntington's disease (Reed et al, 1958), and unsuccessful suicide attempts are common (Dewhurst et al, 1970). The first mental status alterations to occur are usually personality changes, including irritability, untidiness, and loss of interest. Personality changes occur before the onset of chorea in a majority of cases, and major mood disturbances or schizophrenia-like syndromes are manifest prior to the chorea in one-third of patients (Bruyn, 1968; Lishman, 1978; Trimble, 1981). Dewhurst and colleagues (1969, 1970) found that, of 102 patients with Huntington's disease, 57 presented with predominantly psychiatric disturbances, 29 with mixed neurologic and psychiatric syndromes, and 16 with principally neurologic findings.

Episodic mood disorders resembling unipolar or bipolar affective illness and a delusional hallucinatory state with paranoia resembling schizophrenia are frequent in Huntington's disease (Caine and Shoulson, 1983; McHugh and Folstein, 1975). In a group of patients studied by Lieberman and associates (1979b) 53 percent had an affective illness and 25 percent had a schizophrenia-like disorder. The affective illness is usually depression, but alternating periods of depression and mania may occur. Psychotic features, particularly persecutory delusions, are common (Dewhurst et al, 1969; Folstein et al, 1979; McHugh and Folstein, 1975; Rosenbaum, 1941; Trimble, 1981). The prevalence of depressive illness among patients with Huntington's disease correlates with the high rate of suicide and attempted suicide in this population. McHugh and Folstein (1975) argue that the mood changes are an integral feature of Huntington's disease, not a reactive disturbance.

Reactive depression would not explain the episodic nature of the mood changes, the presence of mania as well as depression, or the observation that mood changes and delusional beliefs can appear prior to any knowledge by the patient of the disease or even of its familial nature.

A true schizophrenic thought disorder is more rare than affective disturbances, but exceeds the prevalence expected for schizophrenia and Huntington's disease occurring together coincidentally (Dewhurst et al, 1969; Folstein et al, 1979; Garron, 1973; Lishman, 1978; McHugh and Folstein, 1975; Rosenbaum, 1941; Trimble, 1981).

The dementia syndrome associated with Huntington's disease has the features characteristic of subcortical dementia. Slowing of cognition, impairment of intellectual function, and memory disturbances typically become apparent soon after the chorea begins (Brandt et al, 1990; McHugh and Folstein, 1975). Rarely the dementia may exist without chorea (Curran, 1930). Conspicuously absent are the aphasic and agnosic disturbances typical of cortical dementias (Bruyn, 1968).

Alterations of verbal output include poor performance on tests of verbal fluency (naming as many objects as possible in a given category in one minute), mild word-finding difficulties, and dysarthria. Impaired verbal fluency is among the earliest measurable abnormalities of cognitive function in Huntington's disease and precedes failure of memory and other aspects of cognition (Butters et al, 1978). Language tests that require organization, sequencing, and linguistic elaboration, and naming tests that demand retrieval of low-frequency words are failed by patients in middle and advanced stages of the illness (Kennedy et al, 1981; Podoll et al, 1988). These tasks go beyond language and require memory and cognitive abilities as well. Paraphasic errors and other language changes typically associated with cortical disturbances do not occur; dysarthria, on the other hand, is a prominent feature. Choreiform movements frequently involve the lips and tongue, disrupting timing, pronunciation, and articulatory agility. Diaphragmatic movements disturb speech volume, rate, spacing, and phrase length and impart an explosive quality to the output (Darley et al, 1975).

Memory disturbance is prominent in the dementia of Huntington's disease and usually occurs early (Butters et al, 1978). The pattern of memory impairment differs from the amnesia found in early stages of DAT or in Korsakoff's syndrome where new learning is preferentially disrupted and recall of older information is relatively preserved. Patients with Huntington's disease have as much difficulty recalling remote information as they have recalling recently learned material (Albert et al, 1981; Beaty et al, 1988b; Butters et al, 1979; Butters and Cermak, 1980). Careful analysis of the memory deficit reveals that the initial registration of information is only mildly impaired, but there is a significant difficulty with elaborating information for effective encoding and a marked deficit in retrieval (Butters et al, 1986; Caine et al, 1977; Weingartner et al, 1979). Recall in Huntington's disease patients is substantially improved by priming (prior exposure to the material), encoding enrichment (such as embedding the material to be recalled in a story), and semantic retrieval cues (telling the patient the category to which the target word belonged) (Butters et al, 1983, 1986; Granholm and Butters, 1988). Memory performances of DAT patients are not facilitated by these maneuvers. Motor skill learning, however, is more impaired in Huntington's disease than it is in DAT (Heindel et al, 1988).

As Huntington's disease progresses, other cognitive disturbances occur (Aminoff et al, 1975). Concentration and judgment are progressively impaired. Patients fail to initiate problem-solving behavior; have particular difficulty with cognitive tasks that require organization, planning, and sequential arrangement of information; are overwhelmed by excessive information; and perform badly on some visuospatial tasks (Brandt et al, 1988; Caine et al, 1978). They have difficulty with frontal systems tasks that demand sequential motor programming (serial hand sequences and so forth), and the deficits go beyond what could reasonably be ascribed to their movement disorder. Formal psychological testing reveals maximum deficits in the arithmetic, digit span, digit symbol, and picture arrangement subtests of the Wechsler Adult Intelligence Scale (Josiassen et al, 1982). The behavioral and neuropsychological disturbances exhibited by patients with Huntington's disease resemble those of patients with frontal lobe lesions. All intellectual abilities deteriorate as the disease advances, and in the final stages the patients are mute and intellectually devastated.

Clinical Features

The first manifestations of the choreic movement disorder include transient facial grimacing, head nodding, and flexion-extension movements of the fingers. The movements resemble tics but are slower and less stereotyped. Initially, the patient seems nervous or fidgety and may be able to incorporate the movements into quasi-intentional acts, but as the disease progresses the involuntary nature of the movements becomes obvious. The face, neck, limbs, and trunk are affected. Opening and closing the mouth, elevation of the eyebrows, and head flexion are typical. The hands go through alternating extension-pronation and flexion-supination postures particularly while the patient is walking, and the gait acquires a dancing appearance when these changes are superimposed on the irregular lurching, halting, and faltering movements of the trunk and legs. In advanced stages of disease, the speed of the movements slows and they acquire an athetotic or dystonic character. Terminally the patient may be in a fixed double hemiplegic posture with little involuntary movement (Bruyn, 1968; Denny-Brown, 1962; McDowell et al, 1978). In typical cases the muscle tone is diminished until late phases of the disease. Muscle stretch reflexes are increased in one-third of patients, and a few have extensor plantar responses. Sensation is unaffected. Some patients manifest abnormal eye movements including supranuclear disturbances of voluntary gaze, impaired optokinetic nystagmus, and the fast ocular movements of rapid eye-movement sleep (Starr, 1967).

Although chorea is the typical motor disturbance of Huntington's disease, a minority of patients present with an akinetic rigid variety (the Westphal variant) that may mimic Parkinson's disease. Twelve to 14 percent of patients have this predominantly rigid form (Bird and Paulson, 1971; Bittenbender and Quadfasel, 1962; Bruyn, 1968; Low et al, 1974) and rigidity is particularly common among patients with juvenile-onset Huntington's disease. The juvenile type (onset before age 20) accounts for 5 to 10 percent of all cases of Huntington's disease, and one-third to one-half of these patients have prominent rigidity and little chorea. Contrary to adult cases, the juvenile form also has an increased incidence of epilepsy, with up to 50 percent of patients manifesting generalized seizures (Bruyn, 1968; Byers et al, 1973; Jervis, 1963; Oliver and Dewhurst, 1969).

Laboratory Evaluation

Results of routine serum, urine, and cerebrospinal fluid (CSF) studies are unremarkable in Huntington's disease. Neurochemical analysis of CSF may reveal decreased levels of gamma-aminobutyric acid (GABA) (Enna et al., 1977; Bala Manyam et al, 1978). Electroencephalograms (EEGs) are abnormal in symptomatic patients; the alpha activity is poorly developed or absent and the record is of low voltage (Kiloh et al, 1972; Scott et al, 1972). The EEG remains normal in presymptomatic cases (Bruyn, 1968). Visual evoked potentials show diminished amplitude, but the latency of initial wave components is normal (Ellenberger et al, 1978). Auditory evoked potential latencies—N1, P2, N2, P3—are prolonged in most patients compared to normal subjects and to patients with DAT (Goodin and Aminoff, 1986).

Computerized axial tomography (CT) can demonstrate atrophy of the caudate nuclei with loss of the convex bulge into the lateral aspect of the frontal horns of the lateral ventricles (Fig. 4–1). The atrophy is usually evident on gross inspection of the scan, but can be corroborated by determining the frontal horn: intercaudate ratio or the bicaudate index (ratio of the width of both lateral ventricles at the level of the head of the caudate nuclei to the distance between the outer tables of the skull of the same level). A frontal horn: intercaudate ratio of less than 2 or a bicaudate index of less than 0.18 is indicative of caudate atrophy consistent with Huntington's disease (Barr et al, 1978a; Neophytides et al, 1979; Terrence et al, 1977). Correlations have been established between the severity of dementia, performance on tests of frontal systems functions such as trailmaking tasks, and the bicaudate ratio on CT scans (Bamford et al, 1989; Starkstein et al,

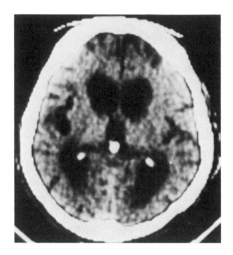

FIGURE 4–1.   CT scan in Huntington's disease shows dilated ventricles with loss of bulge of the caudate nucleus into the lateral aspect of the frontal horns.

1988). Individuals at risk for Huntington's disease but without chorea have normal scans. Enlarged ventricles are also demonstrable by pneumoencephalography in affected patients (Gath and Vinje, 1968), but there is now little justification for performing this study.

PET (Fig. 4–2) reveals markedly decreased glucose metabolism in the caudate areas whereas cortical metabolism usually remains normal (Benson

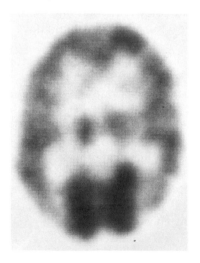
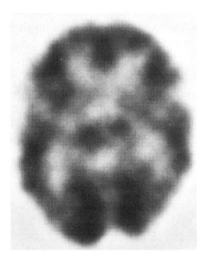

FIGURE 4–2.   PET in Huntington's disease reveals profoundly diminished metabolism in the region of the caudate nuclei. Cortical metabolism is normal.

et al, 1981b; Kuhl et al, 1982). With positron emission tomography, decreased metabolic activity can be demonstrated before caudate atrophy is visible on conventional CT scans (Hayden et al, 1986) and is abnormal in some presymptomatic individuals carrying the Huntington's disease gene (Hayden et al, 1987; Mazziotta et al, 1987). The degree of caudate hypometabolism demonstrated by PET correlates with changes in memory, functional capacity, and bradykinesia/rigidity; putamen metabolism correlates with chorea, oculomotor abnormalities, and fine motor skills (Berent et al, 1988; Young et al, 1986).

Single PET reveals decreased perfusion of the caudate nuclei, and xenon inhalation studies demonstrate diminished fronto-temporal blood flow in Huntington's disease (Nagel et al, 1988; Tanahashi et al, 1985).

Neuropathology

Grossly, the brains of Huntington's disease patients show nonspecific mild to moderate atrophy affecting primarily the frontal and parietal regions. Dramatic changes are usually evident when coronal sections are prepared. The head of the caudate is reduced from a robust structure, imparting a convex shape to the lateral wall of the frontal horn of the lateral ventricle, to a thin ribbon of tissue as little as 2 or 3 mm thick (Fig. 4–3). The putamen and to a lesser extent the globus pallidus are also shrunken (Corsellis, 1976; Dreese and Netsky, 1968).

Histologic changes are also most prominent in the neostriatum. There is a marked loss of the small internuncial neurons and a conspicuous increase in glial cells. The larger neurons may be shrunken and pyknotic. The pallidum, particularly the outer segments, shows neuron loss and gliosis that is less pronounced than that found in the caudate and putamen. The claustrum and subthalamic nuclei have mild to moderate neuronal depletion whereas the cerebellum, brainstem, and spinal cord are little affected (Bruyn, 1968; Corsellis, 1976; Dreese and Netsky, 1968; McCaughey, 1961). Small cells of the thalamus are also involved; the microneuronal population of the ventrobasal thalamic nuclei is reduced by approximately 50 percent in cytometric studies (Dom et al, 1976). More severe striatal changes are seen in patients with more rapid deterioration and younger age at onset (Myers et al, 1988).

Histologic changes in the cerebral cortex in Huntington's disease have long been the subject of controversy and disagreement. Some patients have no detectable cortical alterations while others may have severe disturbances. In affected cases, the frontal cortex is most involved while the occipital lobes tend to be spared. The neuronal depletion is patchy and involves the deeper cortical layers; only a mild degree of gliosis is evident (Bruyn, 1968; Corsellis, 1976; Dreese and Netsky, 1968). The hippocampus shows changes similar

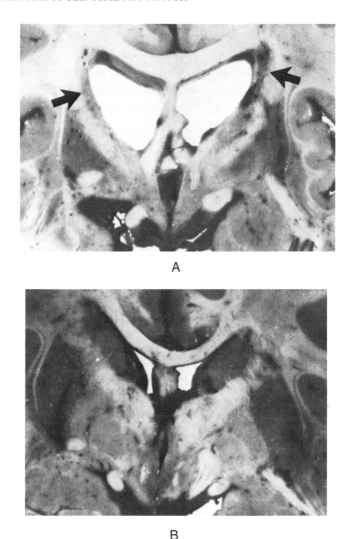

A

B

FIGURE 4–3.   Coronal section of the brain in Huntington's disease (A) shows loss of caudate substance (arrows) when compared with a normal brain (B). (Reprinted by permission of the publisher from W Haymaker et al, Extrapyramidal motor disorders. In: W Haymaker, ed. Bing's local diagnosis in neurological diseases, 15th ed. St. Louis: CV Mosby, 1969:404–440; and courtesy of Dr. Richard Lindenberg.)

to those occurring in other cortical regions, including moderate loss of cells and astrocytosis in the pyramidal cell layer (Bruyn, 1968; McCaughey, 1961).

Electron microscopic studies of the affected neurons in Huntington's disease reveal a marked heterogeneity, polymorphism, and metamorphosis of the chromatic granules and neuronal filaments (Roizin et al, 1979). Forno and Norville (1979) found unmyelinated axons containing synaptic vesicles and axonal dilatations stuffed with vesicles and suggested that these are functional neurons deprived of synaptic contact with the neostriatum.

Neurochemical alterations have also been identified in Huntington's disease. GABA, an inhibiting neurotransmitter, and glutamic acid decarboxylase, an enzyme responsible for GABA synthesis, are reduced by 70 to 90 percent in the striatum, pallidum, and substantia nigra (Bird et al, 1973; McGeer et al, 1973; Perry et al, 1973; Sourkes, 1976; Stahl and Swanson, 1974). Acetylcholine transferase, cysteic acid decarboxylase, succinic dehydrogenase, dopamine, cholecystokinin, neurokinin A, neuropeptide k, neurokinin B, angiotensin-converting enzyme, and substance P are reduced to a lesser extent (Arai et al, 1987; Arregui et al, 1977; Emson et al, 1980; Kanazawa et al., 1979; Spokes, 1979; Stahl and Swanson, 1974; Wu et al, 1979). The enzyme reductions do not reflect simple loss of tissue, since levels of acetylcholinesterase, monoamine oxidase and tyrosine hydroxylase in the basal ganglia are normal (McGeer et al, 1973; Stahl and Swanson, 1974). Serotonin, neuropeptide Y, and somatostatin concentrations are increased in the basal ganglia in Huntington's disease (Beal et al, 1988; Kish et al, 1987). Investigations of cortical levels of GABA, glutamic acid decarboxylase, cysteic acid decarboxylase, and choline acetyltransferase reveal normal levels or depletions less severe than those noted in the basal ganglia (Kremzner et al, 1979; Stahl and Swanson, 1974; Wu et al, 1979).

Neurotransmitter receptor studies have also revealed several abnormalities in Huntington's disease. Receptors of the following types are reduced in the basal ganglia: muscarinic cholinergic, benzodiazepine, GABA, dopamine, glutamate, N-methyl-D-aspartate (NMDA), phencyclidine, and quisqualate (Greenmayre et al, 1985; Whitehouse et al, 1985; Young et al, 1988). Cortical receptors are unchanged or minimally affected.

Pathophysiology

The basic defect in Huntington's disease appears to be the loss of small spiny neurons from the corpus striatum. These cells have an inhibitory function in movement mechanisms and their primary transmitter is GABA (Dom et al, 1976). This system is dynamically balanced with dopaminergic and cholinergic mechanisms so that dopamine agonists increase chorea, whereas cholinergic substances and GABA-ergic compounds diminish spontaneous movements (Aquilonius and Sjostrom, 1971; Klawans, 1970; Perry et al, 1973; Sourkes, 1976). The intermediate steps by which the genetic abnormality is translated into loss of spiny striatal neurons remain to be revealed. The involved neurons have high densities of NMDA receptors, suggesting that NMDA receptor mediated toxicity of an endogenous neurotoxin may play an important role in the pathogenesis of the disorder (Young et al, 1988).

The pathophysiology of the dementia in Huntington's disease is debated. Many authors have attributed the decline in mental status to changes in the cerebral cortex. The inconsistency of neuropathologic alterations in the cortex, increasing recognition of the role of subcortical structures in cognition, and the presence of normal cortical glucose metabolism on positron emission tomograms in Huntington's disease all suggest that the dementia is primarily a consequence of the subcortical changes. This conclusion is supported by the correlation of striatal glucose metabolism and neuropsychological function demonstrated by neuropsychometric tests and positron emission tomography (Berent et al, 1988; Young et al, 1986). Clinically the dementia lacks the linguistic and gnostic disturbances characteristic of cortical degeneration and closely resembles other subcortical dementias.

Diagnosis

Preclinical and prenatal diagnosis of Huntington's disease depends on being able to determine the likelihood that the individual is carrying the abnormal gene. The gene itself has not yet been identified, and predictive diagnosis entails studying DNA from relatives of the at-risk individual to determine which genetic markers are closely associated with the Huntington's disease gene in that particular family. Thus the accuracy of the test depends on the availability of DNA from family members. The test is based on linkage analysis and can never be 100 percent accurate since recombinations can occur (Martin and Gusella, 1986). Given these uncertainties and the current costs of performing these studies, preclinical diagnosis has not been widely applied.

In most cases, the diagnosis of Huntington's disease depends on clinical recognition of the typical choreiform movement disorder and dementia occurring on a familial basis. The diagnosis can be supported by demonstrating diminished caudate volume on CT scans, by diminished caudate perfusion on single photon emission computed tomograms, and by decreased caudate glucose metabolism on positron emission tomography.

Other means of identifying incipient disease in patients known to be at risk have been explored. The knowledge that levodopa increases chorea in symptomatic patients led to a provocative test for at-risk individuals (Klawans et al, 1970). Follow-up studies have shown that the patients in whom levodopa-induced chorea occurred were more likely to develop the disease than were those in whom it did not. The test is not completely validated, however, and false negative responses have occurred (Klawans et al, 1980). Changes in the blink reflex after a levodopa load, decreased levels of GABA in CSF, and subtle cognitive deficits on neuropsychological tests have also been found in individuals at risk for Huntington's disease, but the predictive value of these abnormalities has not been established (Bala Manyam et al, 1978; Esteban et al, 1981; Lyle and Gottesman, 1979). Disturbances in cell density and metabolic demands in skin fibroblast cultures and abnormalities in the membrane properties of lymphocytes and erythrocytes have been discovered in patients with symptomatic Huntington's disease and may eventually contribute to the diagnosis of presymptomatic individuals (Barkley et al, 1977; Goetz et al, 1975; Menkes and Hanoch, 1977; Noronha et al, 1979; Pettegrew et al, 1980). Demonstration on positron emission tomography of decreased glucose metabolism in the caudate may also predate other findings in affected individuals.

Differential Diagnosis

Table 4–1 presents the differential diagnosis of choreic syndromes. Most of these conditions lack dementia and positive family history and cause little confusion with Huntington's disease. Systemic illnesses, endocrinopathies, inflammatory disorders, and drug intoxications are discussed in other chapters of this volume and spinocerebellar degenerations are presented later in this chapter. Choreic syndromes that may be confused with Huntington's disease—including benign familial chorea, Sydenham's chorea, choreoacanthocytosis, adult dystonic lipidosis, and tardive dyskinesia—are discussed briefly.

The clinical syndrome of benign familial chorea typically begins in infancy or early childhood following a period of normal motor development. After its onset, the chorea is nonprogressive and remains present throughout life. Dementia is not a component of the syndrome. The condition is hereditary, and families with both autosomal dominant and autosomal recessive patterns of inheritance have been reported (Chun et al, 1973; Damasio et al, 1977; Haerer et al, 1967; Nutting et al, 1969; Pincus and Chutorian, 1967).

The outstanding clinical features of Sydenham's chorea are spontaneous movements, incoordination, and weakness. Sydenham's chorea occurs primarily between the ages of 5 and 15 years and is twice as common in females as it is in males. The original attack usually lasts less than six months and recurrences occur in one-third of patients. The movements are more abrupt, brusque, jerky, and ticlike than are the typical choreiform movements of Huntington's disease, and they lack the stereotyped patterns of the tic disorders. Compared with Huntington's disease, fewer muscle groups are involved in the lightninglike twitches and distal muscles are more prominently affected. Lability and irritability are common but dementia is rare. Other manifestations of rheumatic fever such as carditis or arthritis may be present, and the erythrocyte sedimentation rate or antistreptolysin O titer

TABLE 4–1.   Differential diagnosis of chorea.

Degenerative diseases	Systemic illnesses
Huntington's disease	Hypoglycemia
Wilson's disease	Hypernatremia
Idiopathic calcification of the basal	Uremia
ganglia	Hepatocerebral degeneration
Benign familial chorea	Remote effect of cancer
Choreoacanthocytosis	Drug-induced
Ataxia telangiectasia	Tardive dyskinesia
Spinocerebellar degeneration	Levodopa
Hallervorden-Spatz's syndrome	Amphetamines
Dystonia musculorum deformans	Tricyclic antidepressants
Adult dystonic lipidosis	Isoniazid
Familial myoclonus epilepsy with	Lithium
chorea	Organophosphates
Multisystem atrophies	Antihistamines
Vascular conditions	Methylphenidate
Posthemiplegic choreoathetosis	Pemoline
Internal cerebral vein thrombosis	Mercury
Lacunar infarction	Methadone
Infections and inflammatory diseases	Phenytoin
Systemic lupus erythematosus	Ethosuximide
Sydenham's chorea	Carbamazepine
General paresis (neurosyphilis)	Cimetidine
Viral encephalitides	Miscellaneous conditions
Endocrine disorders	Postanoxic (including choreoathetotic
Hyperthyroidism	cerebral palsy)
Hypoparathyroidism	Kernicterus
Pregnancy (chorea gravidarum)	Neoplasm
Oral contraceptive administration	Subdural hematoma
	Lupus anticoagulant disorder
	Propionic acidemia

may be elevated (Aaron et al, 1965; Thiebaut, 1968). Many cases of chorea gravidarum and chorea induced by use of oral contraceptives occur in patients with previous episodes of Sydenham's chorea (Gamboa et al, 1971; Nausieda et al, 1979, Pulsinelli and Hamill, 1978).

Tardive dyskinesia refers to a movement disorder that develops in some individuals chronically exposed to neuroleptic drugs. The most prominent movements usually involve the mouth and tongue, but hands, legs, trunk, and respiratory muscles may also develop choreoathetosis. The disorder is presumed to be secondary to hypersensitivity of dopamine receptors in the basal ganglia produced by chronic dopamine receptor blockade (Marsden et al, 1975). Preliminary observations suggest that patients developing tardive dyskinesia may have more intellectual impairment than do comparison groups of patients with similar treatment histories (Famuyiwa et al, 1979; Ivnik, 1979). Identification of such a tardive dementia is complicated by difficulties in evaluating the effects of continuing treatment with major tranquilizers and anticholinergics as well as a variety of other psychoactive drugs, the effects of chronic institutionalization and social isolation, and the late intellectual deterioration that occurs in some psychotic patients (Chapter 9). Huntington's disease can usually be distinguished from tardive dyskinesia by the tendency of the movements of the former to involve the upper, as well as the lower, face and the proximal, as well as the distal, limbs, to be subject to less voluntary control, and to be suppressed less with voluntary action of the involved body part (Cummings and Wirshing, 1989).

A disorder that shares many of the features of Huntington's disease is familial degeneration of the basal ganglia with acanthocytosis-choreoacanthocytosis. This syndrome begins with chorea and prominent orofacial dyskinesias between ages 15 and 35 years. Peripheral neuropathy is common (Vita et al, 1989). The movement disorder leads to progressive disability and death in the fifth to sixth decade. It occurs sporadically or is inherited in an autosomal recessive fashion. Severe conduct disorders and affective changes occur along with decreased concentration and attention, apathy, and impaired abstraction (Medalia et al, 1989). The CT scans and pneumoencephalograms reveal caudate atrophy. Regional glucose metabolism is diminished in the caudate and putamen (Dubinsky et al, 1989). Blood smears reveal that 5 to 50 percent of erythrocytes show acanthocytosis. Levels of serum creatine phosphokinase and lactic dehydrogenase may be elevated. In contrast to Bassen-Kornzweig syndrome with acanthocytosis, serum beta-lipoproteins are not decreased. Electromyograms and muscle biopsies are consistent with neurogenic atrophy. Autopsy studies demonstrate atrophy of the caudate and putamen with loss of small cells and preservation of large neurons similar to the changes of Huntington's disease. Glutamic acid decarboxylase activity, however, is not preferentially reduced. Clinically, choreoacanthocytosis is distinguished from Huntington's disease by the recessive pattern of inheritance, lack of prominent dementia, evidence of neurogenic atrophy, and presence of acanthocytosis (Bird et al, 1978; Kito et al, 1980; Sakai et al, 1981; Yamamoto et al, 1982).

Adult dystonic lipidosis is a very rare neurovisceral storage disorder with supranuclear ophthalmoplegia, mild dementia, choreoathetosis, dystonia, and ataxia. Foam cells and sea-blue histiocytes are found in the bone marrow (Longstreth et al, 1982).

Treatment

There is no treatment that changes the course of Huntington's disease, but the choreic movements can be limited. Major tranquilizers such as phenothiazines or haloperidol are the mainstay of treatment, and tetrabenazine, another dopamine antagonist, is also reported to control the choreiform movements (Asher and Aminoff, 1981; Swash et al, 1972). Neuroleptic doses in excess of 10 mg per day of haloperidol are rarely necessary or beneficial and may increase confusion (Barr et al, 1988).

The demonstration that levels of GABA are decreased in basal ganglia in Huntington's disease led to attempts to treat the disorder with GABA-ergic agents. Isoniazid raises central GABA levels and has led to mild to moderate improvement in some patients (Manyam et al, 1981; Perry et al, 1979, 1982), but other GABA-ergic compounds including glutamate, muscimol, and dipropylacetic acid have had no significant effect (Barr et al, 1978b; Shoulson et al, 1976, 1978).

Identification of low levels of enzymes related to cholinergic metabolism suggested treatment with cholinergic compounds. Intravenous injection of physostigmine, a central anticholinesterase agent, reduces choreiform movements (Aquilonius and Sjostrom, 1971), but oral cholinergic compounds have no beneficial effect or exacerbate the movements (Aquilonius and Eckernas, 1977; Growdon et al, 1977; Nutt et al, 1978a; Tarsey and Bralower, 1977).

A variety of other agents including sodium valproate (Pearce et al, 1977), opiate antagonists (Nutt et al, 1978b), bromocriptine (Kartzinel et al, 1976), and propranolol (Nutt et al, 1979) has been given to patients with Huntington's disease with no consistent benefit.

Levodopa generally exacerbates the choreiform movements, but it has been useful in alleviating the parkinsonian symptoms of the rigid variant of Huntington's disease (Barbeau, 1969).

The dementia of Huntington's disease is not improved by drugs that effectively suppress choreiform movements. The affective component of the mental status changes, however, does respond to treatment. Depression improves with tricyclic antidepressants, lithium, and electroconvulsive therapy (Leonard et al, 1974; McHugh and Folstein, 1975; Whittier et al, 1961). Irritability and angry outbursts may be treated with a neuroleptic agent or a combination of a neuroleptic and lithium carbonate (Leonard et al, 1974). Likewise the psychosis of Huntington's disease is most appropriately treated with low doses of neuroleptic medications.

PROGRESSIVE SUPRANUCLEAR PALSY (PSP)

Steele, Richardson, and Olszewski (1964; Richardson et al, 1963) were the first to call attention to this unique extrapyramidal syndrome characterized by supranuclear gaze paresis, pseudobulbar palsy, axial rigidity, and dementia. Progressive supranuclear palsy (PSP) typically has its onset in the sixth or seventh decade and progresses to death in 5 to 10 years. The disease is sporadic and occurs more commonly in males than it does in females (Steele, 1972; Steele et al, 1964). The prevalence of PSP is approximately 1.4/100,000 (Golbe et al, 1988).

Dementia

Vague changes in personality including apathy and slowness may be among the first features of PSP, but typically intellectual deterioration is mild until the late phases of illness. The characteristic neuropsychological changes are forgetfulness, slowness of thought processes, alterations of personality with apathy or depression, and impaired ability to manipulate acquired knowledge (Albert et al, 1974). These are now regarded as the cardinal features of subcortical dementia. Disorders reflecting cortical involvement such as agnosia or apraxia do not occur. Similarly aphasia is not evident although abnormalities in word selection have been noted in the verbal output of some patients (Obler et al, 1979). In contrast, alterations of speech (voice) are severe. Hypophonia, slurred articulation, and eventually mutism are consistently seen.

Neuropsychological studies of PSP have demonstrated deficits in learning, memory consolidation, and information retrieval (Litvan et al, 1989). Performance on frontal system tasks such as wordlist generation is also compromised, and the rate of central information processing is slowed (Dubois et al, 1988; Maher et al, 1985; Pillon et al, 1986).

Clinical Characteristics

Pseudobulbar palsy, axial rigidity, dementia, and a supranuclear paresis of gaze are the four principal clinical characteristics of PSP. The most common presenting manifestations are postural instability and falling, gait abnormalities, depression, dysarthria, and memory disturbances (Jackson et al, 1983; Maher and Lees, 1986).

Pseudobulbar palsy is manifested by a masklike facies, increased jaw and facial jerks, exaggerated palatal and pharyngeal reflexes, dysphagia, and drooling. As noted, dysarthria is usually severe and may progress to complete anarthria or mutism in the late stages. Forced laughter and crying are unusual (Steele, 1972; Steele et al, 1964; Behrman et al, 1969).

Rigidity is more evident in midline structures such as the neck and trunk than it is in the limbs, thus the term *axial rigidity*. In contrast to the stooped posture noted in those with Parkinson's disease, patients with PSP assume an erect or hypererect posture with neck extension. Behrman and associates (1969) suggested that this position is a partial manifestation of decerebrate rigidity secondary to the extensive changes at the mesencephalic level.

The neuro-ophthalmic abnormalities of PSP have been studied intensively. The type of ophthalmoplegia varies according to the stage of the disease. Loss of volitional downgaze is the most common disturbance early in the course, and it may be the first manifestation of the disease (Steele, 1972; Steele et al, 1964). Oculocephalic reflexes remain intact so that the patient cannot voluntarily look down, and the eyes deviate upward when the head is bent forward. This leads to frequent falls and to the telltale "dirty-tie sign" since the patient cannot look down while walking or eating (Dix et al,1971; Pfaffenbach et al, 1972). As the disease progresses, upward gaze is progressively impaired and volitional horizontal gaze is eventually lost (David et al, 1968). In the final stages, reflex eye movements are abolished along with the other extraocular movements. Electro-oculograms have revealed a variety of more subtle defects. Pursuit movements are broken into a series of short steps or cogwheel movements, the fast component of oculocephalic and vestibular nystagmus is lost, and spontaneous square-wave jerks are present in some patients during attempted fixation (Dix et al, 1971; Kase et al, 1976; Newman et al, 1970; Troost and Daroff, 1977; Troost et al, 1976). Other neuro-ophthalmic abnormalities observed in PSP patients include poor convergence, bilateral exophoria, bilateral lid retraction, apraxia of lid opening, internuclear ophthalmoplegia, blepharospasm, and loss of Bell's phenomenon (Mastaglia and Grainger, 1975; Messert and Van Nuis, 1966; Pfaffenbach et al, 1972).

Patients with PSP develop a profound bradykinesia during the course of the illness that imparts a superficial resemblance to Parkinson's disease. Tremor of either the resting or action type may occur but is unusual (Steele, 1972; Steele et al, 1964).

Laboratory Investigations

Results of blood, serum, urine, and cerobrospinal fluid studies are within normal limits. EEGs are usually normal in the early stages of the disease, but serial EEGs reveal progressive abnormality as the disease advances. Most common is slowing of the background rhythm or excessive theta activity distributed diffusely or bitemporally. High-voltage, bilateral monorhythmic delta waves with their highest voltage frontally occur in some cases (Fowler and Harrison, 1986; Su and Goldensohn, 1973).

Pneumoencephalography, although rarely necessary for diagnostic purposes, reliably demonstrates severe atrophy of the dorsal midbrain and superior colliculi in the late stages of the disorder (Bentson and Keesey, 1974), and diminished midbrain size may be evident on X-ray computed tomography (Ambrosetto and Kim, 1981; Haldeman et al, 1981).

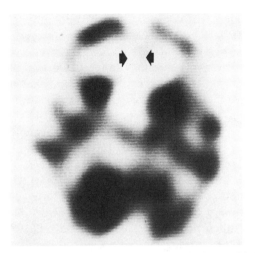

FIGURE 4–4. Single photon emission CT of a patient with PSP demonstrating bilateral frontal lobe hypoperfusion (arrows show regions with diminished flow) (AJ Lees, Progressive supranuclear palsy (Steele-Richardson-Olszcwski syndrome). In: Subcortical dementia. JL Cummings, ed. Oxford University Press, New York, 1990, pp 123–131; reproduced with permission of the publisher.)

PET studies of glucose metabolism reveal marked metabolic reductions in the superior frontal lobes and milder decrements in the caudate nucleus, putamen, thalamus, and pons (D'Antona et al, 1985; Foster et al, 1988; Goffinet et al, 1989). PETs measuring cerebral blood flow and oxygen usage exhibit a similar hypofrontal pattern, and scans using fluorodopa demonstrate diminished striatal dopamine formation and storage (Leenders et al, 1988). Likewise single photon emission tomography reveals bilateral frontal lobe hypoperfusion (Figure 4–4).

Neuropathology

Profound neuropathologic alterations are noted in the subthalamic nucleus, red nucleus, substantia nigra, pedanculopontine nucleus, superior colliculus, periaqueductal gray matter, globus pallidus,and dentate nucleus of the cerebellum (Ishino et al, 1975; Steele et al, 1964; Zweig et al, 1987). As expected from the loss of reflex oculomotor movements late in the disease, the oculomotor, trochlear, and abducens nuclei are also affected (Blumenthal and Miller, 1969; Ishino et al, 1974). The thalamus, globus pallidus, and putamen are involved only to a limited extent. The hypothalamus is not routinely affected, and most investigators report that the cortex is normal (Steele et al, 1964).

The most striking histologic finding in the affected regions is the presence of neurofibrillary tangles. Granulovacuolar degeneration occurs in some of the neurons; nerve cell loss is seen in involved areas; and fibrillary gliosis is present in areas of neuronal change. Demyelination is evident in the brainstem tegmentum, superior cerebellar peduncle, and medial longitudinal fasciculus. Torpedoes are occasionally seen in the axons of Purkinje cells in the cerebellum (Steele, 1972; Steele et al, 1964). Unlike the twisted tangles of DAT, the neurofibrillary tangles that accumulate in PSP are composed of straight tubules measuring 150 Å in diameter (Powell et al, 1974; Roy et al, 1974; Tellez-Nagel and Wisniewski, 1973; Tomonaga, 1977).

Neurochemical alterations in PSP include a marked nigrostriatal dopamine deficiency and a moderate impairment of the cholinergic system (Kish et al, 1985; Ruberg et al, 1985). Glutamic acid, taurine, and GABA are all increased in subcortical structures (Perry et al, 1988). Cortical concentrations of corticotropin-releasing factors are diminished (Whitehouse et al, 1987), and cortical nicotinic cholinergic receptors and subcortical D2-type dopamine receptors are also reduced (Bokobza et al, 1984; Pierot et al, 1988; Whitehouse et al, 1988).

Treatment

There is no cure for PSP, and once the disease has begun, its course is relentlessly progressive. The remarkable response of patients with Parkinson's disease to levodopa suggested that dopamine precursors or dopaminergic-receptor agonists should be tried in PSP. Several investigators found no response (Donaldson, 1973; Gilbert and Feldman, 1969; Gross, 1969; Jenkins, 1969), but other reports have been more optimistic. Akinesia improves in some patients treated with levodopa, and rigidity and extraocular movements improve in a few, whereas the dementia is consistently unaffected (Dehaene and Bogaerts, 1970; DeRenzi and Vignolo, 1969; Donaldson, 1973; Klawans and Ringel, 1971; Mastaglia et al, 1973; Mendell et al, 1970; Neophytides et al, 1982; Wagshul and Daroff, 1969). Similar variable improvement has been reported with amantadine. Benztropine mesylate has been reported to improve gait and speech abnormalities (Haldeman et al, 1981), and methysergide has sometimes been helpful particularly for patients with severe dysphagia (Rafal and Grimm, 1981). Patients may respond favorably to amitriptyline therapy (Kvale, 1982; Newman, 1985). The treatable aspects of the disorder become less responsive to pharmacotherapy as the disease advances.

Differential Diagnosis

The main disorder from which PSP must be distinguished is Parkinson's disease. Both conditions are akinetic rigid states with dementia and abnor-

TABLE 4–2.   Features that distinguish PSP from Parkinson's disease.

Characteristic	PSP	Parkinson's disease (Paralysis agitans)
Clinical features		
Rigidity	Axial > limb	Limb > axial
Posture	Extended	Bowed
Tremor	Uncommon	Common
Ophthalmoplegia	Downgaze lost first	Upgaze and converge lost first
Response to levodopa	Little improvement	Substantial improvement
Pathology		
Location	Subthalamic nucleus, red nucleus, substantia nigra, dentate nucleus	Substantia nigra, locus ceruleus, ventral tegmental area
Type of change	Neurofibrillary tangles, granulovacuolar degeneration, cell loss, gliosis	Lewy bodies, cell loss, gliosis

malities of extraocular movements. Table 4–2 summarizes the features that distinguish the two disorders. In PSP, the posture is extended; rigidity involves primarily the axial structures; downgaze is usually the first neuroophthalmic disturbance to occur; and tremor is unusual. In Parkinson's disease, the posture is bowed; rigidity involves the limbs; upgaze and convergence are impaired early; and tremor is prominent. The characteristic pathologic change in PSP is the occurrence of neurofibrillary tangles in nuclear structures of the mesodiencephalic junction. Parkinson's disease produces Lewy bodies in the substantia nigra and other pigmented brainstem nuclei.

The clinical features of PSP may also be simulated by lacunar state with multiple subcortical infarctions, progressive subcortical gliosis, bilateral intracerebral hemorrhages involving the basal ganglia, cerebral sarcoidosis, and normal pressure hydrocephalus (Dubinsky and Jankovic, 1987; Hankey and Stewart-Wynne, 1987; Morariu, 1979; Schlegel et al, 1989; Will et al, 1988).

PARKINSON'S DISEASE

Paralysis agitans (idiopathic Parkinson's disease) is a degenerative disorder of unknown etiology affecting mainly the pigmented brainstem nuclei and producing a complex motor system disturbance including bradykinesia, cogwheel rigidity, tremor, masked facies, loss of associated movements, and disturbances of gait, posture, and equilibrium. The disease has a prevalence of approximately one per thousand. It is usually a sporadic disorder with onset between the ages of 50 and 65 years, but juvenile and inherited forms of paralysis agitans have been reported (Allen, 1937; Martin et al, 1971; Spellman, 1962). The disease is more common among men than it is among women. The mean duration of the illness is 8 years (range, 1 to 30 years), and death results from aspiration pneumonia, urinary tract infection, or unrelated conditions of the elderly such as cardiovascular disease or cancer (Hoehn and Yahr, 1967; McDowell et al, 1978; Selby, 1968).

Dementia

The study of dementia in Parkinson's disease had an inauspicious beginning in the writing of James Parkinson himself and has continued to be an area of controversy. In his description of the disease, Parkinson specifically denied the presence of mental changes and noted that "the senses and intellect [are] uninjured"; in his case histories, however, he clearly detailed the presence of neuropsychiatric disturbances (Mayeux et al, 1981b). Charcot, on the other hand, believed the intellect was definitely impaired in Parkinson's disease and noted that cognition and memory deteriorated as the disease advanced (Boller, 1980). Early reports of Parkinson's disease concentrated on the motor disturbances and neglected changes in mental status, but recent studies have reestablished dementia as an integral part of the illness. Estimates of the prevalence of dementia in Parkinson's disease vary according to the population studied, the definition of dementia used, and the sensitivity of assessment techniques. Thus estimates as low as 4 percent and as high as 93 percent have been reported (Benson, 1984; Boller, 1980; Cummings, 1988). A majority of studies, accounting for a large number of parkinsonian patients, indicate that dementia is present in 35 to 55 percent of patients examined by standardized mental status assessment techniques (Boller, 1980; Boller et al, 1980; Brown and Wilson, 1972; Celesia and Wanamaker, 1972; Lieberman et al, 1979a; Loranger et al, 1972b; Martilla and Rinne, 1976; Mayeux et al, 1981b; Pirozzolo et al, 1982; Pollock and Hornabrook, 1966; Selby, 1968; Sweet et al, 1976). Longitudinal studies are lacking, but the increased occurrence of dementia in the older patient together with more severe rigidity and hypokinesia suggests that dementia becomes more prevalent and severe as the disease advances (Huber et al, 1989; Mortimer et al, 1982).

   The principal features of the dementia of Parkinson's disease include failure to initiate activities spontaneously, inability to develop a successful approach to problem solving, impaired and slowed memory, impaired visuospatial perception, impaired concept formation, poor wordlist generation, impaired set shifting, and reduced rate of information processing (Albert, 1978; Bowen et al, 1975; Levin et al, 1989; Levita et al, 1964; Loranger et al, 1972b; Marsh et al, 1971; Matison et al, 1982; Mayeux et al, 1981b; Pirozzolo et al, 1982; Talland, 1962; Talland and Schwab, 1964; Warburton, 1967b; Wilson et al, 1980). The dementia is usually of mild to moderate severity; most apparent are the slowness of response, poor wordlist generation, impaired constructions, deterioration in abstraction and concept formation, and poor performance on more complicated mathematical word problems. Cortical features such as aphasia, agnosia, and severe amnesia are unusual in the dementia of Parkinson's disease.

Controversy has arisen concerning the co-occurrence of DAT and Parkinson's disease. Several autopsy studies of demented parkinsonians have found neuropathological changes identical to those found in DAT along with the typical findings of Parkinson's disease (Alvord et al, 1974; Boller, 1980; Boller et al, 1980; Hakim and Mathieson, 1978, 1979). The Alzheimer-type cortical changes have been found in patients who manifest a more severe dementia. DAT increases in frequency with advancing age (Chapter 3) and can be expected to occur in any population of elderly patients, including a parkinsonian group. It is not known if the two conditions occur simultaneously by chance, if one disease predisposes the individual to develop the other, or if both disorders are manifestations of a single predisposition to CNS degeneration. Epidemiologic and pathologic studies by Heston (1981) suggest that the changes of the Alzheimer type among patients with Parkinson's disease can be accounted for on the basis of the patient's age.

There may be several separate but overlapping varieties of mental impairment in Parkinson's disease based on distinct neuropathological and neurochemical changes. The majority show mild cognitive impairment featuring psychomotor retardation, forgetfulness, dilapidated cognition, and depression or apathy. This ubiquitous clinical syndrome is likely related to the common dopaminergic deficiency; more severe intellectual impairment may be related to superimposition of cholinergic deficits and Alzheimer-type pathological alterations (Cummings, 1988).

Depression is frequent in subcortical dementia and is a prominent feature in the symptomatology of Parkinson's disease. It may be the presenting feature of the illness (Jackson et al, 1923; Santamaria et al, 1986), occurs in 40 to 60 percent of patients during the course of idiopathic parkinsonism (Brown and Wilson, 1972; Celesia and Wanamaker, 1972; Mayeux et al, 1981b), and is present in 90 percent of parkinsonian patients referred for psychiatric care (Mindham, 1970). Depressed mood is significantly more common among patients with Parkinson's disease than it is among those with other chronic medical and neurologic disorders, and the severity of the depression does not correlate well with the degree of disability (Celesia and Wanamaker, 1972; Horn, 1974; Marsh and Markham, 1973; Mayeux et al, 1981b; Warburton, 1967a). Depression is more common in patients with other manifestations of mental status impairment (Mayeux et al, 1981b). These observations imply that the depression is not a psychogenic reaction to the physical disability caused by the motor disturbance, but is an integral part of the basal ganglion disorder.

The difficulties created by the mental status changes in Parkinson's disease are exaggerated and compounded by abnormalities of speech and writing. Voice changes of some degree occur in nearly all parkinsonian patients. Speech volume is reduced, inflection is lost, and the voice acquires a monotonous quality without variations in pitch. An increased number of pauses, hesitation at the beginning of a sentence, and progressive dysarthria occur (Cummings et al, 1988; Darkins et al, 1988). The range of mouth and tongue movements is diminished. The rate of speech may be either decreased or increased, with some patients displaying festination of speech. The vocal output may eventually become entirely inaudible and unintelligible (Critchley, 1981; Darley et al, 1975; Nakano et al, 1973; Selby, 1968). Despite these changes in the motoric aspects of speech, there are few alterations in language function. Naming and linguistic comprehension remain intact until the dementia becomes severe late in the course of the illness (Cummings et al, 1988). Micrographia is the initial complaint and harbinger of Parkinson's disease in about 5 percent of cases, and severe micrographia occurs in 10 to 15 percent of patients at some time during their illness. Affected patients are unable to sustain normal-sized writing for more than a few letters. Except for the change in size there may be few changes in the morphology of letters unless tremor and rigidity induce a deterioration in caligraphy (McLennan et al, 1972). The combination of increasingly unintelligible speech and progressive micrographia may make communication nearly impossible.

Neuropsychological assessment of patients with Parkinson's disease is fraught with difficulties, and the many problems encountered explain some differences of opinion regarding the prevalence and typology of the dementia. Timed tests or tests requiring manual dexterity penalize parkinsonian patients because of their motor deficits; on the other hand, it is not safe to assume that all retardation is based solely on the motor disturbance. Only careful comparisons between the degree of motor impairment and the severity of the slowing on psychological tests will reveal the different components of psychomotor retardation. The effects of aging, depression, and chronic disability must also be considered before attributing particular deficits to the effects of Parkinson's disease per se. Relatively specific testing may be required to demonstrate deficits in these patients; adequate performance on tests of general intelligence may mislead the clinician into believing that no intellectual impairment is present.

The intelligence tests of parkinsonian patients usually reveal them to be functioning in the normal or mildly impaired range (Asso, 1969; Hardyck and Petrinovich, 1963; Levita et al, 1964; Loranger et al, 1972a, b; Reitan and Boll, 1971). Even when the scores are in the normal range, ancillary evidence suggests a decline from previous levels of intellectual functioning (Diller and Riklan, 1953). The lowest scores are on the performance subtests, but scores often correlate poorly with the actual degree of motor impairment, and tests requiring little motor speed or coordination are also affected (Loranger et al, 1972b; Mortimer et al, 1982).

Memory tests and tests of intellectual function independent of motor disturbance also demonstrate deficits in parkinsonian patients (Levita et al, 1964; Mayeux et al, 1981b; Reitan and Boll, 1971; Talland, 1962; Warburton, 1967b). The memory abnormalities are typical of those occurring in patients with subcortical dementia syndromes. Recognition memory is preserved, whereas effort-demanding memory, spontaneous recall, temporal ordering of learned information, and procedural memory are impaired (Flowers et al, 1984; Huber et al, 1986b; Sagar et al, 1988a; Saint-Cyr et al, 1988; Weingartner et al, 1984). Memory disturbances are demonstrable early in the clinical course of the disease (Levin et al, 1989). The pattern of memory deficits of demented parkinsonians differs from that of patients with DAT (Sagar et al, 1988a, b).

Visuospatial skills are also compromised in Parkinson's disease (Boller et al, 1984; Stern et al, 1984). Abnormalities are demonstrable on motor-free tests and occur early in the course of the illness in some patients (Hovestedt et al, 1987).

Tests assessing function of frontal-subcortical systems also reveal abnormalities in Parkinson's disease. Deficits are demonstrable on the Wisconsin Card Sorting Test and other tasks that require shifting performance sets (Bowen et al, 1975; Brown and Marsden, 1988; Cools et al, 1984; Flowers and Robertson, 1985; Talland and Schwab, 1964; Taylor et al, 1986, 1987). Tests that demand integration of postural and visual information are compromised in parkinsonian patients, and their deficits resemble those observed in patients with frontal lobe lesions (Danta and Hilton, 1975; Teuber and Proctor, 1964).

Clinical Characteristics

In addition to changes in mental status, the principal clinical features of Parkinson's disease are bradykinesia, rigidity, tremor, loss of associated movements, and neuroophthalmic abnormalities. Disorders of autonomic function are also frequent.

Movement disorder is the hallmark of Parkinson's disease. Bradykinesia or hypokinesia is the primary symptom and accounts for many of the characteristic features of the disease. Hypokinesia is the underlying abnormality of the difficulty with initiation of movement, the expressionless face and diminished blinking, the loss of associated movements, and micrographia. Loss of spontaneous swallowing results in accumulation of saliva in the mouth and the consequent drooling. Hypokinesia is frequently associated with rigidity but the two can be dissociated, and the psychomotor retardation is not a result of rigidity (Selby, 1968). Parkinsonian rigidity involves the limb and trunk musculature, producing a lead-pipe resistance to passive manipulation. When tremor is present, the combination of tremor and rigidity imparts a ratchet or cogwheel character to the rigidity (Lance et al, 1963; Selby 1968). As rigidity increases, postural changes become apparent. A simian-like stance with slight flexion of ankles, knees, hips, elbows, back, and neck develops (McDowell et al, 1978). The common tremor of Parkinson's disease is a four- to eight-cycle-per-second resting tremor that usually develops in one upper extremity and may spread to involve all four limbs, face, and tongue. The tremor is absent or minimal when the patient is relaxed and is exacerbated by stress. Severe rigidity may abolish the tremor. A minority of parkinsonian patients have a six- to twelve-cycle-per-second action tremor in addition to the resting tremor (Lance et al, 1963; McDowell et al, 1978; Selby, 1968). In addition to hypokinesia, rigidity, and tremor, a few patients develop a dystonic foot response during ambulation. The movement consists of tonic extension of the great toe, arching or inversion of the foot, or extension of the ankle (Nausieda et al, 1980). The muscle stretch reflexes are normal in Parkinson's disease and sensation is intact. Autonomic symptoms include postural hypotension, impotence, atony of the large bowel with constipation, and esophageal spasm (Langston and Forno, 1978; McDowell et al, 1978; Selby, 1968). Decreased volitional upgaze and impaired convergence are the most frequent extraocular motor abnormalities. Pursuit movements are performed more rapidly than are voluntary movements, and oculocephalic reflex movements remain intact. Decreased downgaze may also occur. Rapid volitional eye movements are fragmented into multiple saccades, and pursuit movements are also broken into a series of small-amplitude saccadic steps (cogwheel eye movements). Lid abnormalities include decreased spontaneous blinking, increased blepharospasm, and lid retraction or ptosis. Pupillary changes may involve accommodation or light reaction (Corin et al, 1972; Glaser, 1978; Walsh and Hoyt, 1969).

Laboratory Evaluation

Laboratory studies are of little use in the identification of Parkinson's disease, and diagnosis depends entirely on clinical criteria. Results of routine blood, urine, and cerebrospinal fluid tests are normal. Specialized assays of neurotransmitter metabolites in CSF reveal decreased concentrations of homovanillic acid, the product of dopamine metabolism, and of 5-hydroxyindoleacetic acid, a metabolite of serotonin (Sourkes, 1976). EEG findings are nonspecific. In most cases the EEG is normal, but 40 percent of patients have abnormally slow background rhythms (Neufeld et al, 1988). Diffuse theta activity may be seen over the frontal and temporal regions (Green, 1966; Hughes, 1966; Selby, 1968). Electroretinograms are abnormal with diminished response amplitudes (Nightingale et al, 1986). Visual evoked response studies reveal a longer latency and lower amplitude of evoked potentials (Bodis-Wolner and Yahr, 1978; Gawel et al, 1981). Long-latency auditory evoked potentials are prolonged in Parkinson's disease and the abnormalities are more marked in those with dementia than in those without it (Gawel et al, 1981; Goodin and Aminoff,1 987; Hansch et al, 1982).

Computerized cranial tomography reveals that enlarged sulci and dilated ventricles become more evident in elderly patients. As is the case with other demented patients. Parkinson's disease patients with dementia usually have atrophic changes, but many with normal intellect show similar changes, and the CT findings have no specific predictive value concerning the presence or severity of dementia (Inzelberg et al, 1987; Sroka et al, 1981). Pneumoencephalographic studies reveal enlarged ventricles in a majority of patients and cortical atrophy in approximately half (Gath et al, 1975).

Magnetic resonance imaging is capable of revealing reductions in size of the substantia nigra in advanced Parkinson's disease (Duguid et al, 1986). Xenon inhalation studies of cerebral blood flow demonstrate reduced cerebral blood flow and loss of the normal predominance of perfusion anteriorly (Bes et al, 1983; Lavy et al, 1979; Wolfson et al, 1985). PET investigations show diffusely reduced cerebral glucose metabolism (Kuhl et al, 1984), and studies using fluorodopa reveal markedly diminished uptake in the striatum (Leenders et al, 1988). Some demented parkinsonian patients exhibit diminished parietal lobe glucose metabolism bilaterally similar to the characteristic pattern of DAT (Kuhl et al, 1984; Pizzolato et al, 1988).

Neuropathology

At autopsy, the brain of the parkinsonian patient may show widened sulci particularly in the frontal region (Alvord, 1971; Turner, 1968). Horizontal sections of the brainstem reveal prominent depigmentation of the substantia nigra (Fig. 4–5).

Histologically the substantia nigra is the site of the most severe changes. There is extensive neuron loss in the pars compacta and a fibrous glial reaction is present in the area of cell loss (McDowell et al, 1978; Oppenheimer, 1976b; Turner, 1968). Less pronounced changes are evident in a variety of other brainstem and diencephalic nuclei, and there is a predilection for involvement of pigmented nuclei including the locus ceruleus, dorsal vagal nucleus, and sympathetic ganglia (Den Hartog Jager and Bethlem, 1960). The ventral tegmental area and the hypothalamus may also be involved (Javoy-Agid and Agid, 1980; Langston and Forno, 1978). Atrophy

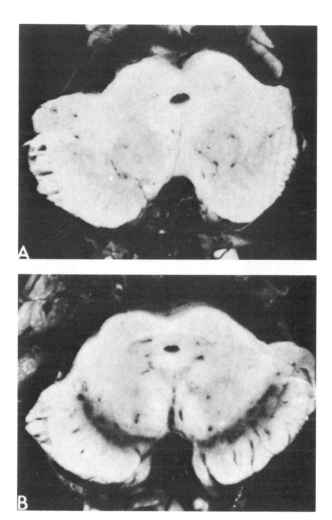

FIGURE 4–5.   Horizontal section of the midbrain reveals depigmentation of the substantia nigra in a patient with Parkinson's disease (A) compared with a normal brain (B). (Reprinted by permission of the publisher from F.H. McDowell et al., Extrapyramidal disease. In: AB Baker, LH Baker, eds. Clinical neurology. New York: Harper & Row, 1978: 1–67.)

of the nucleus basalis of Meynert is evident in some cases (Whitehouse et al, 1983). The caudate and putamen have no consistent changes beyond those associated with normal aging (Greenfield and Bosanquet, 1953; Oppenheimer, 1976b). As noted, in some cases the cerebral cortex has extensive neuronal changes of the Alzheimer type, including senile plaques and neurofibrillary tangles (Boller et al, 1980; Hakim and Mathieson, 1978, 1979).

The most distinctive histologic feature in paralysis agitans is the presence of Lewy bodies in many remaining neurons of the involved nuclei (Den Hartog Jager and Bethlem, 1960). The Lewy bodies are round hyaline bodies with a pale peripheral halo. They may be single or multiple, and they occur in the cell cytoplasm. They are composed of protein and sphingomyelin (Alvord, 1971; Turner, 1968). Electron microscopy reveals that the Lewy bodies consist of loosely packed filaments in the outer zone and densely packed filaments mixed with granular material in the central core (Oppenheimer, 1976b). As the cells die, the bodies are liberated into adjacent tissues.

Neurochemical analysis of the basal ganglia in Parkinson's disease reveals that the normally high dopamine content of these structures is markedly diminished (McDowell et al, 1978; Sourkes, 1976). Dopamine losses are most marked in the caudal putamen (Kish et al, 1988b); dopamine receptor densities are unaffected (Pierot et al, 1988). Dopamine concentrations are lowest in patients manifesting severe akinesia. Norepinephrine, glutamate decarboxylase, GABA, methionine-enkephalin cholestokinin, and serotonin and its metabolite 5-hydroxyindoleacetic acid are also decreased in the substantia nigra of parkinsonian patients compared to controls though reductions are less marked than for dopamine (McDowell et al, 1978; Sourkes, 1976; Studler et al, 1982; Taquet et al, 1982).

Pathophysiology

The pathophysiologic basis of the motor disturbance of Parkinson's disease is ascribed primarily to the dopamine deficiency of the substantia nigra. Dopaminergic neurons in the nigral pars compacta project by way of the comb bundle to synapses in the corpus striatum. Striatal dopamine receptors are deprived of nigral input, and the activity of the basal ganglia in coordinated movement is disrupted (Kornhuber, 1974; Sourkes, 1976). This hypothesis provides a rationale for the use of levodopa in the treatment of Parkinson's disease.

Increased rigidity in Parkinson's disease is a consequence of decreased inhibition of spinal segmental mechanisms. The resting tremor is produced by 4 to 8 Hz alternating contractions of agonist and antagonist muscles. The ratchet or cogwheel rigidity results from superimposition of tremor mechanisms on the rigidity (Lance and McLeod, 1975).

The pathophysiology of intellectual impairment in Parkinson's disease is controversial, and ill understood. Several lines of evidence suggest that the marked dopamine deficiency may contribute to the intellectual deterioration (Cummings et al, 1988). First, mild mental status changes are ubiquitous in Parkinson's disease and dopamine loss is present in all changes with that disease. Second, there is modest restitution of intellectual function following dopamine replacement therapy (Broe and Caird, 1973; Halgin et al, 1977; Loranger et al, 1972a; Marsh et al, 1971; Meier and Martin, 1970). Third, cognitive abnormalities occur in PSP and 1-methyl-4-phenyl-1, 2, 3, 6-tetrahydropyridine (MPTP) parkinsonism (Albert et al, 1974; Stern and Langston,1985) where dopamine disturbances occur in the absence of other types of pathology. Fourth, experimental studies indicate that striatal dysfunction results in visuospatial impairments, set maintenance abnormalities, and deficits in recent memory (Iversen, 1979; Oberg and Divac, 1979) similar to those observed in Parkinson's disease. Fifth, dementia has been observed in parkinsonian patients whose pathology is limited to the classic monoaminergic systems (Helig et al, 1985). Sixth, there is a correlation between cell loss in the medial substantia nigra (projecting to the medial frontal lobes) and the severity of dementia (Rinne et al, 1989). Seventh, the characteristics of the dementia syndrome closely resemble those of other subcortical and frontal lobe disorders (Danta and Hilton, 1975; Teuber and Proctor, 1964). Anatomically there is a prominent dopaminergic projection from the ventral tegmental area to the medial frontal lobe (Javoy-Agid and Agid, 1980; Johnson et al, 1968; Nauta, 1971; Rosvold, 1972; Truex and Carpenter, 1969). Interruption of this circuitry by dopaminergic deficiency could contribute to the cognitive abnormalities. In some cases, the dopamine loss is accompanied by a superimposed cholinergic deficiency, and this combined neurochemical abnormality may exaggerate the mental status changes (Cummings, 1988). In others, these disturbances are further complicated by the presence of Alzheimer-type changes, and the patients could be expected to manifest both cortical and subcortical neuropsychological deficits.

Treatment

Treatment of Parkinson's disease was revolutionized by the discovery of a central dopamine deficiency. Until then, ventrolateral thalamotomy and administration of anticholinergic agents had been the principal means of treatment. Both these interventions had an ameliorating effect on tremor and reduced rigidity but did little to relieve akinesia (Adams and Victor, 1977; McDowell et al, 1978). Anticholinergic compounds remain a useful adjunct to therapy and may be the sole treatment in patients unable to tolerate levodopa. Side effects include dry mouth, blurred vision, constipation, and urinary retention as well as delirium, agitation, and hallucinations.

Amantadine, an agent that releases dopamine from intact neurons and inhibits its reuptake, is also a useful adjunct in the therapy of Parkinson's disease (Sourkes, 1976). Its beneficial effects last for only one to three months and the principal side effects encountered are edema, livedo reticularis, hallucinations, and confusional states (Schwab et al, 1972; Timberlake and Vance, 1978).

The mainstay of current Parkinson's disease therapy is levodopa. Dopamine itself will not cross the blood-brain barrier whereas its precursor, levodopa, is readily transported into the CNS. There it is incorporated into remaining neurons of the substantia nigra, converted to dopamine, and becomes the synaptic transmitter for striatal dopaminergic receptors. To inhibit peripheral side effects, levodopa is frequently administered in combination with a dopa-decarboxylase inhibitor (carbidopa) that does not cross the blood-brain barrier. A daily dose of 1000 to 1500 mg of levodopa combined with 100 to 150 mg of carbidopa in four divided doses usually produces the desired effect. Side effects of levodopa include nausea, choreoathetotic dyskinesias, postural hypotension, palpitation, and cardiac dysrhythmias (Bianchine, 1976; McDowell et al, 1978). Psychiatric side effects are not uncommon and include acute psychosis, delirium, anxiety, depression, and hypomania (Celesia and Barr, 1970; Damasio et al, 1971; Goodwin, 1971; Jenkins and Groh, 1970; Lin and Ziegler, 1976).

Sixty percent of patients who are started on levodopa therapy show symptomatic improvement in their movement disorder. Akinesia responds better than does rigidity or tremor. Micrographia improves in many parkinsonian patients, and levodopa often benefits the quality of speech articulation (Knopp et al, 1970; Leanderson et al, 1971; McLennan et al, 1972; Rigrodsky and Morrison, 1970). Unfortunately the effects of the disease are merely postponed, and incapacitating symptoms reemerge in one to four years (McDowell et al, 1978). This loss of response most likely results from progressive loss of neurons and advancing inability of the remaining cells to convert the administered levodopa into active dopamine. Drugs such as bromocriptine, lisuride, and pergolide are direct dopamine receptor agonists whose action is independent of the integrity of nigrostriatal dopaminergic pathways. They can be useful alone or in combination with levodopa when response to levodopa becomes inadequate. Side effects are similar to those of levodopa, but nausea and neuropsychiatric reactions are more common, and lisuride can cause excessive somnolence (Gopinathan et al, 1981; Lieberman et al, 1976, 1980; McDowell et al, 1978).

In addition to the relief of symptoms, specific types of therapy may slow progression of the disorder. Deprenyl, a monoamine oxidase inhibitor, defers the need for dopaminergic therapy and may retard the pathologic alterations in the substantia nigra (Parkinson Study Group, 1989; Tetrud and Langston, 1989).

Cognitive impairment in parkinsonian patients also improves with treatment (Broe and Caird, 1973). Measurable improvement occurs on subtests of the Wechsler Adult Intelligence Scale measuring perceptual organization skills, visuospatial abilities, and sequencing (Loranger et al, 1972a; Meier and Martin, 1970). Memory and performance on tests of planning and problem solving also improve (Halgin et al, 1977; Marsh et al, 1971; Meier and Martin, 1970), but as the disease advances these improvements are not maintained (Halgin et al., 1977). The beneficial results correlate poorly with improved motor function. Cortical dementias of the Alzheimer type do not respond to levodopa or its precursors (Kristensen et al, 1977; Meyer et al, 1977). Demented parkinsonian patients appear to be more susceptible to levodopa-induced neuropsychiatric disturbances and must be managed with caution (Lieberman et al, 1979a; Sacks et al, 1970a, 1972).

Depression in Parkinson's disease is not altered by levodopa therapy despite marked motor improvement and may progress despite levodopa treatment (Cherington, 1970; Marsh and Markham, 1973; Mindham et al, 1976). Tricyclic antidepressants, however, often successfully elevate the patient's mood and even have a mild ameliorating effect on the motor symptoms (Mandell et al, 1961; Strang, 1965). Similarly electroconvulsive therapy can improve both depression and the motor disability in Parkinson's disease (Asnis, 1977; Lebensohn and Jenkins, 1975).

Differential Diagnosis

Paralysis agitans (idiopathic Parkinson's disease) must be distinguished from other conditions that can produce a parkinsonian syndrome. Numerous conditions produce akinetic rigid states that must be considered in the differential diagnosis of parkinsonism, and most of these illnesses have distinguishing features that allow them to be identified clinically. Table 4–3 lists the principal diseases that cause parkinsonian syndromes.

Postencephalitic Parkinsonism

Von Economo's encephalitis, or encephalitis lethargica, was a condition of presumably viral origin that reached epidemic proportions in the years 1919 to 1926 (Duvoisin and Yahr, 1965; Duvoisin et al, 1963). The incidence of the disease diminished rapidly after 1926, but rare cases with similar clinical features continue to occur (Espir and Spalding, 1956; Hunter and Jones, 1966). In the acute stage, the disease took a lethargic-somnolent or an excited-psychotic form. Various motor disturbances including rigidity, akinesia, catatonia, cataplexy, chorea, or tremor occurred, and ophthalmoplegia and pupillary changes were common (Hall, 1929; Riley, 1930). In some patients the postencephalitic parkinsonian syndrome appeared immediately as the acute illness resolved; in others the extrapyramidal syndrome did not become manifest until 10 or even 20 years later. More than half of the survivors of encephalitis lethargica eventually developed postencephalitic parkinsonism (Duvoisin and Yahr, 1965). Once it appeared, the syndrome remained stable or progressed very slowly with little increasing disability. Clinically the syndrome of postencephalitic parkinsonism is not as stereotyped as is paralysis agitans. Neurologic findings can include ocular and

TABLE 4–3.   Differential diagnosis of parkinsonism.

Degenerative disorders	Infectious illnesses
Paralysis agitans	Postencephalitic Parkinson's disease
Progressive supranuclear palsy	(von Economo's encephalitis)
Striatonigral degeneration	Other viral encephalitides (rare)
Shy-Drager syndrome	Jakob-Creutzfeldt disease
Guamanian ALS-parkinsonism-	Syphilis
dementia complex	AIDS
Huntington's disease (rigid variant)	Bilateral abscesses
Wilson's disease	Vascular disorders
Idiopathic calcification of the basal	Lacunar state (arteriosclerotic
ganglia	parkinsonism)
Hallervorden-Spatz syndrome	Metabolic conditions
Olivopontocerebellar atrophy	Hypoparathyroidism
Neuroacanthocytosis	Hypothyroidism
Primary pallidal atrophy	Hepatocerebral degeneration
Corticodentatonigral degeneration	Miscellaneous conditions
Azorean disease	Normal-pressure hydrocephalus
Diffuse Lewy body disease	Basal ganglia neoplasms
Toxic agents	Dementia pugilistica
Neuroleptics	Post-traumatic encephalopathy
Metoclopramide	Syringomesencephalia
Diazepam	Coroid lipofuscinosis
Reserpine	Neuronal intranuclear inclusion body
Methyldopa	disorder
Lithium	Mitochondrial encephalopathy
Manganese	Type 3 GM1 gangliosidosis
Organophosphates	Subdural hematomas
Cyanide	Taurine deficiency
Carbon disulfide	Paraneoplastic syndrome
Mercury	Psychiatric syndromes
Carbon monoxide	Depression with psychomotor
Methanol	retardation
MPTP	Schizophrenia with catatonia
Calcium channel blockers	
Cytosine arabinoside	

bulbar palsies, hemiparesis, torticollis and other dystonic phenomena, tics, respiratory dysrhythmias, compulsive movements, seborrhea, kyphoscoliosis, and sleep disturbances. Oculogyric crises are virtually pathognomonic of postencephalitic parkinsonism unless the patient is receiving major tranquilizers (Duvoisin and Yahr, 1965; Jelliffe, 1929; Shrubsall, 1927).

Dementia and depression occur with about equal frequency in postencephalitic parkinsonism and paralysis agitans. Forty to 60 percent of patients will manifest intellectual impairment and depressed mood. There is a much higher prevalence of personality disorders, behavioral changes, and conduct disturbances in the postencephalitic population (Bebb, 1925; Brown and Wilson, 1972; Celesia and Wanamaker, 1972; Fairweather, 1947).

The pathology of postencephalitic Parkinson's disease differs from paralysis agitans in both nature and extent. Loss of neurons in the substantia nigra is more severe in postencephalitic cases, and the entire nigral cell population is involved. The locus ceruleus, nucleus basalis, and globus pallidus may also be involved. Inflammatory changes may be found many years after the acute illness and small multifocal glial scars occur in the involved areas. The remaining neurons in affected parts of the nervous system contain abundant neurofibrillary tangles. Few Lewy bodies are present (Alvord, 1971; McAlpine, 1923; Oppenheimer, 1976b).

Treatment of postencephalitic Parkinson's disease is approached with the same agents as those used in paralysis agitans. The improvement in motor disability may be spectacular but is less predictable, and the occurrence of neuropsychiatric complications during treatment is more frequent than it is in idiopathic parkinsonism (Sacks, 1976; Sacks et al, 1970a, b, 1972).

Parkinsonism is a rare consequence of other types of viral encephalitis but has been observed during and after encephalitis due to the arboviruses and to measles, varicella, poliomyelitis, Japanese B, and western equine virus (Duvoisin and Yahr, 1965). Jakob-Creutzfeldt disease, an unconventional viral infection of the CNS, frequently involves the basal ganglia and may present as a parkinsonian syndrome. Parkinsonism has also been observed as part of the encephalopathy of human immunodeficiency virus encephalopathy with or without superimposed opportunistic infection (Nath et al, 1987). These illnesses are discussed in more detail in Chapter 6.

Drug-Induced Parkinsonism

Neuroleptic agents (phenothiazines, thioxanthenes, and butyrophenones) used in the treatment of psychotic disturbances commonly cause a parkinsonian extrapyramidal syndrome. They block dopamine receptors and produce bradykinesia, rigidity, stooped posture, loss of associated movements, festinating gait, masked facies, and drooling. Tremor is usually less prominent than it is in paralysis agitans (Baldessarini, 1977a; Hall et al, 1956; Simpson et al, 1964). At least 10 to 15 percent of patients treated with antipsychotic agents develop parkinsonian complications, and the prevalence is higher in patients on higher-potency neuroleptics. Fifty to 75 percent of patients manifesting parkinsonism become symptomatic within one month of initiating therapy, and 90 percent are symptomatic by three months; thereafter the prevalence decreases. Drug-related parkinsonism is more likely to develop in patients over the age of 40 years (Marsden et al, 1975). The parkinsonian complications of neuroleptic therapy are usually treated with anticholinergic compounds such as benztropine mesylate or trihexyphenidyl or with amantadine. Levodopa is not usually used because of its tendency to exacerbate psychosis (Baldessarini, 1977a; Yaryura-Tobias et al, 1972). Benzamides such as metaclopramide used in the treatment of gastrointestinal disorders are also dopamine blocking agents and may produce parkinsonism (Koller, 1987).

Antihypertensive agents that work by depleting or blocking catecholamine activity can also cause a parkinsonian syndrome and depression. Reserpine and methyldopa are among the antihypertensive drugs known to produce these disturbances (Gordon, 1963; Nickerson, 1970; Strang, 1966). Similarly, calcium channel-blocking agents have been observed to induce a reversible parkinsonian state (Micheli et al, 1987).

Other drugs and toxins capable of producing a parkinsonian type extrapyramidal syndrome include lithium (Reches et al, 1981), organophosphates (Davis et al, 1978), manganese (Mena et al, 1967), high dose diazepam (Suranyi-Cadotte et al, 1985), cytosine arabinoside (Luque et al, 1987), methanol (Koller, 1987), and mercury, cyanide, and carbon disulfide (Schwab and England, 1968). Permanent parkinsonism nearly identical to classic Parkinson's disease has been induced by 1-methyl-4-phenyl-1, 2, 3, 6-tetrahydropyridine (MPTP), a biproduct generated in the synthesis of meperidine analogues. The disorder is nearly completely confined to a group of intravenous drug users in northern California (Ballard et al, 1985). MPTP parkinsonism is accompanied by a dementia syndrome with impaired memory, concentration, and constructional ability (Stern and Langston, 1985).

Other Disorders Associated with Parkinsonism

Many metabolic encephalopathies will also produce psychomotor retardation reminiscent of Parkinson's disease; this is particularly marked in hypothyroidism. Hypoparathyroidism can result in deposition of calcium in the basal ganglia and the production of an akinetic, rigid parkinsonian state (Eraut, 1974; Hossain, 1970).

Until recently, arteriosclerotic parkinsonism was a frequent diagnosis. Multiple small lacunar infarcts in the area of the basal ganglia, thalamus, and internal capsule can give rise to an akinetic rigid state with psychomotor retardation that superficially resembles Parkinson's disease. Bilateral pyramidal signs and limb weakness, hyperreflexia, extensor plantar responses, and pseudobulbar palsy are also present, however, and enable the clinician to identify this syndrome (Eadie and Sutherland, 1964). Tremor is unusual in arteriosclerotic states, and there is usually a history of hypertension and multiple lacunar infarctions. Subcortical dementia is a frequent component of this condition, occurring in 70 to 80 percent of all patients (Brown and Wilson, 1972; Celesia and Wanamaker, 1972). This syndrome is discussed in more detail in the presentation of vascular dementias in Chapter 5.

Other structural disorders involving the basal ganglia, including neoplasms of the subcortical structures (Roth and Bebin, 1958), normal-pressure hydrocephalus (Moore, 1969; Sypert et al, 1973), and carbon monoxide-induced changes may also present with parkinsonian syndromes. The changes caused by carbon monoxide are particularly prominent in the basal ganglia but also involve the hemispheric white matter and the cerebellum. The globus pallidus is most affected (Brierley, 1976; Grinker, 1926; Klawans et al, 1982; Nardizzi, 1979). Other rare conditions associated with parkinsonism include syringomesencephalia, ceroid lipofuscinosis, neuronal intranuclear inclusion body disease, mitochondrial encephalopathy, Type 3 (adult) GM1 gangliosidosis, bilateral subdural hematomas, and paraneoplastic degeneration of the substantia nigra (Koller, 1987).

Various other degenerative disorders are also capable of producing a parkinsonian syndrome. Striatonigral degeneration is a progressive idiopathic degenerative disease that produces clinical findings identical to those of Parkinson's disease. Dementia is a common component of the illness. Pathologically there is marked cell loss and gliosis in the putamen and the substantia nigra with less severe changes in caudate, globus pallidus, and subthalamic nucleus (Adams et al, 1964: Oppenheimer, 1976b).

Shy-Drager syndrome is an illness presenting with features of autonomic dysfunction including impotence, incontinence, and orthostatic hypotension. Anhidrosis, iris atrophy, and decreased tearing may also occur. Several years after the onset of the autonomic dysfunction, an akinetic rigid parkinsonian syndrome develops. In some patients there may be associated cerebellar, upper motor neuron, and/or lower motor neuron findings. Dementia rarely occurs. Pathologic examination reveals cell loss and gliosis in the pigmented brainstem nuclei, striatum, pontine structures, and the intermediolateral cell column of the spinal cord (Bannister and Oppenheimer, 1972; Khurana et al, 1980; Shy and Drager, 1960; Thomas and Schirger, 1970).

Progressive supranuclear palsy, Huntington's disease, Wilson's disease, Hallervorden-Spatz disease, Guamanian amyotrophic lateral sclerosis–Parkinson's disease–dementia complex, olivopontocerebellar atrophy, neuroacanthocytosis, primary pallidal atrophy, corticodentatonigral degeneration, Azorean disease, diffuse Lewy body disease, and idiopathic basal ganglia calcification can also produce akinetic rigid states. Depression causes prominent psychomotor retardation, flattened affect, and bowed posture that may closely mimic Parkinson's disease (Baldessarini, 1977a).

WILSON'S DISEASE

In 1912 Kinnier Wilson reported the clinical and autopsy findings in a small group of patients he had observed personally. The patients were between

18 and 25 years old, and all manifested rigidity, dystonia, dysarthria, and tremor. The three cases autopsied showed extensive alterations in the lenticular nuclei and cirrhosis of the liver (Schulman, 1968; Wilson, 1912). It was later determined that this was the same disorder that Westphal and Strumpell had called pseudosclerosis. Keyser and Fleischer described the corneal rings that bear their names in 1907 and 1903 respectively and in 1930 Haurowitz discovered the pathologic increase in copper content of the brain and liver of patients with Wilson's disease (Schulman, 1968). In retrospect, Wilson's report was of great theoretical importance because it was the first time that abnormal movements were linked to subcortical (basal ganglia) disturbances (Martin, 1968). Wilson's disease was also among the first CNS disorders to be shown to result from an inborn error of metabolism.

Two variants of the disease are described: a juvenile type with onset in youth and relatively rapid evolution and an adult variety beginning between 20 and 30 years of age and following a much slower course (Denny-Brown, 1964). Intermediate and atypical variants are not uncommon, and rare cases with onset in the fourth or fifth decade have been reported (Czlonkowska and Rodo, 1981). The disease is familial with an autosomal recessive pattern of inheritance (Martin, 1968).

Dementia

In his original report, Wilson (1912) commented on the unusual features of the dementia associated with progressive lenticular degeneration. He noted slowness of mental powers, listlessness, emotionalism, and childishness. He recognized that the mental status changes were readily distinguishable from the mental impairment of dementia paralytica and that they shared many features with Huntington's disease.

Failure to make progress in school is often an early sign of the juvenile variant whereas paranoid-hallucinatory psychoses may herald the onset in adults (Beard, 1959; Czlonkowska and Rodo, 1981; Martin 1968). Mood changes and personality alterations are the most common psychiatric manifestations of the illness (Dening, 1985; Dening and Berrios, 1989). As the disease advances, dementia with subcortical-type characteristics become evident. Mental inactivity and inertia, impaired memory, and poor concentration are prominent.

Neuropsychological assessment demonstrates preserved language function and impaired abstraction and concept formation (Knehr and Bearn, 1956). General intellectual levels are decreased from estimated premorbid levels and prominent deficits are noted on the Wechsler Memory Scale and Trail-Making Test (Medalia et al, 1988). The dementia is at least partially reversible if the disorder is identified and treatment is initiated early in its course (Goldstein et al, 1968; Martin 1968; Rossell, 1987).

Clinical Features

Wilson's disease may present as a neurologic syndrome, a psychiatric disturbance, or with hepatic disease, hematologic abnormalities or bone disease (Cartwright, 1978). Neurologic abnormalities include dystonia, rigidity, incoordination, tremor, dysarthria, drooling, dysphagia, and masklike facies (Starosta-Rubinstein et al, 1987). The juvenile variant usually has its onset between ages 7 and 15, and dystonia is often the principal motor disturbance. A set facial expression and dystonic flexion postures of the arms are typical. A rapid finger tremor may be present, but the flapping tremor characteristic of adult Wilson's disease develops late if at all. Choreoathetosis may appear as the disease progresses. The course of the juvenile type is somewhat irregular and fairly rapidly progressive (Denny-Brown, 1964).

The adult variety begins between ages 19 and 35 years with characteristic features of dysarthria and tremor. A flapping tremor of the wrists and so-called "wing-beating" tremor of the shoulders are characteristic. Dystonic posturing is less prominent but laxity of facial expression and decreased blinking are noted in some patients. Cerebellar findings are present in about half the patients and are the principal neurologic abnormality in 25 percent (Denny-Brown, 1964; Dobyns et al, 1979; Starosta-Rubinstein et al, 1987). There is considerable overlap of symptomatology of the two variants.

Liver disease will be detectable in most patients when neurologic abnormalities appear and will antedate the neurologic disturbances in 20 percent of the affected patients. Presentation with hepatic disease is particularly common in children (Cartwright, 1978; Dobyns et al. 1979). Fulminant acute hepatitis, chronic hepatitis, and postnecrotic cirrhosis have all been reported in Wilson's disease. The most common liver condition is chronic hepatitis with an insidiously progressive course leading to weakness, anorexia, jaundice, splenomegaly, and abnormal liver function tests. Nodular cirrhosis and increased copper content in the liver are found on biopsy (Cartwright, 1978; Menkes, 1974).

Kayser-Fleischer rings are the most distinctive clinical clue to the diagnosis of Wilson's disease. They are present in nearly all patients with neurologic abnormalities and are virtually pathognomonic. Rarely Wilson's disease patients without corneal rings have been reported (Bickel et al, 1957; Dobyns et al, 1979), and corneal limbus pigmentation closely resembling Kayser-Fleischer rings have been noted in rare cases of schistosomiasis and primary biliary cirrhosis (Goldstein, 1976; Mozai et al, 1962).

Thrombocytopenia and/or leukopenia are not uncommon in Wilson's disease, and a Coombs-negative hemolytic anemia is occasionally present (Hoaglund and Goldstein, 1978). Various types of bone abnormalities secondary to impaired renal function have been noted, including osteoporosis, osteochondritis, pseudofractures, osteoarthritis, and renal rickets (Cartwright, 1978).

Laboratory Evaluation

Wilson's disease is one of the few extrapyramidal disorders in which a specific laboratory evaluation is an essential step in establishing the diagnosis. A serum ceruloplasmin concentration of less than 20 mg per dl and urinary copper excretion in excess of 100 μg per 24 hours confirm the diagnosis (Cartwright, 1978; O'Reilly, 1967). Several patients with normal serum ceruloplasmin levels have been reported, and therefore this alone is not an absolutely reliable diagnostic test and should be augmented with urinary copper assays.

Routine blood cell counts may reveal thrombocytopenia, leukopenia, or hemolytic anemia as noted. Hypophosphatemia is not unusual and abnormal liver functions may be present, although they are frequently normal even when histologic studies demonstrate hepatic cirrhosis (Cartwright, 1978; Dobyns et al, 1979; Hoaglund and Goldstein, 1978). Examination of the urine reveals elevated copper content, aminoaciduria, peptiduria, glucosuria, uricosurea, and phosphaturia secondary to impaired proximal renal tubular reabsorption (Cartwright, 1978). Results of cerebrospinal fluid studies are unremarkable.

Electroencephalography in Wilson's disease reveals slowing of background frequency and occasional diphasic sharp waves in about half the patients. In general, the degree of EEG abnormality parallels the severity of clinical involvement (Heller and Kooi, 1962). Brainstem auditory evoked potentials are abnormal in symptomatic patients with Wilson's disease but remain normal in asymptomatic cases. Latencies and peak intervals from waves II to VI are increased (Fujita et al, 1981).

CT demonstrates areas of low density in the region of the lenticular nuclei in approximately 50 percent of patients with extrapyramidal symptoms (Williams and Walshe, 1981) (Fig. 4–6). The ventricular system may be dilated, but cerebral sulci are usually not excessively large. The brainstem may appear atrophic, and low-density areas in the region of the cerebellar dentate nuclei are seen in some patients. The abnormal areas are not changed by contrast enhancement (Harik and Post, 1981; Nelson et al, 1979; Selekler et al 1981). Patients without abnormalities have normal CT scans.

Magnetic resonance imaging is more sensitive to the pathological changes in the lenticular nuclei in Wilson's disease than is CT (Metzer and Angtuaco, 1986). Approximately 75 percent of patients have abnormal MRIs, and at least 50 percent have specific basal ganglia changes (Aisen et al, 1985). Correlations have been demonstrated between dysarthria and dystonia and the severity of lesions demonstrated by MRI (Starosta-Rubinstein et al, 1987). Presymptomatic patients exhibit no MRI abnormalities.

PET using fluorodeoxyglucose demonstrates diffusely diminished cerebral metabolism and more marked focal metabolic disturbances in the lenticular nuclei (Hawkins et al, 1987).

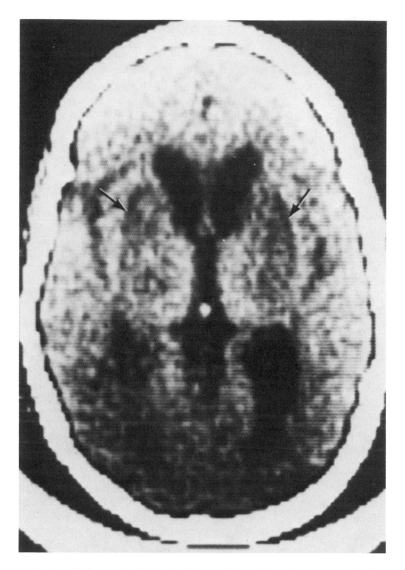

FIGURE 4–6.   CT scan in Wilson's disease shows hypodense areas in the regions of both putamina (arrows). (Reprinted by permission of the publisher from SI Harik and MJD Pool. Computed tomography in Wilson disease. Neurology (Ny) 1981;31:107–110.)

Presymptomatic homozygotes destined to develop Wilson's disease unless treatment is initiated are identifiable by liver biopsy. A concentration of hepatic copper greater than 250 μg per gm dry weight is indicative of the disease (Sternlieb and Scheinberg, 1968). Both presymptomatic homozygotes and heterozygotes not at risk for developing the disease may have low levels of serum ceruloplasmin (Menkes, 1974).

Pathology

Wilson's disease has characteristic histologic changes occurring in a specific topographic distribution. Grossly the brains show no conspicuous abnormalities. Coronal sections reveal that the lenticular nuclei are symmetrically atrophic and have a yellow or brown discoloration. The most severe changes involve the putamen and in advanced cases these nuclei are cavitated (Fig. 4–7). Softening of the white matter of the cerebral hemispheres and in the region of the dentate nucleus of the cerebellum may be evident (Martin, 1968; Schulman, 1968).

Histologically, abnormalities are most prominent in the putamen, but less severe changes are present in the globus pallidus, subthalamic nuclei, caudate, dentate nuclei, cerebral and cerebellar white matter, and frontal cortex. Neuron loss involving both the large and small neurons is evident, and reactive gliosis is present. Alzheimer-type II cells, large astrocytes measuring up to 15 μ in diameter and surrounded by fine yellow-brown granules, and distinctive Opalski cells (large oval or rounded cells without processes and with a finely granular or slightly foamy cytoplasm) are present (Martin, 1968; Schulman, 1968; Smith, 1976a). Giant glial cells (Alzheimer-type I) are seen in a small number of cases in the affected regions. Myelin stains show small amounts of demyelination in the central white matter, and focal areas of neuron loss are occasionally found in the cerebral cortex, particularly in the frontal lobes (Martin, 1968; Schulman, 1968). Electron microscopy of involved tissue reveals exuberant spheroid formation, chromatolytic changes, myelin and axonal degeneration, and alterations of capillary basal lamina (Anzil et al, 1974). The last changes are nonspecific.

The liver has the characteristic changes of multinodular cirrhosis, and studies of the cornea demonstrate granular copper deposition in the Descemet's membrane (Schulman, 1968; Smith, 1976a; Uzman and Jakus, 1957).

Histochemical studies demonstrate increased copper content in the cerebral cortex, basal ganglia, liver, kidney, and cornea when compared to normal controls and to patients with other types of liver disease (Cumings, 1968, Tu et al, 1963).

Pathophysiology

The details of the mechanism of injury in Wilson's disease have not been fully elaborated, but an outline of the disease process can be presented. Copper is absorbed across the intestinal wall where it enters the plasma and

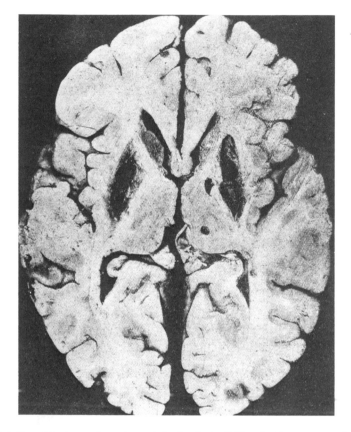

FIGURE 4–7.   Horizontal section of the brain in Wilson's disease reveals bilateral cavitation of the putamen. (Reprinted by permission of the publisher from SAK Wilson, Progressive lenticular degeneration: a familial nervous disease associated with cirrhosis of the liver. Brain 1912;34:295–509.)

is loosely bound to albumin. Under normal circumstances it is then incorporated into ceruloplasmin, a copper-carrying globulin protein, by the liver. In Wilson's disease, ceruloplasmin cannot be synthesized, and unbound copper remains in the serum and is deposited in a variety of tissues including brain, liver, kidney and cornea where levels reach toxic proportions (Hollister et al, 1960; Menkes, 1974; Walshe, 1967). Figure 4–8 summarizes the principal events in the pathophysiologic process.

Treatment

No method for reversing the deficit in ceruloplasmin synthesis has been found, but the destructive effects of tissue copper deposition can be pre-

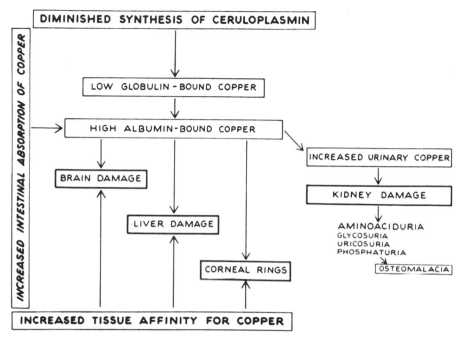

FIGURE 4–8.   Summary of the pathophysiology of Wilson's disease leading to deposition of copper in vulnerable tissues. (Reprinted by permission of the publisher from LE Hollister et al, Hepatolenticular degeneration. Clinical, biochemical and pathologic study of a patient with fulminant course aggravated by treatment with BAL and versenate. Am J Med 1960;28:623–630.)

vented by appropriate treatment. Patients are maintained on a low-copper diet and a cation exchange resin or potassium sulfide is taken with each meal to limit intestinal absorption. The current drug of choice for removing tissue copper and preventing its deposition is a chelating agent, D-penicillamine. This oral agent forms a soluble complex with tissue copper and/or serum copper leading to increased renal excretion (Deiss et al, 1971; Goldstein et al, 1962; Menkes, 1974; Scheinberg and Sternlieb, 1960). In most cases penicillamine will reverse many of the neurologic manifestations, lead to disappearance of the Kayser-Fleischer rings, and normalize renal function. Lifelong treatment is necessary once the disease is diagnosed. Advanced cases may fail to improve, and Denny-Brown (1964) suggested that the juvenile form responded less well to therapy than did the adult variant. Patients with signs of parkinsonism and unresponsive to penicillamine may benefit from levodopa therapy (Barbeau and Friesen, 1970). Penicillamine has proved to be superior to other chelating agents, but possible complications such as fever, rash, adenopathy, nephrotic syndrome, pyridoxine deficiency, thrombocytopenia, and leukopenia must be monitored (Menkes,

1974). In some cases, neurological signs may worsen at the time of initiation of penicillamine therapy (Glass et al, 1990). Asymptomatic patients may be kept symptom free if they are treated with the same regimen of dietary restriction, reduction of intestinal absorption, and penicillamine (Sternlieb and Scheinberg, 1968; Tu et al, 1965).

HALLERVORDEN-SPATZ SYNDROME

In 1922, Hallervorden and Spatz reported an unusual extrapyramidal syndrome that appeared in 5 of 12 siblings of an unfortunate family. The disorder began between ages 7 and 9 and included dementia, dysarthria, and a variety of pyramidal and extrapyramidal signs. Death occurred between 16 and 27 years of age after a steadily progressive course. On macroscopic inspection the globus pallidus and substantia nigra showed a rusty brown discoloration, and on histologic examination there was extensive pigment accumulation and axonal changes (Wigboldus and Bruyn, 1968). Unhappily there was insufficient appreciation of the fact that the histopathologic abnormalities found by Hallervorden and Spatz were relatively nonspecific, and the syndrome was progressively expanded to include cases that bore little or no clinical resemblance to the original patients. The nosology is now thoroughly confused, and the term "syndrome" reflects the possibility that the clinical entities presented here may not be etiologically homogeneous. Three clinical variants of Hallervorden-Spatz syndrome are described: a late-infantile type with onset in the second year of life, the classic juvenile type usually starting between ages 7 and 12, and a rare adult variant that becomes manifest in middle age or later. An infantile type of neuroaxonal dystrophy beginning between ages one and three or presenting with mental retardation from birth is included in some classifications (Indravasu and Dexter, 1968; Smith, 1976a). We present the clinical characteristics of the juvenile and adult forms of Hallervorden-Spatz syndrome—the two variants in which an acquired mental impairment is present.

Dementia and Clinical Characteristics

The dementia of Hallervorden-Spatz syndrome has received little systematic attention. Changes in mental status typically follow the appearance of abnormalities of the motor system but may occasionally be the initial complaints. Depression, rage, moodiness, and personality changes have been reported early in the course (Rozdilsky et al, 1968; Sacks et al, 1966) followed by progressive intellectual deterioration as the disease advances. Psychomotor retardation becomes apparent, and disturbances of memory, attention, concentration, abstraction, visuospatial skills, and calculation gradually develop (Dooling et al, 1974). Aphasia has not been described, but patients may have difficulty with naming tasks late in their course, and most become mute during the terminal stages (Dooling et al, 1974).

A heterogeneous group of motor system abnormalities may occur during the course of Hallervorden-Spatz syndrome. Abnormalities of posture or movement, often interfering with walking, are the presenting symptoms in a majority of patients. Equinovarus foot deformity may be an early finding. Rigidity is present in most cases, producing fixed facial expressions and increased limb tone. Early in the course some asymmetry of the rigidity may be present. Dystonic and/or choreoathetotic movements occur in half the patients, and slightly fewer have pyramidal tract signs including spasticity, hyperreflexia, and extensor plantar responses. Dysarthria is a nearly constant feature, and facial grimacing may occur. Myoclonus is not unusual and postural tremor occurs in one-third of the cases. Adult-onset cases often have a parkinsonian appearance (Alberca et al, 1987; Jankovic et al, 1985). Seizures are rare. Retinitis pigmentosa is seen in a minority of cases, and optic atrophy has been reported in a few. Sensation is intact (Dooling et al, 1974; Smith, 1976a; Wigboldus and Bruyn, 1968).

Laboratory Evaluation

Results of routine serum, blood, urine, and cerebrospinal fluid studies are unremarkable in Hallervorden-Spatz syndrome. Radioactive ferrokinetic studies have shown increased uptake in the basal ganglia in the few patients studied with this technique (Vakili et al, 1977).

The EEGs are frequently normal early in the course but show progressive slowing as the disease advances. Spike- and sharp-wave discharges are not unusual (Dooling et al, 1974). CT demonstrates loss of basal ganglia bulk, a finding that may cause confusion with Huntington's disease. Mineralization of the basal ganglia may occur (Tennison et al, 1988). More extensive cortical atrophy as well as atrophy of the brainstem and cerebellum may be evident (Dooling et al, 1980).

MRI has been abnormal in most cases of Hallervorden-Spatz syndrome. On T2-weighted images, the globus pallidus appears hypodense; in some patients the putamen and substantia nigra also exhibit diminished signal intensity (Littrup and Gebarski, 1985; Schaffert et al, 1989). Occasional patients have shown areas of hyperintensity within the hypodense lenticular nuclei giving rise to the "eye of the tiger" sign (Sethi et al, 1988).

Neuropathology

Widened sulci and narrowed gyri may be visible on gross inspection of the brain particularly in the frontal and temporal regions. Coronal sections reveal reddish brown discoloration of the globus pallidus and the ventral substantia nigra bilaterally (Dreese and Netsky, 1968; Smith 1976a).

Microscopic examination shows that the most severe histologic changes occur in the discolored areas. The involved regions sustain considerable neuron loss, and there is moderate fibrillary gliosis and demyelination. Iron-containing pigment granules are scattered throughout the affected tissues, and numerous axonal swellings (spheroids) are evident. The caudate, putamen, and thalamus show few changes. Axonal swellings are present in the cerebral cortex, but neuron loss and gliosis are minimal. Cortical neurons may show excessive lipochrome accumulation, and cerebellar Purkinje cells are depleted in some cases (Dooling et al, 1974; Dreese and Netsky, 1968; Sacks et al, 1966; Smith 1976a).

Biochemical studies confirm the presence of increased iron concentrations in the affected areas (Vakili et al, 1977). In addition, cystine is elevated and cysteine dioxygenase is reduced in the globus pallidus consistent with an enzymatic block in the metabolic pathway from cysteine to taurine. Gamma-aminobutyric acid content is also reduced in the globus pallidus and substantia nigra (Perry et al, 1985).

Differential Diagnosis

Classic Hallervorden-Spatz syndrome is an autosomal recessive condition in which the characteristic clinical features and criteria for diagnosis are (1) onset at a young age, (2) mixed extrapyramidal and pyramidal motor system disturbances, (3) dementia, and (4) relentlessly progressive course to death in early adulthood. Pathologically one finds (1) discoloration and partial destruction of the globus pallidus and pars reticulata of the substantia nigra, (2) numerous axonal spheroids concentrated in the affected regions, and (3) accumulation of iron-containing pigment in the involved areas (Dooling et al, 1974). The differential diagnosis includes dystonia musculorum deformans, Huntington's disease, juvenile paralysis agitans, postencephalitic parkinsonism, atypical familial tremor, and dyssynergia cerebellaris myoclonica. Neuropathologic changes similar to those of Hallervorden-Spatz syndrome are found in a large number of other conditions particularly vitamin E deficiency and infantile neuroaxonal dystrophy (Sacks et al, 1966; Wigboldus and Bruyn, 1968).

Treatment

There is currently no treatment that halts the progressive course of Hallervorden-Spatz disease. Iron-chelating agents have been used without success and a variety of antiparkinsonian agents has been administered with little clinical benefit. Temporary amelioration of motor symptoms has resulted from levodopa therapy (Dooling et al, 1974).

AMYOTROPHIC LATERAL SCLEROSIS (ALS)–
PARKINSONISM-DEMENTIA COMPLEX

Guam, one of the Mariana Islands in the western Pacific, is the site of several varieties of endemic neurologic illness. Among the native Chomorro population in particular, 10 percent of adult deaths resulted from ALS and 7 percent were the consequence of a parkinsonism-dementia complex. Epidemiologic evidence suggested that in the Chomorros the two conditions were variants of a single disease process (Hirano et al, 1961a; Lessell et al, 1962). Among the Chomorros, the disease is known as Lytico-Bodig (Lepore et al, 1988). Although the disease is rare in other populations, typical examples have been found in non-Chomorro residents of the Mariana Islands, among inhabitants of the Kii Peninsula of Japan, in Auyu and Takai people of western New Guinea, in Chomorros living in the United States, and sporadically in other patients (Elizan et al, 1966a; Gajdusek and Salazar, 1982; Hirano et al, 1967; Lessell et al, 1962; Malamud, 1968; Staal and Went, 1968). The frequency is now declining among the Guamanian Chomorros and is no longer highly prevalent (Garruto et al, 1985; Plato et al, 1986).

Between 1940 and 1970, the prevalence of the parkinsonism-dementia complex on Guam was 118 per 100,000. The average age of onset was 50 with a range of 32 to 77 years. The disease was insidiously progressive and led to death in 4 to 5 years. The ratio of male to female involvement was 2.5:1. Inheritance of the disease was suspected, but common environmental exposure of family members was a more likely explanation of the familial occurrence (Elizan et al, 1966b; Hirano et al, 1961a; Lessell et al, 1962; Plato et al, 1986).

Dementia and Clinical Characteristics

The dementia of the parkinsonism-dementia complex is prominent in nearly all cases. It occurs early in the clinical course, is profound, and may be the most prominent neurologic disability. Mental slowness, poor memory, apathy, irritability, and depression are early features. The patients become disoriented, have difficulty with calculation and abstraction, and lose their ability to reason logically. Terminally they are in a mute, immobile, vegetative state. Although comprehensive examinations have been few, no evidence of aphasia, apraxia, or agnosia has been recognized (Elizan et al, 1966b; Hirano et al, 1961a; Lessell et al 1962; Rodgers-Johnson et al, 1986).

Supranuclear ocular and lid disturbances occur in most patients (Lepore et al, 1988). Nearly all patients show a striking bradykinesia with masklike, expressionless face, diminished blinking, loss of associated movements, and paucity of motor activity. Rigidity occurs later in the clinical course and is usually a plastic-type increase in tone. A postural tremor that increases with directed activity or postural adjustments eventually occurs in two-thirds of the patients. Dementia is much less common when ALS dominates the clinical syndrome, occurring in approximately 10 percent of Guamanian ALS patients (Rodgers-Johnson et al, 1986). Upper motor neuron signs such as hyperreflexia and extensor plantar responses are not uncommon, and 40 percent of patients develop upper and lower motor neuron signs typical of ALS in addition to the parkinsonism dementia complex. The course of the disease is relentlessly progressive and death eventually results from hypostatic pneumonia (Elizan et al, 1966b; Hirano et al, 1961a; Lessell et al 1962; Rodgers-Johnson et al, 1986).

Laboratory Evaluation

Results of routine serum, urine, blood, and cerebrospinal fluid studies are unrevealing in the parkinsonism-dementia complex. Defective cellular and humoral immunity has been demonstrated by appropriate laboratory studies. Affected Guamanians have elevated levels of immunoglobulin A and diminished levels of immunoglobulin M. In addition, there is a diminished response to skin test antigens, lymphopenia, and decreased numbers of T cells (Hoffman et al 1978, 1981). Cerebrospinal fluid monoamine metabolities (homovanillic acid and 5-hydroxyindoleacetic acid) are diminished in patients with parkinsonism-dementia (Brody et al, 1970).

Electroencephalography often reveals a loss of alpha activity with dominant posterior rhythms in the theta range. Frontal and temporal slowing may also be evident (Elizan et al, 1966b; Hirano et al, 1961a; Lessell et al, 1962).

Neuropathology

Grossly the brains of patients with parkinsonism-dementia complex have moderate cortical atrophy with widened sulci and narrowed gyri affecting primarily the frontal and temporal lobes. Brain sections reveal depigmentation of the substantia nigra and locus ceruleus, or the normal black color of the nigra may be replaced by brown pigment. The globus pallidus is often conspicuously atrophic (Hirano et al, 1966; Hudson, 1981).

Histologic changes include severe neuron loss in the substantia nigra, locus ceruleus, substantia innominata, nucleus basalis, and globus pallidus. Neurofibrillary tangles are abundant in the pyramidal cells of the hippocampus, presubiculum, remaining cells of the substantia nigra, hypothalamus, anterior perforated substance, substantia innominata, and amygdaloid nucleus. Less severely involved areas include frontal and temporal cortex and ganglion cells surrounding the third and fourth ventricles and the aqueduct of Sylvius. Granulovacuolar inclusions occur occasionally in the same areas as do the neurofibrillary tangles and are common in the Sommer sector of the hippocampus. Gliosis and microglial reaction occur in affected areas. Inflammatory cells, Lewy bodies, and neuritic plaques are not found in affected brains (Hirano et al, 1961b, 1966; Nakano and Hirano, 1983). Examination of the spinal cords of patients with parkinsonism-dementia reveal that many have loss of anterior horn cells and mild to moderate neurofibrillary changes. Likewise study of Guamanian ALS cases also demonstrates changes involving the substantia nigra, hippocampus, amygdala, hypothalamus, and other regions similar to those occurring in parkinsonism-dementia (Chen, 1981; Hirano et al, 1966; Malamud et al, 1961). These overlapping pathologic changes add support to the hypothesis that the ALS and parkinsonism-dementia on Guam are two expressions of a similar underlying disorder.

Cholinergic system marker enzymes are profoundly depleted in the neocortex and hippocampus (Chen and Yase, 1985), the deficiency has been associated with atrophy of the nucleus basalis of Meynert (Nakano and Hirano, 1983).

The etiology of parkinsonism-dementia is not understood. Genetic, infectious, and environmental causes have been postulated but remain unproved (Chen, 1981; Hirano et al, 1966). Attempts to transmit the disease to primates have been unsuccessful (Gibbs and Gajdusek, 1971). Ingestion of the excitotoxic amino acid beta-N-methylamino-L-alanine present in the cycad nuts that comprised part of the native Chomorro diet may be responsible for the neuronal degeneration (Steele and Guzman, 1987; Weiss and Choi, 1988).

Differential Diagnosis

Dementia or parkinsonism may occur in classic ALS. Dementia has been observed in approximately 2 percent of sporadic ALS patients and 15 percent of patients with familial ALS (Hudson, 1981; Mackay, 1963; Vejjajiva et al, 1967). The dementia has frontal-subcortical characteristics including poor abstraction, decreased wordlist generation, and impaired constructions (Gallassi et al, 1989). Intellectual deterioration may precede evidence of motor neuron dysfunction by many months, and bulbar symptoms are the most common evidence of motor neuron disease in patients manifesting the dementia syndrome (Horoupian et al, 1984; Wikstrom et al, 1982). In some cases, mental status alterations are combined with both ALS and parkinsonism, imitating the Guamanian form of the disorder (Gilbert et al, 1988; Hirano et al, 1967; Schmitt et al, 1984). At autopsy, patients with ALS and dementia exhibit diffuse loss of neocortical and hippocampal neurons, spongiform changes in the frontal cortex, and neuronal loss in the substantia nigra as well as marked involvement of motor neurons (Gilbert et al, 1988; Horoupian et al, 1984; Schmitt et al, 1984; Wikstrom et al, 1982). Neurochemical studies reveal marked loss of nigrostriatal dopamine and normal levels of gamma-aminobutyric acid, cholinergic marker enzymes, and serotonin (Gilbert et al, 1988; Horoupian et al, 1984).

Two other conditions that may cause motor neuron disturbances, extrapyramidal signs, and dementia are chronic mercurialism (Kantarjian, 1961) and Jakob-Creutzfeldt disease (Myrianthopoulos and Smith, 1962). These diseases are discussed in Chapters 6 and 7.

Treatment

No cure has been found for parkinsonism-dementia, but the clinical course may be modified by the use of levodopa. At least half the patients show substantial improvement of tremor and rigidity following levodopa treatment (Schnur et al, 1971).

SPINOCEREBELLAR DEGENERATIONS

The spinocerebellar degenerations are a heterogenous group of neurologic disorders. Many nosologic schemes based on either clinical or pathologic features have been proposed, but none satisfactorily accounts for all the variations observed (Currier, 1984; Greenfield, 1954; Harding, 1984; Konigsmark and Weiner, 1970; Locke and Foley, 1960; Netsky, 1968; Oppenheimer, 1976b; Refsum and Skre, 1978). Several clinical variants may appear in a single family, patients with similar pathologic changes may have different clinical presentations, and patients resembling each other clinically may be found to have dissimilar underlying abnormalities of the CNS. Recently initiated investigations into the biochemistry of these disorders may eventually lead to a classification based on more etiologically relevant information but are not yet comprehensive (Blass et al, 1976; Kark and Rodriguez-Budelli, 1979; Perry et al, 1977; Richards et al, 1974). Despite the current problems in developing an acceptable classification for this evolving area, the disorders under consideration have several important features in common. Each is predominantly a syndrome of progressive ataxia, and abnormalities in cerebellar connections at spinal, cerebellar, or brainstem levels

TABLE 4–4.   Classification of the spinocerebellar degenerations.

Predominantly affecting the spinal cord	Predominantly affecting the cerebellum	Predominantly affecting brainstem and cerebellum
Friedreich's syndrome Friedreich's syndrome variants Hereditary spastic ataxia	Cerebellar cortical degeneration Cerebellar nuclear degeneration (dentatorubral atrophy)	Olivopontocerebellar atrophy

are present in all. A simplified classification that will facilitate discussion of the principal types of spinocerebellar degenerations is presented in Table 4–4.

Alan & Sides

Friedreich's Syndrome and Predominantly Spinal Degenerations

Dementia

Mental status changes in Friedreich's syndrome have received little systematic attention, and some standard neurologic references deny that mental status abnormalities occur, while others state that progressive mental deterioration is not uncommon. Greenfield (1954), in his classic monograph on the spinocerebellar degenerations, noted that mental regression occurred in many patients during the course of Friedreich's syndrome, and several reviews of the available information concluded that neuropsychiatric abnormalities, including mild dementia, were not uncommon among these patients (Lishman, 1978; Tyrer, 1975). Detailed epidemiologic information is not available, but Sjøgren (quoted by Davies, 1949a) found that 58 percent of his large series of patients with Friedreich's syndrome exhibited progressive dementia. Dementia appears to be more common in those families that manifest several variants of spinocerebellar degeneration, suggesting more variable and more widespread CNS involvement.

The characteristics of the dementia have not been well described, but most reports emphasize personality changes, slow cognition, and memory disturbances similar to the disruption of neuropsychological function described in other subcortical disorders (Pfeiffer, 1922, Schut, 1950; Tyrer, 1975). Neuropsychological assessment has demonstrated visuospatial abnormalities, slowed cognitive processing, and impairment in complex mental rotation tasks (Fehrenbach et al, 1984; Hart et al, 1985). Schizophrenia-like psychoses, depression, and conduct disorders have been reported as expressions of disturbed neuropsychiatric function in patients with Friedreich's syndrome (Davies 1949b; Davison and Bagely,1969; Shepherd, 1955).

Hereditary spastic ataxia, another degenerative disorder characterized primarily by spinal cord signs, has been associated with dementia in a small number of cases, and psychometric assessment also suggests compromised intellectual function (Bouchard et al, 1978; Landau and Gitt, 1951).

Clinical Characteristics

There are two clinical variants of Friedreich's syndrome. The more common is an autosomal recessive type with onset between 11 and 12 years of age, whereas the more rare autosomal dominant form begins at age 18 to 22 years (Menkes, 1974). The sexes are equally affected. The disease advances slowly, and most patients die within 20 years of the onset of symptoms.

The disease first becomes manifest as a gait disturbance with truncal ataxia, broad-based gait, clumsiness, and positive Romberg sign. Dysmetria of the upper extremities and dysarthria occur later. Skeletal deformities including pes cavus, hammer toes, and kyphoscoliosis occur in 60 to 80 percent of patients. Loss of vibration and position sense, absent muscle stretch reflexes in the lower extremities, nystagmus, and limb weakness and atrophy eventually develop in a majority of patients (Brain and Walton, 1969; Menkes, 1974). Optic atrophy, pigmentary retinal degeneration, and vestibular involvement are present in a few patients. Electrocardiographic evidence of myocardial degeneration is not uncommon, and some patients with Friedreich's syndrome die of intractable congestive heart failure associated with myocarditis (Boyer et al, 1962; Harding, 1981; Heck, 1963; Menkes, 1974).

Laboratory Evaluation

Except for an abnormally high incidence of diabetes mellitus among patients with Friedreich's syndrome, routine studies of blood, urine, serum, and CSF are usually unremarkable. EKGs may show T-wave abnormalities or conduction block (Boyer et al, 1962; Heck,1963). In some patients, nerve conduction studies reveal that digital nerve action potentials cannot be recorded from median and ulnar nerves after stimulation of afferent fibers. Muscle action potentials and motor fiber conduction velocities are normal or slightly reduced (Dyck and Ohta, 1975). Electroencephalography may reveal excessive slow-wave activity in the late stages of the disease.

Specialized biochemical investigations reveal low activities of pyruvate and oxoglutarate dehydrogenase in fibroblasts and/or white blood cells (Blass et al, 1976), and partial lipoamide dehydrogenase deficiencies have been found in some patients (Kark and Rodriguez-Budelli, 1979).

Neuropathology

Degeneration of the large myelinated sensory fibers, posterior roots and dorsal root ganglion cells is a constant feature. Examination of the spinal cord shows shrunken and degenerated posterior columns and severe involvement of the posterior spinocerebellar tracts. The anterior spinocerebellar tracts are less affected, and the corticospinal tracts show progressive involvement as they descend through the spinal cord. Cell loss and gliosis are common in the dentate nuclei and cerebellar white matter, vestibular and auditory nuclei, and the optic tracts. The globus pallidus and subthalamic nuclei are involved in approximately half the cases, but the cerebral cortex and thalamus are spared (Netsky, 1968; Oppenheimer, 1976b; Pfeiffer, 1922). Interstitial myocarditis is present in many cases.

Treatment

No specific treatment for Friedreich's syndrome is available. Two ataxic patients with pyruvate dehydrogenase deficiency improved on ketogenic diets (Falk et al, 1976) and oral physostigmine produced minimal improvement in another group of ataxic patients including several with Friedreich's syndrome (Rodriguez-Budelli et al, 1978), but definitive and specific clinical intervention is not available. Amantadine hydrochloride provides symptomatic relief in some patients, particularly those who are still in an ambulatory phase of the illness (Peterson et al, 1988). Supportive measures to maximize mobility are of the utmost importance.

Cerebellar and Olivopontocerebellar Degeneration

Dementia

Chronic progressive dementia with subcortical type characteristics is a frequent if not uniform part of the cerebellar and olivopontocerebellar atrophies (Akelaitis, 1937–1938; Carter and Sukavajuna, 1956; Critchley and Greenfield, 1948; Locke and Foley, 1960; Naito and Oyanagi, 1982; Neff, 1894–1895; Nino et al, 1980; Plaitakis et al, 1980; Richter, 1940; Thorpe, 1935; Weber and Greenfield, 1942). Skre (1974) compared autosomal dominant and autosomal recessive forms of olivopontocerebellar atrophy and found dementia in 36 percent with the dominantly inherited disease and in 81 percent with the recessive form. The patients were still living at the time of reporting, and further progression would undoubtedly increase the number with intellectual deterioration. Similarly, Berciano (1982) compared patients with sporadic olivopontocerebellar atrophy with those manifesting familial forms of the disease and found dementia in 57 percent of the latter and 35 percent of the former. Harding (1982) found that 5 of 11 families with late onset autosomal-dominant cerebellar ataxia included some members with dementia. Dementia appears to be more prominent in hereditary ataxias in which degeneration of the cerebellar system is combined with clinical evidence of involvement of other structures such as the basal ganglia or visual system (Chandler and Bebin, 1956; Halsey et al, 1967; Harding, 1982; Jampel et al, 1966; Lambie et al, 1947; Sears et al, 1975; Smith et al, 1958; Trauner, 1985; Wadia and Swami; 1971; Weiner et al, 1967; Woodworth et al, 1959). The intellectual deterioration is slowly progressive and has the features characteristic of subcortical dementia. Memory disturbances, slowing of cognition, frontal system disturbances, and apathy are prominent. Cognitive disturbances characteristic of cortical dysfunction (aphasia, agnosia) are not observed (Kish et al, 1988). In addition to dementia, neuropsychiatric disorders including depression, psychosis, and delinquency have been noted in association with the cerebellar atrophies (Parker and Kernohan, 1933; Patrick, 1902; Thorpe, 1935).

Clinical Characteristics

Cerebellar degenerations are typically sporadic disorders that present between ages 43 and 60 years with evidence of progressive cerebellar dysfunction. Familial cases are occasionally encountered, and onset of the illness in childhood has been reported. Ataxic gait, hypotonia, action tremor, limb unsteadiness, and dysarthria are the most prominent clinical features (Brown, 1971). Neuroophthalmic disturbances, vestibular dysfunction, deafness, optic atrophy, retinal degeneration, hyperreflexia, and extensor plantar responses may occur in combination with the cerebellar signs in some cases although the presence of extracerebellar signs is usually more indicative of olivopontocerebellar atrophy (Brown, 1971; Halsey et al, 1967; Jampel et al, 1966; Sears et al, 1975; Wadia and Swami, 1971; Weiner et al, 1967). Routine laboratory investigations are generally unhelpful. The EEG may show nonspecific slowing, and cerebellar atrophy may be visible on CT scans or pneumoencephalograms. Studies using PET scans have found correlations between reductions in cerebellar and brainstem glucose metabolic rates and severity of ataxia and dysarthria (Kluin et al, 1988; Rosenthal et al, 1988).

Olivopontocerebellar degeneration may be distinguished clinically from most cases of cerebellar atrophy by the presence of ophthalmoplegia and pyramidal tract signs. Gait ataxia, limb incoordination, and dysarthria are the core symptoms of the illness. Titubation of the head and trunk is often severe and the limbs tend to be hypotonic. Extrapyramidal disturbances including parkinsonian features and choreoathetosis may be observed, and spasticity, hyperreflexia, and extensor plantar responses occur in some cases (Adams and Victor, 1977; Brown, 1971; Brain and Walton, 1969). The condition usually begins between ages 30 and 50 years and may be sporadic or inherited in an autosomal recessive or autosomal dominant pattern. The disease is slowly progressive and may have a 25-year course. In the late stages of illness, slowing may be evident on the EEG and brainstem and cerebellar atrophy may be demonstrable by CT scanning, but these laboratory tests are not diagnostic. Glutamate dehydrogenase is reduced in some patients with sporadic olivopontocerebellar atrophy. These patients are also distinguished by a peripheral sensory neuropathy and auditory nerve dysfunction (Chokroverty et al, 1985).

Neuropathology

Cerebellar degenerations are characterized pathologically by nearly complete disappearance of Purkinje cells, proliferation of Bergmann glia, and fibrous gliosis of the molecular layer of the cerebellum. The granule cell layer is less involved. The inferior and accessory olivary nuclei are frequently atrophic (Netsky, 1968; Oppenheimer, 1976b).

Olivopontocerebellar atrophy produces grossly evident shrinkage of the ventral pons. The cerebellum shows loss of Purkinje cells, and the white matter of the pons and cerebellum is deficient. The inferior olives and posterior columns of the spinal cord are abnormal, and the putamen and substantia nigra frequently show cell loss and gliosis. The anterior horn and dorsal root ganglia cells are atrophic and myelinated fibers of peripheral nerves may be reduced (Chokroverty ct al, 1984).

The cholinergic marker enzyme, choline acetyltransferase, is reduced in the cerebral cortex, thalamus, head of caudate, globus pallidus, red nucleus, and medial olfactory area. Levels in the amygdala and hippocampus are mildly reduced (Kish et al, 1989).

Treatment

No specific treatment is available and intervention is directed at limiting the secondary complications of the disorders.

Differential Diagnosis

Table 4–5 lists the disorders that may present with a progressive ataxia and dementia that must be distinguished from the spinocerebellar degenerations. Most of these conditions are discussed in other chapters and are not elaborated on here, but a few particularly important diseases are presented.

Ataxia telangiectasia. Ataxia telangiectasia is an autosomal recessive disorder with a characteristic triad of clinical findings including ataxia, conjunctival telangiectasia, and recurrent sinopulmonary infections. The ataxia appears in infancy or early childhood and is accompanied by choreoathetosis, nystagmus, oculomotor abnormalities, and impaired vibration and position sense (Baloh et al, 1978; Bodensteiner et al, 1980; McFarlin et al, 1972; Menkes, 1974; Stell et al, 1989). Mild progressive mental deterioration is a common feature of the syndrome. Telangiectasia appears on the bulbar conjunctivae, bridge of the nose, ears, neck, and antecubital pulmonary

TABLE 4–5.   Differential diagnosis of progressive ataxia with concomitant dementia

Degenerative disorders	Toxic conditions
Spinocerebellar degenerations	Mercury intoxication (other heavy
Ataxia telangiectasia	metals rarely)
Myoclonic epilepsy	Phenytoin intoxication
Azorean disease	Alcohol-induced cerebellar degenera-
Dentatorubral-pallidoluysian	tion with alcoholic dementia
atrophy	Infections of the CNS
Demyelinating disorders	Jakob-Creutzfeldt disease
Multiple sclerosis	Neoplastic and related syndromes
Metabolic conditions	Paraneoplastic cerebellar degeneration
Hereditary (inborn) errors of	Cerebellar tumors plus hydrocephalus
metabolism	
Metachromatic leukodystrophy	
Adrenoleukodystrophy	
Adult dystonic lipidosis	
Wilson's disease	
Idiopathic vitamin E	
deficiency	
Adult GM2 gangliosidosis	
Acquired metabolic disturbances	
Hypothyroidism	
Acquired vitamin E deficiency	

fossae between three and six years of age. Recurrent infections, particularly pulmonary infections, reflect the compromised immune status of the patients. Laboratory investigations reveal reduced levels of immunoglobulins A and E, increased serum levels of carcinoembryonic antigen and alpha-fetoprotein, and impaired delayed hypersensitivity (Bodensteiner et al, 1980; Gutmann and Lemli, 1963; McFarlin et al, 1972). The patients also exhibit a tendency to neoplastic transformation of lymphoid tissue (Hecht et al, 1973; Saxon et al, 1979). At autopsy there is extensive loss of neurons in the cerebellum including both Purkinje cells and the internal granular cells. Demyelination of the posterior columns and dorsal spinocerebellar tracts of the spinal cord is also evident (Menkes, 1974; Solitare and Lopez, 1967).

Azorean disease.   This disorder has been referred to by a variety of names including Azorean disease, nigro-spino-dentatal degeneration with nuclear ophthalmoplegia, Machado disease, Joseph's disease, autosomal dominant striatonigral degeneration, autosomal dominant system degeneration, and Machado-Joseph's disease (Coutinho and Andrade, 1978; Lima and Coutinho, 1980; Nakano et al, 1972; Romanul et al, 1977a; Rosenberg et al, 1976; Woods and Schaumburg, 1972). The condition is inherited in an autosomal dominant pattern and occurs primarily in Portuguese families originating from the Azores. An identical disorder has been reported in Japan and India and a worldwide distribution seems likely (Bharucha et al, 1986; Kitamura et al, 1989; Yuasa et al, 1986). Rare sporadic cases phenotypically identical to the autosomal dominant form have also been described (McQuinn and Kemper, 1987). The age of onset varies from 20 to 55 years, and the disease lasts for 15 to 25 years. The clinical manifestations are heterogeneous and include cerebellar ataxia and pyramidal signs, a dystonic-rigid extrapyramidal syndrome, or peripheral amyotrophy (Lima and Coutinho, 1980). Ataxia, nystagmus, and dysarthria are the usual cerebellar signs. Progressive external ophthalmoplegia and fasciculations are common findings. Three clinical phenotypes have been identified within the disease complex. Type I combines extrapyramidal and pyramidal signs including dystonia, athetosis, rigidity, and spasticity; type II has cerebellar and pyramidal signs; and type III manifests cerebellar deficits and peripheral amyotrophy (Rosenberg and Fowler, 1981). Intellectual function is usually spared and dementia is evident only late in the disease if at all. Pathologically there is neuron loss and gliosis in the substantia nigra, striatum, subthalamic nucleus, brainstem motor nuclei, pontine and dentate nuclei, columns of Clarke, and the anterior horns of the spinal cord (Fowler, 1984; Romanul et al, 1977a; Rosenberg et al, 1976; Sachdev et al, 1982; Woods and Schaumburg, 1972).

Dentatorubral-pallidoluysian atrophy.   This disease is an autosomal dominant multisystem degenerative disorder clinically resembling Azorean disease. The manifestations include a wide range of neurological symptoms—ataxia, myoclonus, epilepsy, ocular motor disturbances, chorea, dementia (Goto et al, 1982; Iizuka et al, 1984; Takahashi et al, 1988). At autopsy, neuronal loss is evident in the subthalamic nuclei, pallidum, dentate nuclei of the cerebellum, and red nuclei (Goto et al, 1982; Takahashi et al, 1988).

Paraneoplastic cerebellar degeneration.   Subacute cerebellar degeneration can be the initial manifestation of a neoplasm remote from the nervous system. The neoplasm is usually a lung carcinoma, most often of the oat cell type, but cerebellar degeneration has also been reported with neoplasms of the ovary, breast, and fallopian tube, and with the reticuloses (Brain et al, 1951; Brain and Wilkinson, 1965; Currie et al, 1970; Greenfield, 1934). In some cases, the carcinoma may not be identified until after the patient's death. The major features are cerebellar ataxia involving gait and limbs, dysarthria, and nystagmus. Dementia is common and is usually manifested by diminished attention, poor memory, impaired concentration, and personality alterations. Muscle weakness, peripheral neuropathy, hyporeflexia, and extensor plantar responses occur in some patients. The CSF is normal or shows mild lymphocytic pleocytosis and elevation of protein content. A majority of patients have antineural antibodies directed against Purkinje cells detectable in the serum (Cunningham et al, 1986; Tsukamoto et al, 1984). The major pathologic change is loss of Purkinje cells from the cerebellum and perivascular lymphocytic infiltration involving the posterior roots and dorsal columns, the brainstem, and the medial temporal lobes (Brain et al, 1951; Brain and Wilkinson, 1965). No treatment is available, but cerebellar symptoms may remit following removal of the neoplasm (Paone and Jeyasingham, 1980).

IDIOPATHIC CALCIFICATION OF THE BASAL GANGLIA (ICBG)

ICBG is a progressive extrapyramidal syndrome manifesting dementia, parkinsonism or choreoathetosis, and extensive calcification of the basal ganglia. It is a familial disorder with autosomal dominant and autosomal recessive modes of inheritance (Moskowitz et al, 1971). A childhood form of the disease with onset in infancy and death within the first few years of life is recognized in addition to the adult onset variety (Babbitt et al, 1969; Melchior et al, 1960). Among adults with ICBG, two clinical patterns have been identified: an early-onset type with onset between 20 and 40 years of age and manifesting a schizophrenia-like psychosis as the initial presentation and a later-onset variety presenting between the ages of 40 and 60 with dementia and a movement disorder (Cummings et al, 1983a; Francis, 1979). Mood disorders of either depressed or manic type are also common in ICBG (Trautner et al, 1988). Dementia and a motor disturbance eventually appear in those with psychosis (Francis, 1979; Kalambonkis and Molling, 1962; Kasanin and Crank, 1935; Neumann, 1963). The dementia of ICBG has the characteristics typical of subcortical dysfunction, including poor attention and concentration, impaired calculation and abstraction, and poor recent memory. Aphasia does not occur, but palilalia and dysarthria may be prominent (Boller et al, 1973). The usual motor system disturbance is an akinetic-rigid parkinsonian syndrome and/or choreoathetosis, and a few patients have pyramidal signs or ataxia (Friede et al, 1961).

Routine laboratory studies in ICBG are normal including serum calcium and phosphate levels. The EEGs may be normal or may have diffuse slowing in the theta range. Calcification of the basal ganglia and of the dentate nuclei of the cerebellum is evident on skull X-rays and on X-ray CTs (Fig. 4–9). Pathologic examination reveals extensive calcium deposits in the globus pallidus, putamen, thalamus, corona radiata, dentate nuclei, and cerebellar white matter (Adachi et al, 1968; Bruyn et al, 1964; Friede et al, 1961; Kalambonkis and Molling, 1962; Kasanin and Crank, 1935; Neumann, 1963; Pilleri, 1966; Strassman, 1949). The calcium, along with considerable quantities of other minerals, is deposited in an organic matrix containing large quantities of protein (Bruyn et al, 1964; Friede et al, 1961; Smyers-Verbeke et al, 1975).

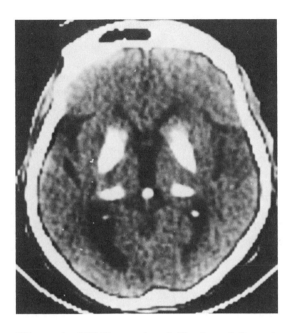

FIGURE 4–9.   CT scan in ICBG reveals calcification of the putamen and lateral nuclei of the thalamus (Reprinted by permission of the publisher from JL Cummings et al., Neuropsychiatric manifestation of idiopathic calcification of the basal ganglia: case report and review. Biol Psychiatry: 1983;18:591–601.)

The differential diagnosis of ICBG includes a number of disorders that can present with impaired intellect and basal ganglia calcification (Table 4–6). The most common cause of basal ganglia calcification and dementia is hypoparathyroidism (Eraut, 1974; Robinson et al, 1954; Slyter, 1979). Calcium deposition in the basal ganglia also occurs in pseudohypoparathyroidism and hyperparathyroidism (Bronsky et al, 1958; Knuth and Kisner, 1956; Margolin et al, 1980). Serum calcium levels are abnormal in hyperparathyroidism, hypoparathyroidism, and pseudohypoparathyroidism. The CT findings in ICBG are indistinguishable from the intracranial calcification noted by CT in cases of hypoparathyroidism and pseudohypoparathyroidism (Berger and Ross, 1981; Cohen et al, 1980; Cummings et al, 1983a; Klawans et al, 1976). Other hereditary disorders that appear in adult life with basal ganglia calcification and as neurologic disturbances include a syndrome with ataxia and pigmentary macular degeneration (Strobos et al, 1957), membranous lipodystrophy (Bird et al, 1983; Hakola, 1972), mitochondrial encephalomyopathy (Talley and Faber, 1989), non-Wilsonian familial apoceruloplasmin deficiency (Miyajima et al, 1987), Hallervorden-Spatz syndrome (Tennison et al, 1988), familial dystonia (Larsen et al, 1985), biotinidase deficiency (Schulz et al, 1988), Down's syndrome, HIV encephalopathy,

TABLE 4–6.   Conditions producing mineralization of the basal ganglia.

Abnormal calcium metabolism	Inflammatory and infectious conditions
Hypoparathyroidism	Cytomegalic inclusion disease
Pseudohypoparathyroidism	Encephalitis
Pseudopseudohypoparathyroidism	Toxoplasmosis
Hyperparathyroidism	Cysticercosis
Adult-onset hereditary disorders	HIV encephalopathy
Idiopathic calcification of the basal ganglia	Toxic and anoxic disorders
	Carbon monoxide exposure
Pigmentary macular degeneration and ataxia	Lead intoxication
	Birth anoxia
Membranous lipodystrophy	Radiation therapy
Mitochondrial encephalomyopathy	Methotrexate therapy
Familial apoceruloplasmin deficiency	
Hallervorden-Spatz syndrome	
Familial dystonia	
Biotinidase deficiency	
Osteopetrosis	
Congenital hereditary disorders	
Cockayne syndrome	
Tuberous sclerosis	
Progeria-like syndrome	
Kearns-Sayre syndrome	
With hydrotic ectodermal dysplasia	
Down's syndrome	

Adapted from Cohen et al., 1980 and Cummings et al., 1983.

and osteopetrosis (Ellie et al, 1989). A variety of congenital syndromes and acquired disorders can also result in extensive basal ganglia calcification (Table 4-6), but these disorders have identifying somatic features or historical antecedents (Bennett et al, 1959; Cohen et al, 1980; Cummings et al, 1983).

5

Vascular Dementias

The concept of vascular dementia has changed dramatically as more information has become available about the many types of dementing illnesses (Hachinski et al, 1974). At one time, most dementias were ascribed to "hardening" of the cerebral vessels causing poor perfusion of the cortex. It was suspected that the neurofibrillary tangles and senile plaques frequently found in the brains of older patients resulted from cerebral ischemia and tissue hypoxia. When no correlation was found between the extent of vascular involvement and the abundance of plaques and tangles, the idea of vascular dementia fell into disrepute and was seldom invoked as a cause of dementia. More recently it has been shown that multiple cerebral infarctions can result in dementia and that, with careful attention to historical details, general physical and neurologic examination, mental status testing, and appropriate neuroimaging, the vascular dementias can be recognized clinically and are not uncommon.

Terminology regarding vascular dementia is variable and confusing. "Multi-infarct dementia" was the term originally used by Hachinski and colleagues (1974) to describe the dementia associated with multiple cerebrovascular occlusions. They made the important point that it was tissue destruction and not cerebral hypoperfusion that accounted for most of the mental status changes in patients with vascular dementia. Multi-infarct dementia is often used interchangably with "vascular dementia." Vascular dementia, however, is a more inclusive term and encompasses dementia syndromes associated with small strategically located single strokes (as is discussed below), dementias following hemorrhagic events, and dementias associated with ischemic tissue changes that do not meet the usual pathologic criteria for infarction. In this chapter we will use the term "vascular dementia" and will specify individual subtypes of the disorder as outlined below.

Vascular dementia is most often associated with ischemic cerebral injury resulting from occlusion of cerebral blood vessels in thrombotic or embolic disorders but may also be seen with hypotensive ischemic injury or hemorrhagic disorders (Sulkava and Erkinjuntti, 1987). In the course of evaluating patients with suspected vascular dementia, it must be remembered that they frequently have cardiovascular conditions that may secondarily compromise cognitive function (for example, cardiac failure and renal failure) and are often under treatment with medications that have adverse effects on intellectual function. Depression is a common complication of cerebrovascular disease and may contribute to the dementia syndrome. Table 5–1 summarizes the conditions to be considered in the patient with evidence of vascular disease and a dementia syndrome.

CHARACTERISTICS OF VASCULAR DEMENTIA

The intellectual impairments of vascular dementia result primarily from occlusions of multiple vessels with infarctions in the corresponding areas of cerebral tissue. The clinical characteristics of the ensuing dementia depend on the specific distribution of the involved vessels. There is only a rough, imprecise correlation between the total amount of infarcted tissue and the severity of the dementia syndrome (Tomlinson et al, 1970). Identification of vascular dementia depends on recognizing characteristic historical, clinical, and neuroimaging findings.

Although vascular dementia is a heterogenous syndrome, a few generalizations applicable to most patients with the condition are possible. Epidemiologic factors that distinguish vascular dementia from DAT include an earlier age of onset of vascular dementia and its tendency to affect men more than it does women (Morimatsu et al, 1975; Tomlinson et al, 1970). Most studies suggest that the duration of survival after onset of mental status changes is approximately 20 percent less in vascular dementia than it is in DAT (Barclay et al, 1985b).

Historical features that aid in the identification of vascular dementia include an abrupt onset, stepwise deterioration, fluctuating course, nocturnal exacerbation of confusion, previous hypertension, and a history of neurological symptoms of transient ischemic attacks (Erkinjuntti et al, 1988; Hachinski et al, 1975). In some cases, however, the disease may progress gradually, imitating the course of a degenerative condition, and the absence

TABLE 5–1.   Differential diagnosis of etiologic and contributing factors in vascular dementia.

Etiologic conditions
   Thrombo-embolic disorders
      Multiple infarction dementia
      Single stroke dementia syndromes
   Anoxic-ischemic disorders
      Cardiopulmonary arrest
      Recurrent hypotension with syncope
      Cardiac arrhythmia
      Marked anemia
      Sleep apnea syndromes
      Arteriovenous malformations with local "steal" ischemia
   Mechanical-vascular conditions
      "Pipestem" basilar artery with obstructive hydrocephalus
      Giant cerebral aneurysm with brain tissue compression
   Hemorrhagic disorders
      Aneurysmal rupture with local brain injury
      Posthemorrhagic normal pressure hydrocephalus
      CNS hemosiderosis with recurrent intracranial bleeding
Conditions exacerbating vascular dementia
   Comorbid conditions
      Cardiac failure
      Renal failure
   Toxic disorders
      Antihypertensive agents
      Cardiac agents
   Depression

of typical historical features does not exclude the diagnosis of vascular dementia (Hershey et al, 1986; Weisberg, 1982). Risk factors of vascular dementia include hypertension, heart disease, cigarette smoking, diabetes mellitus, alcohol consumption, and hyperlipidemia (Meyer et al, 1988a).

On examination, the patient with vascular dementia usually has evidence of multifocal CNS disease (Bucht et al, 1984; Ladurner et al, 1982). Bilateral, asymmetric pyramidal and extrapyramidal signs comprise the classical clinical syndrome. Most patients exhibit some degree of limb rigidity, spasticity, hyperreflexia, extensor plantar responses, gait abnormality, and incontinence (Thompson and Marsden, 1987). Pseudobulbar palsy with pathological laughter or weeping may be present, and at least mild dysarthria is common (Powell et al, 1988). The blood pressure may be elevated, and up to 85 percent of vascular dementia patients have abnormal EKGs revealing arrhythmias, coronary ischemia, or cardiac hypertrophy (Bucht et al, 1984; St. Clair and Whalley, 1983; Tresch et al, 1985).

The neuropsychological syndrome of vascular dementia is characterized by a "patchy" distribution of intellectual deficits that may differ among patients (American Psychiatric Association, 1987). Deficits in orientation, recent memory, abstraction skills, and calculation are common (Erkinjuntti et al, 1986). Language may be impaired with abnormalities in writing, following complex commands, and grammatical complexity (Powell et al, 1988). Patients tend to use short, simplified sentences with limited lexical diversity (Hier et al, 1985). Depression and psychosis are common neuropsychiatric manifestations, and personality changes are ubiquitous (Cummings et al, 1987; Dian et al, 1990; Raskin and Ehrenberg, 1958; Rothschild, 1941). Most of the commonly used neuropsychological batteries are insensitive to the differences in performance deficits between vascular dementia and DAT patients, and they often fail to distinguish between the two dementias (Erkinjuntti et al, 1986; Tierney et al, 1987).

In 1975 Hachinski and colleagues introduced an ischemia scale with elements typical of the history and examination of patients with multifocal vascular disease (Table 5–2). Its components were chosen on the basis of clinical experience and not subjected to extensive psychometric verification (Liston and La Rue, 1983 a, b), but the overall accuracy and utility of the scale has been supported by both post mortem and imaging studies (Table 5–2) (Loeb and Gandolfo, 1983; Rosen et al, 1980).

TYPES OF VASCULAR DEMENTIA

Vascular dementias can be subclassified according to the predominant location of the cerebral infarctions or the etiology of the underlying vascular disease. The localization approach is summarized in Table 5–3 and will be discussed first: the etiologic classification is presented in Table 5–5 and is considered later in this chapter.

The principal vascular dementia syndromes are: (1) subcortical disorders such as lacunar state and Binswanger's disease resulting from occlusion of arteriole-sized vessels irrigating the deep gray and white matter structures, and (2) cortical disorders involving extracranial (carotid) or intracranial vessels or the small vessels supplying the cortical mantle. Lacunar infarctions are present in approximately 70 percent of patients with vascular dementia; white matter ischemia, in 60 to 100 percent; and cortical infarctions, in 20 percent (Erkinjuntti, 1987; Meyer et al, 1988a). Mixtures of cortical and subcortical infarctions are present in approximately 30 percent of patients. Atrial fibrillation is significantly more common in patients with cortical infarctions whereas other risk factors are approximately equally frequent in the two syndromes (Erkinjuntti, 1987).

TABLE 5–2. Ischemia Scale introduced by Hachinski and colleagues (1975) and modifications suggested by Rosen and colleagues (1980) on the basis of a postmortem investigation and Loeb and Gandolfo (1983) on the basis of radiologic studies.

Ischemia Scale*	Rosen et al (1980)	Loeb and Gandolfo (1983)
Abrupt onset (2)	+	+
Stepwise deterioration (1)	+	
Fluctuating course (2)		
Nocturnal confusion (1)		
Relative preservation of personality (1)		
Depression (1)		
Somatic complaints (1)	+	
Emotional incontinence (1)	+	
History of hypertension (1)	+	
History of strokes (2)	+	+
Associated atherosclerosis (1)		
Focal neurological symptoms (2)	+	+
Focal neurological signs (2)	+	+
		Single stroke on CT (2)
		Multiple strokes on CT (3)
Diagnosis suggested by total score:		
Degenerative dementia <5	<3	<3
Vascular dementia >6	>3	>4

Note: Original scale elements introduced by Hachinski and colleagues (1975) with relative weight assigned to each element in parentheses.
Sources: VC Hachinski et al, Cerebral blood flow in dementia, Arch Neurol 1975; 32:632–637; C Loeb, C Gandolfo, "Diagnostic evaluation of degenerative and vascular dementia," Stroke 1983; 14:399–401; and WG Rosen et al, Pathological verification of ischemic score in differentiation of dementias, Ann Neurol 1980;7:486—488.

Lacunar State

Lacunes are small, deep ischemic infarcts 0.5 to 15 mm in diameter and located predominantly in the basal ganglia, thalamus, and internal capsule (DeReuck and Vander Eecken, 1976; Fisher, 1965a, 1969; Hughes et al, 1954). The usual vessels involved are the lenticulostriate branches of the middle cerebral artery or the thalamogeniculate, choroidal, and thalamo-perforator branches of the posterior communicating and posterior cerebral arteries (Fig. 5–1), vessels measuring 50 to 150 mm in diameter (Adams and Victor, 1977; Davison and Brill, 1939; Gillilan, 1968). The infarcts are most commonly ischemic, although local hemosiderin deposits suggest that some have an initial hemorrhagic component. The occluded vessels usually

TABLE 5-3. Classification of multi-infarct dementias according to the predominant location of the infarctions, size of vessels involved, and characteristics of the dementia.

Pattern of infarctions	Size of occluded vessel	Structures involved by the infarctions	Principal features of the associated dementia
Deep hemispheric infarctions			
Lacunar state	Arterioles	Basal ganglia, thalamus, internal capsule	Subcortical dementia
Binswanger's disease	Arterioles	Subcortical white matter	Subcortical dementia
Superficial cortical infarctions			
Intracranial occlusions	Medium-sized arteries	Distribution of anterior, middle, and/or posterior cerebral arteries or their branches	Cortical dementia
Extracranial occlusions	Large (carotid) arteries	Border-zone territory between anterior, middle, and posterior cerebral artery distributions	Cortical dementia
Microangiopathy	Small arterioles	Superficial cerebral cortex	Cortical dementia
Combined deep and superficial infarctions	All sizes	Cortical and subcortical structures	Mixed features

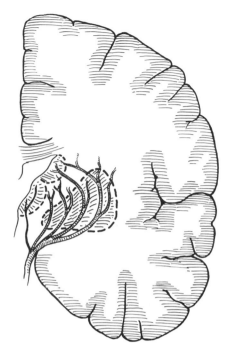

FIGURE 5–1.   Distribution of the lenticulostriate arteries as they penetrate upward from the base of the middle cerebral artery to supply the basal ganglia and the internal capsule.

have segmental arterial disorganization and replacement of the normal vascular architecture with fibrinoid deposits (Fisher, 1969). A single asymptomatic lacune may be an incidental autopsy finding in some patients, but when as many as 10 to 15 infarctions involve the deep structures of the hemispheres, the term "lacunar state" is applied. The vascular lesions are the product of sustained hypertension, and up to 40 percent of patients with chronic hypertension have lacunar infarctions at autopsy (Yates, 1976). Similar small, deep, lacunar infarcts can also result from atherosclerosic emboli or diabetes (Donnan et al, 1982; Pullicino et al, 1980) as well as from the fibrinoid necrosis associated with prolonged hypertension. Many patients have changes of the larger cerebral vessels and superficial cortical infarctions in addition to deep lacunar lesions (Tomlinson et al, 1970). Nearly all patients with lacunar states have mild to severe ischemic injury to hemispheric white matter (Roman, 1987). When both lacunes and white matter ischemia are prominent, the disorder might be considered lacunar/Binswanger complex or angiopathic dementia (Erkinjuntti et al, 1984).

   Clinically the patient with lacunar state has a history of chronic hypertension punctuated by discrete episodes of mild neurologic disability.

The initial events may conform to well-known lacunar syndromes such as pure motor hemiplegia, pure sensory stroke, dysarthria–clumsy hand syndrome, or homolateral ataxia and crural paresis (Fisher 1965b, 1967; Fisher and Cole, 1965; Fisher and Curry, 1965). Recovery from the initial episodes is the rule, but the neurologic deficits gradually accumulate to produce a state of dementia combined with multifocal motor, reflex, and sensory disturbances. Rigidity, spasticity, pseudobulbar palsy, limb weakness, exaggerated muscle stretch reflexes, and extensor plantar responses are common in the fully developed syndrome. The rigidity, extrapyramidal features, and bradykinesia of some patients with lacunar state creates a superficial resemblance to Parkinson's disease, and the term "arteriosclerotic parkinsonism" was used until recently to describe this condition (Parkes et al, 1974).

Dementia is a prominent feature of lacunar state, occurring in 70 to 80 percent of patients (Brown and Wilson, 1972; Celesia and Wanamaker, 1972). The characteristics of the dementia are variable and not well defined; most patients show personality changes including apathy and loss of tact; and many have memory disturbances. Preservation of insight is common in the early stages (Hughes et al, 1954). Mood changes and emotional lability frequently accompany the apathetic behavior and subcortical dementia (Ishii et al, 1986). Associated cortical disturbances such as aphasia may be present and fluctuations in the mental state are common.

Bilateral lacunar infarctions involving the paramedian thalamic nuclei produces a dementia syndrome characterized by apathy, memory deficits, impaired mental control, and psychomotor retardation (Guberman and Stuss, 1983; Katz et al, 1987). The median nuclei of both thalami may be supplied by branches from a single thalamoperforator vessel, allowing a single vascular occlusion to produce bilateral damage and a dementia syndrome.

Investigation of patients with lacunar state frequently reveals evidence of cardiac or renal disease in addition to the neurologic findings. Focal or generalized slowing may be demonstrated on the EEG (Parkes et al, 1974), and CT scanning frequently demonstrates one or more lucencies consistent with infarctions deep in the cerebral hemispheres (Fig 5–2) (Donnan et al, 1982; Nelson et al, 1980; Pullicino et al, 1980; Weisberg, 1982) although the lesions may be too small to be visualized by CT. MRI is more sensitive to ischemic brain injury than is X-ray CT scanning. Lacunes appear as areas of diminished signal intensity on T_1 images and increased intensity of T_2 images (Brown et al, 1988). Metabolic imaging using positron emission tomography and (F-18)-fluorodeoxyglucose reveals regions of local hypometabolism at the site of the cortical infarctions and may demonstrate diminished cortical metabolic activity in areas receiving projections from the affected subcortical structures (Metter et al, 1985).

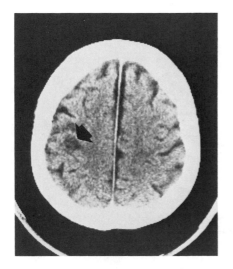 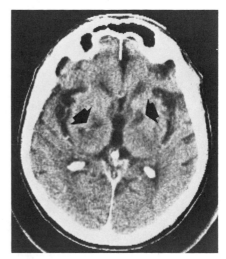

FIGURE 5–2.   CT scan shows multiple areas of cerebral infarction (arrows) in a patient with multi-infarct dementia.

Binswanger's Disease

In 1894, in a series of papers discussing the differential diagnosis of general paresis of the insane, Otto Binswanger briefly described eight patients with dementia who were found at autopsy to have pronounced atrophy of the white matter. All eight patients had severe atherosclerosis of the cerebral arteries, and Binswanger dubbed the syndrome "encephalitis subcorticalis chronica progressiva" (Olszewski, 1962). A more detailed description of the cases was promised but never appeared. Alzheimer, Nissl, and van Bogaert published similar cases and associated Binswanger's name with the condition. European and American investigators continued to report cases through the first half of the twentieth century, and most authors emphasized the role of vascular disease (Davison, 1942; Farnell and Globus, 1932). In 1947 Neumann challenged the concept of Binswanger's disease as a vascular dementia and suggested that the condition was a primary demyelinating process similar to Schilder's disease. Most clinicians abandoned the diagnosis, and the disease was rarely discussed. More recently, attention was refocused on subcortical arteriosclerotic encephalopathy by the results of brain imaging studies, and Binswanger's disease has been reborn (Roman, 1987).

Pathologically, the brains of patients with Binswanger's disease show multiple infarcts in the white matter of the cerebral hemispheres. In some cases the posterior temporal and occipital white matter is more involved than are the more anterior white matter areas, but in other cases essentially all white matter is markedly atrophic. Lacunar infarctions are usually present

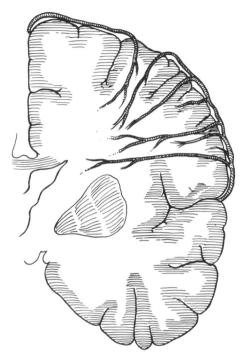

FIGURE 5–3.   The white matter of the cerebral hemispheres is supplied by long penetrators arising from stem vessels, whereas the cortex is supplied by superficial penetrators. The long penetrators are preferentially affected in Binswanger's disease, resulting in ischemic injury and white matter infarctions.

in the basal ganglia and thalamus, but the cortex and subcortical arcuate fibers are largely spared. Demyelination, loss of axons, gliosis, and infiltration by macrophages are noted in the involved regions (Burger et al, 1976; Caplan and Schoene, 1978; DeReuck et al, 1980; Jelgersma, 1964). The long, penetrating vessels of the white matter show advanced arteriosclerotic changes. These vessels do not supply the cortex but instead course through the cortical mantle and converge near the corner of the lateral ventricle (Fig. 5–3). The long, penetrating medullary branches are the same size as vessels supplying basal ganglia, thalamus, and pons and share the same propensity for developing hypertensive changes (DeReuck, 1972).

The clinical features of Binswanger's disease may include a history of persistent severe hypertension and systemic vascular disease, a history of acute strokes, a lengthy clinical course with long plateau periods and a gradual accumulation of focal neurologic symptoms and signs, dementia, and prominent motor disturbances including pseudobulbar palsy (Caplan and Schoene, 1978). Clinically, the disease usually resembles lacunar state, but patients with gradually progressive deficits resembling degenerative de-

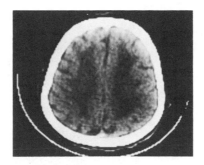

FIGURE 5–4. CT of a patient with autopsy-proven Binswanger's disease reveals increased lucency of the cerebral white matter.

mentias may also be encountered. The EEG usually demonstrates diffuse slowing with minor focal disturbances; periodic complexes have been reported occasionally (Biemond, 1970; White, 1979). The CT scan reveals enlarged ventricles and may show periventricular lucency consistent with ischemic injury of the hemispheric white matter (Fig. 5–4) (Rosenberg et al, 1979). Lacunar infarctions may also be seen in the basal ganglia and thalamus. MRI is very sensitive to white matter injury and usually reveals extensive abnormalities in Binswanger's disease. Smooth periventricular rims and limited capping of the anterior and posterior ventricular horns may be seen on T_2-weighted MRI images in elderly individuals without cognitive impairment (Kertesz et al, 1988); patients with Binswanger's disease typically evidence thickened irregular periventricular margins, prominent ventricular capping, and large or coalesced lesions in the hemispheric white matter (Fig. 5–5) (Brant-Zawadzki et al, 1985; Erkinjuntti et al, 1984).

Cortical Infarctions

The pattern of neurologic deficits resulting from embolic or thrombotic occlusion of large and/or medium-sized vessels will depend on the cortical territory irrigated by the involved vessel. When a number of focal infarctions have occurred, the resulting clinical picture commonly includes dementia. As a general rule when dementia is the product of cortical infarction, the infarcts are multiple and bilateral. In contrast, single, unilateral infarctions usually produce relatively well-defined focal syndromes.

Occlusions of the middle cerebral artery stem or branches are among the most commonly observed of the cortical insults (Fig. 5–6). If the left hemisphere is affected, the resulting deficit typically includes aphasia and apraxia (Benson, 1979a; Benson and Geschwind, 1975; Geschwind, 1975). Infarctions anterior to the rolandic fissure produce nonfluent aphasias, whereas

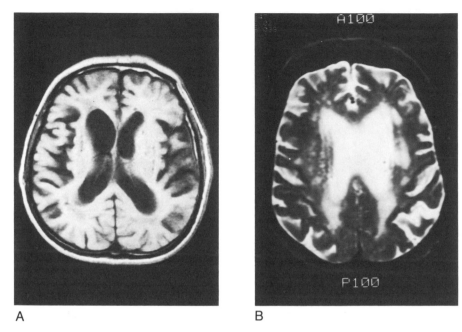

A   B

FIGURE 5–5.   MRI of a patient with lacunar state/Binswanger's disease reveals large, irregular, and asymmetric ventricular caps; uneven periventricular margins; and lesions in the hemispheric white matter: (A) T_1-weighted image, (B) T_2-weighted image.

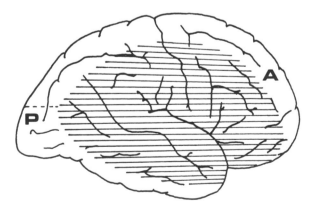

FIGURE 5–6.   Territory of the anterior cerebral artery (A), posterior cerebral artery (P), and middle cerebral artery (lines) on the lateral aspect of the cerebral hemisphere.

fluent aphasic output is associated with lesions posterior to the central fissure. Infarctions immediately adjacent to the sylvian fissure disrupt repetition, whereas the ability to repeat is preserved (transcortical pattern of aphasia) when the perisylvian area is spared. Global aphasia occurs when the entire dominant middle cerebral artery territory is infarcted. Right middle cerebral artery infarcts produce less well-defined cognitive deficits but may cause abnormalities in language melody, dressing disturbances, and problems with visuospatial orientation and visuo-motor performance (Hemphill and Klein, 1948; Ross, 1981). Unilateral neglect, denial of weakness, and constructional disturbances may occur after lesions of either hemisphere (Benson and Barton, 1970; Cutting, 1978a; Piercy and Smyth, 1962), and bilateral infarcts may produce Balint's syndrome with optic ataxia and "sticky" visual fixation (Hecaen and de Ajuriaguerra, 1954; Luria, 1959; Tyler, 1968b).

The angular gyrus syndrome, a symptom complex resulting from lesions in the posterior portion of the middle cerebral artery territory, deserves special emphasis because of the difficulties involved in distinguishing it from DAT (Table 5–4) (Benson et al, 1982). The complete angular gyrus syndrome includes fluent aphasia, alexia with agraphia, Gerstmann syndrome (acalculia, right-left disorientation, dysgraphia, and finger agnosia), plus constructional disturbances (Benson, 1979a). Focal motor and/or sensory signs may be absent, and the lesion may be too small for detection by CT scanning. Clinically the syndrome closely resembles DAT, but careful attention to historical details, mental status examination, and laboratory studies will usually lead to the correct diagnosis. As emphasized in Chapter 3, memory impairment and visuospatial disturbances are among the earliest signs of DAT. While patients with angular gyrus syndrome frequently complain of memory problems, they usually refer to word-finding difficulties (they cannot remember names). Intact memory and preserved visuospatial skills are evident in daily behavior. Differences in language function also exist. Patients with DAT are often unaware of their language problems and become difficult to engage in conversation (Albert, 1981), whereas those with angular gyrus syndrome tend to be frustrated and apologetic about their performance. Verbal paraphasias occur in both conditions but tend to be closer to the target word in patients with angular gyrus syndrome. Paradoxically, reading aloud may be better preserved in DAT, but reading comprehension is impaired in both conditions. Subtle right-sided neurologic findings, asymmetric EEG abnormalities, or minor asymmetries on the CT scan may provide supportive evidence for the presence of a focal left-sided lesion. Single photon emission tomography or positron emission CT scanning may demonstrate a striking focal abnormality (Figs. 5–7 and 5–8).

Posterior cerebral artery occlusion also produces neurologic deficits determined by the laterality and extent of the infarctions. A contralateral hemianopia is a common finding, and right-sided lesions may be associated with visual hallucinations, palinopsia, abnormalities in facial recognition,

TABLE 5–4.   Factors that distinguish DAT from the angular gyrus syndrome.

Characteristic	Angular gyrus syndrome	DAT
History	Abrupt onset	Insidious onset
	Hypertension or cardiac disease	Progressive course
Mental status		
Memory	Intact (except for verbal tests)	Impaired
Topographic orientation	Intact	Impaired
Language		
Aware of deficit	Yes	No
Engaged in conversation	Yes	No
Paraphasias	Within category	Little relation to target word
Reading aloud	Impaired	May be preserved until late in course
Neurologic examination	Right-sided abnormalities may be present	No focal findings
EEG	Normal or left-sided slowing	Normal or bilateral slowing
X-ray CT	Normal or left-sided abnormalities	Normal or evidence of diffuse atrophy
Positron CT	Left posterior hypometabolism	Bilateral frontal and parietal hypometabolism

and environmental disorientation (Cummings et al, 1983b; DeRenzi et al, 1969; DeRenzi and Spinnler, 1966; Landis et al, 1986; Lessell, 1975). Contralateral hemiparesis and hemisensory loss, mild anomia, and the syndrome of alexia without agraphia have been reported following left posterior cerebral artery occlusion (Benson and Tomlinson, 1971). Bilateral posterior cerebral artery territory infarctions may produce severe amnesia, cortical blindness, achromatopsia, visual object agnosia, or prosopagnosia depending on the extent and location of the lesions (Albert et al, 1979; Benson, 1978; Benson et al, 1974a, b; Damasio et al, 1980; Green and Lessell, 1977; Meadows, 1974).

The anterior cerebral arteries supply most of the medial portion of the frontal lobes, and the anterior four-fifths of the corpus callosum. Occlusion of the anterior cerebral artery produces contralateral leg weakness and may cause sensory loss in the same distribution. An interhemispheric disconnection syndrome may occur with destruction of callosal fibers (Geschwind and Kaplan, 1962). When the left anterior cerebral artery is occluded, transient

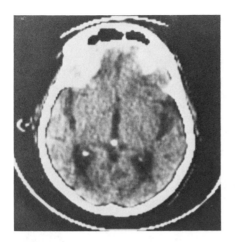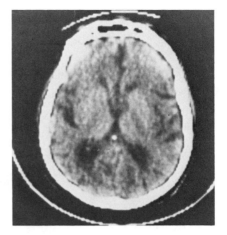

FIGURE 5–7.   CT scan from a patient with angular gyrus syndrome. The lesion is too small to be visualized by conventional X-ray tomography, but PET (Fig. 5–8) reveals a hypometabolic area in the posterior left hemisphere. (Reprinted by permission from DF Benson, JL Cummings, SY Tsai, Angular gyrus syndrome simulating Alzheimer disease. Arch Neurol; 1982;39:616–620. Copyright, 1982, American Medical Association.)

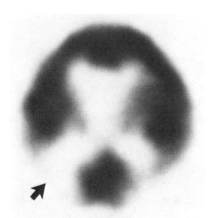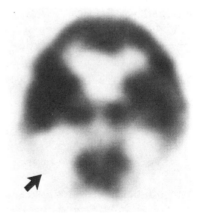

FIGURE 5–8.   Positron emission scan of a patient with angular gyrus syndrome (same patient as in Fig. 5–7). There is an area of hypometabolism in the posterior left hemisphere (arrows). (Reprinted by permission from DF Benson, JL Cummings, SY Tsai, Angular gyrus syndrome simulating Alzheimer disease. Arch Neurol; 1982;39:616–620. Copyright, 1982, American Medical Association.)

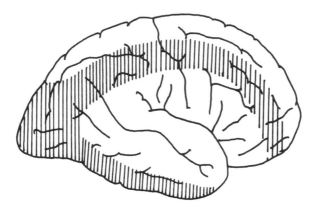

FIGURE 5–9.   The cortical areas affected most in border-zone infarctions.

mutism followed by transcortical motor aphasia is often seen (Alexander and Schmitt, 1980; Rubens, 1975).

Border-zone Infarctions

Carotid artery occlusion results in maximal ischemia and infarction in the region between the distributions of the middle, anterior, and posterior cerebral arteries, often called the border zone or watershed region (Fig. 5–9) (Romanul, 1970; Romanul and Abramowicz, 1964). The maximal weakness and sensory loss involve the proximal portions of arm and leg with relative preservation of hand and face function. When the dominant hemisphere is affected, transcortical aphasia may occur featuring echolalic verbalizations (Geschwind et al, 1968). Carotid artery occlusion may be asymptomatic if collateral circulation is available, but when alternative sources are insufficient, bilateral carotid occlusion produces a multi-infarct dementia syndrome (Fisher, 1951; Paulson et al, 1966; Shapiro, 1959).

Multiple Small Cortical Infarctions

A few patients with multiple small cortical infarctions resulting from thrombotic or embolic occlusions of the small leptomeningeal arterioles have been reported (Jellinger 1976; Kaplan et al, 1985; Monteiro et al, 1985; Torvik et al, 1971). The resulting dementia is slowly progressive and may or may not be associated with episodes of focal neurologic dysfunction. Hearing loss and retinal arteriole occlusions may co-occur with dementia (Monteiro et al, 1985).

Mixed Cortical and Subcortical Infarctions

Most commonly the infarctions producing a multi-infarct dementia are not limited to subcortical or cortical locations but involve both deep and superficial structures. The resulting dementia has features characteristic of both cortical and subcortical dysfunction.

ETIOLOGIES OF VASCULAR DEMENTIA

Multiple vascular occlusions with resulting multi-infarct dementia can occur with either widespread thrombotic or embolic cerebrovascular disease. The number of conditions that can affect the cerebral vessels is enormous and cannot be exhaustively presented. Table 5–5 lists the principal disease categories and some of the specific disease entities that can produce multi-infarct dementia.

Thrombotic Vascular Occlusions

The most common intracerebral occlusive diseases are atherosclerosis, arteriosclerosis, and diabetic vasculopathy. Atherosclerotic vessels have multilayered lesions with organized thrombus overlying subintimal deposits of cholesterol. The arterial media undergoes degenerative changes, and the muscularis and internal elastic membrane are weakened (Toole and Patel, 1967; Yates, 1976). These changes affect the aorta, carotid arteries, and large intracerebral vessels. Arteriolosclerosis (or arteriosclerosis) refers to fibrinoid necrosis of arterioles induced by sustained hypertension (Robbins, 1967). Diabetes can also produce an occlusive vascular disease involving the smaller arteries and arterioles. Cocaine accounts for an increasing number of cerebrovascular events among younger individuals by precipitating vasoconstriction, hypertension, or intracerebral hemorrhage (Klonoff et al, 1989). Many other conditions including Fabry's disease, homocystinuria, amyloidosis, moya-moya disease, pseudoxanthoma elasticum, fibromuscular dysplasia, radiation-induced vascular occlusion, and neoplastic angioendotheliosis are rare causes of intracerebral vascular occlusion that may produce multi-infarct dementia (Dolman et al, 1979; Iqbal et al, 1978; Kramer and Lee, 1974; Mandybur, 1979; Menkes, 1974; Okazaki et al, 1979; Paulson et al, 1978; Petito et al, 1978; Suzuki and Takaku, 1969; Toole and Patel, 1967).

Inflammatory vascular disorders are well-known causes of altered mental states. They usually present acutely with a clinical syndrome resembling acute confusional state, but they may produce a slowly progressive dementing illness. Systemic lupus erythematosus (SLE) is the best known collagen-vascular disorder; it most commonly affects young women and frequently

TABLE 5–5.   Etiologies of multi-infarct dementia.

Thrombotic	Embolic
Atherosclerosis	Cardiac disease
Arteriosclerosis	Myocardial infarction with mural
Diabetes	thrombus
Fibromuscular dysplasia	Atrial fibrillation
Amyloidosis	Rheumatic endocarditis
Fabry's disease	Postrheumatic valvular disease
Homocystinuria	Congenital heart disease
Moya-moya disease	Cardiac surgery
Pseudoxanthoma elasticum	Subacute bacterial endocarditis
Radiation-induced vasculopathy	Marantic endocarditis
Neoplastic angioendotheliosis	Libman-Sacks endocarditis
Inflammatory (noninfectious) vascular	Prosthetic valves
disorders	Septal defect with paradoxical
Systemic lupus erythematosus	embolization
Giant cell arteritis (temporal arteritis)	Cardiomyopathy
Sarcoidosis	Atrial myxoma
Polyarteritis nodosa	Mitral valve prolapse syndrome
Granulomatous arteritis	Endocardial fibroelastosis
Wegener's granulomatosis	Atherosclerotic ulcerative plaques with
Hypersensitivity angiitis	cholesterol emboli
Scleroderma	Atherosclerotic stenosis with distal
Rheumatoid arthritis with arteritis	embolization
Thrombotic microangiopathy	Metastatic deposits
Takayasu's aortitis	Parasites and ova
Cogan's syndrome	Septic emboli
Behçet's syndrome	Air emboli
Vogt-Koyanagi-Harada syndrome	Fat emboli
Dermatomyositis	Nitrogen bubble emboli
Kohlmeier-Degos disease	
Chemical arteritis	
Amphetamines	
"Crack" cocaine	
Carbon monoxide	
Arsenic	
Ergot	
Oral contraceptives	
Hematologic disorders	
Leukemia	
Sickle cell disease	
Waldenstrom's macroglobulinemia	
Polycythemia vera	
Dysproteinemias	
Idiopathic thrombocytosis	
Hyperlipidemia	
Disseminated intravascular	
coagulation	

TABLE 5–5.   *(continued)*

Thrombotic

Cryoglobulinemia
Antibody-mediated thrombosis
Anticardiolipin antibodies
Lupus anticoagulant
Meningovascular infections (infectious
arteritis)
    Bacterial arteritis
        Syphilis
        Tuberculosis
        Miscellaneous
    Yeast and fungal arteritis
    Rickettsia arteritis
    Viral arteritis
    Cysticercosis

involves the central nervous system. Many neurologic disorders including neuropsychiatric disturbances, seizures, focal weakness, chorea, and visual symptoms have been reported in the course of SLE (Brandt et al, 1975; Feinglass et al, 1976; Kaell et al, 1986; Lusins and Szilagyi, 1975; O'Connor and Musher, 1966, Sergent et al, 1975). Manifestations of dementia include focal cortical deficits, poor work performance, impaired concentration, and failing memory (Strub and Black, 1981). Pathologically the brains show multifocal areas of encephalomalacia and the vessels have an inflammatory infiltrate or fibrinoid degeneration with endothelial proliferation (Devinsky et al, 1988; Johnson and Richardson, 1968; Mintz and Fraga, 1965).

Awareness of giant cell arteritis (temporal arteritis) as a cause of dementia is particularly important because it occurs in the elderly age group where inflammatory vascular disorders can easily be overlooked (Caselli, 1990; Hamilton et al, 1971). The condition involves a giant cell reaction affecting the elastic tissue of the arterial media and adventitia (Wilkinson and Russell, 1972). The arteritis is most intense in the extracranial arteries of the head and neck and largely spares the intracranial vessels. Neuropsychiatric manifestations include impaired memory, depression, and progressive intellectual deterioration (Cochran et al, 1978; Grant and McMenemey, 1966; Pascuzzi et al, 1989; Paulley and Hughes, 1960; Vereker, 1957; von Knorring et al, 1966). Polymyalgia rheumatica often coexists with temporal arteritis to produce muscle pain, stiffness, and fatigue (Hunder et al, 1969). These symptoms may draw attention away from the arteritis and are frequently misinterpreted as being functional.

Sarcoidosis usually has prominent systemic manifestations, but in some instances the disease is almost entirely confined to the CNS. It may be present as a single inflammatory tumor, as multiple mass lesions, as hydrocephalus, or as a syndrome of progressive dementia with memory disturbance, aphasia, and cognitive impairment (Cares et al, 1957; Cordingly et al, 1981; Douglas and Maloney, 1973; Ho et al, 1979; Luke et al, 1987; Matthews, 1965; Silverstein et al, 1965; Stern et al, 1985; Wiederholt and Siekert, 1965). Elevated CSF protein may be an important clue to the diagnosis (Cordingly et al, 1981). Angiotensin converting enzyme is elevated in the serum of approximately two-thirds of cases and may help support the clinical diagnosis (Crystal, 1987).

Other types of inflammatory arteritis are considerably more rare but must be considered in any patient presenting with a progressive multifocal syndrome with dementia. Systemic inflammatory disorders that may affect the brain include polyarteritis nodosa, thrombotic microangiopathy. Wegener's granulomatosis, hypersensitivity angiitis, dermatomyositis, scleroderma, Kohlmeier-Degos' disease, and rheumatoid arthritis with vasculitis (Drachman, 1963; Estey et al, 1979; Ferris and Levine, 1973; Ford and Siekert, 1965; Glaser, 1963; McFarland et al, 1978; Ramos and Mandybur, 1975; Susac et al, 1979; Winkelman and Moore, 1950; Yates, 1976). Granulomatous giant cell angiitis affects small leptomeningeal and cortical vessels with little symptomatic extracerebral involvement. The disease often presents as a progressive dementia with periods of confusion (Hughes and Brownell, 1966; Kolodny et al, 1968; Nurick et al, 1972; Rajjoub et al, 1977; Vauderzant et al, 1988; Younger et al, 1988). Takayasu's arteritis is a disease primarily affecting young women and producing obliterative inflammatory occlusion of the large cervical and brachial branches of the aorta (Judge et al, 1962; Riehl, 1963). Three uncommon inflammatory encephalopathies with vascular involvement are Behçet's syndrome, Cogan's syndrome, and Vogt-Koyanagi-Harada syndrome (Bicknell and Holland, 1978; Kozin et al, 1977; Pallis and Fudge, 1956; Pattison, 1965; Reed et al, 1958a; Wadia and Williams, 1957; Serdaroglu et al, 1989; Vollersten et al, 1986). Chemical arteritis has been induced by ergot compounds, carbon monoxide, arsenic, and intravenous amphetamine administration (Citron et al, 1970; Ferris and Levine, 1973; Margolis and Newton, 1971). Intimal hyperplasia has been demonstrated in the vessels of young women with oral contraceptive-induced stroke syndromes (Irey et al, 1978).

Hematologic disorders must also be considered in the adult presenting with an unexplained dementia and clinical features suggesting multifocal infarction. Included in this broad category are leukemia. Waldenström's macroglobulinemia, hemoglobinopathies such as sickle cell disease, polycythemia vera, dysproteinemias, idiopathic thrombocytosis, cryoglobulinemias, hyperlipidemia, and disseminated intravascular coagulation (Collins et al, 1975; Haruda et al, 1981; Levine and Swanson, 1969; Logothetis et al, 1960; Mueller et al, 1983; Reagan and Okazaki, 1974; Reik and Korn, 1981).

Disseminated intravascular coagulation may follow cerebral trauma or may occur with systemic malignancies or bacterial sepsis.

Antibody-mediated thromboses have also been identified. Elevated anticardiolipin antibody levels and lupus anticoagulant are associated with recurrent cerebral infarction and ischemic encephalopathies (Briley et al, 1989; Goodnight et al, 1974; Hardin, 1987; Keimowitz and Annis, 1973; Preston et al, 1974; Young et al, 1989).

Finally, infectious meningovascular processes may invade arterial walls from the subarachnoid space and produce multiple vascular occlusions. Such conditions include meningovascular syphilis, tuberculous meningitis, cat-scratch disease, bacterial arteritis, yeast and fungal arteritis, rickettsial vasculitis, viral arteritis, and cysticercosis vascular lesions (Ferris, 1974; Ferris and Levine, 1973; Selby and Walker, 1979).

Embolic Vascular Occlusions

Embolic occlusion of multiple cerebral vessels is the other major category of conditions producing multi-infarct dementia. The two principal embolic sources are (1) the heart and (2) the atherosclerotic plaques of the aorta and the carotid arteries. The latter give rise to cholesterol and fibrin emboli that travel distally to occlude intracranial vessels. Cardiac conditions that produce emboli include myocardial infarction with mural thrombosis, congenital heart disease, septal defects allowing paradoxical embolization, cardiomyopathy, and endocardial fibroelastosis (Frederick, 1971; Toole and Patel, 1974). Atrial fibrillation may cause embolization, and cerebral emboli can occur with cardiac valvular disease including rheumatic endocarditis and postrheumatic valvular abnormalities, cardiac surgery, subacute bacterial endocarditis, mitral valve prolapse syndrome, marantic endocarditis, Libman-Sacks endocarditis in SLE, and prosthetic valves (Fox et al, 1980, Frederick, 1971; Toole and Patel, 1974).

Atrial myxoma can produce a progressive dementing condition through recurrent embolization (Frank et al, 1979; Hutton, 1981a). Myxomas may closely imitate collagen-vascular disease and escape detection until autopsy (Joynt et al, 1965; Yarnell et al, 1971; Yufe et al, 1976).

The most common sources of cerebral emboli are ulcerative plaques in the aortic arch and carotid arteries. Cholesterol and fibrin debris are carried into the cerebral vessels where they lodge at bifurcations or in distal arborizations, giving rise to multiple infarctions (Beal et al, 1981b). Significant carotid stenosis may produce flow abnormalities that facilitate clotting and produce distal embolization.

Finally in specific situations, metastatic emboli, ova and parasites, septic particles, air, fat, or nitrogen bubbles may produce multiple cerebrovascular occlusions (Toole and Patel, 1974).

CEREBRAL HYPOPERFUSION AS A CAUSE OF DEMENTIA

Vascular dementia most often results from multiple cerebrovascular occlusions causing infarctions in local vascular territories. The occurrence of dementia induced by chronic cerebral hypoperfusion secondary to stenosis of the large vessels supplying the brain is considerably more controversial. Dramatic reversal of apparent dementia has occasionally followed carotid endarterectomy (Levin et al, 1976a), and improvement in neuropsychological test performance has been documented in groups of endarterectomized patients (Goldstein et al, 1970; Kelly et al, 1980). Endarterectomized patients, however, have fewer transient ischemic attacks postoperatively and experience less anxiety and depression. These changes might significantly influence behavior and test performance (Asken and Hobson, 1977; Williams and McGee, 1964). Minor infarctions can also occur during transient ischemic attacks, and gradual improvement of function follow as a product of spontaneous recovery independent of surgical intervention.

Cerebral blood flow studies suggest that there may be at least limited dynamic aspects of vascular dementia. Changes in cognitive deficits appear to correlate with fluctuations in cerebral blood flow, and intellectual ability may show modest improvement with appropriate intervention (Kitagawa et al, 1984; Meyer et al, 1986, 1988b, 1989).

Abrupt cerebral hypoperfusion with ischemic cerebral injury may also occur with systemic hypotension associated with cardiopulmonary arrest, transient arrhythmias, hypovolemia, and chronic severe anemia.

EVALUATION OF VASCULAR DEMENTIA

Adequate evaluation of the patient with vascular dementia includes studies of blood pressure, cardiac function, hematologic variables, and inflammatory conditions. Hematocrit, hemoglobin, white cell, and platelet counts are part of the standard work-up along with erythrocyte sedimentation rate and serologic test for syphilis or fluorescent treponemal antibody absorption. If SLE is suspected, antinuclear antibodies represent a sensitive screening test, but they are not completely specific and may be present in other disorders; antibodies to dsDNA and Sm are relatively specific for the diagnosis and should be obtained in patients with positive screening studies (Hahn, 1987). Serum protein electrophoresis and lipoprotein electrophoresis will reveal conditions producing serum dysproteinemias and hyperlipidemia. Multiple blood pressure measurements, an EKG, and a chest X-ray are essential parts of the examination. More elaborate studies of cardiac function such as echocardiography may be necessary if valvular disease or an atrial myxoma is suspected. Cerebrospinal fluid studies can demonstrate infectious and inflammatory meningovascular processes.

An anamnesis eliciting the features listed in Table 5–2 will help establish the diagnosis of vascular dementia, and use of the Hachinski Ischemia Scale, where each characteristic is assigned a numeric value of one or two, enhances the clinician's diagnostic certainty. A score of four or less is most consistent with a degenerative process, whereas a score of seven or more correlates with vascular dementia (Hachinski et al, 1975; Rosen et al, 1980).

Electrophysiologic studies do not give etiologically specific information, but help confirm the diagnosis of a multifocal process. The EEG may demonstrate generalized or multifocal slowing and late components of visual evoked response studies are delayed compared to normal controls (Straumanis et al, 1965). The CT scan may show multiple hemispheric lucencies consistent with infarctions (Ladurner et al, 1982). Many lacunar infarcts are too small to be revealed by CT, but loss of substance deep in the hemispheres results in ventricular dilatation. Recent infarctions or areas of cerebritis in cerebral vasculitis may be enhanced by administration of contrast medium during CT scanning (Weisberg, 1980). MRI is highly sensitive to ischemic change and often reveals abnormalities in patients with normal CT scans (Brown et al, 1988; Erkinjuntti et al, 1984).

As expected, cerebral blood flow is diminished in vascular dementia (Hachinski et al, 1975; O'Brien, 1977), and there is a correlation between the severity of dementia and the extent of diminished circulation (Judd et al, 1986; Kitagawa et al, 1984). Blood flow is also decreased in active cerebral vasculitis (Weinberger et al, 1979).

Positron emission tomographic scanning of patients with vascular dementia reveals multiple areas of cerebral hypometabolism (Benson et al, 1983), and single photon emission computed tomograms demonstrate multiple regions of cerebral hypoperfusion.

TREATMENT OF VASCULAR DEMENTIA

Vascular dementia is not a curable condition, but recognition and diagnosis of the underlying condition may lead to specific treatment that may halt progression and allow limited recovery to occur. When hypertension is discovered, adequate treatment is essential to stop the advancement of hypertensive cerebrovascular disease and the occurrence of additional infarctions. Treatment must be cautious, however, since rapid lowering of blood pressure may produce cerebral ischemia (Editorial, *British Medical Journal*, 1979; Meyer et al, 1986). Treatment with aspirin to engage its platelet antiaggregation effect is indicated in patients with thrombotic vascular occlusions (Meyer et al, 1986). Recognition of hematologic, inflammatory, or infectious processes will lead to specific treatment of the underlying condition. Each cardiac condition requires individual consideration, but anticoagulant therapy will be necessary for most cardiac diseases that result in multiple cerebral emboli.

A wide variety of drugs has been administered in an attempt to improve cognitive function in multi-infarct dementia, and extravagant claims have been made for some treatments. Unfortunately the claims have not been substantiated, and no consistently effective therapy has been found (Cook and James, 1981; Hier and Caplan, 1980). This failure is not surprising since the condition is thought to result primarily from multiple vascular occlusions, and restoration of function would depend on revival of infarcted cerebral tissue. Among the treatments that have been attempted but not found to be consistently effective are anticoagulants (Ratner et al, 1972; Walsh, 1969a, b; Walsh and Walsh, 1974), several different types of cerebral vasodilators (Affleck et al, 1961; Ball and Taylor, 1967; Branconnicer and Cole, 1977; Fine et al, 1970; Forster et al, 1955; Gaitz et al, 1977; Hall 1976; Rivera et al, 1974; Smith et al, 1968; Treptow et al, 1963; Westreich et al, 1975), precursor amino acids (Meyer et al, 1977), and agents that increase cyclic adenosine monophosphate (AMP) levels (Shimamoto et al, 1976). Surgical interventions such as carotid endarterectomy would not be expected to benefit vascular dementia patients except in situations where transient ischemic episodes complicate the clinical syndrome.

The course of multi-infarct dementia fluctuates and some spontaneous improvement may occur if progression of the disease can be halted. Aphasic patients should have language evaluated and may benefit from speech therapy. General supportive measures such as prevention of limb contractures, treatment of spasticity, gait retraining, attention to bladder function and urinary tract infections, and speech therapy for dysarthria are also indicated. Depression and psychosis are common among these patients and may require treatment with antidepressant or neuroleptic agents.

Vascular dementia associated with recurrent hypotension or hypoxemia may improve following disease-specific intervention. Likewise, appropriate management of post-hemorrhagic hydrocephalus and optimization of treatment of associated systemic conditions may contribute to improved mental function in vascular dementia.

6

HIV Encephalopathy, Jakob-Creutzfeldt Disease, and Other Infectious Dementias

Investigation of infectious causes of dementia has significantly influenced ideas of mental illness, treatability of dementia, and types of biologic agents capable of invading the brain. General paresis of the insane, a syphilitic dementia, was one of the first mental illnesses to be shown to be produced by an organic condition. Identification of the specific pathologic changes produced in the brain by the organism allowed its separation from mania, melancholia, dementia praecox, and degenerative dementias. The discovery that penicillin frequently halted progression of the disease and could lead to partial recovery of intellectual function in some patients demonstrated that syphilis was a treatable cause of mental status impairment and established a precedent for optimism in the search of reversible dementias. More recently, demonstration that Kuru and Jakob-Creutzfeldt disease were caused by infectious agents that could be transmitted from species to species as well as the appearance and spread of the human immunodeficiency virus (HIV) and the acquired immunodeficiency syndrome (AIDS) has reinforced the importance of the role of infectious agents in dementia. Currently, HIV encephalopathy is the most common infection-related dementia and the most common nontraumatic etiology of dementia in young individuals. In this chapter, the principal infectious dementias will be reviewed.

TABLE 6–1.   Viral infections producing dementias.

Slow virus infections
  Unconventional viruses
    Jakob-Creutzfeldt disease
    Kuru
    Gerstmann-Straussler-Scheinker disease
    Alper's disease
  Conventional viruses
    HIV encephalopathy
    Subacute sclerosing panencephalitis
    Progressive rubella panencephalitis
    Progressive multifocal leukoencephalopathy
    Paraneoplastic limbic encephalitis
Post encephalitic dementias following acute encephalitis
  Herpes encephalitis
  Post encephalitic parkinsonism with dementia
  Other viral encephalitides

VIRAL AND PRION DEMENTIAS

Acute viral encephalitis characteristically produces a fulminating clinical syndrome with rapid onset and progression followed by death or partial to complete resolution. Only the chronic postencephalitic states enter the differential diagnosis of a dementia syndrome. Slow virus infections, on the other hand, are viral (or prion, see below) infections that progress slowly over months or years and must be considered in the evaluation of the patients with subacute or chronic mental status changes. Slow viral infections can be divided into those produced by conventional viruses and those caused by unconventional agents or prions (Harter and Petersdorf, 1987). Conventional viruses are responsible for subacute sclerosing panencephalitis, progressive multifocal leukoencephalopathy, progressive rubella encephalitis, paraneoplastic limbic encephalitis, and HIV encephalopathy (Table 6–1). Unconventional agents are responsible for Kuru, Jakob-Creutzfeldt disease, GSSD, and Alper's disease. Prion is the term used to designate unconventional agents consisting of small proteinaceous infectious particles that are resistant to inactivation by many disinfectants, contain no nucleic acid, and produce spongiform tissue changes in the brain.

HIV Encephalopathy

Infection of the brain with the HIV produces a dementia syndrome. The disorder is known as HIV encephalopathy and has also been called the AIDS dementia complex (ADC). HIV encephalopathy is used preferentially here because not all patients with the condition have evidence of immunologic abnormalities at the time the dementia becomes evident. AIDS was first recognized in the United States in 1978, the dementia was observed in 1983, the responsible virus was isolated and characterized in 1984, and the characteristics of the dementia were described in detail in 1986 (Enlow, 1984; Navia et al, 1986b, 1990). In less than a decade, AIDS has reached epidemic proportions, increasing from a nearly unknown disease to a major public health challenge costing billions of dollars per year and posing a health threat of global proportions (Rosenblum et al, 1988).

The principal risk factors for AIDS and HIV encephalopathy are homosexual behavior and intravenous administration of illicit drugs with contaminated needles. Seventy-two percent of AIDS patients are homosexual or bisexual men, 17 percent are intravenous drugs abusers, 2 percent were infected with the virus through blood transfusions prior to thorough screening of blood supplies, 1 percent are hemophiliacs regularly receiving concentrated blood products, 1 percent are children of women infected with the HIV virus, 1 percent are heterosexual sexual partners of HIV-infected individuals, and 2 percent have no known risk factors (Rosenblum et al, 1988).

Nearly all patients with AIDS will develop an HIV encephalopathy at some time in the course of their illness although there is wide variability in its severity and time of occurrence. Seventy percent of patients with HIV dementia have overt AIDS when the mental status changes become evident, but in at least 10 percent the dementia and other evidence of AIDS are recognized simultaneously, and in 20 percent the mental status changes precede the immunologic abnormalities (Price et al, 1988a,b). In children, HIV encephalopathy occurs in 50 percent of those with HIV infection, and dementia in the absence of immunodeficiency is more common in children than it is in adults. Children infected *in utero* or in the perinatal period may become symptomatic as early as two months or as late as five years after delivery (Epstein and Sharer, 1988).

The HIV virus appears to enter the nervous system soon after exposure occurs. During this period of initial infection and seroconversion, a monophasic illness may occur in the form of acute encephalitis, aseptic meningitis, ataxia, or myelopathy (Price et al, 1988a). The virus then remains latent in the nervous system in asymptomatic seropositive individuals for several years, although aseptic meningitis may occur during this period. Virus may often be cultured from the CSF of asymptomatic seropositive individuals, indicating that the CNS is infected, but the virus produces no symptoms (Resnick et al, 1988). Finally the dementia syndrome appears either before or after the virus affects the immune system (Price et al, 1988a). Death usually occurs within nine months of onset of the manifest dementia syndrome, and some cases progress from onset to severe dementia in as little

TABLE 6–2.   Centers for Disease Control classification of HIV infection.

Group I	Initial infection
Group II	Chronic asymptomatic infection
Group III	Persistent generalized lymphadenopathy
Group IV	Other diseases
Subgroup A	Constitutional disease
Subgroup B	Neurologic disease
Subgroup C	Secondary infectious diseases
Subgroup D	Secondary cancers
Subgroup E	Other conditions

Source: Centers for Disease Control, CDC classification system for human T-lymphocytes virus Type III/lymphadenopathy associated virus infection. Mortal Morbid Weekly Report 1987;36 (Suppl):1–9.

as two months (Navia et al, 1986b). This course of events is reflected in the Centers for Disease Control Classification of HIV infection (Table 6–2) (Centers for Disease Control, 1987a).

HIV encephalopathy is far from the only cause of mental status changes in patients with AIDS, and the differential diagnosis of dementia in this group of patients is extensive (Table 6–3). AIDS patients may also develop cytomegalovirus encephalitis (15–30 percent), toxoplasmosis (3–30 percent), cryptococcus infection (2–11 percent), progressive multifocal leukoencephalopathy (1–6 percent), primary CNS lymphoma (1–5 percent), herpes simplex encephalitis (2–3 percent), varicella-zoster encephalitis (1–2 percent), amoebic infections, Epstein-Barr virus encephalitis, candida albicans brain abscesses, aspergillus infections, systemic lymphomas with secondary brain involvement, cerebrovascular accidents, syphilis, or Kaposi's sarcoma of the brain (Dix and Bredesen, 1988; Levy et al, 1985, 1988; McArthur, 1987; Nielsen and Davis, 1988). Thus the differential diagnosis of dementia in AIDS patients entails a thorough evaluation for a variety of brain diseases, and several neurological disorders may coexist in the same patient.

Dementia

HIV encephalopathy is the most common neurological disturbance associated with HIV infection and eventually occurs in a majority of infected patients. The dementia syndrome characteristic of HIV infection is relatively stereotyped and is dominated by features indicative of subcortical dysfunction (Navia et al, 1986b). Early in the clinical course, the patients manifest forgetfulness and poor concentration. Losing the train of thought and slowed thinking are common. Apathy and social withdrawal are observed in many individuals, and a few exhibit delusions and hallucinations. Memory abnor-

TABLE 6–3.   Principal conditions to be considered in the differential diagnosis of the seropositive individual with mental status changes.

HIV encephalopathy
Opportunistic infections
   Cytomegalovirus
   Toxoplasmosis
   Cryptococcal meningitis
   Progressive multifocal leukoencephalopathy
   Herpes encephalitis
   Varicella-zoster encephalitis
   Epstein-Barr virus encephalitis
   Candida albicans microabscesses
   Aspergillus infections
   Amoebic infections
   Syphilis
Neoplasms
   Primary CNS lymphoma
   Lymphoma with secondary CNS involvement
   Kaposi's sarcoma
Depression
Cerebrovascular accident
Metabolic encephalopathy
   Pneumonia
   Other infection
   Drug and medication intoxication
   Drug withdrawal (particularly in AIDS patients with a history of substance abuse)

malities become more obvious as the disease progresses, and disturbances of visuospatial function, abstraction, and calculation also occur. Language abilities are preserved throughout the illness. The disease progresses slowly, and as it approaches the preterminal state, patients exhibit more severe psychomotor retardation, indifference, and quiet confusion. Terminally many are in an awake state with a wide-eyed stare but are akinetic and mute (Navia et al, 1986b). Agitation and psychosis occur in a small number of patients.

    Neuropsychological assessment of patients with HIV encephalopathy reveals that they exhibit diminished verbal, performance, and full-scale intelligence test scores; poor verbal and nonverbal learning and memory; and impaired motor speed and cognitive flexibility (Van Gorp et al, 1989). Simple reaction time tests reveal no performance deficits, whereas choice times are prolonged, reflecting abnormalities in speed of cognitive processing (Perdices and Cooper, 1989). The profile of performance is similar to that seen in normal aged individuals and patients with subcortical degenerative dementias and contrasts sharply with that of DAT (Van Gorp et al, 1989).

The neuropsychological status of asymptomatic seropositive individuals is controversial. Some investigators suggest that neuropsychological impairment is present in a substantial number (Grant et al, 1987), whereas others have found little evidence of neuropsychological compromise (Janssen et al, 1989; McArthur et al, 1989; Miller et al, 1990; Perry et al, 1989; Selnes et al, 1990).

Clinical Features of AIDS

HIV encephalopathy is usually accompanied by other evidence of neurological dysfunction. Gait ataxia, dysarthria, disrupted smooth pursuit eye movements, action tremor, and lower limb hyperreflexia are common, and headache and seizures may occur (Navia et al, 1986b). In the final phase of the illness, the principal neurological signs include ataxia, rigidity, motor weakness, incontinence, tremor, myoclonus, and seizures (Navia et al, 1986b). Other complications include cytomegalovirus retinitis, inflammatory demyelinating neuropathy, sensory neuropathy, cranial neuropathy, multiple mononeuropathies, herpes zoster myeloradiculitis, myopathies, and myelopathy (Fischer and Enzensberger, 1987; McArthur, 1987; Snider et al, 1983). Metabolic encephalopathies with delirium resulting from systemic illnesses, infections, or the use of medication may be superimposed on the underlying dementia.

Laboratory Features and Diagnosis

In the presence of laboratory evidence of HIV infection, any of the following conditions indicates a diagnosis of AIDS: disseminated coccidioidomycosis, HIV encephalopathy, disseminated histoplasmosis, isosporiasis with diarrhea persisting for longer than one month, Kaposi's sarcoma, primary CNS lymphoma, other non-Hodgkin's lymphoma of B-cell or unknown immunologic phenotype and small noncleaved lymphoma or immunoblastic sarcoma histologic type, disseminated nontuberculous mycobacterial disease, extrapulmonary tuberculosis, recurrent *Salmonella* septicemia, HIV wasting syndrome, or multiple or recurrent bacterial infections in a child under age 13 (Centers for Disease Control, 1987b). Individuals who have positive antibody tests and are symptomatic with fever, weight loss, diarrhea, fatigue, night sweats, lymphadenopathy, or immunologic abnormalities but who do not fulfill the above criteria for AIDS are diagnosed as suffering from AIDS-related complex (ARC) (Fauci and Lane, 1987). Clinical criteria for HIV encephalopathy include disabling cognitive or motor dysfunction or loss of developmental milestones in a child, progressing over weeks or months, and the absence of any concurrent illness or condition other than HIV infection that could explain the alterations (Center for Disease Control, 1987b).

A number of tests have been developed for the identification of the presence of the immunodeficiency virus. The most common screen for the presence of serum HIV antibodies is an enzyme-linked immunoabsorbent assay (ELISA); positive results are confirmed by Western blot techniques (Steckelberg et al, 1988). Other available tests include HIV culture confirmed by reverse transcriptase detection, *in situ* hybridization using a nucleic acid probe, HIV radioimmunoprecipitation, or immunoassays constructed from molecularly cloned and expressed viral envelope polypeptide (Burke et al, 1988; Center for Disease Control, 1987b).

The principal immunologic defect in AIDS is an abnormality in cell-mediated immunity that produces increased host susceptibility to opportunistic infections, Kaposi's sarcoma, and specific lymphomas. HIV is a retrovirus that selectively affects T_4 helper/inducer lymphocytes causing a leukopenia. T_8 suppressor/cytotoxic lymphocytes are spared and an abnormal T_4/T_8 ratio emerges in the course of the illness (Bowen et al, 1985; Fauci and Lane, 1987). Normally there is a predominance of T_4 helper cells and a low helper/suppressor ratio or an absolute number of T_4 cells of less than 400/cu. mm. are usually regarded as abnormal (Enlow, 1984).

Abnormalities in the CSF of patients with AIDS and HIV encephalopathy are common. Approximately 60 percent of seropositive asymptomatic individuals have CSF alterations, particularly elevated white cell counts (Marshall et al, 1988). Elevated IgG levels and increased CSF IgG synthesis is observed in some patients (Elovaara et al, 1987; Marshall et al, 1988). In one study of patients with HIV encephalopathy, 66 percent of the patients had elevated CSF protein, 43 percent had oligoclonal bands, and 20 percent had a mononuclear pleocytosis (Navia et al, 1986b). HIV can be cultured from the CSF of approximately 20 percent of seropositive individuals even prior to the occurrence of neurological or immune-related symptoms (Resnick et al, 1988).

Neurodiagnostic studies play a crucial role in the evaluation of the seropositive patient with mental status changes (Fig. 6–1). These investigations are often the first step in deciding if the behavioral alterations reflect HIV encephalopathy or an opportunistic infection and then in constructing an appropriate diagnostic and management strategy. HIV usually produces no changes on X-ray CTs; at most there may be mild cortical atrophy, ventricular enlargement, and nonspecific periventricular lucencies. Calcification of the basal ganglia has been observed in infants and children with HIV encephalopathy (Belman et al, 1986). MRI often reveals cerebral atrophy and ventricular enlargement; in some patients with HIV encephalopathy, there are high-signal periventricular white matter lesions that progress as the dementia worsens; and patients with opportunistic infections, focal encephalitis or lymphoma may have solitary high-signal lesions. Large symmetrical lesions occur in cytomegalovirus and in HIV encephalopathy while isolated high-signal lesions are more indicative of toxoplasmosis, pro-

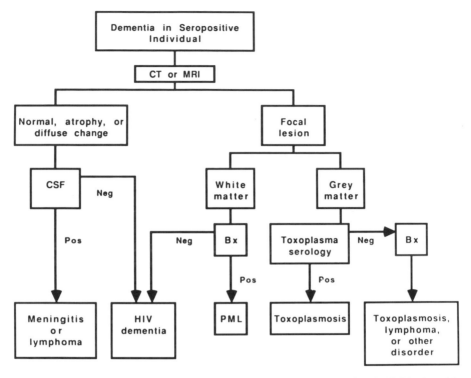

FIGURE 6-1.   Decision guide to the evaluation of seropositive individuals with mental status changes (modified from Snider et al, Neurological complications of acquired immune deficiency syndrome: Analysis of 50 patients, Ann Neurol 1983; 14:403-418, with permission of the publisher).

gressive multifocal leukoencephalopathy, or other opportunistic infections (Figs. 6-2 and 6-3) (De La Paz and Enzmann, 1988; Ekholm and Simon, 1988; Jarvik et al, 1988; Shabas et al, 1987).

PET with fluorodeoxyglucose reveals subcortical hypermetabolism in the early phases of HIV encephalopathy and combined cortical and subcortical hypometabolism in the late phases of the illness (Rottenberg et al, 1987). Electroencephalography is abnormal in approximately two-thirds of patients with AIDS, and brainstem auditory evoked responses and spinal cord conduction somatosensory responses may be slowed even before neurological symptoms become evident (Gabuzda et al, 1988; Smith et al, 1988c).

Neuropathology

Seventy to 90 percent of the brains of AIDS patients are histologically abnormal at the time of autopsy. Pathological abnormalities in patients with

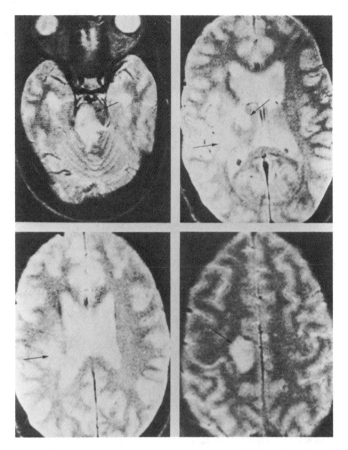

FIGURE 6–2.   MRI scans in a 34-year-old patient with AIDS. Focal high signal lesions indicative of toxoplasmosis are seen (from Jarvik et al, Acquired immunodeficiency syndrome. Magnetic resonance patterns of brain involvement with pathologic correlation, Arch Neurol 1988;45:731–736, reproduced with permission of the publisher).

HIV encephalopathy without opportunistic infections affect primarily the hemispheric white matter and subcortical nuclear structures. Inflammatory changes with perivascular and parenchymal lymphocytic infiltrates are seen in most brains although the abundance of inflammation is limited. In patients with advanced dementia at the time of death, foamy macrophages, and multinucleated giant cells are seen particularly in the white matter (Fig. 6–4). Reactive astrocytosis occurs in areas of inflammation. Other prominent white matter abnormalities include areas of pallor, focal rarefaction with macrophages, and vacuolation (Navia et al, 1986b).

    Microglial nodules and intranuclear inclusion bodies consistent with

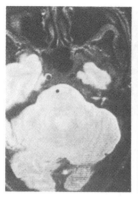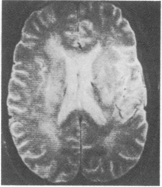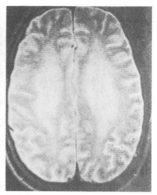

FIGURE 6–3. MRI scan of a 27-year-old man with HIV encephalopathy. Symmetrical periventricular high-signal lesions are demonstrated (from Jarvik et al, Acquired immunodeficiency syndrome. Magnetic resonance patterns of brain involvement with pathologic correlation, Arch Neurol 1988;45:731–736, reproduced with permission of the publisher).

cytomegalovirus infection are also common (Fig. 6–5). These typically occur in the cortex and basal ganglia and are less frequent in the white matter (Navia et al, 1986a; Nielsen and Davis, 1988). Other opportunistic infection (for example, progressive multifocal leukoencephalopathy and toxoplasmosis) exhibit characteristic pathologic abnormalities.

Vacuolar myelopathy is found in the spinal cord in approximately half of the post mortem examinations of HIV encephalopathy patients (Navia et al, 1986a). Cytomegalovirus-related inflammatory changes account for many of the inflammatory peripheral neuropathies in AIDS (Grafe and Wiley, 1989).

Pathophysiology

HIV enters the nervous system soon after infection. The virus has the capacity to induce cell lysis and fusion resulting in syncytial or multinucleated cells and preferentially affects cells of the immune system including macrophages (Navia, 1990). The virus may be transported to the CNS in macrophages (Trojan horse hypothesis) or may enter the brain directly after infection. The cell replicates in the immunologically privileged environment of the brain. The predominant distribution of the virus in the basal ganglia and deep hemispheric white matter is unexplained but correlates well with the subcortical features of the dementia syndrome. HIV has also been

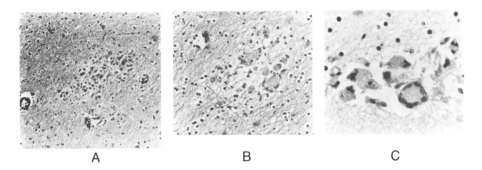

A   B   C

FIGURE 6–4.   A collection of macrophages and lymphocytes in white matter (A), macrophages and multinucleated giant cells (B), and multinucleated cells with scattered macrophages (C) (from Navia et al, The AIDS dementia complex: II, Ann Neurol 1986a;19:525–535, reproduced with permission of the publisher).

identified in microglia and vascular endothelial cells, but involves these cells less frequently than it does the macrophages. Thus the dementia results from disturbances of the supporting elements of the brain or local metabolic alterations rather than from primary neuronal death. HIV may produce dementia through brain invasion without associated immunocompromise, but most HIV encephalopathy patients have immunological deficits and immunosuppression may facilitate CNS viral replication and emergence of the dementia (Price et al, 1988a). Leukopenia accounts for the limited inflammatory response noted in the brains of patients with HIV encephalopathy.

Treatment

Therapy for dementia syndromes is determined by the etiology of the mental status changes. HIV encephalopathy, depression, opportunistic infections, and toxic-metabolic dysfunction may all respond at least partially to specific therapeutic interventions. Infections are treated with antibiotics and toxic-metabolic encephalopathies are managed through minimization of toxic exposure and optimization of medical care.

Treatment of HIV encephalopathy has two goals: (1) suppress the activity of the virus and (2) maximize the remaining intellectual function. Azidothymidine (AZT), an antiretrovirus agent, has beneficial effects for both AIDS and HIV encephalopathy. Patients with moderately severe dementia may have substantial recovery of intellectual function as well as

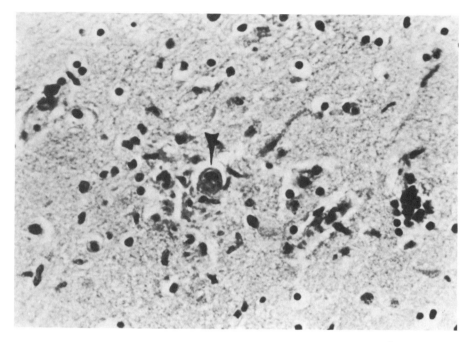

FIGURE 6–5.   Intranuclear inclusion in neuron in brain of an AIDS patient consistent with cytomegalovirus infection (from Snider et al, Neurological complications of acquired immune deficiency syndrome: Analysis of 50 patients, Ann Neurol 1983;14:403–418, reproduced with permission of the publisher).

improvement in cerebral glucose metabolism as measured by PET when treated with AZT (Yarchoan et al, 1987). Patients with milder intellectual impairment likewise exhibit improved attention, memory, motor skills, mental speed, and general cognitive acuity when treated chronically with AZT (Schmitt et al, 1988). AZT is accompanied by substantial adverse side effects including anemia, leukopenia, rash, vomiting, headaches, insomnia, myalgia, and hepatitis, and its administration must be carefully monitored. AZT usually produces clinical benefit for several months before the virus reasserts itself and the disease progresses (Dournon et al, 1988; Yarchoan et al, 1987).

Depression in AIDS patients is treated with conventional antidepressant agents. Psychomotor retardation, poor motivation, and attentional deficits may respond to psychostimulants such as methylphenidate or dextroamphetamine (Fernandez et al, 1988).

JAKOB-CREUTZFELDT DISEASE

In 1921, Jakob reported clinical and pathologic findings in three patients suffering from a disorder he called spastic pseudosclerosis. The disease started in adulthood, had a rapidly progressive course leading to death in less than one year, and had degenerative type neuropathologic changes involving the cortical, pyramidal, and extrapyramidal systems. A report of a fourth case was published later in 1921, and a fifth case was described in his book on movement disorders published in 1923 (Jakob, 1977; Kirschbaum, 1968). In discussing similar conditions described previously in the literature, Jakob referred to a case reported by Creutzfeldt in 1920. Creutzfeldt's patient was 16 years old when she first manifested behavioral changes, and the disease had a remitting course lasting five years. The patient had two retarded sisters who were cared for in an institution. At autopsy the patient had several congenital malformations of the nervous system as well as noninflammatory disintegration of neurons in the hemispheres. The white matter was largely spared (Creutzfeldt, 1977; Kirschbaum, 1968). Jakob's cases closely resemble the dementing illness we now know to be caused by a transmissible agent, whereas Creutzfeldt's case differs in many respects from the disease under consideration. For this reason, it seems appropriate to credit Jakob and to use the previously more popular eponym Jakob-Creutzfeldt disease.

Clinical Characteristics

Jakob-Creutzfeldt disease is an uncommon disorder with a worldwide incidence of approximately one per million. Onset is usually in the sixth or seventh decade of life, although patients as young as age 20 and as old as 79 have been reported (Goldhammer et al, 1972; Harries-Jones et al, 1988; Packer et al, 1980; Roos et al, 1973). Ten to 15 percent of cases have a family history of the illness (Brown et al, 1979; Davison and Rabiner, 1940; Masters et al, 1981b; May et al, 1968). The disease is approximately equally prevalent in men and women (Brown et al, 1986; Roos and Johnson, 1977). Jakob-Creutzfeldt disease is rapidly progressive; 50 percent of patients die within six months and 75-90 percent are dead one year after onset (Brown et al, 1986; Kirschbaum, 1968). Familial cases have a significantly earlier age of onset than do sporadic cases (Masters et al, 1981b) and tend to have a more protracted course. Cases with a sudden, strokelike onset and progression to death in less than two months have been observed, but a few patients have had unusually long courses lasting 2 to 16 years (Brown et al,

1979; Cutler et al, 1984). Long duration cases are characterized by a higher proportion of familial representation (30 percent), younger age at onset, and lower frequency of myoclonus and periodic EEG changes than classic short-duration cases (Brown et al, 1984). There is suggestive evidence that previous surgery, physical trauma, or preexisting neurologic disease may be associated with an increased risk of developing Jakob-Creutzfeldt disease (Davanipour et al, 1985; Kondo and Kuriowa, 1982; Masters et al, 1979; Will and Matthews, 1982).

Although the usual clinical features and course of Jakob-Creutzfeldt disease are fairly stereotyped, there is some variability in the presentation of the disease, its duration, underlying pathologic changes, and transmissibility. Some investigators speculate that these differences indicate that at least two disease processes (transmissible and nontransmissible) are included in the condition currently considered as Jakob-Creutzfeldt disease (Christensen and Brun, 1963; Nevin et al, 1960). Nontransmissible disease has had a somewhat longer duration, more evidence of lower motor neuron disease, and less tendency to exhibit characteristic EEG changes (Roos et al, 1973; Traub et al, 1977). In other respects the two groups are indistinguishable, and they are considered together here.

Jakob-Creutzfeldt disease progresses through three identifiable stages: The first stage lasts weeks and consists of the ingravescent buildup of symptoms. In the second stage, there is evidence of widespread hemispheric involvement with diverse signs of neurologic disturbance. Finally there is a terminal vegetative state leading to death (Kirschbaum, 1968; Nevin et al, 1960). The initial manifestations consist of a short prodromal period during which the patient complains of vague physical discomfort, is mildly apprehensive and fatigued, has difficulty with sleep and changes in appetite, and is unable to concentrate. Forgetfulness and depression may be prominent (Brown et al, 1986; McAllister and Price, 1982). After several weeks, dementia becomes evident along with cortical, pyramidal, and extrapyramidal signs. A full cortical dementia syndrome often occurs with aphasia, agnosia, amnesia, apraxia, hallucinations, delusions, and devastating intellectual disintegration. Aphasia is the single most commonly identified cognitive deficit in this stage. The neurobehavioral features coexist with an array of primary neurologic abnormalities including pyramidal tract signs, myoclonus, cerebellar disturbances, rigidity, tremor, choreoathetosis, somatosensory and visual disturbances, and cranial nerve palsies (Brown et al, 1986; Fisher, 1960; Jones and Nevin, 1954; Kirschbaum, 1968; Mandell et al, 1989; Roos et al, 1973; Siedler and Malamud, 1963). Virtually all patients eventually have dementia, myoclonus, and pyramidal and extrapyramidal signs in addition to evidence of involvement of other CNS functions. The stage of rapidly accumulating neurologic deficits leading to neurologic

TABLE 6–4. Clinical varieties of Jakob-Creutzfeldt disease based on their mode of presentation

Clinical variant	Principal structures involved
Amyotrophic type	Spinal cord
Ataxic (Brownell-Oppenheimer) type	Cerebellum
Extrapyramidal type	Basal ganglia
Occipital (Heidenhain) type	Occipital cortex
Frontopyramidal (Jakob) type	Frontal cortex
Panencephalopathic (Mizutani) type	Gray and white matter
Miscellaneous manifestations	
Autonomic dysfunction	Sympathetic ganglia
Supranuclear ocular disorders	Frontal cortex

devastation usually lasts several months, gradually merging into a vegetative akinetic state with stupor, mutism, myoclonus, seizures, autonomic disturbances, and decerebrate rigidity (Kirschbaum, 1968). Urinary tract infections, aspiration pneumonia, and decubitus ulceration are increasingly difficult to prevent, and the patient eventually dies.

Several clinical variants distinguished primarily by their mode of presentation have been identified (Table 6–4). An amyotrophic form with prominent lower motor neuron signs indicating involvement of the spinal cord has been described (Davison, 1932; Myrianthopoulos and Smith, 1962). Lower motor neuron signs more characteristically occur late in the course of Jakob-Creutzfeldt disease in conjunction with fulminate cerebral and cerebellar involvement (Salazar et al, 1983). The ataxic form of disease presents primarily as a cerebellar syndrome and can be difficult to distinguish from subacute cerebellar degeneration associated with an occult carcinoma. The ataxic variant comprises 10 percent of cases of Jakob-Creutzfeldt disease (Brownell and Oppenheimer, 1965; Gomori et al, 1973; Jones et al, 1985). When the condition affects primarily the posterior cerebral cortex and produces cortical blindness early in the clinical course, it is designated Heidenhain's syndrome (Meyer et al, 1954). In the panencephalopathic type, there is diffuse involvement of both gray and white matter of the cerebral hemispheres (Mori et al, 1989). Rarely patients have been reported whose initial or outstanding clinical abnormality has involved supranuclear disturbances of eyelid function (Russell, 1980) or autonomic disorders (Khurana and Garcia, 1981). As the disease progresses, the clinical variants lose their separate identities and merge into the common clinical syndrome characterized by dementia, pyramidal and extrapyramidal disturbances, and myoclonus.

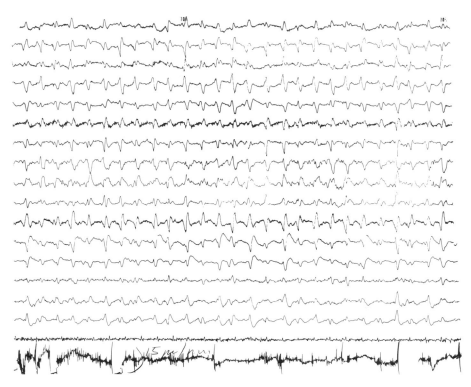

FIGURE 6-6.   EEG in Jakob-Creutzfeldt disease reveals diffuse sharp and slow-wave activity.

Laboratory Evaluation

Routine studies of urine and blood are unremarkable and do not aid in the diagnosis of Jakob-Creutzfeldt disease. The cerebrospinal fluid is normal in 80 percent of cases whereas 20 percent show minor elevations in protein content, slight lymphocytosis, or a small increase in gamma globulins (Kirschbaum, 1968).

The EEG changes are not pathognomonic but are highly characteristic and provide considerable diagnostic support in identifying the disease. Patterns undergo a progressive deterioration as the condition advances. In the early stages, there is a gradual slowing of the background rhythm. Approximately one-third of patients show intermittent periodic bursts early in the disease. Asymmetric slowing is not uncommon, and occasional patients show periodic lateralized epileptiform discharges (PLEDs). With progression into the second stage of disease, the background rhythm falls into the theta or delta range, and periodic discharges occur in most patients (Fig. 6-6). The discharges are complex and are usually initiated by sharp waves that are predominantly triphasic. Occasional monophasic, biphasic, and polyphasic sharp waves are noted. High-voltage rhythmic slow waves follow the preliminary sharp-wave activity. The bursts last 200 to 600 msec and are separated by intervals usually lasting less than 2.5 seconds. Resting background activity may appear between periodic bursts or the background rhythms may be suppressed. As the disease progresses, the bursts become more symmetric, and 75 to 90 percent of patients with Jakob-Creutzfeldt disease eventually show the periodic burst pattern during the course of the illness. Terminally, the scalp EEG may become diffusely flat (Au et al, 1980; Brown et al, 1986; Burger et al, 1972; Chiofalo et al, 1980; Furlan et al, 1981; Lee and Blair, 1973). Casual inspection may reveal no immediate relationship between periodic complexes and myoclonic jerks, but jerk-locked averaging techniques reveal a close temporal association between periodic electrocerebral events and contralateral myoclonic activity (Shibasaki et al, 1981). Periodic EEG patterns resembling those seen in Jakob-Creutzfeldt disease are also observed in postanoxic brain damage, in patients with toxic or metabolic encephalopathies, in SSPE, in postviral encephalitides, and in cerebral lipidoses (Evans, 1975; Gloor et al, 1968; Kirschbaum, 1968; Kuroiwa and Celesia, 1980).

Visual evoked potentials in one patient showed markedly enlarged responses early in the clinical course followed by an increase in latency and a decrease in amplitude of the early components and reversal of polarity of the late responses as the disease advanced (Lee and Balir, 1973).

Computerized tomographic scanning may reveal no change or may show enlarged sulci and dilated ventricles. MRI in Jakob-Creutzfeldt disease may be normal, may reveal nonspecific atrophy, or may demonstrate areas of increased signal intensity corresponding to involved brain regions (Gertz et al, 1988). Positron emission tomography demonstrates multifocal areas of cortical and subcortical hypometabolism (Fig. 6–7) (Horowitz et al, 1982). Single photon emission CT studies reveal multifocal areas of diminished cerebral perfusion (Shih et al, 1987).

Neuropathology

On gross inspection, the brains show mild nonspecific atrophy or are normal. Coronal sections may be normal or atrophy of the basal ganglia may be evident. Three principal neuropathologic features affecting gray matter are seen on microscopic examination: degeneration and loss of neurons, proliferation of astrocytes, and development of a spongiform state (Corsellis, 1976). The neuron loss occurs singly or in groups and involves all areas of the cortical mantle, the basal ganglia, the thalamus, the brainstem, and the spinal cord in varying degrees. Golgi stains of pyramidal neurons demonstrate a striking loss of dendritic spines and focal spheric distentions of dendritic

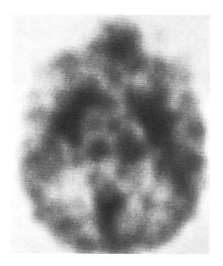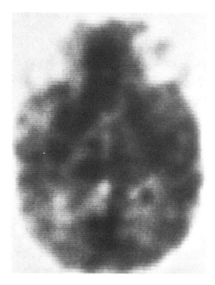

FIGURE 6–7.   PET reveals multiple diffuse hypometabolic areas in a patient with Jakob-Creutzfeldt disease.

and axonal processes (Landis et al, 1981). Astrocytic hypertrophy is even more ubiquitous. Large fibrous astrocytes are prominent; fibrous gliosis is extensive in affected regions (Fig. 6–8); and moderate microglial reaction is evident. There are no appreciable inflammatory changes. Myelin loss is usually minor and there is little gliosis of the white matter, although in occasional cases axon loss and demyelination are severe (Corsellis, 1976; Kirschbaum, 1968; Macchi et al, 1984; Mizutani et al, 1981). Amyloid plaques similar to those occurring in Kuru are found in the cerebellum in 10 percent of cases (Roos and Johnson, 1977), and some patients have both cerebral and cerebellar amyloid deposits (Adam et al, 1982). The neuropathologic feature that has attracted most attention is the spongy state of the cerebral cortex (Fig. 6–9). Not all patients develop this change, but careful neuropathologic examination will reveal it in most of those with clinical findings consistent with Jakob-Creutzfeldt disease. Masters and Richardson (1978) pointed out that there are two types of spongy changes in Jakob-Creutzfeldt disease. The first, called spongiform change and characteristic of the spongiform encephalopathies, is comprised of intracellular vacuoles within the processes of astrocytes and neurons and is prominent in patients dying within five months of onset. The second, called status spongiosus, is a nonspecific extracellular alteration characteristic of end-stage gliosis and is found in many disorders. Spongiform change may be found in the cerebral cortex, thalamus, caudate, and putamen. Electron microscopic studies confirm the intracytoplasmic location of the vacuoles (Gonatas et al, 1965; Landis et al, 1981).

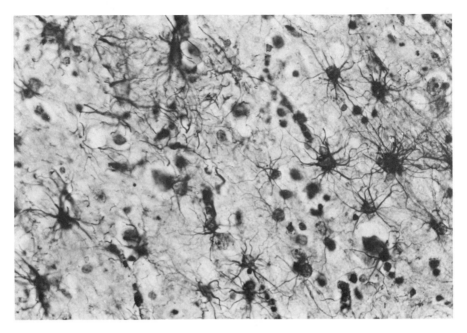

FIGURE 6–8.   Light microscopy demonstrates exuberant fibrous gliosis in cortex of patient with Jakob-Creutzfeldt disease. (Holzer stain: original magnification ×400.) (Courtesy of LW Duchen, Department of Neuropathology, National Hospital for Nervous Diseases, Queen Square, London.)

Neurochemical analyses reveal decreased phosphatides, decreased gangliosides, and depletion of cellular RNA. These changes reflect ongoing neuronal disintegration (Bass et al, 1974; Suzuki and Chen, 1966).

Etiology and Transmissibility

Originally considered a degenerative or possibly vascular process, Jakob-Creutzfeldt disease is now regarded as a transmissible infectious disorder. Although the agent has been labeled as a virus, it is unlike other known viruses; Gajdusek (1977) has suggested that the word unconventional be used to describe the agents responsible for Jakob-Creutzfeldt disease, Kuru and Gerstmann-Straussler-Scheinker syndrome. Prusiner (1987) invoked the label "prion" for these small *pro*teinaceous *in*fectious particles that contain little or no nucleic acid. These agents differ from conventional slow viruses in that they do not evoke an inflammatory response, there is no evidence of an immune response, no recognizable virions or inclusion bodies have been identified by electron microscopy, and they have unusual resistance to

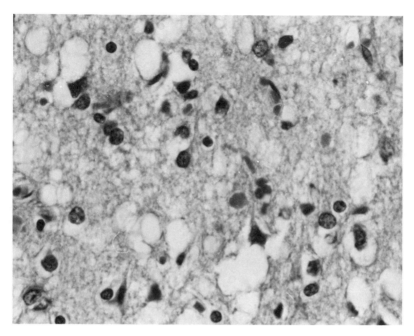

FIGURE 6–9.   Microscopic examination reveals spongiform appearance of cortex in patient with Jakob-Creutzfeldt disease. (Hematoxylin and eosin: original magnification ×400.) (Courtesy of LW Duchen, Department of Neuropathology, National Hospital for Nervous Diseases, Queen Square, London.)

most traditional physical and chemical disinfectant techniques (Gajdusek, 1977). The unconventional viruses are moderately sensitive to most membrane-disrupting agents. Although infection of the nervous system is responsible for the symptomatology of Jakob-Creutzfeldt disease, the agent has been recovered from a variety of tissues including lymph nodes, lung, liver, kidney, and cerebrospinal fluid (Gibbs and Gajdusek, 1978).

Transmission of spongiform encephalopathy from humans with Jakob-Creutzfeldt to several species of primates, cats, pigs, and mice has been achieved (Gajdusek, 1977; Gibbs and Gajdusek, 1978; Traub et al, 1977). Not all attempts at transmission have been successful, suggesting species-specific and/or individual variations in susceptibility. The occurrence of familial cases also suggests an inherited susceptibility to the disease (Masters et al, 1981b).

Human-to-human transmission has been documented. One patient developed Jakob-Creutzfeldt disease after receiving a corneal transplant from an affected donor (Duffy et al, 1974), and two others were infected when depth electrodes previously used in a patient with Jakob-Creutzfeldt disease were used for recording purposes (Bernoulli et al, 1977). A dramatic instance of human-to-human transmission occurred when human cadaveric pituitary glands were harvested to produce human growth hormone to treat children with idiopathic hypopituitarism. Sources of the hormonal extract included unrecognized cases of Jakob-Creutzfeldt disease, and several children treated with the material subsequently developed the fatal dementia (Marzewski et al, 1988; Rappaport, 1987; Tintner et al, 1986). This example of transmission by consumption of human products tragically recapitulates the transmission of kuru by natives practicing cannibalism in New Guinea that is discussed below. Reports of transmissibility have given rise to fear that health professionals and others in contact with affected patients may be at increased risk for developing the disease. Systematic population studies do not indicate an increased rate among health professionals, conjugal partners, or other close personal contacts (Brown et al, 1979). The current practice of some clinicians, surgeons, and pathologists to refuse to obtain and process material from these patients is unsupported by data concerning the risk of transmissibility of the disease and should not be condoned. Objects contaminated by infected tissues should be autoclaved (1 hour at 120 degrees C at 15 pounds per square inch) or disinfected with 5 percent sodium hypochlorite (immersed for two hours). Tissues and disposable equipment should be incinerated, and electrodes and needles coming in contact with the patient should be disinfected or incinerated. There is no evidence that stool, urine, saliva, and other secretions are infectious, and no isolation procedures are currently recommended (Baringer et al, 1980; Gajdusek et al, 1977).

Treatment

Recognition of the viral etiology of Jakob-Creutzfeldt disease has not led to effective therapy. Idoxyuridine was tried without benefit (Goldhammer et al, 1972). Amantadine hydrochloride was reported to halt the disease and restore function in one patient (Braham, 1971), but this report has not been confirmed. Amantadine may produce transient improvement in arousal and attention (Terzano et al, 1983). Supportive care and family counseling remain the mainstays of management.

Differential Diagnosis

The principal condition from which Jakob-Creutzfeldt disease must be distinguished is the rapidly progressive form of DAT. Occasional cases of pathologically typical DAT progress to death in a few months' time and have EEG and clinical features including dementia and myoclonus, identical to those of Jakob-Creutzfeldt disease (Ehle and Johnson, 1977; Watson, 1979). Such cases can be differentiated only at autopsy.

Another disorder or group of disorders that may closely imitate Jakob-Creutzfeldt disease are the thalamic dementias (McDaniel, 1990). These conditions have a subacute course leading to death in six months to two years. Dementia, psychomotor slowing, and myoclonus are the principal clinical features. In some cases, the disease is inherited in an autosomal dominant pattern (Little et al, 1986); others are sporadic. At autopsy there are marked degenerative changes in the dorsomedial and midline thalamic nuclei. A greater tendency toward somnolence early in the clinical course, family history, and absence of periodic EEG changes characteristic of Jakob-Creutzfeldt disease help distinguish the two disorders.

OTHER INFECTIOUS DEMENTIAS

Kuru

Kuru is a progressive fatal disease of the CNS found primarily among the Fore tribe in the eastern highlands of Papua, New Guinea. When its prevalence was highest, it affected 1 percent of the population and was the leading cause of death among the Fore people. The disease progressed through ambulant, sedentary, and terminal stages and led to death in less than one year. It primarily affected adult women and children and produced a stereotyped clinical syndrome. Kuru began with gait ataxia, followed by truncal and limb ataxia. There was a characteristic shiverlike tremor and dysarthria. Dementia was a late finding and was rarely severe, but behavioral changes and psychomotor retardation were common (Gajdusek, 1977; Traub et al, 1977).

Kuru is caused by an unconventional slow virus that shares many of the features of the Jakob-Creutzfeldt agent and may be identical (Gajdusek, 1977). Pathologically there is loss of neurons, a great excess of hypertrophied astrocytes, an increase in rod-shaped microglial cells, and mild spongiform changes. In the cerebellum there is a conspicuous loss of granule cells, loss and disturbance of Purkinje cells (torpedo formation, antlerlike swellings of dendrites), and formation of amyloid plaques (Adams, 1976; Traub et al, 1977).

Kuru is thought to have been transmitted by endocannibalistic consumption of dead kinsmen, and the disease is disappearing as cannibalism is abolished in New Guinea (Gajdusek, 1977). A similar disorder has occasionally been reported in non-Fore individuals in other parts of the world (Horoupian et al, 1972).

Gerstmann-Straussler-Sheinker Disease (GSSD)

GSSD, also known as Gerstmann-Straussler disease, Straussler's disease, and spinocerebellar ataxia with dementia and plaque-like deposits, is a disease first described clinically by Gerstmann in 1928. Later the pathology of the propositus and clinical information on seven affected family members was reported by Gerstmann, Straussler, and Sheinker (quoted from Masters et al, 1981a). The patients manifested a cerebellar syndrome and dementia; at autopsy they were found to have distinctive plaque-like structures in the cerebellum and to a lesser extent in the brainstem and cerebrum. The disease was assumed to be a heredofamilial degenerative disorder until 1981 when Masters and colleagues showed that inoculation of brain material from affected individuals into spider and squirrel monkeys was followed in 20 to 30 months by development of a typical spongiform encephalopathy similar to that of Jakob-Creutzfeldt disease.

GSSD typically begins between age 40 and 70 and progresses to death in 4 to 10 years. Most cases are familial and exhibit a pattern consistent with autosomal dominant inheritance, although sporadic cases have been observed (Farlow et al, 1989; Masters et al, 1981a; Pearlman et al, 1988). Ataxia, lack of coordination, dysarthria, supranuclear gaze palsy, and impaired smooth pursuit eye movements are usually prominent early in the clinical course, and parkinsonian features have been reported in several families. Muscle stretch reflexes are typically diminished, particularly in the lower limbs, but there is no peripheral neuropathy. Rigidity, Babinski signs, and bradykinesia become more pronounced as the disease progresses. Myoclonus is rare (Farlow et al, 1989; Kuzuhara et al, 1983; Pearlman et al, 1988).

Mental status changes become evident in the middle and late stages of the illness and include dementia, depression, and psychosis. Memory impairment, psychomotor retardation, mild naming disturbances, disorientation, and poor judgment are the principal features of the dementia syndrome (Farlow et al, 1989).

X-ray CT scans are normal or reveal cerebellar atrophy. T_2-weighted MRIs demonstrate cerebellar atrophy and lucencies in the caudate, putamen, pallidum, substantia nigra, and red nucleus (Farlow et al, 1989). In most cases, EEG studies have been unremarkable or show only mild slowing.

At autopsy, neuronal loss, gliosis, and spongiform change are noted in the brains of GSSD patients. The most remarkable pathological feature of GSSD is the occurrence of amyloid plaques often surrounded by smaller daughter plaques but without the halo of degenerating neuritis typical of DAT. The plaques are not immunodecorated by polyclonal antibodies against the protein of DAT amyloid plaques but do contain epitopes recognized by antibodies directed against prion protein (Ghetti et al, 1989). The plaques are most abundant in the cerebellum but are seen throughout the neuraxis (Hudson et al, 1983; Masters et al, 1981a; Vinters et al, 1986). Neurofibrillary tangles are present in the neurons in some GSSD patients.

Alper's Disease

Alper's disease is a progressive dementing illness of infants and children. It was recently shown to be transmissible to laboratory animals where it produces a spongiform encephalopathy (Manuelidis and Rorke, 1989). The disease is characterized clinically by loss of developmental milestones and seizures. At autopsy, the principal histologic alterations include spongiform changes with marked vacuolation of the neuropil, neuronal loss, and astrocytic proliferation (Manuelidis, and Rorke, 1989).

Subacute Sclerosing Panencephalitis (SSPE)

SSPE, also known as subacute sclerosing leukoencephalitis and Dawson's encephalitis, is a slow virus dementia produced by measles virus that occurs in children and adolescents. The principal clinical features are intellectual deterioration, myoclonus, and a characteristic burst-suppression EEG pattern (Weil, 1974). The disease usually has its onset between ages 5 and 15, although occasional cases with onset in the early 20s have been recorded. More boys than girls are affected and the disease usually leads to death in 3 to 10 months (Haddad et al, 1977; Lorand et al, 1962; Osetowska and Torck, 1962; Weil, 1974). Fulminating cases lasting only a few months and chronic relapsing cases lasting 8 to 10 years have been reported (Dubois-Dalcq et al, 1974; Gilden et al, 1975; Landau and Luse, 1958; Silva et al, 1981).

Clinical Features

The disease course progresses through three stages. Initially there are behavioral changes and intellectual deterioration; myoclonus occurs late in the first stage. In the second phase there is further intellectual impairment along with extrapyramidal disturbances, rigidity, and cortical blindness. In the final stages, intellectual impairment is profound, and there is hypothalamic dysfunction and decerebrate posturing (Freeman, 1969; Weil, 1974). Although the clinical course is reasonably stereotyped, variations of the common sequence are not unusual (Risk and Haddad, 1979).

The earliest behavioral changes include an insidious decrease in school performance, forgetfulness, disobedience, and outbursts of temper. Distractibility, sleeplessness, and hallucinations may occur (Freeman, 1969). As the disease progresses, disturbances in writing, reading, and visuomotor performance and constructional impairment become evident. Dressing disturbances, apraxia, agnosia, and Balint's syndrome may be seen (Begeer et al, 1986; Lorand et al, 1962).

The myoclonic jerks initially involve the head and subsequently spread to the trunk and limbs. There is a sudden flexion movement followed by a one- to two-second relaxation period. Initially they are infrequent, but as the disease advances the myoclonus occurs every 5 to 15 seconds (Freeman, 1969; Weil, 1974). With further progression, extrapyramidal disorders occur. There is an expressionless face, paucity of spontaneous movement, and appearance of dystonic movements. Athetosis and/or chorea are occasionally observed. Decerebrate rigidity becomes manifest in the final phase of illness. Papilledema, chorioretinitis, cortical blindness, and abnormal eye movements occur in some patients (Freeman, 1969; Vignaendra et al, 1978). Terminally death results from aspiration pneumonia or irreversible autonomic abnormalities.

Laboratory Evaluation

Results of routine blood, serum, and urine studies are unremarkable. Special techniques reveal an increased level of measles antibodies (Weil, 1974). CSF may have a slightly elevated protein content and minimal pleocytosis. The concentration of immunoglobulin G in the CSF is strikingly increased and may account for up to 60 percent of the protein concentration. The abnormal globulins have been shown to be produced within the central nervous system (Cutler et al, 1967; Tourtellotte et al, 1981).

The EEG is particularly helpful in confirming the diagnosis of SSPE. Nearly all patients develop periodic high-amplitude complexes with the following characteristics: (1) They are bilateral, usually synchronous, and symmetric; (2) they are remarkably stereotyped; (3) they usually consist of two or more delta waves and are diphasic, triphasic, or polyphasic; (4) the amplitude of the complexes is usually around 500 μV; (5) the complexes repeat every four to five seconds; and (6) when myoclonus is present, there is a one-to-one relationship between the jerks and the EEG complexes (Cobb, 1966; Markand and Panszi, 1975). The periodic complexes may be more evident during sleep or in response to afferent stimuli in some patients (Westmoreland et al, 1977, 1979). Evoked potential studies may be useful in confirming the clinical impression of cortical blindness (Celesia, 1973).

X-ray CT in SSPE demonstrates cortical atrophy, cerebellar and brainstem atrophy, ventricular enlargement, and lucency of the hemispheric white matter (Krawiecki et al, 1984). MRI reveals high signal areas on T_2-weighted scans, particularly in the subcortical basal ganglion areas most affected by the disease (Huber et al, 1989a). Glucose metabolism, assessed with PET, is notable for early subcortical hypermetabolism and cortical hypometabolism followed by a more generalized increase in glucose metabolism later in the course (Huber et al, 1989a).

Etiology and Pathology

SSPE is produced by a conventional paramyxovirus that is similar to or identical with measles virus. In addition to high serum and CSF measles antibody titers, measles antigen and measles-specific IgG have been identified in the brain, and measles virus has been isolated from brain biopsy tissue of patients suffering from SSPE (Adams, 1976; Mehta et al, 1978). Reduction in measles-virus specific cytotoxic T lymphocytes and consequent impairment in cell-mediated immunity to the organism may account for the postinfectious persistence and late recrudescence of the virus in SSPE patients (Dhib-Jalbut et al, 1989).

Grossly the brain may appear normal or slightly atrophic. On microscopic examination, there are abnormalities of variable intensity in both gray and white matter of all levels of the central neuraxis. Perivascular spaces in the gray and white matter are infiltrated with lymphocytes and plasma cells. Where the cortex is severely affected there is neuron loss and astrocytic and microglial hyperplasia. Neurofibrillary tangles are seen in cortical and subcortical neurons, and type A intranuclear inclusion bodies are seen in neurons and oligodendroglial cells (Adams, 1976; Mandybur et al, 1977). The intensity of involvement of the white matter is variable, and gliosis is much more conspicuous than is myelin destruction (Adams, 1976; Lorand et al, 1962).

Treatment

Remissions and plateau periods are not unusual in SSPE, making it difficult to determine the effect of treatment on the natural history of the disorder. No therapeutic agent has been found that completely reverses or cures SSPE, but length of survival and induction of temporary remissions seem to be increased by both amantadine (Robertson et al, 1980) and isoprinosine (Dyken et al, 1982; Haddad and Risk, 1980; Huttenlocher and Mattson, 1979; Streletz and Cracco, 1977). A trial of these agents is indicated in any patient with SSPE. Intraventricular interferon may produce a temporary remission in some patients (Panitch et al, 1986). Efforts should also be directed to family counseling and preventing complications of chronic debility.

Progressive Rubella Panencephalitis

Progressive rubella panencephalitis is a subacute viral encephalitis that is clinically similar to SSPE. It usually occurs in children or young adults with congenital rubella but has been reported as a late complication of childhood rubella (Wolinsky et al, 1976). The disease typically has its onset between the ages of 10 and 12 and pursues a course of gradual neurologic deterioration, terminating in death in 2 to 5 years. Intellectual deterioration, ataxia, spasticity, and seizures are the principal clinical features (Townsend et al, 1975; Weil et al, 1975). Rubella antibody titers are usually elevated in the serum and CSF, and the CSF has increased protein content and gamma globulin (Coyle and Wolinsky, 1981). EEGs reveal generalized slowing without the classic burst-suppression pattern observed in SSPE. Rubella virus has been isolated from the brains of affected patients (Cremer et al, 1975; Weil et al, 1975). At autopsy, there is widespread destruction of white matter with loss of myelin, axonal fragmentation, gliosis, and perivascular lymphocytes and plasma cells. In the cortex, there is diffuse neuron loss and intracortical gliosis. The brainstem and cerebellum are similarly involved. Amorphous perivascular deposits are present in the white matter, but no intranuclear inclusion bodies are present (Townsend et al, 1976, 1982). No treatment is currently available for progressive rubella panencephalitis.

Progressive Multifocal Leukoencephalopathy (PML)

PML is a progressive subacute viral disorder produced by papova viruses and occurring primarily in patients with chronic lymphoproliferative, myeloproliferative, or granulomatous diseases (Richardson, 1970) and in immunocompromised individuals (Krupp et al, 1985).

Clinical characteristics

PML is a disease of adults who are suffering from an underlying systemic illness. Typically the predisposing condition has been present for months or years before the onset of the viral encephalopathy. The disease usually progresses to death in 2 to 4 months, but cases lasting 6 to 12 months or even longer and occasional patients with remissions have been observed. The disease has rarely been observed in children with immunodeficiency disorders or in adults with AIDS (Krupp et al, 1985; Zu Rhein et al, 1978). Table 6–5 lists the conditions that have been associated with PML. The most common underlying disorders are AIDS, chronic lymphocytic leukemia, Hodgkin's disease, lymphosarcoma, chronic myelocytic leukemia, sarcoidosis, and tuberculosis (Levy et al, 1988; Richardson, 1970, 1974). Less commonly associated conditions are other lymphoproliferative, myeloproliferative, and granulomatous diseases as well as carcinomatosis, SLE, asthma, liver cirrhosis, hepatosplenomegaly, diabetes mellitus, nontropical sprue, and long-term immunosuppressive treatment (Kepes et al, 1975; Mathews et al, 1976; Richardson, 1970; Sponzilli et al, 1975).

The lesions of PML are distributed randomly in the nervous system and the resulting clinical manifestations are highly variable. Changes in mental status have included behavioral alterations, impaired memory, poor

TABLE 6–5.   Diseases associated with progressive multifocal
leukoencephalopathy.

Lymphoproliferative diseases	Miscellaneous conditions
Chronic lymphocytic leukemia	Acquired immunodeficiency
Hodgkin's disease	syndrome (AIDS)
Plasmacytoma (multiple myeloma)	Carcinomatosis
Reticulum cell sarcoma	Systemic lupus erythematosus
Myeloproliferative diseases	Chronic asthma
Chronic myelocytic leukemia	Liver cirrhosis (with
Acute myelocytic leukemia	hypergammaglobulinemia)
Polycythemia vera	Hepatosplenomegaly (with acute
Non-neoplastic granulomotoses	necrosis of liver and spleen)
Sarcoidosis	Diabetes mellitus
Tuberculosis	Chronic immunosuppressive therapy
Pulmonary anthracosilicosis	in rheumatoid arthritis
Primary hypersplenism	Nontropical sprue (with anemia and
Whipple's disease	hypoproteinemia)
	No relevant disease

Modified from EP Richardson, Jr, Progressive multifocal leukoencephalopathy, In: PJ Vinken, GW Bruyn, eds. *Multiple sclerosis and other demyelinating diseases, Vol. 9, Handbook of clinical neurology.* New York: American Elsevier, 1970:485–499.

concentration, language disturbances, and cognitive decline. Hemiparesis, ataxia, dysarthria, and visual disorders are common elemental neurologic signs. Extrapyramidal disorders and ocular motor disturbances occur in some cases. Progressive dementia, blindness, and impaired motility characterize the advanced stages (Locke, 1973; Richardson, 1970; Woolsey and Nelson, 1965).

No specific abnormalities are found on examination of serum, blood, or urine. A mild elevation of protein or slight pleocytosis may be present in the CSF. No specific EEG changes occur, but there is progressive slowing and multifocal abnormalities may be evident (Farrell, 1969; Richardson, 1970, 1974).

X-ray CT demonstrates areas of lucency in the cerebral white matter. There is little mass effect, and the involved areas do not enhance with contrast agent administration (Krupp et al, 1985). MRIs show multifocal high signal regions in the hemispheric white matter (Jarvik et al, 1988; Kiyosawa et al, 1988). PET studies measuring glucose metabolism reveal multifocal areas of diminished cortical activity at sites related to the underlying white matter changes (Kiyosawa et al, 1988).

Etiology and Pathology

Electron microscopic and fluorescent antibody-staining techniques have led to identification of papova viruses in brain tissue of patients suffering from PML. Simian virus 40 (SV40) and JC virus are the papova viruses found in most cases (Adams, 1976; Narayan et al, 1973; Woodhouse et al, 1967). These viruses do not usually cause disease in humans; the underlying systemic illness appears to compromise the immunocompetence of the host sufficiently to release the pathogenicity of the viral agents.

Externally the brains appear normal or are slightly atrophic. Coronal sections reveal multiple small gray foci distributed widely and asymmetrically, occurring in small groups or coalescing to form cystic areas. The foci are present in both gray and white matter but are much more apparent in the latter. The cerebral hemispheres, brainstem, and cerebellum are affected. The most striking feature on microscopic examination is the presence of abnormal oligodendrocytes. The oligodendrocyte nuclei are large and hyperchromatic, have abnormal chromatin, and contain intranuclear inclusions. Bizarre, multinucleate astrocytes are also found in the lesions. There is demyelination with relative preservation of axons in the involved focus. Neurons are largely spared. Perivascular inflammatory changes are absent or minimal (Adams, 1976; Mancall, 1965; Richardson, 1970). Oligodendrocytes stain intensely with antisera directed at the papova virus (Itoyama et al, 1982).

Treatment

There is controversy over the treatment of PML. Several patients improved following cytarabine therapy (Bauer et al, 1973; Conomy et al, 1974) whereas others continued to deteriorate (Smith et al, 1982; Van Horn et al, 1978). Adenine arabinoside and transfer factor had no impact on the course of the disease (Rand et al, 1977; Van Horn et al, 1978); iododeoxyuridine administered intraventricularly maintained one patient without progression during the period of treatment, but the patient eventually relapsed (Tarsy et al, 1973). Further clinical trials with these antiviral agents are needed before their efficacy can be determined.

Limbic Encephalitis (Paraneoplastic Encephalomyelitis)

Limbic encephalitis is a syndrome of progressive intellectual impairment occurring in patients harboring an occult or apparent carcinoma. Oat cell carcinoma of the lung is the most common underlying malignancy, but the syndrome has been described with a variety of neoplasms and occasionally none has been found (Brierley et al, 1960; Corsellis et al, 1968; Henson et al, 1965; Langston et al, 1975). Although intranuclear inclusion bodies indicative of viral disease have been identified in a few cases (Dayan et al, 1967), they are not present in most patients, and a viral etiology of this syndrome is suspected but not definitely established (Dorfman and Forno, 1972; Shapiro, 1976). The syndrome is discussed in more detail in Chapter 7.

Herpes Encephalitis and Postencephalitic Dementias

Herpes simplex encephalitis is an acute viral encephalitis that typically produces mental status changes, focal neurologic signs, seizures, and coma. Untreated cases have a high mortality (Drachman and Adams, 1962; Rawls et al, 1966). Pathologically the medial temporal and orbitofrontal regions are severely damaged, and the cortex is more involved than is the white matter. Lymphocytic infiltration of the meninges, perivascular aggregation of inflammatory cells, and intranuclear Cowdry type A inclusion bodies in neurons, astrocytes, and oligodendrocytes are seen (Drachman and Adams, 1962). Diffuse or focal slowing may be evident on the EEG, and some patients show periodic, stereotyped sharp- and slow-wave complexes (Ch'ien et al, 1977; Illis and Taylor, 1972; Smith et al, 1975; Upton and Gumpert, 1970). The X-ray CT scan may demonstrate areas of lucency in the temporal lobes (Kaufman et al, 1979). Treatment with adenine arabinoside decreases mortality and improves the outcome (Whitley et al, 1977, 1981).

The onset of herpes encephalitis is acute, lasting at most a few days, and is not likely to be misdiagnosed as dementia. Neurologic sequelae are not unusual, however, and dementia can be a long-term consequence of the disease. Amnesia is the most common intellectual residual and reflects the propensity of herpes encephalitis to involve the medial temporal lobe structures (Drachman and Adams, 1962; Rose and Symonds, 1960). Aphasia is not uncommon during the recovery phase and may be a permanent deficit; the Klüver-Bucy syndrome is evident in some patients with severe bilateral damage of the temporal lobe (Lilly et al, 1982; Marlowe et al, 1975; Shoji et al, 1979). Neuropsychological testing may reveal more subtle deficits in cognitive functions (Rennick et al, 1973; Taber et al, 1977). In some patients, intellect appears to recover completely whereas in others there is a permanent dementia. In rare cases, there is a subacute onset and more gradual progression over several months (Sage et al, 1985).

Other Viral Encephalitides

Almost any of the viral encephalitides can give rise to a postencephalitic dementia. Younger children and infants are the most likely to have permanent sequelae, but older children and adults sometimes show permanent intellectual impairment. Dementia is uncommon but in many cases is a transient feature of the recovery process of adults. Intellectual deficits have been observed in the postencephalitic stages of western equine encephalitis, eastern equine encephalitis, Japanese encephalitis, and St. Louis encephalitis (Bailey and Baker, 1958; Fulton and Burton, 1953; Herzon et al, 1957; Mulder et al, 1951).

TABLE 6–6.   Varieties of chronic meningitis that can present as dementia.

Fungal	Parasitic (protozoan and helminthic)
Cryptococcus	Malaria *(Plasmodium falciparum)*
Coccidioides	Cysticercosis
Histoplasmosis	Cerebral coenurosis
Candida	Toxoplasmosis
Blastomyces	Chronic bacterial
Aspergillosis	*Mycobacterium tuberculosis*
Paracoccidioides	Whipple's disease
Dermatomycosis (chronomycosis)	Syphilis
Clodosporium	Brucellosis
Allescheria	Lyme disease *(borreliosis)*
Cephalosporium	
Sporothrix	
Actinomyces	
Nocardia	

Chronic Meningitis

Acute bacterial meningitis is a fulminating disorder with rapid onset that is not likely to be confused with a dementing process. Chronic meningitides, on the other hand, have an insidiously progressive course that slowly compromises intellectual function. Fluctuations in arousal, apathy, lethargy, impaired concentration, disorientation, and poor memory are among the usual mental status alterations. Focal signs such as aphasia, hemiparesis, and hemianopia may be present if vascular infiltration and occlusion occur or if the meningitis is secondary to parameningeal abscess formation. Cranial nerve abnormalities are common, and hydrocephalus occurs if CSF absorption is disturbed or interventricular communication is obstructed (Chapter 7). Papilledema, headache, stiff neck, and fever complete the clinical picture but may not always be present. Lymphocytic pleocytosis, hypoglycorrhachia, and increased protein content are noted in the CSF. Table 6–6 lists the fungal, parasitic, and bacterial meningitides that must be considered in the differential diagnosis of chronic infectious meningitis with dementia. The clinician must be particularly alert to the potential occurrence of these disorders in immunocompromised patients such as those with AIDS.

Chronic Fungal Meningitis

Cryptococcal meningitis (torulosis) is now the most common form of chronic meningitis in the United States. Half of the cases occur in patients with AIDS, systemic malignancies, renal failure, or other conditions associated with immunosuppression and chronic debilitation (Chernick et al, 1973; Ellner and Bennett, 1976; Mosberg and Arnold, 1950; Pons et al,

1988). Encapsulated yeast forms of *Cryptococcus neoformans* are visible in India ink preparations of CSF in only about 50 percent of cases, so definitive diagnosis often depends on detection of cryptococcal antigen in the CSF (Ellner and Bennett, 1976; Snow and Dismukes, 1975). Cryptococcal meningitis is treated with a combination of amphotericin B and flucytosine (Bennett, 1974; Bennett et al, 1979).

Coccidioidomycosis is a fungal infection that involves skin, subcutaneous tissue, bone, lungs, and CNS. The fungus is endemic in the southwestern United States, Mexico, Argentina, and Paraguay (Utz, 1971) and is known as valley fever or desert fever. In some patients, the preliminary symptoms may be slight and the disease manifests itself solely as a chronic meningitis (Caudill et al, 1970; Jenkins and Postlewaite, 1951; Norman and Miller, 1954).

Histoplasmosis is a systemic fungal infection that originates as a pulmonary infection and spreads to involve the CNS. The disease may progress insidiously, producing a chronic progressive dementia of 7 to 10 years' duration (Bellin et al, 1962; Tynes et al, 1963; Utz, 1964).

Candida fungi (monilia, thrush) are common organisms that usually produce lesions of the skin or mucous membranes. In some cases particularly in the immunocompromised patient, the fungus becomes widely disseminated and may cause a chronic meningitis with dementia (De Vita et al, 1966; Parrillo et al, 1962; Zimmerman et al, 1947).

Blastomycosis is a chronic systemic fungal disease that enters the body through the lungs and becomes widely distributed throughout. The disease occurs almost exclusively in North America from northern Latin America to Canada. Pulmonary infection or skin rash are the usual presenting features, but chronic meningitis may be the principal symptomatic manifestation in some cases (Friedman and Signorelli, 1946; Loudon and Lawson, 1961).

Aspergillus organisms rarely invade the lungs and disseminate, but in special circumstances particularly in patients with debilitating diseases or in those receiving immunosuppressant drugs, the fungus may reach the CNS and produce chronic meningitis (Burston and Blackwood, 1963; Mukoyama et al, 1969). Other fungi including *Paracoccidioides, Cladosporium, Allescheria, Cephalosporium, Sporothrix,* and *Nocardia* and diseases such as chromomycosis and actinomycosis have all been associated with chronic meningitis and concomitant mental status changes on rare occasions (Ellner and Bennett, 1976). In each, the abnormal CSF indicates the presence of an infectious agent, and special stains, cultures, or titers are necessary to determine the specific etiologic agent.

Chronic Parasitic (Protozoan and Helminthic) Meningitis

Several protozoan and helminthic parasitic agents are capable of producing a chronic meningitis with or without an associated cerebritis and vascular infiltration. *Plasmodium falciparum* malaria, cerebral cysticercosis, toxoplasmosis, amebiasis, and coenurosis are among the parasitic conditions that may invade the CNS and cause a dementia syndrome.

Cerebral malaria is not confined to meningitis but can also produce a disseminated inflammatory vasculomyelinopathy with brain edema, perivascular infiltrates, hemorrhages, demyelination, and gliosis. An allergic reaction has been suggested as the basis for the extensive pathologic changes (Toro and Roman, 1978). Cerebral malaria occurs with the *P. falciparum* variety of malarial infection and is completely reversible if antimalarial and steroid therapy is initiated early in the clinical course (Daroff et al, 1967).

Cerebral cysticercosis produces a chronic meningitis associated with parenchymal or intraventricular cysts. Cysticercosis cysts are the encapsulated larvae of *Taenia solium* and can be found in the cortex, meninges, ventricles, and brainstem. Cysticercosis is common in Mexico, South America, Asia, Spain, and eastern Europe. The disease presents with mental status changes, seizures, and symptoms of increased intracranial pressure. The CT scan frequently demonstrates the cysts. There is no effective medical therapy for cerebral cysticercosis, but surgical removal of accessible cysts may significantly ameliorate the course of the disease (Latovitzki et al, 1978; Rosselli et al, 1988; Trelles, 1961).

Chronic Bacterial Meningitis and Encephalitis

Bacterial meningitis is usually an obvious fulminating infection, but a few bacteria are capable of producing a chronic meningeal process with an insidious or subacute dementing syndrome (Udani and Dastur, 1970).

There is frequently a cerebritis associated with tuberculous meningitis. Alterations of consciousness, involuntary movements, and pyramidal, extrapyramidal, and cerebellar signs are the principal clinical manifestations. Prominent memory disturbances, alterations in personality, and impaired insight are the characteristic mental status changes (Williams and Smith, 1954). The CT scan may show contrast enhancement of the involved areas including the brainstem cisterns and parameningeal cortex (Arimitsu et al, 1979; Chu, 1980). In addition to pleocytosis, hypoglycorrhachia, and elevated protein content, the CSF may have identifiable acid-fast tubercle bacilli. Tuberculous meningitis was formerly uniformly fatal, but is now treatable and curable. Combination therapy with isoniazid, streptomycin, and para-aminosalicylic acid or isoniazid and rifampin are the current modes of therapy (Sahs and Joynt, 1981). Postmeningitic neurologic residua are not uncommon, but may be minimal if the disease is recognized and treatment initiated early in its course (Fitzsimons, 1963; Sahs and Joynt, 1981).

Whipple's disease is a rare multisystemic disease manifested by diarrhea and malabsorption, lymphadenopathy, arthritis, anemia, malaise, and fever. When the CNS is involved, there is an indolent inflammatory meningoencephalitis with dementia, supranuclear gaze paralysis, uveitis, myoclonus, and hypothalamic symptoms (Finelli et al, 1977; Koudouris et al, 1963). A number of patients have exhibited a unique oculomasticatory myorhythmia consisting of pendular oscillations of the eyes in concert with contractions of the masticatory muscles (Hausser-Hauw et al, 1988; Schwartz et al, 1986). Multiple low-density contrast-enhancing lesions may be seen on CT scan (Halperin et al, 1982). MRIs may be normal or may show areas of increased signal intensity in the region around the third ventricle including the hypothalamus, uncus, and medial temporal lobes (Adams et al, 1987; Schwartz et al, 1986). The infectious agent responsible for Whipple's disease has not been fully characterized, but bacilli have been identified in macrophages from involved cerebral regions (Romanul et al, 1977b). Pathologically, Whipple's disease is characterized by numerous minute ringlike lesions confined to the cerebral gray matter. The lesions stain deeply with periodic acid-Schiff (PAS) and are particularly evident in the cerebral cortical mantle. Astrocytic hyperplasia is present at the periphery of the lesion and moderate perivascular inflammatory infiltration is common (Lampert et al, 1962; Romanul et al, 1977b). If they are begun early, antibiotics may successfully halt progression of the disease (Feurle et al, 1979). Brain biopsy may be necessary for diagnosis if PAS-positive material is not demonstrated by lymph node or intestinal tract biopsies. Current therapeutic recommendations include a two-week course of parenteral antibiotics (procaine penicillin G plus streptomycin) followed by one year of oral trimethoprim-sulfamethoxazole (Fleming et al, 1988).

Table 6–7 gives the differential diagnosis of dementing disorders that

TABLE 6–7.   Dementias associated with supranuclear gaze palsies.

Progressive supranuclear palsy
Parkinson's disease
Huntington's disease
Corticobasal degeneration
Neuroacanthocytosis
Wilson's disease
Jakob-Creutzfeldt disease
Gerstmann-Straussler-Scheinker disease (GSSD)
Lipid storage diseases (including adult dystonic lipidosis)
Spinocerebellar degenerations
Ataxia telangiectasia
Whipple's disease
Progressive multifocal leukoencephalopathy
Neoplasms involving mesodiencephalic junction

Modified from PF Finelli et al, Whipple's disease with predominantly neuro-ophthalmic manifestations, Ann Neurol 1977;1:247–252.

TABLE 6–8.   Diseases that can produce dementia combined with uveitis.

Infections	Granulomatous disorders
Bacterial	Sarcoidosis
Syphilis	Wegener's granulomatosis
Brucellosis	Collagen-vascular diseases
Psitacosis	Systemic lupus erythematosus
Tuberculosis	Temporal arteritis
Whipple's disease	Polyarteritis nodosa
Parasitic	Rheumatoid arthritis
Toxoplasmosis	CNS malignancies
Amebiasis	Leukemia
Malaria	Metastatic carcinoma
Viral	Reticulum cell sarcoma
Rubeola	Other
Subacute sclerosing panencephalitis	Behçet's syndrome
Vaccinia	Multiple sclerosis
Fungal	Trauma
Aspergillosis	Vogt-Koyanagi-Harada syndrome
Candidiasis	Cogan's syndrome
Cryptococcosis	
Histoplasmosis	

Modified from Finelli et al., Whipple's disease with predominantly neuro-ophthalmic manifestations, Ann Neurol 1977;1:247–252.

may present with supranuclear gaze palsies, and Table 6–8 lists the dementing syndromes that may co-occur with uveitis (Finelli et al, 1977). These disorders must be considered in the differential diagnosis of Whipple's disease.

Lyme disease is a tick-transmitted spirochete infection produced by *Borrelia burgdorferi*. The manifestations of the illness are legion and include a gradually progressive dementia syndrome. Diagnosis is based on serologic tests; low density lesions may be evident on CT images (Reik et al, 1985; Steere, 1989). Neurobrucellosis can also produce a chronic demyelinating encephalopathy (Al Deeb et al, 1989). Other bacteria that may cause chronic meningitis particularly in the immunocompromised host include listeria and syphilis as well as mycobacteria species including *M avium-intracellulare, M kansasii,* and *M tuberculosis* (Pons et al, 1988).

Postmeningitic Dementia

Survivors of acute or chronic meningitis can have some degree of dementia as a permanent consequence of the infectious process. Postmeningitic sequelae are most frequent when the infection occurs in the first two months of life, but meningitis occurring in adolescence or adulthood can

TABLE 6–9.   Dementias associated with neurosyphilis.

General paresis
  Classic dementia paralytica
    Simple dementia
    Expansive, manic type
    Depressed type
    Paranoid, schizophrenia-like form
    Miscellaneous and unclassified forms
  Taboparesis
  Lissauer's dementia paralytica
  Juvenile paresis
Meningovascular syphilis
Symptomatic syphilitic meningitis
Single or multiple syphilitic gummas

produce residual neurologic deficits. The characteristics of the dementia are variable and reflect the pattern of cortical or subcortical involvement, the presence of associated infarctions, or the existence of hydrocephalus.

CNS Syphilis

Syphilis can involve the CNS in a variety of ways including asymptomatic meningitis, gummas, vascular neurosyphilis, symptomatic meningitis, general paresis, tabes dorsalis, and optic atrophy (Luxon et al, 1979; Schmidt and Gonyea, 1980). The forms of syphilis that can manifest as dementia include general paresis, meningovascular neurosyphilis, symptomatic syphilitic meningitis, and gummas (Table 6–9). The dementing processes frequently coexist with other CNS manifestations of the syphilitic infection.

    The infectious nature of syphilis was not established until Metschnikoff and Roux transmitted general paresis to chimpanzees in 1903. Schaudinn and Hoffman demonstrated the *Treponema pallidum* organism in 1905, the Wasserman test was developed 1906, and spirochetes in the brains of fatal cases of paresis were demonstrated by Noguchi and Moore in 1913 (Schmidt and Gonyea, 1980). *Treponema pallidum* is a spirochetal organism transmitted almost exclusively by direct contact with infectious lesions. Transient CNS invasion occurs in 50 to 60 percent of early untreated cases, but the permanent infestation necessary to produce late neurosyphilis is established in only 10 percent (Guthe, 1971; Hotson, 1981). The primary lesion is a chancre occurring at the site of contact. Six to eight weeks later, secondary luetic manifestations occur in the form of generalized lymphadenitis and cutaneous rash. Symptomatic syphilitic meningitis may occur in the early stages of syphilis, but that is unusual. Late syphilitic manifestations include neurosyphilis, skeletal lesions, and cardiovascular disorders (especially aortitis of the ascending aorta) (Guthe, 1971). Meningovascular syphilis becomes manifest 2 to 10 years after the initial infection; general paresis is evident 3 to 40 years following the infection; and tabes dorsalis appears 10 to 20 years after the original infection.

Laboratory diagnosis of neurosyphilis depends on detecting nonspecific reagin antibodies (Venereal Disease Research Laboratory [VDRL] test) and specific treponemal antibodies (fluorescent treponemal antibody absorption [FTA-abs]). The VDRL is a general screening test but is neither particularly sensitive nor specific. As many as one-third of patients with neurosyphilis may have nonreactive serum reagin tests (particularly patients with late syphilis), and the false positives occur in nonsyphilitic conditions such as collagen-vascular disease, after vaccinations and some viral infections, and during pregnancy (Hotson, 1981; Simon, 1985). The serum FTA-abs is more sensitive and more specific than is the VDRL. It has a false positive rate of less than 1 percent in celibate nuns and is positive in more than 97 percent of cases of neurosyphilis (Hotson, 1981; Schmidt and Gonyea, 1980). The CSF VDRL is more reliable than is the serum tests, but it may be nonreactive in rare cases. The CSF FTA-abs reflects the antibody activity of the serum. A CSF pleocytosis usually accompanies active neurosyphilis; the CSF protein is also elevated, and the percentage of gamma globulin is increased. Oligoclonal immunoglobulin G in the CSF appears to represent treponemal antibody manufactured in the CNS in response to the infectious agent (Vartdal et al, 1982). After successful treatment of neurosyphilis, both serum and CSF VDRL usually decline or eventually revert to normal, the pleocytosis subsides, and the CSF protein level returns to normal, but the FTA-abs may remain positive indefinitely (Jaffe, 1975; Schmidt and Gonyea, 1980).

Treatment of neurosyphilis has progressed from the administration of mercury, bismuth, or arsphenamines and deliberate inoculation with malaria to produce fever to the contemporary use of penicillin and other antibiotics. Recommendations concerning the appropriate dose of penicillin are constantly evolving, and current dosage schedules should be consulted prior to initiation of treatment. A standard recommendation has been weekly injections of 2.4 million units of benzathine penicillin G for 3 consecutive weeks (total dose of 7.2 million units) or 600,000 units of aqueous procaine penicillin G daily for 15 days (total dose of 9 million units) (Centers for Disease Control, 1976). Recommended doses of benzathine penicillin may not consistently achieve treponemicidal levels of penicillin in the CSF, however, and some authors recommend more aggressive dosage schedules (Ducas and Robson, 1981; Hotson, 1981). Schmidt and Gonyea (1980) suggest using 600,000 units of aqueous penicillin G given intramuscularly every 12 hours for 15 to 21 days. Simon (1985) recommends 12 to 24 million units of a nonbenzathine penicillin IV daily for 10 to 14 days. A Jarisch-Herxheimer reaction with transient elevation of temperature and exacerbation of neurologic disability may occur during the course of penicillin treatment. This is not an indication for discontinuing therapy and must be distinguished from a penicillin allergic reaction. The CSF and blood reagin tests should be checked every 3 months for the first year after treatment and every 6 months during the second year. Elevation of the CSF cell count or fourfold increase in the VDRL titer indicate that treatment should be repeated.

General Paresis

Prior to the introduction of penicillin, general paresis accounted for between 15 and 30 percent of all mental hospital admissions (Bruetsch, 1959). Since then, the occurrence of paresis has declined dramatically and is now diagnosed in less than one-tenth of one percent of psychiatric inpatients (Schmidt and Gonyea, 1980). The disease has not disappeared, however, and both early and late cases are still observed (Bockner and Coltart, 1961; Steel, 1960).

General paresis usually becomes evident 7 to 15 years after the initial infection and is insidiously progressive. Incubation periods as short as 3 years and as long as 40 years have been reported (Bruetsch, 1959). Ninety percent of patients are between the ages of 30 and 60, and men are more frequently affected than are women (Dodge, 1971). Although grandiose delusional manifestations have received the most attention, they are not the most common expression of paresis. Between 40 and 60 percent will have a "simple" dementia; 20 to 40 percent, the expansive manic variety; 6 percent, prominent depression; 3 to 6 percent, paranoid or schizophrenia-like manifestations; and the remainder, miscellaneous or unclassified characteristics (Bruetsch, 1959; Hahn et al, 1959; Kraepelin, 1913). A variety of intellectual impairments is present together with the neuropsychiatric features. The patients become inattentive and absent-minded, do not grasp events transpiring about them, and have impaired insight and judgment. Memory is disturbed; severely involved patients become disoriented and tend to confabulate. Kraepelin (1913) noted that the memory disorder is not as severe as in Korsakoff's psychosis and attributed the defect in recent memory to disturbed attention. Illusions and hallucinations are not uncommon, and apraxia is frequently present. Anomia and verbal paraphasia occur in some, and speech disturbances and logoclonia (repetition of the final few syllables of a word) may be prominent. The voice is monotonous and tremulous, and there may be visible tremors of the tongue and facial muscles. Articulation is disturbed, speech output may be hesitant, and abnormal contractions of multisyllabic words may occur. Pseudobulbar palsy with forced laughter occurs in some (Kraepelin, 1913). The face is frequently expressionless, coordination is impaired, and a hyperreflexic, spastic weakness of the limbs gradually progresses. Pupillary abnormalities occur in two-thirds of patients with general paresis, but the classic Argyll-Robertson pupillary change is found in a minority (Lishman, 1978; Schmidt and Gonyea, 1980). The reflexes are diminished, vibration and position sense are impaired, and lightning-like root pains occur if the patient is also suffering from tabes dorsalis (taboparesis). Examination of the eye may reveal chorioretinitis and/or optic atrophy (Walsh and Hoyt, 1969). Convulsions, sometimes called paralytic attacks, occur in many patients as the disease advances, and death in status epilepticus was not unusual prior to the advent of penicillin therapy.

Juvenile paresis occurs in children affected with congenital syphilis. Onset of symptoms may be between 6 and 21 years with a mean age of 13 years. Fifty to 80 percent have other stigmata of congenital luetic infection such as interstitial keratitis, chorioretinitis, defective (Hutchinson) teeth, saddle nose, saber shins, Clutton joints, or rhagades. The most prominent manifestations of paresis are regressive behavior, flat affect, cognitive impairment, and confusion (Bruetsch, 1959; Weil, 1974). Cerebellar signs, spasticity, and seizures occur in many patients.

Untreated cases coming to autopsy have thickened, opaque meninges covering an atrophic cortex. Atrophy is most pronounced in the frontal and temporal regions; the ventricular system is dilated. On microscopic examination, the cortical organization is disturbed, neurons are lost or diminished in size, and there is proliferation of astrocytes and microglial cells. *Treponema pallidum* organisms have been identified in appropriately stained sections of the brains of many patients and are most abundant in the frontal cortex. Inflammatory infiltrates surround the penetrating blood vessels, and perivascular deposits of iron are present in the cortex. The most prominent changes are found in the cortex with less advanced disturbances in the striatum and hypothalamus (Harriman, 1976; Schmidt and Gonyea, 1980). In taboparesis, the encephalitic changes are combined with fibrosis and inflammation of the posterior roots and demyelination of the posterior columns of the spinal cord. Lissauer's dementia paralytica is a rare form of dementia paralytica characterized clinically by prominent focal neurologic deficits and pathologically by a combination of paretic and vascular changes (Harriman, 1976; Merritt and Springlova, 1932).

Half of general paretics who receive adequate treatment show substantial improvement, and another 25 percent improve enough to return to the community. Prognosis is best for those with less severe cognitive deficit, younger age, and shorter duration of illness (Hahn et al, 1959; Schmidt and Gonyea, 1980).

Meningovascular Syphilis, Meningitis, and Gumma

Meningovascular syphilis begins 2 to 10 years after the original syphilitic infection and, like general paresis, affects more men than it does women.

It is now a rare cause of stroke but deserves consideration in the differential diagnosis of stroke syndromes including multi-infarct dementia. Gradual behavioral and personality changes frequently antedate the acute or subacute vascular event (Holmes et al, 1984). Pathologically meningovascular syphilis is an inflammatory arteritis with lymphocytic and plasma cell infiltrates in the vascular wall and adventitia. Hyperplasia of subintimal fibrous tissues narrows the vessel lumen and completes the picture of syphilitic (Heubner) arteritis. A CSF pleocytosis is invariably present and elevated protein and increased gamma globulin are almost always evident (Schmidt and Gonyea, 1980). Serologic diagnosis and treatment are the same as those for general paresis.

Syphilitic meningitis is rare and occurs in the first year of infection. Its manifestations are similar to those of other chronic meningitides, including headache, stiff neck, dementia, cranial nerve palsies, and focal neurologic signs. Intracranial pressure may be increased with resulting papilledema. Inflammatory infiltrates are found in the perivascular areas and leptomeninges. Exudate is present in the subarachnoid space and may occlude the basilar cisterns to produce noncommunicating obstructive hydrocephalus. The CSF pressure is elevated and there is mononuclear pleocytosis. Protein is elevated and glucose may be slightly decreased. Serologic tests are positive in serum and CSF. Spontaneous remission occurs in some cases, and treated patients respond promptly to antibiotic therapy (Dodge, 1971; Schmidt and Gonyea, 1980).

Gummas of the brain are now very rare but like other mass lesions may produce dementia when appropriately located. Frontal lobe gummas may cause prominent intellectual impairment with few focal motor or sensory signs. Gummas are usually solitary lesions 1.5 to 6 cm in diameter. They consist of a central necrotic area surrounded by a zone of fibroblasts and an outer core of collagenous fibers (Kaplan et al, 1981). Gummas are corticomeningeal, originating in the pia mater or perivascular extensions of the pia in the Virchow-Robin spaces. Results of CSF studies demonstrate pleocytosis, elevated protein, increased pressure, and positive antibody tests. Treatment includes both surgical removal of the gummas and antibiotic therapy (Oblu, 1975).

7

Dementia in Metabolic Disturbances and Toxic Conditions

Intellectual and emotional activities are undoubtedly the most complex and demanding functions performed by the brain and are the most sensitive to disruption by metabolic and toxic conditions. Although compensatory mechanisms have evolved to minimize the impact of variations in the supply of essential ingredients to the brain and to provide maximum stability to the internal milieu of the CNS, prolonged or recurrent interruption of the availability of metabolic substrates or extended exposure to cellular toxins will eventually compromise cellular function and produce an impairment of intellectual abilities. When the metabolic or toxic condition is acute and overwhelming, an acute confusional state results, and the major behavioral abnormality is a reduction or erratic shifting of attention. Slowness and sluggishness of response, disorientation in time and space, fluctuating arousal, changes in mood, and hallucinations frequently accompany the attention deficit (Chedru and Geschwind, 1972; Lipowski, 1983). When the metabolic disturbance or toxic exposure occurs slowly and insidiously, the corresponding cognitive change is a slowly progressive dementia. The characteristics of the dementia conform most closely to the intellectual disturbances produced by impaired subcortical function (Feldman and Cummings, 1981). Psychomotor retardation, memory impairment, dilapidation of cognition, and mood changes are prominent, and arousal and attention may be impaired. Word-finding abnormalities and misnaming may occur, but frank aphasias or agnosias indicative of cortical impairment are not present. Disturbances of

TABLE 7–1.   Principal metabolic conditions associated with dementia.

Conditions associated with anoxia	Porphyria
Anoxic anoxia	Cerebral effects of systemic malignancies
Pulmonary insufficiency	Metabolic changes
Stagnant anoxia	Structural abnormalities (mass
Cardiac disease	lesions, hydrocephalus)
Hyperviscosity states	CNS infections
Anemic anoxia	Remote effects–limbic encephalitis
Postanoxia dementia	Vitamin deficiency states
Chronic renal failure	Thiamine (B_1)
Uremic encephalopathy	Cyanocobalamin (B_{12})
Dialysis dementia	Folate
Hepatic diseases	Niacin
Portosystemic encephalopathy	Endocrinopathies
Acquired hepatocerebral degeneration	Thyroid disturbances
Pancreatic disorders	Parathyroid abnormalities
Insulinoma and recurrent	Adrenal diseases
hypoglycemia	Panhypopituitarism
Pancreatic encephalopathy	
Electrolyte abnormalities	
Hyponatremia	
Hypernatremia	

motor function including tremor, myoclonus, asterixis, choreoathetosis, tone changes, or bradykinesia may be prominent.

It is important to recognize the toxic or metabolic nature of a dementia syndrome so that timely intervention may restore or significantly improve intellectual function. Dementias associated with potentially reversible metabolic disorders may sometimes show little or no improvement when the underlying illness is correctly identified and treated (Barry and Moskowitz, 1988; Clarfield, 1988). Appropriate intervention, however, halts progression of the intellectual deterioration and may substantially alter the course of the illness. Moreover irreversible dementias may be complicated by superimposed medical conditions that exaggerate underlying cognitive abnormalities, and discovery and treatment of these concomitant disturbances improves intellectual function (Larson et al, 1984).

The number of systemic illnesses and environmental toxins that can impact cerebral function and impair mental abilities is enormous. In this chapter, we review the principal metabolic (Table 7–1) and toxic (Table 7–8) conditions that can present as a dementia syndrome or that have intellectual impairment as a major component.

METABOLIC DISTURBANCES

As was noted in Chapter 1, dementia is largely a problem of the elderly. The incidence of degenerative disorders of the cortex such as DAT and Pick's disease increases dramatically with age, and many of the subcortical degenerative processes such as Parkinson's disease and PSP appear predominantly or exclusively during the later stages of life. Cerebrovascular disease and cardiac disturbances that lead to multi-infarct dementia are rare in young individuals and become progressively more common with age. Similarly, the systemic illnesses that are associated with dementia are most prevalent in the elderly population. Eighty-six percent of individuals over the age of 65 years living in the community (not institutionalized) have at least one chronic illness, and 50 percent have two or more such illnesses (Jarvik and Perl, 1981; Levenson and Hall, 1981). The percentages are higher for persons residing in nursing homes. Jarvik and Perl (1981) found that only 13 percent of their elderly patients with moderate or severe dementia were free of diagnosed systemic illness. Thus, many elderly individuals are suffering from systemic disorders that may compromise intellectual function and produce or exacerbate dementia.

Failure to recognize the intellectual consequences of systemic disturbances may lead the clinician to overlook significant intellectual impairment. The clinician's attention is directed to the identified medical illness, and coexisting mental disturbances may go unrecognized and unaddressed. Use of simple mental status questionnaires, for example, reveals that 20 to 30 percent of all unselected patients admitted to general medical wards score in the impaired range, and the intellectual disturbances are unrecognized by one-third to one-half of the professional hospital staff (Fields et al, 1986; Jacobs et al, 1977; Knights and Folstein, 1977; Roca et al, 1984). On the other hand, when dementia is prominent, the clinician often assumes that the aged individual is suffering from irreversible "senile dementia" without thoroughly evaluating for an underlying physical disease that could account for the intellectual impairment. Furthermore, preexisting cognitive deficits may be exaggerated by concurrent physical illness, leading the physician to overestimate the severity of the dementing process.

Once a systemic process is recognized and treatment is initiated, the impact of therapeutic agents on cognitive function must also be recognized, and the fact that many commonly used drugs can produce or exacerbate dementia must be borne in mind. The dementias associated with systemic diseases and those produced by drugs are discussed separately in this chapter, but the two often appear in conjunction.

TABLE 7–2.   Causes of cerebral anoxia associated with dementia.

Anoxic anoxia	Anemic anoxia
Chronic pulmonary disease	Postanoxic dementia
High-altutude hypoxia	Following cardiopulmonary arrest
Sleep apnea	Folowing carbon monoxide poisoning
Stagnant anoxia	Following strangulation or hanging
Ischemic disturbances	Following anaesthetic accidents
Congestive cardiac failure	Delayed demyelination syndrome
Persistent cardiac arrhythmias	
Hyperviscosity and hypercoaguable	
states	
Polycythemia vera	
Hyperproteinemias	
Hyperlipidemia	

Chronic Anoxia

Chronic cerebral anoxia produces a dementia syndrome. Anoxic anoxia resulting from insufficient oxygenation of the blood, ischemic (stagnant) anoxia secondary to inadequate cerebral perfusion, and anemic anoxia caused by poor oxygen-carrying capacity can all embarrass cerebral metabolism and compromise intellectual function (Table 7–2).

Chronic Pulmonary Insufficiency and Anoxic Anoxia

Dementia is occasionally the principal manifestation of pulmonary disease (Cummings et al, 1980a), and neuropsychological testing of affected individuals reveals that reversible intellectual deficits are common (Greenberg et al, 1985; Krop et al, 1973). Tremulousness and asterixis are frequent accompaniments of chronic pulmonary encephalopathy, although specific testing may be required to reveal their presence (Conn, 1958; Leavitt and Tyler, 1964).

When continuous oxygen deprivation and carbon dioxide retention are severe, dementia may occur as part of a more extensive syndrome consisting of headache, papilledema, tremor and twitching of the extremities, and signs of cardiac and pulmonary decompensation (Austen et al, 1957; Bacchus, 1958; Carter and Fuller, 1957; Hamilton and Gross, 1963). Mental status changes include inattentiveness, drowsiness, lethargy, and forgetfulness. Slowness is apparent, and most patients are disoriented. Chronic hypoxia, hypercapnia, and CSF acidosis have been implicated as etiologically significant factors in producing the neurologic syndrome (Austen et al, 1957; Bulger et al, 1966). The clinical and metabolic abnormalities reverse with improved pulmonary function.

Long-term lack of oxygen at high altitudes may also lead to cognitive impairment (Lishman, 1978). Mountain climbers ascending summits higher than 6500 meters without supplementary oxygen may manifest persistent defects in concentration, memory, naming, mental control, and shifting of mental set (Hornbein et al, 1989; Regard et al, 1989).

Sleep apnea with recurrent nocturnal oxygen desaturation and hyercapnea may also be associated with a chronic confusional-type dementia syndrome. Both the chronic hypoxia and sleep deprivation may contribute to reversible mental status changes (Riley, 1989). Sleep apnea may also increase the risk of vascular dementia through hypertension and cardiac arrhythmias.

Chronic Cardiac Disease and Stagnant Anoxia

Ischemic (stagnant) anoxia secondary to chronic cardiac insufficiency can also lead to a reversible dementia. The brain represents only 2 percent of the total body weight but it receives 15 percent of the cardiac output and accounts for 20 percent of total body oxygen consumption (Hall, 1981; Sokoloff, 1976). Any interruption of the flow of oxygenated blood to the brain will have deleterious effects on mental function. Chronic cardiac encephalopathy may be secondary to congestive heart failure or sustained arrhythmias with impaired cardiac output (Cummings et al, 1980a; Dalessio et al, 1965; Lishman, 1978). The principal clinical characteristics are inanition, irritability, disorientation, impaired memory, and somnolence. The deficits are reversible with improved cardiac function.

Reversible dementia syndromes may occasionally be associated with stagnant anoxia produced by hyperviscosity and hypercoagulable states such as Waldenström's macroglobulinemia, hyperlipidemia, and polycythemia vera (Heilman and Fisher, 1974; Johnson and Chalgren, 1950; Logothetis et al, 1960; Mas et al, 1985; Mathew et al, 1976; Mueller et al, 1983).

Anemia (Anemic Anoxia)

Anemic anoxia, like anoxic and stagnant anoxia, can cause dementia. Low hemoglobin concentration with impaired oxygen-carrying capacity and cerebral anoxia produces intellectual impairment, poor attention, emotional lability, restlessness, and myoclonus. The anemia may be caused by chronic low-grade blood loss, hemoglobinopathies, failure of normal erythropoiesis, or excessive red cell destruction (Haruda et al, 1981; Lishman, 1978). Correction of the anemia and restoration of normal cerebral oxygenation usually reverse the deficit.

Anemic anoxia, stagnant anoxia, and anoxic anoxia, even when they are relatively minor, may all co-occur leading to diminished oxygen availability and intellectual impairment. These conditions should be carefully considered in the elderly individual with dementia since relatively simple measures may improve cognitive function.

Postanoxic Dementia

When oxygen deprivation has been acute and profound, injury to, or death of, neurons may occur, and return of function takes place slowly or not at all when tissue oxygenation is restored. The anoxic insult may result from cardiopulmonary arrest, carbon monoxide intoxication, strangulation, or hanging.

Three categories of postanoxic encephalopathy can be identified. The first and most severe is brain death. In these cases, anoxia is so profound as to destroy all neuronal activity, and bodily functions continue only if maintained by external support (Adams et al, 1966; Neubuerger, 1954; Walker et al, 1975). The second category is characterized by return of the autonomous respiratory and circulatory functions governed by brainstem mechanisms without evidence of higher cortical activity. The patients breathe spontaneously, their eyes may be open, and diurnal variation in eye opening may even be present. Patients may remain in this persistent vegetative state for many years, with death from aspiration pneumonia the usual outcome, but rare cases with late recovery of cognitive function have occurred (Brierley et al, 1971; Dougherty et al, 1981; Jennett and Plum, 1972; Rosenberg et al, 1977). Persistent vegetative state is to be distinguished from akinetic mutism where arousal is maintained but volitional activity is absent, and from locked-in syndrome in which the patient is cognitively intact but paralyzed and anarthric.

The third category of postanoxic encephalopathy is a dementia syndrome with sufficient cortical function to support partial cognitive activity. The severity of postanoxic dementia and the eventual degree of recovery vary greatly. Aphasia, visuospatial disorientation, constructional disturbances, memory disorders, acalculia, and impaired abstraction may be combined with spasticity, paresis, ataxia, and pseudobulbar palsy (Allison et al, 1956; Bell and Hodgson, 1974; Garland and Pearce, 1967; Norris and Chandrasekar, 1971; Richardson et al, 1959). In some cases, a more mild syndrome consisting of memory impairment, apathy, disinhibition, and poor judgment may occur (Reich et al, 1983). Patients coming to postmortem examination usually have widespread anoxic cerebral cortical changes although in a few cases lesions of white matter predominate.

Delayed demyelination is a rare dementing syndrome that occasionally follows an anoxic cerebral insult. The patient recovers from the initial event and improves for 10 to 14 days. Deterioration then begins, leading to death or eventual stabilization and partial recovery. At autopsy, diffuse demyelination is present in the cerebral hemispheres (Dooling and Richardson, 1976; Plum et al, 1962).

TABLE 7–3.   Differential diagnosis of mental status changes in chronic renal failure.

Chronic renal failure
  Uremic encephalopathy
  Electrolyte imbalance
  Anemia
  Hypertensive encephalopathy
  Hypertensive cerebrovascular disease (multi-infarct dementia)
  Hypertensive cardiovascular disease
  Drug accumulation
  CNS effects of underlying disease (lupus, amyloidosis, and so on)
Chronic renal failure with dialysis
  Dialysis dementia
  Subdural hematoma
  Emboli from Scribner shunt
  Disequilibrium syndrome
  Wernicke-Korsakoff syndrome (thiamine depletion)
Chronic renal failure with transplantation and immunosuppression
  Steroid psychosis
  Progressive multifocal leukoencephalopathy
  Chronic meningitis
  Viral encephalitis
  Brain tumors (reticuloendothelial neoplasms)

Chronic Renal Failure

Many conditions associated with chronic renal failure produce a dementia syndrome. Table 7–3 tabulates the major disturbances that occur in patients with renal insufficiency and impair intellectual abilities. Some clinical disorders are associated with the consequences of the renal failure; others are associated with dialysis or transplantation and immunosuppression.

Uremia (Uremic Encephalopathy)

Chronic renal failure is the end product of many different disorders including glomerulonephritis, pyelonephritis, polycystic renal disease, urinary tract obstruction, malignant hypertension, arteritis and granulomatous diseases, amyloidosis, diabetes, and renal toxins (Kerr, 1971). Disruption of renal function results in a variety of metabolic abnormalities, including elevation of blood urea nitrogen (BUN), accumulation of serum creatinine, hyponatremia, hypovolemia, hyperkalemia, hypermagnesemia, metabolic acidosis, hypocalcemia, and other less easily identified changes. The resulting mental status alterations include fatigue, apathy, drowsiness, poor concentration, erratic memory, irritability, hallucinations, and paranoia (Ginn,

1975; Schreiner, 1959). Memory impairment, disorientation, and mood changes are common (Glaser, 1974; Raskin and Fishman, 1976; Tyler, 1968b). Disturbances of motor system function occur in most patients and include increased muscle tone, asterixis, myoclonus, and/or limb tremor. Convulsions occur late in the clinical course (Raskin and Fishman, 1976; Tyler, 1968b). Peripheral neuropathy may occur relatively early in the disease and worsen as renal function deteriorates (Avram et al, 1978; Dyck et al, 1971; Jebsen et al, 1967).

The EEG is conspicuously abnormal in uremia and is a good index of changes in renal function. The most frequently observed changes are disorganization and slowing of the background rhythm. Bursts of paroxysmal, bilaterally synchronous slow waves are also seen (Jacob et al, 1965). The CT scans show enlarged ventricles in end-stage uremia (Passer, 1977).

The differential diagnosis of uremic encephalopathy includes electrolyte imbalance, anemia, CNS compromise by associated cardiovascular disease, and the effects of underlying disorders—hypertension, arteritis, diabetes, and so on. The accumulation of potentially toxic drugs must also be considered and guarded against (Gibson, 1979; Taclob and Needle, 1976). Patients receiving dialysis or those treated with immunosuppressants following transplantation are subject to additional disorders that may impair mental status (reviewed below).

Dialysis and Dialysis Dementia

Dialysis dementia is a fatal neurologic syndrome occurring in patients receiving chronic hemodialysis for treatment of renal failure. It is characterized by progressive intellectual deterioration, distinctive speech abnormalities, myoclonus, and markedly abnormal EEGs (Alfrey et al, 1972; Burks et al, 1976; Lederman and Henry, 1978; Mahurkar et al, 1973; Raskin and Fishman, 1976).

Dialysis dementia (also called dementia dialytica and progressive dialysis encephalopathy) was first reported in 1972 and has since been described from hemodialysis centers around the world. The disease is independent of the cause of the renal failure, the patient's age, or the type of hemodialysis used. Most victims have received dialysis for three to four years at the time of onset although some patients have been treated for as little as nine months or as long as six years (Burks et al, 1976; Lederman and Henry, 1978). The duration of the dialysis dementia is usually between 3 and 12 months with some patients dying within a month and some surviving for as long as 2 years (Burks et al, 1976; Chokroverty et al, 1976; Lederman and Henry, 1978; Weddington, 1978). The first symptoms often appear immediately after a dialysis treatment, and early in the course of the disease transient worsening frequently occurs following dialysis (Lederman and Henry,

1978; Raskin and Fishman, 1976). Death occurs from respiratory arrest after development of a terminal comatose state.

The mental status abnormalities in dialysis dementia appear early in the illness and may be flagrant or remain relatively mild until the terminal stages. Neuropsychiatric symptoms including agitation, paranoid delusions, hallucinations, and bizarre behavior are common during the course of the syndrome (Chokroverty et al, 1976). Intellectual alterations with impaired naming, inattention, forgetfulness, apathy, and perseveration become evident as the disease progresses. Several authors have commented on the presence of what they called apraxia or dyspraxia, but neither term was defined, and the nature of the disability referred to is not clear (Alfrey et al, 1972; Burks et al, 1976).

Speech disturbances are the most distinctive findings in dialysis dementia and are often the earliest to appear. At first, they may occur transiently following dialysis and may antedate any other aspects of the syndrome by several months (Lederman and Henry, 1978). Typically the speech difficulty begins as a stutter. Progressive difficulty with initiation and articulation of speech occurs and temporary periods of anarthria may progress to complete mutism. Measured or syllable-by-syllable speech may be present and sentence production is more impaired than is single word production. Speech abnormalities are more prominent than are language changes, but word-finding difficulties, impaired naming, poor auditory comprehension, occasional paraphasia, and mispellings of written language occur as the disease advances (Baratz and Herzog, 1980; Madison et al, 1977; Rosenbek et al, 1975).

Myoclonus occurs in most patients with dialysis dementia. It may be multifocal, involving the face and limbs independently, or synchronous myoclonic jerks may involve several body areas. Facial grimacing, asterixis, generalized seizures, apneic spells, and loss of limb coordination are not uncommon during the course of the illness (Alfrey et al, 1972; Burks et al, 1976; Chokroverty et al, 1976; Garcia-Bunuel et al, 1980; Lederman and Henry, 1978; Mahurkar et al, 1973).

The EEG shows characteristics changes in dialysis dementia (Hughes and Schreeder 1980; Lederman and Henry, 1978; Mahurkar et al, 1978). Serial studies demonstrate that the first abnormalities to appear are occasional slow-wave bursts in the theta or delta range. Later there is increased slowing of the background rhythms, and slow-wave burst activity increases in amplitude and duration. Next bursts of slow and sharp waves, spikes, and polyspike activity, usually in a bifrontal distribution, appear (Fig. 7–1). Finally the entire record shows slowing in theta and delta ranges with no normal activity (Mahurkar et al, 1978). Slowing is a common feature of the EEGs of uremic patients without dialysis dementia, but paroxysmal activity occurs in over 80 percent of patients with dialysis dementia and less than

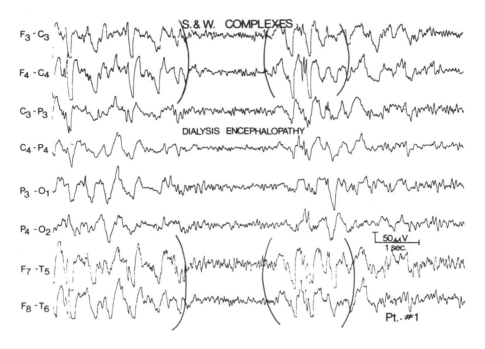

FIGURE 7–1.   EEG in dialysis dementia reveals intermittent bursts of polyspike and slow-wave complexes. (Reprinted by permission of the publisher and the authors from JR Hughes and MT Schreeder. "EEG in dialysis encephalopathy." Neurology 1980;30:1148–1154.)

10 percent of dialyzed patients without the dementia syndrome (Hughes and Schreeder, 1980). In some cases, the characteristic polyspike and wave complexes are detectable before any other evidence of the syndrome is present.

The CT scans in patients with dialysis dementia are normal or show moderate ventricular dilatation and sulcal widening (Lederman and Henry, 1978). Cisternography reveals slow CSF flow with reflux of radionuclide into the ventricular system. The ascent of the tracer substance over the convexities is slow, and parasagittal concentration is delayed or absent (Mahurkar et al, 1978). These findings resemble those of normal-pressure hydrocephalus, but the ventricles are not greatly dilated and ventriculoperitoneal shunting has been of no benefit.

No distinctive gross or histologic changes are seen in the brains of patients dying of dialysis dementia. Nonspecific cellular changes of chronic metabolic encephalopathy are present and hypertensive lacunar infarctions in the basal ganglia and thalamus are common. No differences are evident between the brains of dialysis patients with and without dementia (Lederman and Henry, 1978). Histochemical analyses reveal a significant elevation in levels of brain aluminum in those with dialysis dementia (Alfrey et al, 1976). Biochemical studies reveal 30–50 percent reductions in gamma-aminobutyric acid concentrations and 25–35 percent reductions in hemispheric choline acetyltransferase levels (Sweeney et al, 1985).

The etiology of dialysis dementia remains to be determined. The absence of neuropathologic changes favors a metabolic cause. Numerous factors have been suggested as etiologic agents, including heavy metal or plasticizer accumulation; vitamin, asparagine, or phosphate depletion; viral infection; recurrent hypoglycemia; hypercalcemia; and many others (Cameron et al, 1978; Dunea et al, 1978; Gunale, 1973; Lyle, 1973; Mahurkar et al, 1978; Pierides et al, 1976; Riley, 1973). A consistent, but not yet conclusive, relationship between chronic aluminum intoxication and dialysis dementia has been demonstrated (Alfrey et al, 1976; Arieff et al, 1979; Dunea et al, 1978; Flendrig et al, 1976; Rozas et al, 1978). Alfrey and co-workers (1976) found significant elevations of aluminum content in the brains of dialysis dementia patients compared with nondemented patients receiving long-term dialysis. They suspected that aluminum-containing phosphate-binding gels were the source of the aluminum. More recent studies suggest that parenteral aluminum received during dialysis is a more likely origin of the offending agent (Dunea et al, 1978; Flendrig et al, 1976; Rozas et al, 1978). Since all patients receive similar treatment and only a small number develop dialysis dementia, other unidentified factors must also be playing a role (Arieff et al, 1979).

Treatment of dialysis dementia has so far been unsuccessful, but prevention may be possible. Attempts at treatment have included chelating agents, corticosteroids, increased dialysis, ventriculoperitoneal shunting, and vitamins (Lederman and Henry, 1978). Improvement has occasionally occurred following successful renal transplantation (Sullivan et al, 1977), but most cases progress to death despite transplantation and a few have had onset of initial manifestations after transplantation (Burks et al, 1976; Mattern et al, 1977; Platts et al, 1973). Administration of diazepam often produces a dramatic improvement in the mental status and speech disturbances with normalization of the EEG. Unfortunately, these effects are transient, and relentless deterioration resumes after a few days or weeks (Nadel and Wilson, 1976; Noriega-Sanchez et al, 1978; Snider et al, 1979). The discovery of elevated intracerebral aluminum levels led to attempts to limit the amount of parenteral aluminum received by dialysis patients. The result has been a steady reduction in the number of new patients with the dementia syndrome, and the use of deionized water in the dialysate solution is recommended as a preventive measure (Dunea et al, 1978; Flendrig et al, 1976; Rozas et al, 1978). The incidence of dialysis dementia has dramatically declined in the recent past.

The differential diagnosis of the dialysis dementia syndrome (see Table

TABLE 7–4.   Characteristics of uremic encephalopathy compared with dialysis dementia.

Characteristic	Uremic encephalopathy	Dialysis dementia
History	Renal failure ± dialysis	Renal failure with dialysis
Dementia	Aphasia uncommon	Aphasia common
Speech	Slurred, slow	Stuttering, dysarthria, mutism common
EEG	Slow background with excess theta and delta activity	Slow background with bursts of delta-range slow waves and spikes, polyspikes, and sharp waves
Treatment	Improved by dialysis No change with diazepam	Worsened by dialysis Improved by diazepam

7–3) includes the disorders of chronic renal failure plus a few additional conditions specifically associated with dialysis. The most common diagnostic problem is differentiating increasing uremic encephalopathy from dialysis dementia. Changes in mental status may be similar in the two syndromes, but other features usually allow clinical identification. Table 7–4 summarizes the main distinguishing features. Speech may be slurred, slow, and hypophonic in uremic encephalopathy whereas stuttering, dysarthria, and mutism are characteristic of dialysis dementia. Background slowing is present on the EEGs of both disorders, but paroxysmal slowing with sharp or spike activity is more indicative of the dementia syndrome. Dialysis improves uremic encephalopathy but often produces temporary worsening of dialysis dementia. Diazepam has no effect on uremic encephalopathy and may temporarily cause dramatic improvement in dialysis dementia.

Anticoagulation of dialysis patients is frequently necessary to maintain patency of the dialysis access shunt. Combined with shifts in brain size due to osmotic changes and minor head trauma, the anticoagulation results in an increased incidence of subdural hematomas in dialyzed patients (Bechar et al, 1972; Leonard and Shapiro, 1975; Talalla et al, 1970). Fluctuating alertness, severe headache, and/or focal neurologic signs should alert the clinician to this possibility.

The disequilibrium syndrome is another dialysis-related encephalopathy that must be distinguished from dialysis dementia. It begins during or soon after dialysis and consists of headache, nausea, cramps, irritability, agitation, obtundation, convulsions (Raskin and Fishman, 1976). The syndrome is usually transient, but delirium may persist for several days and is accompanied by generalized slowing of the EEG. It is attributed to cerebral edema following rapid removal from the serum of osmotically active particles and is controlled by slowing and extending the period of dialysis (Peterson and Swanson, 1964; Raskin and Fishman, 1976).

Declotting upper extremity shunts by injection of saline may cause cerebral embolization and focal neurologic deficits with behavioral consequences (Gaan et al, 1969). Behavioral changes may also result from chronic accumulation of poorly dialyzable drugs (Gibson, 1979). Benzodiazepines in particular have been implicated in this regard (Taclob and Needle, 1976). Finally thiamine depletion may occur during the course of chronic dialysis, giving rise to Wernicke-Korsakoff syndrome and severe deficits in recent memory (Faris, 1972; Lopez and Collins, 1968).

Kidney Transplantation and Immunosuppression

Patients receiving kidney transplants are treated with steroids and a wide variety of immunosuppressive compounds that predispose them to illnesses that may impair intellectual function. Steroids produce psychosis and intellectual impairment in some patients. Patients receiving immunosuppressive compounds are more likely to develop progressive multifocal leukoencephalopathy, meningitis, encephalitis, and cerebral neoplasms (Agamanolis et al, 1979; Schneck and Penn, 1970, 1971; Tyler, 1965).

Uretorosigmoidostomy

Another genitourinary disorder capable of producing a dementia syndrome is ureterosigmoidostomy, a urinary diversion procedure performed in patients with congenital urologic deficits or bladder cancer. In rare cases, a hyperammonemic encephalopathy characterized by dysarthria, ataxia, and progressive obtundation complicates the procedure. The mental status changes may reverse after surgical revision (Cascino et al, 1989).

Hepatic Diseases

Cirrhosis and Portosystemic Encephalopathy

Portosystemic encephalopathy (also called hepatic coma and hepatic encephalopathy) is a chronic neuropsychiatric disorder caused by severe impairment of liver function and shunting of portal venous blood through collateral vessels into the peripheral circulation. Alcohol-induced cirrhosis is the most common liver disease associated with hepatic encephalopathy, but other types of chronic hepatic disease can also give rise to the syndrome (Hoffman, 1981, Jeffries, 1971). Occasionally, fistulas occur allowing extrahepatic portacaval shunting and leading to hepatic-type encephalopathy in the absence of liver disease (Russell et al, 1989). The principal clinical manifestations are an altered mental state, a flapping tremor (asterixis), increased muscle tone and hyperreflexia, gait ataxia, and a typical fetor. Neurobehavioral alterations include changes in mood with euphoria or depression, impaired concentration and attention, poor memory, fluctuating level of arousal, and bizarre behavior (Hoffman, 1981; Sherlock et al, 1954). Constructional disturbances and motor impersistence are common. Asterixis (liver flap) is present in nearly all patients. It is usually manifested as intermittent lapse in posture (flap) of the hands when the arms are held outstretched with the hands dorsiflexed at the wrist. Occasionally, the same phenomenon is present in the arms, neck, jaws, protruded tongue, retracted mouth, or tightly closed eyelids (Leavitt and Tyler, 1964; Sherlock et al, 1954). Asterixis is usually accompanied by an irregular postural tremor.

The pathogenesis of portosystemic encephalopathy is not fully understood. Contributing factors may include neurotransmitter changes, abnormal blood-brain barrier function, impaired sodium-potassium-ATPase activity, and elevated levels of ammonia, mercaptans, and short-chain fatty-acids (Conn, 1969; Fraser and Arieff, 1985; Hoffman, 1981; Soeters and Fischer, 1976). Abnormalities of ammonia metabolism have been most studied and show the best correlation with the severity of hepatic encephalopathy. The correlation is not exact, but serum ammonia levels between one and three μg per milliliter are usually associated with mental status impairment (Sherlock et al, 1954), and CSF glutamine, a metabolite of ammonia, is elevated in encephalopathic patients (Hourani et al, 1971). Dietary protein is the principal source of nitrogenous substances metabolized to ammonia, and in some patients, the severity of encephalopathy is exquisitely sensitive to fluctuations in dietary protein. Shakespeare recognized this aspect of the mental disorder (Summerskill, 1955), and in *Twelfth Night* Sir Andrew Aguecheek, a victim of the hepatic consequences of prolonged indiscretion in the use of alcohol, observes of himself:

> Methinks sometimes I have no more wit than a Christian or an ordinary man has. But I am a great eater of beef, and I believe that does harm to my wit. (Act I, Scene 3)

In addition to abnormalities of liver function tests, serum ammonia, and CSF glutamine, there are characteristic EEG abnormalities. Disorganization and slowing of the background alpha activity and generalized slow waves in the theta or delta range occur, and bursts of 2-Hz bilaterally synchronous triphasic waves with frontal predominance are common (Kiloh et al, 1972; Silverman, 1962).

There are few pathologic changes in the brain in hepatic encephalopathy, but hyperplasia of protoplasmic astrocytes is consistently present.

Treatment of portosystemic encephalopathy is directed at minimizing gut protein, modifying intestinal bacterial activity, and limiting protein absorption. Strict control of dietary protein and use of neomycin or lactulose are the mainstays of therapy (Conn, 1969; Hoffman, 1981; Welsh et al, 1974). Improvement in mental status usually occurs when the treatment regimen is instituted. Some patients show improved intellectual function in response to levodopa or bromocriptine when conventional measures fail (Lunzer et al, 1974; Morgan et al, 1977).

The differential diagnosis of portosystemic encephalopathy in patients with advanced liver disease includes subdural hematoma associated with clotting abnormalities, depression of consciousness by poorly metabolized psychotropic medication, and nonwilsonian hepatocerebral degeneration.

Acquired (Nonwilsonian) Hepatocerebral Degeneration

A few patients who survive chronic portosystemic encephalopathy develop a permanent CNS disorder characterized by dementia and a variety of motor system disturbances. In all cases there has been longstanding portosystemic shunting produced by advanced cirrhosis or surgical intervention. The mental status abnormalities of hepatocerebral degeneration include slowness and disorganization of thought, inattention and poor concentration, poor memory, constructional disturbances, emotional lability, paranoia, and hallucinations (Read et al, 1967; Victor et al, 1965). Depressed consciousness is less evident in acquired hepatocerebral degeneration than it is in portosystemic encephalopathy, and agnosia, apraxia, and aphasia are absent (Victor et al, 1965). Motor system abnormalities occur in every case and include dysarthria, cerebellar ataxia, dysmetria and titubation, asterixis and tremor, choreoathetosis and facial grimacing, and mild increase in muscle tone. Some patients have extensor plantar responses (Victor et al, 1965). Once it has been established, the neurologic disorder progresses very slowly or remains stationary, and death is usually a result of the underlying hepatic disorder. Diffuse slowing of the EEG is usually evident and CSF is normal or shows a modest elevation of protein content.

At autopsy, the brain shows patchy cortical laminar or pseudolaminar necrosis and microcavitation at the corticomedullary junction, in the striatum, and in the cerebellar white matter. Microscopically there is an increase in the number and size of protoplasmic astrocytes; degeneration of nerve cells and medullated fibers in the cerebral cortex, cerebellum, dentate nucleus, and lenticular nuclei; and appearance of glycogen-containing intranuclear inclusion bodies in astrocytes (Finlayson and Superville, 1981; Smith, 1976a; Victor, 1974; Victor et al, 1965). Opalski cells may be present but are less numerous than they are in Wilson's disease.

Treatment is directed at controlling recurrent bouts of portosystemic encephalopathy. The main entities considered in the differential diagnosis include Wilson's disease, portosystemic encephalopathy, and subdural hematoma.

Pancreatic Disorders

Insulinoma and Recurrent Hypoglycemia

Chronic or recurrent hypoglycemia results in mental status impairment with personality alterations, aggressive behavior, defective memory, apathy, and emotional lability (Lishman, 1978; Markowitz et al, 1961; Tom and Richardson, 1951). The memory disturbance is often severe and at times may be the major behavioral disorder. Peripheral neuropathy can occur and focal neurologic deficits may be observed during a hypoglycemic episode. The causes of recurrent hypoglycemia capable of producing dementia include insulinoma, postgastrectomy hypoglycemia, overadministration of hypoglycemic agents used in the treatment of diabetes, liver necrosis, and large retroperitoneal tumors (Bondy, 1971; Burton and Raskin, 1970).

Pathologically there is patchy necrosis and loss of neurons in the cerebral cortex, basal ganglia, and cerebellum. Neuronal changes are accompanied by proliferation of microglial cells, astrocytes, and blood vessels. The anterior horn cells of the spinal cord may be severely affected (Tom and Richardson, 1951).

Identification and treatment of the hypoglycemia will halt progression of the dementia, but existing deficits may not be reversible.

Pancreatic Encephalopathy

Acute pancreatitis is sometimes accompanied by an unusual subacute encephalopathy manifested by confusion, agitation, hallucinations, paranoia, lack of insight, and incoherent speech (Pallis and Lewis, 1974; Rothermich and von Haam, 1941). The dementia is associated with dysarthria and extrapyramidal rigidity, and seizures may occur. In some cases, the encephalopathy resolves spontaneously whereas others terminate fatally. Pathologic findings include focal loss of neurons and areas of demyelination. The pancreatitis is manifested by abdominal pain and elevation of serum amylase levels. Although the underlying mechanism of this disorder is unknown, the CNS changes are assumed to be produced by lipases and proteolytic enzymes liberated from the acutely inflamed pancreas, but definitive evidence is lacking (Pallis and Lewis, 1974). Biliary tract disease with gallstones and alcohol-induced pancreatitis are the most common etiologies of the pancreatitis (Kowlessar, 1971).

Electrolyte Abnormalities

Hyponatremia

Chronic or recurrent hyponatremia can occur in diverse clinical circumstances, including inappropriate secretion of antidiuretic hormone, Addison's disease, chronic renal failure, congestive heart failure, cirrhosis of the liver, and idiopathic sodium depletion (Berl et al, 1976; Schwartz, 1971). The inappropriate antidiuretic hormone syndrome with hyponatremia can be produced by bronchogenic carcinoma, cerebral malformation and injuries such as subdural hematomas, and tuberculosis (Epstein et al, 1961). Inappropriate antidiuretic hormone secretion can also be stimulated by oral hypoglycemic agents such as chlorpropamide and tolbutamide, sulfonylurea drugs, antineoplastic agents including vincristine and cyclophosphamide, tricyclic compounds such as carbamazepine and amitriptyline, and diuretics and major tranquilizers (Matuk and Kalyanaraman, 1977; Moses and Miller, 1974). Neuropsychiatric alterations resulting from hyponatremia include weakness, anorexia, lethargy, disorientation, psychosis, and seizures (Arieff et al, 1976; Dubovsky et al, 1973; Welti, 1956). Seizures may occur when the serum sodium gets as low as 110 to 112 mEq per liter, but cerebral edema occurs when the serum sodium concentration is 125 mEq per liter, and behavioral changes could be expected with this degree of hyponatremia. The EEG shows slowing of background rhythms and high-voltage slow waves (Cadilhac and Ribstein, 1961). Fluid restriction and restoration of normal serum sodium concentration result in normalization of intellectual function and improvement in the EEG.

Hypernatremia

Dehydration, hypernatremia, and hyperosmolality are better tolerated by the brain than are hyponatremia and hypoosmolality. Elderly patients, however, may be very sensitive to any fluctuations in serum sodium concentrations, and intellectual impairment may occur with relatively minor degrees of hypernatremia. In some cases, no sensation of thirst is present to indicate the fluid imbalance (Jana and Romano-Jana, 1973). Hypernatremia usually occurs when there is decreased or absent fluid intake or increased water loss; disorders of fluid and electrolyte regulation, particularly diabetes insipidus; or osmotic diuresis (Jana and Romano-Jana, 1973; Schwartz, 1971). The principal neurobehavioral abnormalities are confusion, disorientation, and restlessness. The EEG changes are usually minor, but there may be disorganization of background activity and episodic bursts of slow waves (Cadilhac and Ribstein, 1961). Disorders of serum sodium usually produce acute confusional states and rarely become sufficiently chronic to cause a dementia syndrome.

Serum Calcium and Magnesium Abnormalities

Elevated serum calcium levels usually reflect the presence of a malignant neoplasm (usually breast cancer, lung cancer, or multiple myeloma) or hyperparathyroidism. Mental status changes are common with hypercalcemia, particularly when the serum calcium level exceeds 14 mg/dl, and these changes include confusion, lethargy, and somnolence (Riggs, 1989).

Hypocalcemia is rare in adults but may occur in conjunction with pancreatitis and hypoparathyroidism. Cognitive changes include confusion, irritability, hallucinations, delusions, anxiety, and agitation. Parkinsonism, chorea, and tetany may also occur (Riggs, 1989). Calcification of the basal ganglia may be evident on the CT scan.

Hypomagnesemia rarely occurs in isolation; it has been reported in starvation syndromes, malabsorption, renal disease, chronic alcoholism, and diabetic acidosis. The principal neurological abnormalities accompanying these disorders include confusion, seizures, tremor, myoclonus, and tetany (Riggs, 1989). Hypermagnesemia commonly produces muscle weakness and occasionally results in confusion.

Porphyria

The porphyrias are a complex group of disorders that include hepatic disorders of porphyrin production such as acute intermittent, variegate, and hereditary porphyrias and porphyria cutanea tarda, as well as the erythropoietic porphyrias of both congenital and idiopathic types (Goldberg, 1959; Ridley, 1975). Among these conditions, acute intermittent porphyria is the disorder most likely to have dementia as an important clinical element. This is a dominantly inherited abnormality of porphyrin metabolism manifested by attacks of abdominal pain, gastrointestinal dysfunction, and neurologic disturbances. The disease rarely becomes evident before puberty and females are more affected than are males (Ridley, 1975; Schmid, 1971). The first symptoms of an attack are usually abdominal pain, constipation, nausea, and vomiting. Neuropsychiatric abnormalities follow or occur simultaneously with the abdominal phase, and peripheral neuropathy becomes evident late in the attack. The neuropathy involves motor more than sensory neurons and leads to flaccid weakness, hyporeflexia, dysphonia, and dysphagia. Respiratory paralysis may cause death (Naef et al, 1959). Neurobehavioral changes include personality alterations, agitation, depression, impaired memory, hallucinations, disturbances of consciousness. and convulsions (Goldberg, 1959; Naef et al, 1959; Roth, 1945). Attacks may be short-lived and manifested merely by mild abdominal pain, or they may be severe and protracted, lasting several months. They recur irregularly over months or years and tend to decrease in frequency and severity with age (Schmid, 1971). The episodes may occur spontaneously or may be precipitated by a variety of drugs including barbiturates, sulfonamides, griseofulvin, chlordiazepoxide, meprobamate, phenytoin, methsuximide, glutethimide, imipramine, ergot preparations, and tolbutamide (Tschudy et al, 1975). In some cases, the neuropsychiatric features may dominate the clinical presentation in the absence of gastrointestinal abnormalities or seizures (Tischler et al, 1985).

Laboratory studies are helpful in diagnosing the condition. During attacks, delta-aminolevulinic acid and porphobilinogen are excreted in the urine. In the bladder, porphobilinogen is converted to uroporphyrins that impart a reddish brown color to the urine. Porphobilinogen is often present in the urine between attacks (Ridley, 1975).

Pathologic changes include myelin and axonal damage of peripheral nerves and chromatolysis and vacuolation of anterior horn cells of the spinal cord. In the brain, vascular and anoxic changes are common, but no specific abnormalities are described, and neuropsychiatric disturbances are probably the result of reversible metabolic alterations (Hierons, 1957).

Treatment of porphyria depends on avoiding exposure to compounds that can precipitate attacks and treatment of symptoms and complications. Attacks can sometimes be aborted by a high-carbohydrate diet (Tschudy et al, 1975).

Historical research suggests that King George III and many members of the royal houses of Hanover and Stuart, as well as the royalty of Prussia, suffered from acute intermittent porphyria (MacAlpine and Hunter, 1966; MacAlpine et al, 1968), and it seems likely that this remitting dementia significantly influenced the course of British, European, and American history.

Cerebral Effects of Systemic Malignancies

Extracerebral neoplasms can result in cerebral disturbances by producing metabolic abnormalities, generating secondary CNS deposits, facilitating CNS infections, or producing so-called remote effects (Table 7–5). The effects of cancer treatment may also affect cerebral function and produce chronic encephalopathy.

Metabolic Disturbances Induced by Malignancies

Dementia syndromes and chronic metabolic encephalopathies can be associated with systemic malignancies through a variety of mechanisms. Primary or metastatic tumors may result in organ destruction and metabolic, encephalopathy; anemia and vitamin deficiencies can deprive cerebral metabolism of essential ingredients; and some tumors have secondary endocrine abnormalities that impair cerebral function.

Endocrine abnormalities associated with neoplasms include hypoglycemia, inappropriate antidiuretic hormone production with hyponatremia, parathormone secretion with hypercalcemia, and ectopic adrenocorticotropic hormone (ACTH) production with Cushing's disease. Neoplasms associated

TABLE 7–5.   Encephalopathies associated with systemic malignancies.

Metabolic disturbances	CNS infections
Anemia	Progressive multifocal
Inappropriate antidiuretic hormone and	leukoencephalopathy
hyponatremia	Meningitis
Ectopic adrenocorticotropic hormone	Encephalitis
production	Abscess
Hypercalcemia	Remote effects of cancer
Vitamin deficiency	Limbic encephalitis
Systemic effects of destruction of vital	Effects of treatment
organs	Toxic encephalopathy
Pulmonary insufficiency	Demyelination
Uremia	Radiation necrosis
Hepatic disease	
Hypoglycemia	
Structural abnormalities	
Metastases and infiltrates	
Meningeal carcinomatosis	
Cerebral infarction	
Intravascular coagulation	
Marantic endocarditis	
Neoplastic angioendotheliosis	
Intracranial hemorrhage (secondary to	
thrombocytopenia)	
Subdural hematoma	
Subarachoid hemorrhage	
Intracerebral hemorrhage	

with hypoglycemia include mesenchymal tumors, hepatic malignancies, adrenal carcinomas, and a variety of other organ cancers (Odell and Wolfsen, 1978). Brain tumors, pancreatic carcinomas, and intrathoracic neoplasms (especially oat cell carcinoma of the lung) have all been associated with the syndrome of inappropriate secretion of antidiuretic hormone (Leaf, 1971; Martin et al, 1977a). Similarly oat cell lung carcinoma is the most common tumor associated with ectopic ATCH production, although ACTH may also be secreted by bronchial carcinomas, thymic and pancreatic neoplasms, carcinoid, tumors of neural crest origin, and several other malignancies (Martin et al, 1977). Hypercalcemia can be produced by metastases to bone or by ectopic parathormone elaborated by neoplastic tissue. Lung, kidney, ovarian, uterine, and pancreatic tumors are the malignancies most commonly associated with parathormone production (Odell, 1968).

Structural Abnormalities Produced by Malignancies

The most direct changes induced by extracerebral neoplasms and capable of producing dementia are produced by solid tumor metastases or lymphomatous infiltrates of the brain (Kakulas and Finlay-Jones, 1962; Madow and Alpers, 1951; Marshall et al, 1968). Infiltration of the meninges by leukemic cells, lymphomas, or carcinomatous cells can produce increased intracranial pressure and chronic encephalopathy (Fischer-Williams et al, 1955; Floeter et al, 1987; Gonzalez-Vitale and Garcia-Bunuel, 1976; Griffin et al, 1971; Little et al, 1974; Shaw et al, 1960; Theodore and Gendelman, 1981).

Multiple cerebral infarctions and multi-infarct dementia can occur in association with systemic malignancies as a result of intravascular coagulation (Collins et al, 1975; Reagan and Okazaki, 1974), marantic endocarditis with cerebral emboli (Barron et al, 1960), or neoplastic angioendotheliosis (Dolman et al, 1979; LeWitt et al, 1983; Petito et al, 1978; Strouth et al, 1965). Thrombocytopenia interferes with normal coagulation mechanisms and facilitates intracranial hemorrhage (Groch et al, 1960; Moore et al, 1960; Wells and Silver, 1957).

CNS Infections Associated with Malignancies

Immunologic mechanisms necessary to resist CNS infections may be compromised both by the presence of a systemic malignancy and by many of the drugs used to inhibit the neoplastic process. Bacterial and fungal meningitis, viral encephalitis, and brain abscesses are the principal infections that require consideration in the cancer patient with advancing dementia (Chernik et al, 1973; Wolinski et al, 1977). (Progressive multifocal leukoencephalopathy, a viral encephalopathy that complicates reticuloendothelial malignancies, is discussed in Chapter 6).

Remote Effects of Cancer: Limbic Encephalitis

Limbic encephalitis is a syndrome of obscure origin that occurs almost exclusively in patients with a malignancy. Patients are typically but not exclusively in the sixth to eighth decade of life and men are affected more often than are women. Lung carcinoma is the most common underlying neoplasm, particularly oat cell carcinoma of the bronchus, but the syndrome has been described with a variety of other tumors including carcinoma of the breast, uterus, ovary, kidney, multiple myeloma, lymphosarcoma, reticulum cell sarcoma, acute leukemia, and cerebellar medulloblastoma (Arseni et al, 1978; Brierley et al, 1960; Corsellis et al, 1968; Currie et al, 1970; Dorfman and Forno, 1972; Henson et al, 1965; Nelson et al, 1966).

The course of limbic encephalitis lasts one to two years. Mental status changes include a marked disturbance of affect usually with severe anxiety and depression. Memory impairment is the most prominent cognitive disturbance, and in a few patients, amnesia is virtually the only neuropsychological abnormality. Hallucinations are not uncommon and alertness may be compromised. Gradual dilapidation of other cognitive abilities appears as the disease progresses (Corsellis et al, 1968; Daniels et al, 1969; Dorfman and Forno, 1972; Glaser and Pincus, 1969; Posner, 1989). Other neurologic disorders are often present in patients with limbic encephalitis, including seizures, cerebellar disturbances, myeloradiculoneuropathy, and/or myopathy (Brain, 1963; Fisher et al, 1961).

Pathologically, the principal changes are loss of neurons and perivascular inflammatory infiltrates concentrated in the hippocampi and other medial temporal areas. The changes are not confined to the limbic areas and involve more lateral temporal regions, and there are inflammatory foci in other areas of the cortex (Brierley et al, 1960; Corsellis et al, 1968). Some patients have had widespread changes involving the cerebellum, brainstem, spinal cord ganglia, and peripheral nerves.

The etiology of the paraneoplastic encephalomyelitis is uncertain. The acute nature of the process, the widespread inflammatory changes, the topographic similarity to cerebral involvement by the herpes virus, and the occasional identification of intranuclear inclusions all suggest that it is a subacute viral infection (Brierley et al, 1960; Dayan et al, 1967; Glaser and Pincus, 1969). Inclusion bodies have not been identified in most cases, however, and most viral studies have been unrevealing. Toxic, immunologic, and nutritional theories have been expounded, but none have been verified (Dorfman and Forno, 1972; Wilner and Brody, 1968).

Treatment of limbic encephalopathy is not available. Although paraneoplastic neuropathies and cerebellar syndromes have occasionally remitted following removal of the offending tumor, surgery has not affected paraneoplastic dementia.

Effects of Treatment of Neoplasms

The toxic effects of antineoplastic agents are discussed later in this chapter with other toxic dementias.

Deficiency States

Vitamins are a group of unrelated organic elements that are necessary in small amounts for normal cellular metabolism. They are not manufactured by the body and must be obtained from dietary sources. Vitamins B_1 (thiamine), B_{12} (cyanocobalamin), niacin, and folate are particularly essential for normal cognition; deficiency states result in impaired intellectual function. Clinicians must be particularly aware of possible vitamin deficiency in patients on limited diets such as alcoholics, socially isolated elderly individuals ("tea and toast" diets), and patients anorectic with chronic illness or severe depression.

Thiamine Deficiency: Wernicke-Korsakoff Syndrome

The mental impairment of Wernicke-Korsakoff syndrome does not meet the criteria presented in Chapter 1 for a diagnosis of dementia. The principal neuropsychological deficit is impaired recent memory, and there-fore it is better classified as an amnesia (Benson, 1978). A change in personality with increased placidity often accompanies the amnesia, how-ever, and the effects of chronic alcohol intake (considered below), repeated head trauma, and frequent seizures can combine to produce a dementia syndrome in many patients with Wernicke-Korsakoff syndrome. For this reason, the syndrome is discussed here.

In his three-volume *Lehrbuch der Gehirnkrankheiten* published in 1881–1883, Carl Wernicke described the acute phase of the syndrome that came to bear his name. He called attention to the clinical triad of ophthalmoplegia, ataxia, and disturbance of consciousness. He also recognized the periven-tricular hemorrhages occurring in the gray matter adjacent to the third and fourth ventricles and suggested the name *hemorrhagic superior polioence-phalitis* (Brody and Wilkins, 1968; Wernicke, 1977). The mental changes of the syndrome were described by Russian neuropsychiatrist S. S. Korsakoff in a series of papers appearing in the years 1887 to 1889 (Victor and Yakovlev, 1955). He emphasized the co-occurrence of peripheral neuropathy with the deficit in recent memory and proposed that they represented two facets of the same disorder.

The Wernicke-Korsakoff syndrome usually has an abrupt onset with ocular motor abnormalities, ataxia of gait, and confusional state; not infre-quently, however, patients have repeated subclinical episodes of vitamin B1 deficiency and develop mental status changes (memory loss) in the absence of acute neurologic signs (Harper et al, 1986). If thiamine is administered in the acute stage, the ophthalmoplegia may reverse within a few minutes or hours, and the other abnormalities may improve gradually over the course of several days. Amnesia becomes apparent as the confusional state resolves (Cravioto et al, 1961; Malamud and Skillicorn, 1956; Victor et al, 1971). The amnesia has an anterograde component with inability to learn new material and a retrograde component affecting the recall of information learned years prior to onset of the syndrome. Both recall and recognition of newly presented verbal information are impaired in Korsakoff's syndrome; procedural (motor skill) memory is relatively preserved (Martone et al, 1984). Recall of more remote information is less impaired than is recently acquired knowledge (Albert et al, 1979; Seltzer and Benson, 1974). Con-fabulation is common in the initial phase of Korsakoff's syndrome but becomes less prominent later in the course. The amnesia is not a source of concern, and patients are typically placid and congenial (Lishman, 1978). Nystagmus, ataxia, and/or peripheral neuropathy even if they are mild are detectable in a majority of patients in the chronic phase of the Wernicke-Korsakoff syndrome.

Pathologically the most intense changes are found in the periventricular gray matter surrounding the third and fourth ventricles and the aqueduct of Sylvius, the mammillary bodies, and the dorsomedial nuclei of the thalamus. The involved areas show loss of neurons, intense gliosis, and moderate vascular proliferation. Frank hemorrhage is apparent in a few cases (Liss, 1958; Malamud and Skillicorn, 1956). Grossly the mammillary bodies are shrunken and discolored.

X-ray CT in Korsakoff's syndrome may reveal small areas of hypodensity in the walls of the third ventricle and around the Sylvian aqueduct (Mensing et al, 1984). Sagittal and coronal sections MRI may reveal the mammillary body atrophy (Charness and DeLaPaz, 1987).

Most patients with Wernicke-Korsakoff syndrome are alcoholics whose thiamine deficiency is the result of poor diet. Other causes of dietary deficiencies and gastrointestinal malabsorption syndromes including carcinoma of the esophagus or stomach, excessive vomiting, gastric surgery, and prolonged diarrhea can produce thiamine deficiency and the Wernicke-Korsakoff syndrome (Haid et al, 1982; Lishman, 1978). Wernicke's first case was a 20-year-old woman who had pyloric stenosis resulting from ingestion of sulfuric acid (Brody and Wilkins, 1968). The thiamine deficiency syndrome resulting from polished rice diets (beriberi) produces neuropathy and cardiomyopathy before neurobehavioral abnormalities become evident, but typical cases of Korsakoff's psychosis were noted among some prisoners of war who were fed rice diets (De Wardener and Lennox, 1947; Lishman, 1978). Patients with Wernicke-Korsakoff syndrome may have an inherited abnormality of the thiamine-dependent enzyme transketolase that predisposes them to the development of cellular abnormalities when dietary thiamine is inadequate (Blass and Gibson, 1977).

Once it has been established, the memory deficit does not respond to thiamine administration, but adequate thiamine should be provided to prevent worsening or recurrence of the disorder. Improved performance on memory tests has occasionally been recorded following administration of vasopressin, clonidine, or methylphenidate (McEntee and Mair, 1980; O'Donnell et al, 1986; Oliveros et al, 1978), but no agent consistently produces clinically significant memory recovery. On the other hand, some degree of spontaneous recovery occurs in most Korsakoff's patients. Approximately 25 percent improve sufficiently to return to their previous occupation, 25 percent return to regular employment at a lower level, 25 percent return home but are unable to work, and 25 percent require chronic custodial care (Victor et al, 1971).

The differential diagnosis of the Wernicke-Korsakoff syndrome includes the amnesic syndromes that follow head trauma, temporal lobe surgery, herpes encephalitis, anoxia, and posterior cerebral artery occlusion (Benson, 1978; Symonds, 1966). The Wernicke-Korsakoff syndrome is compared with alcoholic dementia below.

Vitamin B₁₂ Deficiency

Vitamin B_{12} is essential to human nutrition; its absence results in disturbances of function of hematopoietic tissues, epithelial cells, and the nervous system. Neurologic manifestations include peripheral neuropathy, myelopathy, optic neuropathy, and dementia (Pallis and Lewis, 1974). The main features of B_{12} deficiency dementia include slowness of mental reactions, confusion, memory defect, and depression. Agitation, delusions, paranoid behavior, and hallucinations may also occur (Burvill et al, 1969; Fraser, 1960; Holmes, 1956; Smith, 1960). The encephalopathy may have a fluctuating course and can precede any detectable hematologic or marrow changes by months or years (Pallis and Lewis, 1974; Strachan and Henderson, 1965). Approximately 25 percent of patients with cobalamin (B_{12}) deficiency exhibit neither anemia nor macrocytosis when CNS symptoms become evident (Lindenbaum et al, 1988). Cerebral oxygen use is decreased in B_{12} deficiency dementia, and the EEG usually reveals diffuse slowing (Pallis and Lewis, 1974). The typical neuropathy of B_{12} deficiency includes superficial sensory impairment with burning paresthesias, tender peripheral nerves, early loss of ankle jerks, and distal weakness (Abramsky, 1972; Pallis and Lewis, 1974; Victor and Lear, 1956). The myelopathy involves the posterior and lateral columns of the spinal cord (combined systems disease) and produces impairment of vibration sense, limb weakness, spasticity, exaggerated muscle stretch reflexes, and extensor plantar responses (Pant et al, 1968; Victor and Lear, 1956). The spinal cord syndrome is the most common neurologic manifestation of vitamin B_{12} deficiency. Hematologic abnormalities eventually occur in all patients with chronic B_{12} deficiency and include megaloblastic anemia, oval macrocytosis, poikilocytosis, leukopenia with hypersegmented polymorphonuclear leukocytes, and a mild or moderate thrombocytopenia (Jandl, 1971).

The cerebral and spinal lesions of B_{12} deficiency are similar. There is a diffuse though uneven degeneration of the white matter with little proliferation of the fibrous glia. Within the foci of demyelination, histologic changes include fusiform swelling of myelin sheaths and axis cylinders in recent foci followed by destruction of myelin and axons and appearance of lipid-laden macrophages (Adams and Kubik, 1944; Smith, 1976b). In the spinal cord, the white matter changes begin in the posterior columns at the thoracic level of the spinal cord. Demyelination then extends up and down the cord and anteriorly to the lateral columns (Pant et al, 1968; Victor and Lear, 1956). The peripheral nerves are demyelinated in many cases.

Lack of intrinsic factor in the syndrome of pernicious anemia is the most common cause of B_{12} deficiency. The gastrointestinal abnormalities include atrophy of the gastric mucosa with virtual absence of parietal and chief cells. There is gastric achlorhydria and an absence of intrinsic factor necessary for the absorption of dietary B_{12} (Jandl, 1971). Other conditions that can disturb vitamin B_{12} absorption include total and subtotal gastrectomy; ileal resection; gastric carcinoma; gastrointestinal strictures, fistulas, and diverticula; tuberculous ulceration; regional ileitis; idiopathic and tropical sprue; vegetarian diets; atrophic gastritis; and intestinal helminthiasis, particularly the fish tapeworm *Diphyllobothrium latum* (Higginbottom et al, 1978; Lindenbaum et al, 1988; Pallis and Lewis, 1974; Smith, 1976b). The elderly are especially vulnerable to vitamin B_{12} deficiency. In addition to dietary inadequacies that may occur in the aged, there is increased frequency of atrophic gastritis with achlorhydria and lack of intrinsic factor in older patients (Gershell, 1981).

Definitive identification of B_{12} deficiency depends on direct determination of the serum B_{12} level. Serum levels of 200 pg per ml or less indicate that B_{12} intake or absorption are inadequate (Thompson et al, 1987). There is also decreased conversion of methylmalonyl-coenzyme A to succinyl-coenzyme A and urinary excretion of measurable levels of methylmalonic acid ensues (Dreyfus and Geel, 1976). The diagnosis of pernicious anemia is made by demonstrating histamine-fast achlorhydria or by doing the Schilling test to show the absence of intrinsic factor (Jandl, 1971).

Treatment consists of parenteral administration of 100 μg of vitamin B_{12} daily for one week, followed by every-other-day injections until 2000 ug have been administered over a six-week period (Babior and Bunn, 1987). When the deficiency is a result of poor gastrointestinal absorption, 100-μg injections must be given monthly for the rest of the patient's life (Jandl, 1971). Neurologic improvement is usually evident within a few days of initiating therapy and is often complete by one month (Zucker et al, 1981). Partial deficits may remain after treatment particularly when the cobalamin deficiency has been longstanding. Administration of folic acid may reverse the hematologic abnormalities while allowing CNS changes to progress (Baldwin and Dalessio, 1961).

Folate Deficiency

Although folate lack is among the most common vitamin deficiencies in western countries, it rarely produces symptomatic changes in the nervous system. On occasion, however, it closely mimics the syndromes of vitamin B_{12} deficiency, including neuropathy, myelopathy, and dementia (Fehling et al, 1974; Pincus et al, 1972; Reynolds et al, 1973; Strachan and Henderson 1967). Mental status examination of demented patients reveals apathy, disorientation, poor memory and concentration, and perseveration. Diffuse slowing is evident in the EEG (Strachan and Henderson, 1967). Megaloblastic anemia is the most common manifestation of folate deficiency.

The condition may result from poor dietary intake or from malabsorption following jejunal resection, after partial gastrectomy, or in patients with Crohn's disease. Folate absorption is also diminished by phenytoin and primidone (Jensen and Olesen, 1969; Pallis and Lewis, 1974).

A serum folate level of less than 2 μg per ml is abnormally low. Treatment consists of giving 10 to 20 mg per day of folic acid for one week and a maintenance dose of 2.5 to 10 mg per day by mouth (Gershell, 1981).

Most neurologic and mental status symptoms are reversible with treatment (Gotez et al, 1984).

Niacin Deficiency

Nicotinic acid deficiency results in cutaneous lesions, lesions of the gastrointestinal tract, and nervous system abnormalities. The neurologic abnormalities include peripheral neuropathy and myelopathy and neurobehavioral disturbances (Dreyfus and Geel, 1976; Pallis and Lewis, 1974). A pellagrous dementia and an acute niacin-deficient encephalopathy (Jolliffe's syndrome) have been reported. The dementia syndrome includes lassitude, depression, irritability, apprehension, memory impairment and confabulation, and psychomotor retardation (Spillane, 1947; Sydenstricker, 1943). Acute symptoms resulting from lack of niacin include clouding of consciousness, cogwheel rigidity, and marked sucking and grasping responses (Jolliffe et al, 1940). The predominant skin change of pellagra consists of a sunburnlike dermatitis appearing first on the dorsum of the hands. Gastrointestinal lesions include gingivitis, stomatitis, glossitis, and enteritis. Anorexia, abdominal pain, and diarrhea are common. Dermatitis, diarrhea, and dementia (the three D's of pellagra) constitute the typical triad of signs of niacin deficiency.

The most striking histologic alteration produced by niacin deficiency is central chromatolysis of neurons. The change is most evident in Betz cells and in brainstem nuclei. Neurons are rounded with peripheral displacement of the Nissl substance and nuclei. Electron microscopy reveals that RNA granules and lipofuscin pigment deposits are pushed to the periphery of the cytoplasm, whereas the central portion of the cytoplasm is occupied by mitochondria, lysosomes, and dilated vesicles (Nobuyoshi and Nishihara, 1981; Smith, 1976b).

Niacin deficiency results from chronic dietary neglect such as may occur in alcoholics or from a variety of systemic disorders including cirrhosis of the liver, chronic diarrheal disease, diabetes mellitus, neoplasms, chronic infectious disease, and thyrotoxicosis (Scrimshaw, 1971). Other vitamin deficiencies commonly coexist and may account for some of the symptoms.

A diet adequate in niacin is usually sufficient treatment, but in severe cases 300 to 500 mg of niacinamide may be given orally for the first few days. The acute symptoms improve within a few days, and the chronic symptoms show improvement over the course of several weeks (Scrimshaw, 1971).

Endocrine Disturbances

The endocrine system enables cells to adapt to constantly changing environmental circumstances by regulating the rate of cellular biochemical reactions.

TABLE 7–6.   Endocrine disturbances associated with dementia.

Thyroid disturbances
Hyperthyroidism
Classic thyrotoxicosis
Apathetic thyrotoxicosis
Hypothyroidism
Parathyroid disturbances
Hyperparathyroidism (with hypercalcemia)
Hypoparathyroidism (with hypocalcemia)
Adrenal abnormalities
Cushing's disease
Addison's disease
Panhypopituitarism
Inappropriate antidiuretic hormone (with hyponatremia)

Hormones exert profound influences on CNS function, and major deviations in hormone production result in alterations in intellectual activity (Smith et al, 1972; Williams, 1970) (Table 7–6).

Hyperthyroidism

Hyperthyroidism occurs most commonly in the second and third decades of life and affects women more often than it does men (Lishman, 1978). Neurologic manifestations of excessive thyroid production include myopathy, peripheral neuropathy, corticospinal tract disease, chorea, seizures, neurobehavioral disturbances, optic neuropathy, retinopathy, and exophthalmic ophthalmoplegia (Logothetis, 1961; Swanson et al, 1981; Waldenström, 1945). The dementia associated with thyrotoxicosis is typically characterized by subjective feelings of anxiety, restlessness, irritability, and emotional lability. Distractability leads to poor attention, impaired memory, and difficulty with calculation (Abend and Tyler, 1989; Lishman, 1978; Logothetis, 1961; Whybrow et al, 1969). Depression, euphoria, and schizophrenia-like psychoses may also become manifest in the hyperthyroid state (Bursten, 1961; Lishman, 1978). If the thyrotoxicosis becomes more severe, intellectual function is increasingly compromised, apathy and somnolence progress, and coma supervenes (Weaver et al, 1956; Waldenström, 1945).

In the elderly, thyrotoxicosis may present in an atypical or masked form that obscures the diagnosis. Anxiety, tremor, tachycardia, and restlessness may be completely lacking, and the only manifestations may be lethargy, apathy, and psychomotor retardation (Arnold et al, 1984; Gordon and Gryfe, 1981; Ronnov-Jessen and Kirkegaard, 1973; Thomas et al, 1970). The clinician must remain particularly alert to the possibility of apathetic thyrotoxicosis in the aged individual who has what seems to be a simple dementia.

The EEG is abnormal in most patients with hyperthyroidism. Slow-wave activity is present, and approximately half the patients have diffuse, paroxysmal sharp waves and spikes occurring with slow waves (Condon et al, 1954; Olsen et al, 1972). Large-amplitude fast-wave activity may be present, and a few patients have triphasic delta activity (Scherokman, 1980). Cerebral blood flow is increased in thyrotoxicosis (Sensebach et al, 1954).

Typical non-CNS abnormalities of hyperthyroidism are weight loss, tremulousness, skin changes, heat intolerance, tachycardia, palpitations, exertional dyspnea, and menstrual irregularities. The thyroid gland may be palpably enlarged and an orbitopathy with prominent eyes may occur (DeGroot, 1971). Laboratory diagnosis depends on identification of an elevated free thyroxine index and resin triiodothyronine uptake (Lavis, 1981; Stiel et al, 1972) and a low level of thyroid-stimulating hormone (TSH) (Spencer, 1988).

Hyperthyroidism usually results from idiopathic excessive thyroid activity but can also be the result of a toxic thyroid nodule, multinodular goiter, thyroid carcinoma, a TSH-secreting pituitary adenoma, or from ectopic TSH production by carcinomas (DeGroot, 1971). Appropriate management must include attention to the underlying cause of the thyrotoxicosis; some symptoms may be controlled by propranolol hydrochloride. The mental status and EEG changes improve with successful therapy.

Hypothyroidism (Myxedema)

Diminished thyroid activity has profound effects on the nervous system and may cause myopathy, peripheral neuropathy, cranial nerve abnormalities, ataxia and other cerebellar signs, psychosis and dementia, coma, and seizures (Abend and Tyler, 1989; Nickel and Frame, 1958; Sanders, 1962; Swanson et al, 1981). The psychosis of hypothyroidism, so-called myxedema madness, has no single pathognomonic feature, but inattention, disorientation, paranoia, and hallucinations are common (Asher, 1949; Logothetis, 1963). Psychosis occurs in 5 to 15 percent of patients with hypothyroidism and may occasionally be the initial manifestation of thyroid failure. Dementia occurs in approximately 5 percent of hypothyroid individuals and is manifested by psychic retardation, memory impairment, poor attention, and impaired abstraction (Hadden, 1882–1883; Swanson et al, 1981; Whybrow et al, 1969). If the hypothyroidism persists and advances, the patient becomes obtunded and may progress to coma and death. The EEG studies demonstrate slowing of background rhythms with diminished wave amplitude (Olivarius and Roder, 1970), and cerebral flow studies show increased cerebral vascular resistance and reduced blood flow (Sensenbach et al, 1954).

Non-CNS manifestations of myxedema include edema, weight gain, menorrhagia, cold intolerance, coarse hair, thickened skin, and constipation. Pleural and pericardial effusion and abdominal ascites may occur (DeGroot,

TABLE 7–7.   Correlation between mental status changes and serum calcium abnormalities.

Serum Calcium Level (mg/100 ml)	Mental Status Changes
12–16	Loss of initiative, depression, fatigue, mild memory impairment
16–19	Decreased attention, disorientation, poor memory, paranoia, hallucinations
>19	Obtundation, coma

1971). Laboratory studies demonstrate low levels of serum thyroxine and triiodothyronine and elevated levels of TSH and serum cholesterol. Hypothyroidism is treated by administering exogenous thyroid preparations. The neurologic abnormalities are usually reversible, but in some cases, deficits may persist even after adequate hormonal replacement.

Hyperparathyroidism and Hypercalcemia

The most prominent manifestations of hyperparathyroidism are weakness and fatigability; renal lithiasis with weight loss, mental disturbance, constipation, and abdominal pain; anorexia; arthralgias; and bone pain (Mallette et al, 1974). Mental status changes occur in more than half of these patients. Initially patients are apathetic and depressed, but as the condition advances, they become disoriented with poor memory, impaired calculation, limited concentration, depression, paranoia, and hallucinations (Fitz and Hallman, 1952; Gatewood et al, 1975; Henson, 1968; Karpati and Frame, 1964). Catatonia occurs in some patients and may mislead the clinician into considering the problem as primarily psychiatric (Gelenberg, 1976). Obtundation and coma occur in advanced stages of the illness. The changes in mental status correlate roughly with the degree of elevation of the serum calcium (Table 7–7) (Peterson, 1968), and similar neurobehavioral disturbances are noted in hypercalcemic patients without hyperparathyroidism (Lehrer and Levitt, 1960). The EEG in hypercalcemic patients may be normal or may show slowing of the posterior background rhythms, excess theta and delta activity, and high-voltage bilaterally synchronous frontal delta activity (Cohn and Sode, 1971; Allen et al, 1970).

Laboratory abnormalities in hyperparathyroidism include low levels of serum phosphate and high levels of serum calcium. Hypercalciuria is present and serum alkaline phosphatase levels may be elevated (Aurbach, 1971).

In addition to hyperparathyroidism, hypercalcemia may be produced by multiple myeloma, sarcoidosis, multiple bone metastases, milk-alkali syndrome, vitamin D intoxication, hyperthyroidism, acute adrenal insufficiency, hypophosphatasia, and ectopic parathormone production (Aurbach,

1971). Appropriate treatment is determined by discovering the underlying etiology of the hypercalcemia. Mental status abnormalities are reversible with normalization of the serum calcium.

Hypoparathyroidism and Hypocalcemia

Hypoparathyroidism affects many organ systems. Typical manifestations include chronic tetany, low levels of serum calcium and high levels of inorganic phosphate, seizures, dementia, cataracts, coarseness of the skin, and trophic nail changes (Robinson, et al, 1954). Calcification of the basal ganglia and an extrapyramidal motor disturbance with parkinsonian features or choreoathetosis are distinctive features of this metabolic disorder (Hossain, 1970; Muenter and Whisnant, 1968). The dementia is characterized by poor concentration, impaired memory, disorientation, apathy, and hallucinations (Eraut, 1974; Mortell, 1946; Robinson et al, 1954; Slyter, 1979). Extrapyramidal manifestations include bradykinesia, cogwheel rigidity, and choreiform or athetotic movements. Calcification of the basal ganglia may be visible on skull X-rays or CT scans (Klawans et al, 1976; Levin et al, 1961). In some cases, the extrapyramidal syndrome and dementia respond to successful treatment and normalization of the serum calcium levels (Berger and Ross, 1981; Slyter, 1979).

Hypocalcemia in pseudohypoparathyroidism is due to tissue unresponsiveness to parathyroid hormone. Dementia, conduct disorders, seizures, tics, and athetoid movements occur in a significant proportion of patients with pseudohypoparathyroidism, and the basal ganglia may be calcified (Ettigi and Brown, 1978).

The differential diagnosis of intracranial calcification includes toxoplasmosis, cysticercosis, trichinosis, brain abscess, tuberculosis, tuberous sclerosis, arteriovenous malformations, aneurysms, hematomas, brain tumors, idiopathic and postoperative hypoparathyroidism, idiopathic calcification of the basal ganglia, and congenital craniosomatic disorders (Levin et al, 1961).

Cushing's Disease

Cushing's disease results from long-term overproduction of glucocorticoids by the adrenal medulla or from iatrogenic administration of exogenous steroids. The cortisol may be produced directly by adrenocortical tumors (carcinomas, solitary adenomas) or may be secreted in response to ACTH originating from pituitary disorders or nonpituitary neoplasms (lung, thyroid, thymus, pancreas, and so forth). Pituitary adenomas account for 70 to 90 percent of cases of Cushing's disease (Carpenter, 1986). The usual clinical manifestations are obesity, rounding of the face, thickening of the supraclavicular fat pads and abdominal panniculus, thinning and bruisability of the skin, striae formation, hirsutism, acne, oligomenorrhea, limb weakness, osteoporosis, hypertension, diabetes, psychosis, and dementia (Liddle, 1971). The organic mental syndrome associated with Cushing's syndrome is characterized by depression, psychomotor retardation, irritability, poor concentration and memory, and disturbed sleep patterns (Glaser, 1953; Spillane, 1951; Starkman and Schteingart, 1981; Trethowan and Cobb, 1952). The severity of the neuropsychiatric disturbance correlates with the degree of cortisol elevation (Starkman and Schteingart, 1981). Laboratory tests that confirm the diagnosis include elevated serum cortisol levels, increased urinary excretion of 17-hydroxycorticosteroids, and failure to suppress serum cortisol levels following administration of exogenous dexamethasone. High-resolution X-ray CT reveals pituitary abnormalities in 30 to 50 percent of patients with Cushing's disease (Carpenter, 1986). When the cause of the syndrome is identified and treated and levels of serum cortisol return to normal, the mental status alterations resolve.

Addison's Disease

Too little cortisol (Addison's disease) as well as too much (Cushing's disease) can result in a dementia syndrome. The patient becomes languid, weak, and apathetic; there is anorexia, weight loss, and hypotension. Hyperpigmentation of the skin especially in sun-exposed regions occurs in some longstanding cases. Typical abnormalities on laboratory studies include hyponatremia, hyperkalemia, and failure of the adrenal to respond to a standard dose of ACTH (Liddle, 1971). In severe cases, there may be low levels of 24-hour urinary cortisol, 17-hydroxycorticosteroids, and 17-ketosteroids (Williams and Dluhy, 1987). Adrenocortical insufficiency results from idiopathic atrophy of the cortex, granulomatous destruction by tuberculosis or fungal infections, amyloidosis, or metastatic tumor.

Mental status changes in Addison's disease are similar to those observed in other endocrinopathies. The principal features are apathy, irritability, depression, suspiciousness, agitation, and memory impairment (Cleghorn, 1951; Lishman, 1978). Treatment of the adrenal insufficiency normalizes mental status in most cases.

Addison's disease may also accompany an inherited leukodystrophy (adrenoleukodystrophy) (Chapter 10), and in such cases, cortisol replacement has no effect on the dementia.

Panhypopituitarism

The combined hypothyroidism and adrenal insufficiency associated with panhypopituitarism can produce a dementia syndrome. The patients are apathetic, depressed, and lethargic. They have impaired concentration and poor memory and may have hallucinations and delusions (Cleghorn, 1951; Hanna, 1970). Endocrine replacement therapy reverses the dementia.

Panhypopituitarism can result from a chromophobe adenoma, postpartum necrosis (Sheehan's disease), idiopathic fibrosis, granulomas (idiopathic, syphilitic, or tuberculous), acute infection, skull fracture, surgical manipulation in the region of the third ventricle, or septic cavernous sinus thrombosis (Christy, 1971).

Inappropriate Antidiuretic Hormone Syndrome

The syndrome of inappropriate antidiuretic hormone and the intellectual deficits associated with chronic hyponatremia are discussed above with the electrolyte abnormalities.

TOXIC DEMENTIAS

We live in an age of "better living through chemistry" with constant industrial and domestic exposure to potentially harmful chemical agents. Insect and rodent poisons, additives to both fresh and processed foods, cosmetic products, household cleaners, airborne pollutants, and a myriad of additional toxins are constantly present. The wide variety of these compounds and their ubiquitous distribution and potential neurotoxicity, combined with inadequate consumer and worker safety measures produce an increasing number of toxic dementias. In addition to unknowing and unintentional exposure to environmental toxins, we purchase large quantities of potentially toxic over-the-counter and prescription medications that can adversely affect CNS function. When he or she is evaluating the demented patient, the clinician must be alert to the possible role of toxins and drugs in producing or exaggerating intellectual impairment (Table 7–8).

The elderly are more at risk for developing toxic dementias induced by drugs than are any other age group. Chronic diseases of all types are more prevalent in the aged, and medical treatment is required more frequently in this population. People over 65 years comprise only about 10 percent of the population, but they consume 25 percent of all prescription drugs (Burks, 1979; Thompson et al, 1983). In addition, equivalent dosages of drugs may not have equivalent effects in different age groups. Loss of body mass, age-related decrease in drug-binding serum proteins, differences in drug disposition, and alterations in cellular metabolism all make the elderly more susceptible to adverse consequences of drug ingestion (Dorsey, 1979; Greenblatt et al, 1982, Jenike, 1985; Ouslander, 1981). In his study of patients over the age of 65 admitted to a psychogeriatric service, Learoyd (1972) found that 16 percent had disorders directly attributable to the ill effects of psychoactive drugs. Prescribing practices must be modified for these individuals, and in some cases, a trial period without medication may be necessary to determine the role of drugs in dementia.

TABLE 7–8.   Toxic agents associated with dementia.

Drugs	Industrial agents and pollutants
Psychotropic agents	Perchloroethylene
Anticholinergic compounds	Toluene
Antihypertensive agents	Carbon tetrachloride
Anticonvulsants	Methyl chloride
Antineoplastic therapies	Ethylene glycol
Antibiotics	Methyl alcohol
Miscellaneous drugs	Acrylamide
Polydrug abuse	Trichlorethane
Alcohol	Trichloroethylene
Metals	Carbon disulfide
Lead	Organophosphate insecticides
Mercury	Organochlorine pesticides
Manganese	Ethylene oxide
Arsenic	Formaldehyde
Nickel	Hydrogen sulfide
Cadmium	Jet fuels
Thallium	Carbon monoxide
Aluminum	
Gold	
Tin	
Bismuth	

Drugs Associated with Dementia

Nearly any drug taken in excess can produce CNS toxicity manifested by impaired concentration, poor attention, memory disturbance, fluctuating arousal, and agitation. In higher dosages, stupor, coma, or death may occur. In many cases of drug toxicity, however, excessive doses have not been ingested and the patient demonstrates an idiosyncratic susceptibility to what are expected to be therapeutic amounts of medication (Table 7–9). The toxic effects are usually reversible by discontinuation of the drug.

Psychotropic Agents

All major classes of psychotropic agents are capable of producing intellectual impairment. Among psychoactive drugs, lithium carbonate, widely used in the treatment of manic-depressive illness, occasionally produces a dementia syndrome. Disorientation, poor attention and concentration, and impaired comprehension have been noted at serum levels within the usual therapeutic range (Shopsin et al, 1970). Lithium may disturb thyroid function (Fieve and Platman, 1968), and continuous use of the agent can induce a hypothyroid encephalopathy. The hypothyroidism can easily be misdi-

TABLE 7–9.   Therapeutic agents associated with dementia.

Psychotropic agents	Antibiotics
Lithium carbonate	Penicillin
Tricyclic antidepressants	Chloramphenicol
Phenothiazines	Griseofulvin
Butyrophenones (haloperidol)	Polymyxins
Anticholinergic compounds	Rifampin
Antihypertensive agents	Sulfonamide
Methyldopa	Metronidazole
Clonidine	Miscellaneous drugs
Propranolol hydrochloride	Disulfiram
Diuretics	Digitalis
Anticonvulsants	Bromides
Phenytoin	Steroids
Mephenytoin	Amphetamines
Barbiturates	Ergot
Ethosuximide	Oral contraceptives
Antineoplastic therapies	Antidiabetic agents
Mcthotrexate	Levodopa
Vincristine	
Asparaginase	
Hexamethylamine	
Interferon	
Cytosine arobinoside	
X-radiation	

agnosed as recurrent depression. The combination of lithium and haloperidol has been reported to produce an irreversible dementia (Cohen and Cohen, 1974), but the syndrome described had characteristics similar to those of the neuroleptic malignant syndrome that has been produced by haloperidol alone.

Tricyclic antidepressants produce chronic confusional states in as many as 10 to 15 percent of all patients receiving them and as many as 35 percent of the elderly (Hollister, 1979). CNS toxicity of the antidepressants is attributed to their anticholinergic activity. Acute toxic effects of tricyclic antidepressants can be reversed rapidly by intravenous administration of physostigmine (Granacher and Baldessarini, 1975). In addition to direct effects, the anticholinergic action delays gastrointestinal motility and may interfere with the absorption of other essential drugs (Morgan et al, 1975). Tricyclics have also been reported to cause inappropriate secretion of antidiuretic hormone and to produce chronic hyponatremia (Matuk and Kalyanaraman, 1977).

Major tranquilizers of both the phenothiazine and butyrophenone types can produce syndromes of intellectual impairment. Neuroleptic medications are widely used in nursing homes where approximately 40 percent of residents may receive one or more of these drugs (Avorn et al, 1989). Phenothiazines produce chronic confusional states that must be carefully distinguished from the endogenous psychoses for which whose agents are prescribed (Chaffin, 1964; Lang and Moore, 1961; Van Putten et al, 1974). Similarly, haloperidol can cause dementia, and the combination of haloperidol and methyldopa has been reported as etiologically significant in a syndrome of intellectual compromise (Thornton, 1976). Haloperidol and phenothiazines can produce a potentially lethal syndrome characterized by fever, rigidity, and stupor (Henderson and Wooten, 1981; Morris et al, 1980), and the combination of haloperidol and lithium has produced a similar syndrome with irreversible dementia (Cohen and Cohen, 1974). Major tranquilizers have also induced inappropriate secretion of antidiuretic hormone and hyponatremia (Matuk and Kalyanaraman, 1977). The risk of falling and hip fracture is increased among elderly patients receiving neuroleptic medications (Ray et al, 1987).

Anticholinergic Compounds

Acetylcholine is an essential neurotransmitter, and disruption of cholinergic synaptic function results in intellectual impairment. Pharmacologic studies show that anticholinergic compounds impair recent memory abilities, whereas cholinergic-enhancing drugs may improve performance on tests of memory and other intellectual functions (Drachman and Leavitt, 1974; Drachman and Sahakian, 1980; Katz et al, 1985). Many drugs that produce reversible dementing conditions have anticholinergic properties. Phenothiazines, haloperidol, and tricyclic antidepressants all have anticholinergic effects, and atropine and the nondopaminergic antiparkinsonian drugs exert powerful anticholinergic actions (De Smet et al, 1982; Longo, 1966; Syndulko et al, 1981). Patients may simultaneously receive more than one drug with anticholinergic properties (for example, an antidepressant, a neuroleptic, and an antiparkinsonian agent); toxic effects are additive. Up to 60 percent of nursing home residents receive drugs with anticholinergic effects and potential behavioral toxicity (Blazer et al, 1983). The CNS toxicity can be reversed rapidly by intravenous administration of physostigmine (Granacher and Baldessarini, 1975), and this response serves as an important diagnostic test for identifying toxic anticholinergic effects.

Antihypertensive Agents

Many antihypertensive agents exert their blood pressure lowering effects by disrupting function of catecholaminergic synapses and may have concomitant effects on mental function. Methyldopa produces dementia with depression, impaired concentration, poor memory, disturbed calculating abilities, and lethargy (Adler, 1974). A similar syndrome has been reported following clonidine administration (Allen and Flemenbaum, 1979; Lavin and Alexander, 1975), and depression, dementia and memory loss have occurred after treatment with propranolol hydrochloride (Cummings et al, 1980b; Kurland, 1979; Remick et al, 1981; Solomon et al, 1983; Voltoline et al, 1971). The mental status changes are not associated with systemic hypotension or cerebral hypoperfusion. Another class of antihypertensive agents, the diuretics, facilitate excretion of sodium and may lead to chronic hyponatremia. The intellectual impairment associated with low serum sodium is reviewed above with electrolyte abnormalities.

Anticonvulsants

Most of the major anticonvulsants have been associated with chronic encephalopathy. In some cases, the dementias have been induced by excessive intake of anticonvulsants, but careful psychometric assessment indicates that some patients have mild cognitive impairment even when serum levels are in the therapeutic range and other signs of toxicity are absent (Reynolds and Travers, 1974; Trimble and Reynolds, 1976). Lennox (1942) found that approximately 15 percent of patients had symptomatic mental deterioration after treatment with anticonvulsants despite improved seizure control. Therapeutic levels of phenobarbital almost invariably produces at least mild slowing of mentation and impaired concentration. Phenytoin can also produce cognitive slowing and several cases of chronic reversible phenytoin dementia have been reported (Ambrosetto et al, 1977; Glaser, 1973; Roseman, 1961; Vallarta et al, 1974). Other neurologic signs of phenytoin toxicity that may be present include nystagmus, ataxia, choreoathetoid movements, ophthalmoplegia, peripheral neuropathy, and asterixis (Glaser, 1973; Kutt et al, 1964; Murphy and Goldstein, 1974; Vallarta et al, 1974). In addition to direct toxic effects, phenytoin produces low levels of serum folate that may also impair neuropsychological function (Trimble et al, 1980).

Chronic encephalopathies have also been produced by barbiturates, ethosuximide, and mephenytoin (Isbell et al, 1950; Trimble and Reynolds, 1976; Vallarta et al, 1974). Except in high doses, carbamazepine does not directly impair cerebral function, but it can stimulate antidiuretic hormone to produce chronic hyponatremia (Moses and Miller, 1974).

The toxic effects of anticonvulsants are additive and conversion from multiple-drug treatment regiments to monotherapy has been associated with improved cognition.

Antineoplastic Therapies

Antineoplastic therapies depend on differential tissue responsiveness to biologically destructive agents such that tumor cells are selectively more vulnerable than are nonneoplastic tissues. In the course of treatment or after a latent period, CNS damage induced by chemotherapy or radiotherapy may become evident, and dementia may be one manifestation (Goldberg et al, 1982; Weiss et al, 1974).

L-asparaginase is an antineoplastic agent used in the treatment of acute leukemia and of some solid tumors. It hydrolyzes L-asparagine, which sensitive tumor cells cannot synthesize (Whitecar et al, 1970). Two types of encephalopathy have been reported following L-asparaginase administration: an acute confusional syndrome that usually resolves within a few days of discontinuing therapy and a more insidious dementia that begins soon after stopping therapy and lasts several weeks (Haskell et al, 1969; Weiss et al, 1974). The EEG is usually slow during the encephalopathic period.

Methotrexate is a folic acid antagonist useful in treating acute leukemia, choriocarcinoma, and solid tumors. It has been administered intrathecally to treat meningeal leukemia and meningeal carcinomatosis. Continuous intrathecal therapy occasionally results in an irreversible dementia syndrome. At autopsy the patients have had multiple small infarctions in the cerebral hemispheres or diffuse demyelination of hemispheric white matter (Norrell et al, 1974; Weiss et al, 1974). Seizures, myelopathy, and/or subacute meningeal irritation may also be manifestations of intrathecal methotrexate toxicity. Long-term survivors of combined antineoplastic therapy involving methotrexate, other chemotherapeutic agents, and irradiation may develop a delayed dementia syndrome with progressive intellectual impairment, ataxia, and seizures (Goldberg et al, 1982).

Nitrogen mustard can produce a chronic dementia and cerebral degeneration when high dosages are administered by way of intracarotid and regional perfusion techniques (Weiss et al, 1974).

Neuropsychological deficits are uncommon during procarbazine therapy, but occasional patients manifest hallucinations, agitation, poor attention, and lassitude (Weiss et al, 1974). Vincristine also affects the peripheral nervous system and tends to spare the CNS, but on rare occasions seizures and mental changes have been reported during the course of vincristine therapy (Weiss et al, 1974).

Hexamethylamine commonly produces a peripheral neuropathy and is also toxic to the CNS. Encephalopathic manifestations include dementia, depression, anxiety, and hallucinations (Goldberg et al, 1982).

Interferon, used in the treatment of multiple myeloma and other malignancies, has also been associated with production of a dementia syndrome. The encephalopathy begins during treatment and is manifested by intellectual deterioration, lethargy, and anorexia. Partial resolution follows discontinuation of therapy (Suter et al, 1984).

Cytosine arabinoside (Ara-C) is also neurotoxic. Reversible encephalopathies are encountered with low-dose therapy, whereas high dose treatment may result in irreversible mental status changes (Hwang et al, 1985). Dementia and cerebellar signs are the common toxic manifestations.

Irradiation of intracranial or extracranial cephalic neoplasms (usually with total doses in excess of 6000 rad) may damage the fine vasculature of the brain and produce a delayed degeneration syndrome with damage occurring primarily to the cerebral white matter. The delayed syndrome may present as a focal mass lesion, as multifocal neurologic deficits, or as a slowly progressive dementia syndrome (Kramer and Lee, 1974; Rottenberg et al, 1980; So et al, 1987).

Antibiotics

Numerous antibiotic agents have been implicated in the production of reversible dementia syndromes. Penicillin, chloramphenicol, griseofulvin, polymyxins, rifampin, sulfonamides, and metronidazole have been reported as responsible agents (Goetz et al, 1981; Johnson, 1979). Often the mental status changes are short-lived and occur only during the period of drug administration. Long courses of antibiotic therapy can produce reversible chronic confusional states under unusual circumstances such as uremia, individual predisposition, or underlying intellectual deficit.

Miscellaneous Drugs

In addition to the major classes of drugs presented above, a number of other agents used in a variety of therapeutic situations can produce reversible dementia syndromes. Disulfiram, a compound used to discourage the use of alcohol, produces an organic psychosyndrome in a small percentage of recipients, even when given in low dosages. The dementia is characterized by disorientation, paranoia, impaired memory, and hallucinations. Dysarthria, the appearance of primitive reflexes, and abnormal slowing of the EEG are also present (Hotson and Langston, 1976; Knee and Razani, 1974). The dementia reverses when the drug is discontinued. Disulfiram inhibits dopamine betahydroxylase, and the neuropsychiatric syndrome may reflect central dopamine excess.

Gastrointestinal and cardiac side effects usually precede the neurologic manifestations of digitalis toxicity, but neurologic complications occur in approximately 9 percent of patients receiving excessive amounts of the drug. Digitalis-induced dementia includes disorientation, impaired attention, and hallucinations (Sagel and Matisonn, 1972). Bromides are now rarely used, but occasional cases of bromism continue to be reported. Depression, disorientation, hallucinations, and impaired memory develop insidiously and progress to marked mental deterioration unless the bromide exposure is identified and corrected (Bucy et al, 1941; Carney, 1971; Zatuchni and Hong, 1981). Levodopa can cause chronic confusional states in the course of its use in the treatment of Parkinson's disease and related syndromes. Several drugs are capable of producing irreversible multi-infarct dementia by inducing the blood to clot or by causing a cerebrovascular arteritis. These agents include oral contraceptives, amphetamines, and ergot derivatives

(Citron et al, 1970; Ferris and Levine, 1973; Kessler et al, 1978; Margolis and Newton, 1971; Shafey and Scheinberg, 1966). A variety of drugs have been reported to stimulate inappropriate secretion of antidiuretic hormone and may induce a hyponatremic dementia. Agents known to cause hyponatremia include chlorpropamide and tolbutamide, sulfonylurea drugs, vincristine and cyclophosphamide, carbamazepine, amitriptyline, diuretics, and major tranquilizers (Matuk and Kalyanaraman, 1977; Moses and Miller, 1974). Use of long-acting oral hypoglycemic agents or recurrent excessive insulin administration may deprive the brain of glucose and produce irreversible CNS damage with dementia. Finally, administration of exogenous steroids may induce Cushing's disease with dementia.

Chronic Polydrug Abuse

Long-term excessive use of barbiturates or intake of combined barbiturates and analgesics can produce a chronic dementia that may not reverse with abstinence (Judd and Grant, 1978). Neuropsychological assessment after several drug-free months shows that some patients have persisting deficits in nonverbal abstracting ability, perceptuomotor integration, and memory (Grant and Judd, 1976; Grant et al, 1976; Murray et al, 1971). Forty percent of polydrug abusers continue to have EEG abnormalities three to five months after cessation of drug use (Judd and Grant, 1978), and persistence and severity of neuropsychological and EEG abnormalities correlate with the amount of drug use.

Other syndromes occurring in drug abusers that may lead to dementia syndromes include amphetamine-induced cerebral arteritis, multi-infarct dementia associated with infective endocarditis (resulting from unsterile intravenous injections), and chronic complications of alcohol use if drugs and alcohol are used concurrently. AIDS and HIV encepholopathy may occur in individuals with a history of intravenous drug abuse (Chapter 6).

Chronic Solvent Vapor Abuse ("Glue Sniffing")

Inhalation of the vapor from toluene-based products such as spray paint and glue is associated with a transient euphoria and has become a popular form of drug abuse. Chronic solvent vapor inhalation (for example, for periods exceeding 2 years of regular use) is associated with neurologic abnormalities including dementia, pyramidal and cerebellar dysfunction, and brainstem and cranial nerve signs (Hormes et al, 1986). CT reveals atrophy of the cerebral hemispheres, cerebellum, and brainstem in a majority of patients (Hormes et al, 1986). MRI demonstrates diffuse structural atrophy, attenuation of the difference between white matter and gray matter throughout the CNS, and increased signal intensity on T_2 weighted images in the periventricular region (Rosenberg et al, 1988). Postmortem examination

TABLE 7–10.   Organic psychosyndromes associated with chronic excessive alcohol use.

Alcoholic dementia	Acute alcohol-associated
Marchiafava-Bignami disease	psychosyndromes
Dietary deficiency syndromes	Acute inebriation
Korsakoff's psychosis (thiamine	Delirium tremens
deficiency)	Alcoholic blackouts
Pellagra (niacin deficiency)	Withdrawal seizures
Subacute and chronic alcohol-related	Pathologic intoxication
encephalopathies	Alcoholic hallucinosis
Posttraumatic encephalopathy	
Subdural hematoma	
Hepatic encephalopathy	
Acquired hepatocerebral degeneration	
Meningitis	
Central pontine myelinolysis	

reveals diffuse myelin pallor with few other histologic abnormalities (Rosenberg et al, 1988).

A similar encephalopathic syndrome has been described among house painters chronically exposed to solvents used as paint thinners (Arlien-Soborg et al, 1979).

Dementias Associated with Chronic Excessive Alcohol Use

Chronic overindulgence in the use of alcohol can affect the CNS and produce dementia in a variety of ways. Table 7–10 summarizes the major forms of dementia associated with alcoholism as well as other organic psychosyndromes occurring in alcoholic patients that must be distinguished from dementia.

Alcoholic Dementia

Despite the large number of alcoholics in public institutions, remarkably few sophisticated studies of the effects of long-continued alcohol use on intellectual function have been reported (Cutting, 1978b, 1982; Lishman, 1981). The diagnosis of alcoholic dementia fell into disrepute as the more specific amnesic Korsakoff's syndrome was identified and gained popularity (Lishman, 1981). Recently, attention has again turned to question the effects of chronic alcohol abuse on the brain, and the accumulated evidence suggests that alcoholics have intellectual deficits distinct from the amnesia of Korsakoff's syndrome. The idea of an alcoholic dementia is also supported by serial neuropsychological and radiologic studies, although the exact etiology of the syndrome remains obscure.

Clinically obvious dementia occurs in 3 percent of alcoholic in-patients and is responsible for approximately 7 percent of dementias among patients admitted for evaluation of progressive intellectual impairment (Cutting, 1982; Marsden and Harrison, 1972). Dementia is more common among elderly alcoholics than it is among younger individuals drinking for a similar period of time: It occurs in up to 45 percent of alcoholics over age 65 (Finlayson et al, 1988). Neuropsychological investigations suggest that as many as 50 percent of chronic alcoholic patients have some intellectual impairment (Carlen et al, 1981; Cutting, 1982; Lee et al, 1979). Alcoholic dementia is more apparent in elderly than it is in young subjects and appears earlier and with less alcohol consumption in women than it does in men (Cutting, 1982). For most studies, excess alcohol intake is defined as a daily intake of 150 ml or 120 gm of absolute alcohol—equivalent to two bottles of wine, seven pints of beer, or half a bottle of distilled spirits. The duration of consistent excessive intake is usually 10 to 15 years, and dementia is more likely to occur if the drinking is continuous than if it is interrupted by periods of withdrawal and abstinence.

Clinically, the dementia is mild and nonprogressive or only slowly progressive. Forgetfullness, psychomotor retardation, circumstantiality, perseveration, poor attention, and disorientation are typical (Lee et al, 1979; Lishman, 1981). Most neuropsychological studies show impaired abstracting abilities, poor short-term memory, and disturbed verbal fluency (Blusewicz et al, 1977; Carlen et al, 1981; Cutting, 1978c; Fitzhugh et al, 1965; Jones and Parsons, 1971, 1972). Nonverbal performance is usually more affected than are verbal skills, and aphasia is not present (Goldstein, 1985). Unless the patient has had head trauma, alcohol-related cerebellar or peripheral nerve damage, or focal CNS injury, elementary neurologic abnormalities are absent.

CT scans show enlargement of the lateral ventricles and widening of the cortical sulci in a majority of chronic alcoholics (Carlen et al, 1978; Fox et al, 1976; von Gall et al, 1978). The apparent shrinkage (atrophy) demonstrated by CT correlates with age but does not predict intellectual impairment (Cala et al, 1978; Carlen et al, 1981). The abnormalities demonstrable on scans may reverse if the patient remains abstinent (Carlen et al, 1978). Demented alcoholics over the age of 60 have a high incidence of EEG abnormalities, and EEG slowing is more common than is CT scan evidence of atrophy in this age group (Newman, 1978). Studies using pneumoencephalography also demonstrate atrophy in most chronic alcoholics (Brewer and Perrett, 1971; Haug, 1968; Ron, 1977). Glucose metabolism measured by PET is significantly reduced in chronic alcoholism and region-to-region correlations normally present are lost (Sachs et al, 1987).

Autopsy studies of patients with chronic alcoholism demonstrate mild cortical atrophy and disproportionate white matter atrophy suggesting that alcohol has its major effect on myelin (de la Monte, 1988).

Alcoholic dementia is at least partially reversible. If the patient remains abstinent, improvement in neuropsychological function occurs although full return to nonalcoholic levels is unusual (Bennett et al, 1960; Brandt et al, 1983; Guthrie and Elliott, 1980; Grant et al, 1984a; O'Leary et al, 1977; Page and Linden, 1974).

Marchiafava-Bignami Disease

Marchiafava-Bignami disease is an idiopathic syndrome involving demyelination of the corpus callosum and other midline white matter structures; it occurs almost exclusively in alcoholics (Ironside et al, 1961; Merritt and Weisman, 1945). Originally described in middle-aged Italian males with a history of excessive intake of red wine, it has been observed in other nationalities, in females, and rarely in nonalcoholics.

Clinically the disorder may start with stupor or coma; on recovery, the patients are demented and show a combination of amnesia, aphasia, disorientation, and personality change. Most have had seizures (Hathaway and Ch'ien, 1971; Ironside et al, 1961; Koeppen and Barron, 1978; Merritt and Weisman, 1945). Signs of callosal disconnection including left-hand tactile anomia, left-sided apraxia, and left-hand agraphia have been reported in clinically observed cases (Lechevalier et al, 1977; Lhermitte et al, 1977). Alcohol-induced neuropathy and other signs of chronic alcoholism have been present in some patients (Novak and Victor, 1974). The dementia may be progressive and intellectual changes have usually been present for several weeks to several months prior to death. The patient dies of aspiration pneumonia or intractable seizures.

X-ray CT reveals increased lucency in the region of the genu of the corpus callosum between the anterior horns of the lateral ventricles (Kawamura et al, 1985). MRI is notable for an area of diminished signal intensity on T_1-weighted images in the region of the corpus callosum (Kawamura et al, 1985).

At autopsy the primary lesion is demyelination continuing to complete necrosis of the central portion of the corpus callosum. The demyelination is accompanied by a variable amount of axonal degeneration. Gliosis is minimal. In some cases, there is demyelination of the anterior commissure, optic chiasm, hippocampal commissure, white matter of the cerebral hemispheres, cerebellar peduncles, and/or regions of the central pons (Ghatak et al, 1978; Ironside et al, 1961; Koeppen and Barron, 1978; Merritt and Weisman, 1945).

Alcohol-related Encephalopathies

Alcoholic dementia and Marchiafava-Bignami disease must be distinguished from a variety of chronic, subacute, and acute psychosyndromes that also occur in the alcoholic population (see Table 7–10). Dietary deficiency syndromes such as Korsakoff's psychosis and pellagra are presented above. Alcoholics are susceptible to head trauma; posttraumatic encephalopathy and subdural hematomas are important considerations in any alcoholic presenting with altered mental status. The long-term effects of alcohol on the liver make alcoholics vulnerable to hepatic encephalopathy and acquired hepatocerebral degeneration as discussed above. Infectious diseases, particularly meningitis, enter the differential diagnosis of acute acquired mental status changes among alcoholics. Central pontine myelinolysis is a subacute demyelinating syndrome of unknown etiology. The demyelination may be confined to the midpontine region or may affect widespread areas of the brainstem and cerebral hemispheres. Clinically there is progressive paralysis of bulbar function and the limbs, leading to coma and death (Adams et al, 1959; Goebel and Zur, 1972; McCormick and Danneel, 1967; Tomlinson et al, 1976).

Acute alcohol-related syndromes to be considered in alcoholic patients with altered intellectual function include inebriation, withdrawal phenomena such as delirium tremens and seizures, alcoholic blackouts, pathologic intoxication, and alcoholic hallucinosis (Charness et al, 1989; Sellars and Kalant, 1976; Victor, 1979; Victor and Hope, 1958).

Dementias Associated with Exposure to Metals

Many metallic agents interfere with cellular metabolism and produce dementia when exposure is prolonged. The principal dementias associated with metal exposure are listed in Table 7–8.

Lead

Lead enters the body by way of the gastrointestinal tract, lungs, or skin and is excreted by the liver, kidneys, and integument. Sources of lead in the environment include lead-based paints, vapors from gasoline and industrial compounds, lead-lined containers, glazes used in ceramics, and exhaust fumes from motor vehicles (Graef, 1979). Lead powder (azarcon) is used by some folkhealers in the treatment of gastrointestinal disorders. Neuropathy is the most common neurologic manifestation of lead intoxication in the adult, whereas encephalopathy is the primary neurologic complication in children. Encephalopathy has been reported in adults, however, and deserves consideration in the demented adult with a history of continuous exposure involving either organic or inorganic lead. Gasoline sniffing and ingestion of lead-contaminated "moonshine" whiskey are the most common sources of lead-induced encephalopathy in the adult (Graef, 1979; Valpey et al, 1978). Mental status manifestations are diverse but include impaired attention and memory, hallucinations, paranoia, delusions, and agitation. Headaches and convulsions may also occur and evidence of increased intracranial pressure may be present (Akelaitis, 1941; Whitfield et al, 1972). Asymptomatic children with elevated lead levels show permanent intellectual deficits when they are compared to those with no history or evidence of lead exposure (de la Burde and Choate, 1975; Landrigan et al, 1975; Needleman et al, 1979). At autopsy, the brains of patients with acute encephalopathy have cerebral edema, petechial hemorrhages, partial demyelination, and astrocytic hyperplasia. Chronic exposure results in extensive tissue destruction, cavity formation, and astrocytic and microglial proliferation (Popoff et al, 1963). Non-neurologic abnormalities of lead intoxication include anemia, abdominal pain, aminoaciduria, and bone changes. Blood levels of lead below 50 µg per 100 ml are not considered toxic and most clinically significant exposure produces lead levels in excess of 80 µg per 100 ml (Goetz et al, 1981). Chelation therapy with ethylenediaminotetraacetic acid (EDTA) or penicillamine is used to reduce the body's lead burden and reverse the acute toxic manifestations (Boyd et al, 1957; Graef, 1979). Permanent sequalae including mental status deficits are common in individuals with severe encephalopathy (Perlstein and Attala, 1966).

Mercury

Mercury intoxication occurs during the manufacture of paper or thermometers, in the preparation of chlorine, from ingestion of seafood or grain containing alkyl mercury, or from excessive use of calomel laxatives (David et al, 1974; Goetz et al, 1981). The principal manifestations are paresthesias, visual field constriction, ataxia, dysarthria, and deafness (Kurland et al, 1960; Marsh, 1979; Rustam and Hamdi, 1974). Choreoathetosis and a syndrome resembling amyotrophic lateral sclerosis have been described in some cases (Kantarjian, 1961; Snyder, 1972). Inorganic mercury poisoning is less severe and usually produces stomatitis, erethism (irritability in response to stimulation), and tremor whereas organic mercury intoxication causes paresthesias, ataxia, blindness, and dementia (Vroom and Greer, 1972). Mental status abnormalities produced by mercury poisoning include impaired short-term memory, insomnia, agitation, depression, and hallucinations (Evans et al, 1975; Okinaka et al, 1964; Ross et al, 1977). Visual agnosia in a case of inorganic mercury poisoning was extensively investigated by Landis and associates (1982). EEG abnormalities are found in many cases of mercury intoxication (Brenner and Snyder, 1980).

Pathologically the major areas of involvement include the calcarine cortex, insular cortex, and cerebellum. Severe cases show more widespread changes. Nerve cell degeneration with edema, small hemorrhages, and reactive gliosis are the usual histologic changes (Kurland et al, 1960; McAlpine and Araki, 1958; Shiraki, 1979). Diagnosis of mercury intoxication can be confirmed by measuring mercury levels in blood, saliva, or hair samples (Kark, 1979; Marsh, 1979). Many of the CNS abnormalities are manifestations of permanent structural changes, but chelation with penicillamine facilitates the excretion of mercury and produces at least partial amelioration of symptoms (Kark et al, 1971; Smith and Miller, 1961).

Manganese

Manganese toxicity is unusual but is a well-documented cause of dementia and extrapyramidal signs. It occurs primarily in mine workers but follows manganese exposure in the course of manufacturing chlorine gas, storage batteries, paints, varnish, enamel, linoleum, colored glass, and soaps (Goetz et al, 1981). Extrapyramidal manifestations of excessive manganese exposure include gait disturbance, dysarthria, clumsiness, tremor, increased muscle tone, masked facies, and bradykinesia (Mena, 1979; Mena et al, 1967). Neurobehavioral features occurring in patients with manganese intoxication are memory disturbance, compulsive phenomena, euphoria, hallucinations, poor concentration, irritability, and aggressiveness (Abd el Naby and Hassanein, 1965; Penalver, 1955; Saric et al, 1977; Schuler et al, 1957). Levodopa is partially effective in ameliorating the extrapyramidal symptoms, and EDTA produces improvement in some patients (Cook et al, 1974; Mena, 1979).

Arsenic

Arsenic is used in many insecticide sprays, as a disinfectant in animal hides and furs, and in the manufacture of paints, prints, and enamels (Goetz et al, 1981). Its availability results in occasional use as a suicidal or homicidal agent. Chronic organic ingestion results in a dementia syndrome characterized by somnolence, poor attention, impaired memory, difficulty with calculation, and disorientation (Freeman and Couch, 1978; Glaser et al, 1935; Hartman, 1988; Schenk and Stolk, 1967). Other manifestations of arsenic intoxication include myelopathy and peripheral and optic neuropathy. Hyperpigmented skin lesions, transverse white lines (Mees lines) on the nails, as well as gastrointestinal, respiratory, and cardiac abnormalities may occur (Chhuttani and Chopra, 1979; Goetz et al, 1981; Jenkins, 1966). Punctate hemorrhages concentrated in the white matter and chromatolysis of the neurons is the usual pathology of fatal cases. Laboratory diagnosis depends on identification of arsenic concentrations above 0.1 mg per 100 gm in the hair or nails or above 0.01 mg per 100 ml of blood (Chhuttani and Chopra, 1979). Reversal of the clinical manifestations depends on eliminating continuing exposure. Dimercaprol therapy may be useful in some patients (Jenkins, 1966).

Thallium

Thallium is not common in the environment, but it is used in the manufacture of sulfuric acid, as a rodenticide, as a depilatory, and therapeutically in the treatment of dysentery, ringworm, and malignancies (Goetz et al, 1981). Neurologic manifestations are frequent in thallium poisoning and include dysesthesia, neuropathy, choreoathetosis, ataxia, tremor, cranial nerve abnormalities, dementia, convulsions, and death (Bank et al, 1972; Domnitz, 1960). Mental disturbances may be early manifestations of thallium poisoning. Irritability, anxiety, somnolence, hallucinations, memory impairment, and confabulation may occur (Prick, 1979). The most prominent nonneurologic abnormality is alopecia, but gastrointestinal symptoms are also frequent (Grunfeld and Hinostroza, 1964; Reed et al, 1963). Vacuolar foamy degeneration of neurons especially in the hypothalamic region and edema of the white matter are found in the CNS of fatal cases. Treatment is directed primarily at eliminating exposure and increasing diuresis. Some cases may require hemodialysis.

Other Metals Associated with Dementia

In addition to the agents already discussed, numerous other metals have occasionally produced dementia. Aluminum is implicated as an etiologic agent in dialysis dementia and is discussed with disorders of renal function. The possible role of aluminum in the genesis of DAT is presented in Chapter 5 on cortical dementias. Excessive occupational exposure to aluminum may also result in a dementia syndrome. Hearing loss, ataxia, tremor, and fatigue accompany the neuropsychological defects (Hartman, 1988).

Gold is used in the treatment of arthritic conditions, and gold-induced neuropathy is an occasional complication; encephalopathy with apathy, disorientation, and poor memory has occurred in some cases (Goetz et al, 1981; McAuley et al, 1977).

Tin poisoning may produce mental abnormalities including insomnia, poor attention and memory, and apathy. Headache, pseudotumor cerebri, and spinal cord involvement also occur (Foncin and Gruner, 1979). Generalized slowing and epileptiform discharges are evident on EEG (Prull and Rompel, 1970).

Bismuth exposure results in a prominent dementia with alterations of intellectual function and emotional behavior. Depression, anxiousness, hallucinations, delusions, and intellectual impairment are common. Seizures and myoclonic jerks occur in more advanced stages of the disorder (Buge et al, 1981; Goetz and Klawans, 1979).

Dementia syndromes have also been described in individuals exposed chronically to nickel (Hartman et al, 1988) and to cadmium (Hart et al, 1989).

Industrial Agents and Pollutants

An enormous variety of compounds are being used in industry and many of them are potentially toxic to the nervous system. An alarming number of these agents have been linked to encephalopathies and peripheral neuropathies (see Table 7–8), and no doubt many more will be identified in the future (Rall and Tower, 1977). The largest group of potential toxins are the organic volatile substances used as solvents (Prockop, 1979). Among the organic solvents and related compounds known to produce encephalopathy after prolonged exposure are trichloroethylene, trichlorethane, perchloroethylene, toluene, carbon disulfide, methyl alcohol, carbon tetrachloride, ethylene glycol, methyl chloride, and acrylamide (Allen, 1979; Berger and Ayyar, 1981; Feldman, 1979; Feldman and Cummings, 1981; Hartman, 1988; Stevens and Forster, 1953; Vigliani, 1954). Most patients exposed to toxic amounts of these substances develop irritability, lethargy, poor concentration, and impaired memory (Allen, 1979; Chalupa et al, 1960; Salvini et al, 1971; Vernon and Ferguson, 1969). Workers with these symptoms may be accused of malingering to obtain compensation, so-called occupational neurosis. Many have a peripheral neuropathy, and nerve conduction studies may help document the occurrence of toxic exposure.

Insecticide exposure is another source of toxic dementia. The organochlorine compounds (DDT, kepone, telone, and so on) produce anxiety and irritability, but cognitive impairment is unusual (Taylor et al, 1979; Hartman, 1988). Organophosphate insecticides, widely used as pesticides, have powerful anticholinesterase activity (Namba et al, 1971), and exposure produces a dementia syndrome characterized by irritability, forgetfulness, anxiety, and sleep disturbances (Gershon and Shaw, 1961; Hartman, 1988; Levin et al, 1976b). Neuropsychological assessment confirms the presence of distractability and poor memory (Metcalf and Holmes, 1969). Increased random slow-wave activity is evident on EEGs of affected subjects.

Prolonged exposure to carbon monoxide can occur when poorly functioning motorized machinery is operated in a badly ventilated area (Gilbert and Glaser, 1969; Katz, 1958). Dullness, lethargy, forgetfulness, and irritability are common manifestations of carbon monoxide intoxication. The symptoms reverse when the cause is identified and eliminated.

Chronic exposure to methylene oxide (a gas used to sterilize heat-sensitive materials), formaldehyde, hydrogen sulfide, and jet fuels have all been associated with persistent neuropsychological defects (Crystal et al, 1988; Estrin et al, 1987; Hartman, 1988; Wasch et al, 1989).

DEMENTIA AND PERIPHERAL NEUROPATHY

Peripheral neuropathy can be an important clue in the diagnosis of dementia; the co-occurrence of dementia and peripheral neuropathy is uncommon,

TABLE 7–11.   Major conditions manifesting dementia and peripheral
neuropathy.

Metabolic and toxic disorders	Systemic disorders
Chronic renal failure	Inflammatory conditions (mononeuritis
Recurrent hypoglycemia	multiplex)
Porphyria	Degenerative disorders
Remote effects of malignancy	Spinocerebellar degenerations (some)
Vitamin deficiency state	Choreoacanthocytosis
B complex deficiency (Korsakoff's	Denny-Brown disease (progressive
syndrome and alcoholic	sensory radiculopathy)
dementia)	
Cyanocobalamin (B_{12}) deficiency	
Endocrinopathies	
Hypothyroidism	
Drugs	
Antineoplastic agents	
Antibiotics	
Disulfiram	
Heavy metals	
Industrial agents	
Endogenous metabolic disturbances	
Cerebrotendinous xanthomatosis	
Metachromatic leukodystrophy	
Leigh's disease	
Fabry's disease	
Membranous lipodystrophy	

except in the toxic-metabolic disorders. Degenerative disorders affecting
cortical or subcortical structures are rarely seen in combination with peripheral neuropathy, and most nondegenerative CNS processes—trauma, neoplasm, stroke, hydrocephalus, viral infection, multiple sclerosis—entirely
spare the peripheral nerves. Inflammatory disorders may affect the brain
and peripheral nerves, but the peripheral pattern is an asymmetric mono-
neuropathy multiplex. Thus the presence of symmetric distal peripheral
neuropathy in a demented patient should direct investigative efforts toward
the identification of a toxic or metabolic condition causing or exacerbating
the intellectual deficits. Table 7–11 summarizes the principal conditions
producing dementia and peripheral neuropathy.

8

Hydrocephalic Dementia

Literally, *hydrocephalus* means "water in the head." The term is ancient and almost without question, observations of hydrocephalus predate medical reporting. It has long been recognized that considerable mental abnormality (mental retardation) can accompany early-onset hydrocephalus, but only in more recent times has an acquired impairment of intellect been associated with late-onset hydrocephalus—hydrocephalic dementia. Hydrocephalus is not a common cause of dementia in adults, but some of the conditions that produce it can be corrected and the intellectual deficit reversed.

Although it was known in antiquity, little of consequence was written about hydrocephalus until the time of Vesalius. It was generally believed that a collection of water between the brain and the skull produced the skull enlargement, but Vesalius (1725) demonstrated that hydrocephalus produced enlargement of the ventricular system apparently without accumulation of fluid outside the brain.

All early studies of hydrocephalus concerned children. This is logical as the massive enlargement of the skull caused by accumulation of fluid in the ventricles of young children produces an obvious abnormality. Whytt (1768) studied a number of childhood hydrocephalic brains and described consistent enlargement of the ventricular system but no enlarged channels between the brain and the skull. Morgagni (1769) was the first to note that enlargement of the ventricles could also be present in an adult whose head was not enlarged, but his observation was not accepted by most eighteenth-century physicians. The next advances were made by anatomists who demonstrated the major foramina of the ventricular system and traced the flow of cerebrospinal fluid. While most of these major anatomic discoveries date from the nineteenth century, it was not until the twentieth century that the formation and absorption of cerebrospinal fluid was clearly outlined (Dandy, 1919; Schaltenbrand and Putnam, 1927).

Why hydrocephalus develops has long been the subject of debate. Oversecretion by the choroid plexi was proposed by some (Claisse and Levy, 1897; Davis, 1924); others suggested that hydrocephalus resulted from obstruction in the CSF pathway. Scrutiny of accumulated neurosurgical and pathologic data supports the latter theory. CSF flow may be obstructed either within the ventricular system or prior to its absorption in the sagittal sinus. Many published cases of hydrocephalus originally thought to be secondary to excessive choroid plexus secretion are probably due to obstructive hydrocephalus; in some cases, choroid plexus papillomas may produce hydrocephalus by CSF hypersecretion (Bell and McCormick, 1972; Russell and Rubinstein, 1977). A third cause is also recognized—secondary enlargement of the ventricular system due to wasting or atrophy of cerebral tissues producing so-called hydrocephalus *ex vacuo*.

A relationship between hydrocephalus and impaired intelligence is well documented (Laurence and Coates, 1962a, b; Laurence and Tew, 1967). Most studies demonstrate both a lower mean IQ for patients with hydrocephalus and a considerable range of standard deviation. This great variability in intellectual abilities suggests that influences other than hydrocephalus are present. For instance, the etiology of hydrocephalus, its severity and degree, age at onset and at initial examination, gender (boys develop more favorably than do girls with an equivalent disease), and finally the presence and nature of associated abnormalities such as spina bifida—all are factors that influence mental status. That the native intelligence of patient and parents is pertinent has also been considered.

Until the last decade and a half, all discussion of mental impairment secondary to hydrocephalus concerned children. While the adult-onset condition was recognized and a correlation with mental impairment was acknowledged, it was not until Hakim (1964) demonstrated a reversible condition based on an obstructive but communicating variety of hydrocephalus that hydrocephalic dementia was investigated. Foltz and Ward (1956), in an elegant study of the residuals of subarachnoid hemorrhage, clearly demonstrated enlarged ventricular size and decreased mentation, but it was the work of Hakim and colleagues (Hakim, 1964; Adams et al, 1965) that aroused interest in adult hydrocephalus and hydrocephalic dementia.

The cause of ventricular enlargement remains a topic of debate. Spiller (1902) stated: "It is not necessary to study the different works on hydrocephalus very exhaustively to find that actually observed lesions are much rarer than theories explanatory of the causes of hydrocephalus." Most

TABLE 8–1. Classification of hydrocephalus.

Obstructive	Nonobstructive
Noncommunicating (obstruction of ventricular CSF outflow channels) Communicating (obstruction of extraventricular CSF flow channels)	Hydrocephalus *ex vacuo* (ventricular enlargement secondary to focal or widespread loss of brain tissue) Hypersecretion hydrocephalus (rare disorder associated with choroid plexus papilloma)

theories focus on one of two causes—obstruction or atrophy. Separation of the two is not always obvious, and a specific diagnostic approach has been sought. Dandy and Blackfan (1913) introduced the widely used classification of communicating or noncommunicating hydrocephalus based on the presence or absence of obstruction of the ventricular outflow system. The former was automatically thought to represent hydrocephalus *ex vacuo,* whereas the latter implied obstruction to the ventricular outflow system. The demonstration of normal-pressure hydrocephalus (NPH) by Hakim (1964) and others proved this approach inadequate. Characteristically NPH has free communication between the ventricular system and the spinal subarachnoid space, but there is obstruction of CSF flow upward to the sagittal area. A revised classification of hydrocephalus is presented in Table 8–1.

Obstructive hydrocephalus can be subdivided into communicating and noncommunicating types. Obstructive noncommunicating hydrocephalus refers to those instances in which a lesion (tumor, glial scar) obstructs ventricular outflow (see Fig. 8–1). Obstructive communicating hydrocephalus refers to instances with free flow through and out of the ventricular system but with obstruction to flow of CSF upward along the subarachnoid channels to the sagittal sinus area.

Nonobstructive hydrocephalus refers to enlargement of the ventricular system secondary to atrophic changes of cerebral tissue (and possibly rare cases of hydrocephalus produced by overproduction of CSF), producing compensatory enlargement. Dementia can be associated with any of these disorders, but treatment and prognosis are distinctly different.

PATHOPHYSIOLOGY OF HYDROCEPHALUS

Basic to an understanding of hydrocephalus is knowledge of the body's third system of circulation, CSF. While some variations and exceptions occur, the basic principles of the circulation of CSF are well established. Following the presentation by Dandy and Blackfan (1913), it is generally agreed that most

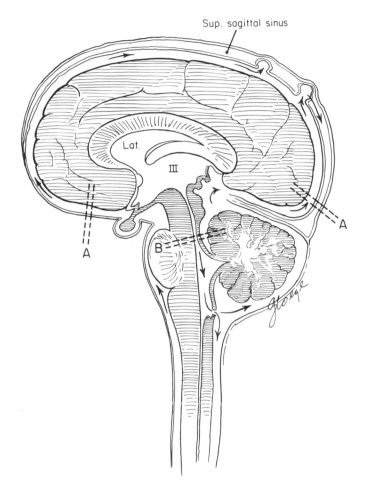

FIGURE 8–1.   The normal flow of CSF from its production by the choroid plexus in the ventricles to its absorption in the superior sagittal sinus. Dotted lines A indicate obstruction in the extraventricular channels; dotted lines B represent intra-ventricular blockage.

CSF is formed by the ventricular choroid plexi, organs with cuboidal cells resembling the cells of the renal proximal tubule. Considerable evidence indicates that CSF is formed by an active transport mechanism, not by a simple exudative process, and that the transport of ions across the membranes of the choroid plexus is an energy-requiring process (Held et al, 1964).

There is less agreement concerning the production of CSF by extrachoroidal sources. Some data suggest that a small portion of the fluid and certain constituents of the CSF do come from sources other than the choroid cells, and a dual origin of CSF is generally accepted, but "the anatomical structures responsible for extrachoroid fluid formation remains unknown" (Pollay, 1972).

The flow of CSF formed within the ventricles is fixed and unidirectional from the lateral ventricles through the foramen of Monro into the third ventricle, from the third ventricle through the aqueduct of Sylvius to the fourth ventricle, and thence through the foramina of Magendie and Luschka into the cisterna magna and subarachnoid space. CSF is accumulated during this flow as active choroid plexi are present in both lateral ventricles, the third ventricle, and the fourth ventricle. Almost all CSF emanates from the ventricular system and passes through the foramina of Luschka and Magendie into the subarachnoid channels at the base of the brain.

From the basal cisterns, two directions of circulation are possible. One is a continuation of CSF flow downward into the spinal subarachnoid space along the spinal cord into the lumbar sac. This is probably a limited circulation with two-way diffusion of CSF contents into spinal tissues (particularly veins) and only a limited return of CSF or contents to the upper circulation.

The second and more important flow is upward through the subarachnoid spaces of the posterior fossa cisterns to the cisterns at the base of the forebrain and into the subarachnoid spaces over the cortical convexity, eventually arriving in the area of the superior sagittal sinus. Most spinal fluid is absorbed through the pacchionian villi of the sagittal sinus, but there is evidence suggesting that small amounts may be absorbed into venous protrusions located along the spinal venous network (Dandy and Blackfan, 1913; Key and Retzius, 1875; Weed, 1935). In both instances, CSF is absorbed into the venous circulation through macroscopic arachnoid granulations or microscopic arachnoid villi protruding into the venous channels.

Figure 8–1 illustrates the principal directions of cerebrospinal fluid flow. Pollay (1972) has described the entire system: "CSF is almost entirely produced within the ventricular system from a dual source at a rate related to the surface area of the choroid plexus and ventricular wall." He goes on to describe the removal of CSF: "The bulk drainage of this fluid into blood has been shown to be primarily through open tubes in the arachnoid villi under the influence of the hydrostatic gradient existing between CSF and the blood in the cranial venous sinuses."

Although this system appears relatively simple and straightforward, several bothersome questions remain. First, how is CSF pressure maintained? Second, how is ventricular size maintained? Both questions become even more difficult to answer in the context of selected pathologic conditions. For instance, in some instances CSF pressure can become very high without enlargement of the ventricles (for example, pseudotumor cerebri) while in others the ventricular system can become extremely large despite normal or even low CSF pressure (for example, normal-pressure hydrocephalus). Much has been written on these questions and, while they are still unresolved, many of the comments are relevant. One obviously pertinent factor in maintenance of CSF pressure is the elasticity of tissues surrounding the ventricles. This periventricular elasticity has been considered a function of the ependyma (Geschwind, 1968) or the entire brain acting as a viscoelastic structure (Hakim, 1972). Whatever the mechanism, an intrinsic elasticity of the periventricular structures is an important factor in the determination of ventricular size and CSF pressure.

In understanding CSF pressure/volume relationships, considerable stress has been given to Pascal's principle that force is the product of pressure times area ($F = P \times A$). Over an enlarged ventricular area, a given degree of force would sustain a lower pressure. To produce the initial enlargement of the ventricular system, however, an increase in pressure appears essential. Hakim (1972) states flatly: "In order to reach a state of NPH it is necessary for the ventricles to have been dilated previously." He goes on to say that to start the hydrocephalic process an increase in CSF pressure or a decrease in the pressure of the intracranial venous system is necessary because, "it is not the CSF pressure alone that determines the size of the ventricles; instead, it is the difference between the forces of the CSF and the venous systems." He surmises that venous collapse is necessary for production of hydrocephalus, the collapse reducing blood flow, inducing hypoxia and metabolic alteration in the choroid plexus with further ventricular enlargement resulting from loss of lipids and proteins. Two possible causes are suggested for increased ventricular size in true hydrocephalus: (1) an alteration of the venous absorption mechanism or (2) an obstruction to CSF outflow producing a temporary increase in both CSF volume and pressure.

What is the explanation of increased ventricular size in NPH in the face of normal CSF pressure and no ventricular outflow obstruction? Hakim's theory that increased pressure is necessary to initiate ventricular dilatation is widely accepted, but pressure elevation is often not demonstrated. One of the more plausible alternative explanations is Fishman's (1966) suggestion of a simple pressure gradient, the normal CSF pressure within the ventricular system being far greater than is the nonexistent pressure in the newly established potential space over the subarachnoid membrane, thereby producing ventricular enlargement. Most investigators, however, suggest that considerably greater pressure gradients would be needed. One early thought was that pulsations of the carotid arteries at the base of the brain produced a water-hammer effect that enlarged the ventricles (Ekbom et al, 1969a). These pulsations originate outside the ventricular system, however, and Hakim (1972) suggested that a more likely mechanism was pulsation of the choroid plexus, occurring within the comparatively rigid water column created by obstructed CSF flow and producing a water-hammer effect sufficient to enlarge the ventricles. None of the explanations is totally satisfactory, but hydrocephalus does appear in individuals without evidence of either increased pressure or demonstrable cerebral atrophy.

In contrast to the complex mechanical and physiologic alterations of normal-pressure hydrocephalus, both noncommunicating and nonobstructive varieties produce predictable changes in CSF dynamics. In the former, the ventricles enlarge in the face of increased pressure; in the latter, the enlargement is passive as cerebral tissue is lost.

While hydrocephalus can result from a variety of causes and can show a variety of effects, an almost universal accompaniment is mental impairment, a hydrocephalic dementia.

PATHOLOGIC STATES PRODUCING HYDROCEPHALIC DEMENTIA

Spontaneously Arrested Hydrocephalus

Not infrequently, individuals born with cerebral maldevelopment who sustain an early acquired insult develop hydrocephalus and then undergo a spontaneous arrest of the condition. They often have moderately enlarged heads and, not infrequently, some degree of mental impairment. Even more pertinent, however, these individuals are at high risk for further intracerebral complications. A minor cranial insult can produce an overwhelming dementia. Any individual with spontaneously arrested hydrocephalus who survives to adulthood is at risk to develop hydrocephalic dementia eventually.

The etiologic factors producing hydrocephalic disturbances of childhood are multiple and have been well described. In her classic monograph, Russell (1949) outlined five major causes:

1. Maldevelopment such as aqueductal stenosis, spina bifida, platybasia, and lissencephaly
2. Gliosis of the aqueduct
3. Inflammatory disturbances (the most prevalent in Russell's series was tuberculosis)
4. Dural sinus thrombosis and thrombophlebitis (often associated with so-called otitic hydrocephalus)
5. Neoplasm

In a study using operative rather than pathologic data, Foltz and Shurtleff (1963) described 113 children with hydrocephalus and found:

1. Communicating (obstructive) hydrocephalus (basal arachnoiditis secondary to infection, bleeding, and so on)
2. Aqueductal stenosis

3.   Mass of the third ventricle
4.   Obstruction of the fourth ventricle outflow channels (Dandy-Walker syndrome)
5.   Encephalocele
6.   Arnold-Chiari malformation
7.   Multiple anomalies
8.   Cystic brain disease
9.   Undiagnosed

Many causes of childhood hydrocephalus are recognized but the exact cause in the adult with an arrested hydrocephalus may be difficult to discern in retrospect.

The number of individuals with hydrocephalus who enjoy a spontaneous arrest appears limited. The largest study, that of Laurence and Coates (1962a), suggested a 10-year survival rate of only 27 percent and did not take into consideration the degree of intellectual impairment. Foltz and Shurtleff (1963) and Foltz alone (1966) projected that only about 5.5 percent of those hydrocephalics who survived without surgical intervention enjoyed an IQ of 75 or better, with another 16.7 percent alive but seriously impaired mentally, a total survival of only 22.2 percent. With the advent of shunting as a treatment for developmental hydrocephalus, this grim picture has improved. Foltz and Shurtleff (1963) and Foltz alone (1966) projected a 61.4 percent 10-year survival rate of surgically treated cases, over half of whom would have an IQ above 75. Thus it is now likely that arrested hydrocephalus in an adult reflects successful surgical intervention, also these individuals are susceptible to decompensation and hydrocephalic dementia in later years.

Obstructive Noncommunicating Hydrocephalus

The onset of specific symptomatology, including mental impairment, caused by obstruction to ventricular outflow has been recognized by neurosurgeons for most of this century. If the obstruction occurs acutely, a dramatic alteration in clinical status occurs. The individual develops severe headache, nausea and vomiting, lethargy and drowsiness, and eventually drifts into stupor and coma. Bilateral sixth nerve palsy, paraparesis or quadriparesis, and respiratory depression are often present. Surgical intervention becomes essential. If the outflow obstruction is subacute, however, with stenosed but not fully obstructed ventricular outflow, the onset of symptomatology may be far less dramatic, with development of a considerable degree of hydrocephalus before symptoms appear and the patient comes to appropriate medical attention. In either situation, significant mental impairment (dementia) is almost inevitably present.

The etiology of obstructed ventricular communication can be any disorder capable of blocking the ventricles, the exit foramina, or the sylvian

TABLE 8–2.   Causes of obstructive hydrocephalus.

Noncommunicating obstructive	*Communicating obstructive (NPH)*
Aqueductal blockade	Posttraumatic
Congenital aqueductal stenosis	Posthemorrhagic
Aqueductal compression	Postinfectious
(tumors, vascular	Idiopathic
malformations, cysts)	Neoplastic
Inflammatory aqueductal	Sagittal sinus meningioma
stenosis	Carcinomatous meningitis
Hemorrhagic obstruction	Lymphomatous meningitis
Intraventricular obstructive lesions	Tentorial tumor
Tumors	Partial obstruction
Meningiomas	Intraventricular tumors
Papillomas	Colloid cysts
Ependymomas	Pituitary tumors
Vascular malformations	Aqueductal stenosis
Compressive lesions	Posterior fossa mass lesions
Astrocytomas	Basilar impression
Oligodendrogliomas	Ectatic basilar artery
Colloid cysts	
Hemorrhagic obstruction	
Obstruction of outlet foramina	
Posterior fossa neoplasms	
Posterior fossa vascular	
malformations	
Inflammatory processes in	
basilar cisterns	
Dandy-Walker malformation	
Arnold-Chiari malformation	
Hemorrhagic obstruction	

aqueduct (Table 8–2). The aqueduct is the most vulnerable to stenosis, compression, or plugging. Congenital aqueductal stenosis may present with hydrocephalic dementia (Drachman and Richardson, 1961; Nag and Falconer, 1966; Vanneste and Hyman, 1986; Wilkinson et al, 1966). Neoplasms are the most common cause of noncommunicating hydrocephalus and may obstruct one or both lateral ventricles, the aqueduct, or the outlet foramina in the posterior fossa.

    Inflammation, particularly ependymitis, arachnoiditis, and pachymeningitis due to acute or chronic intracranial inflammatory disorders, is a relatively common cause of hydrocephalus. The high incidence of tuberculosis as a cause of hydrocephalus in the past has decreased with the advent of antibiotic therapy; similarly, syphilitic pachymeningitis as a cause of ventricular obstruction is now rare. On the other hand, parasitic and fungal disorders are increasingly recognized to cause CSF flow obstruction. Opportunistic infections in immunosuppression (for example, AIDS, steroid therapy for organ transplant, or tumor therapy) are increasingly common. In one of the most common helminthic disorders, cysticercosis, only seizures are a more common clinical presentation than hydrocephalus and dementia. Focal paresis and the pathognomonic constriction of visual fields of cysticercosis almost invariably appear in individuals with hydrocephalus and mental impairment. Among viral inflammatory disorders, mumps encephalitis appears to have a predilection for producing an obstructing ependymitis of the cerebral aqueduct (Bell and McCormick, 1972).

Aqueductal kinks and obstructions can be produced by the greatly dilated lateral ventricles of communicating hydrocephalus, converting from a communicating to a noncommunicating pattern and creating a continued shunt dependency (Nugent et al, 1979). Intracranial hemorrhage can easily produce acute or subacute obstruction of the ventricular outflow system particularly when blood clots form within the ventricles or posterior fossa. The hemorrhage may result from trauma, blood dyscrasias, ruptured aneurysm, tumors, or vascular malformations. Similarly, tumors within the ventricles—ependymomas, intraventricular meningiomas, papillomas, cysticercosis cysts, and colloid cysts—can obstruct interventricular flow and produce hydrocephalic dementia (Little and MacCarty, 1974). The Arnold-Chiari malformation, Dandy-Walker malformation, and congenital or acquired basilar impression may remain asymptomatic until adulthood and then produce an insidiously progressive hydrocephalus and intellectual impairment (Banerji and Millar, 1974; Culebras et al, 1974; Gardner et al, 1972; Hart et al, 1972). While acute ventricular outflow obstructions are more common and far more readily diagnosed, subacute obstruction deserves consideration in any adult with the clinical picture of hydrocephalic dementia.

Obstructive Communicating (Normal-Pressure) Hydrocephalus

As described earlier, CSF flow can be obstructed even though ventricular outflow remains patent, a state originally called occult hydrocephalus (McHugh, 1964) but now termed normal-pressure hydrocephalus (NPH). The most common basis for NPH is subarachnoid hemorrhage (Ellington and Margolis, 1969; Foltz and Ward, 1956; Kibler et al, 1961). Katzman (1977) reported that about 35 percent of reported patients had a history of subarachnoid bleeding, most often due to ruptured aneurysm but in some cases due to bleeding from an arteriovenous malformation or trauma. Multiple studies (Bergvall and Galera, 1969; Galera and Greitz, 1970) have demonstrated that about one-third of all subarachnoid hemorrhages produce a hydrocephalic state, but the incidence of persistent, symptomatic hydrocephalus is closer to 10 percent (Theander and Grenholm, 1967; Yasargil et al, 1973). Head trauma, in addition to causing bleeding into the subarachnoid space, can produce scarring and subsequent fibrosis in the subarachnoid space, leading to obstructed CSF flow. Inflammatory disease, particularly meningitis that involves the subarachnoid tissues, can produce a fibrosis capable of obstructing the subarachnoid CSF channels (Heck et al, 1971; Voris, 1955). All of these entities (hemorrhage, trauma, and infections) tend to produce meningeal thickening at the base of the brain plus fibrosis in the subarachnoid channels over the cortical surface. A variety of tumors has been reported to cause normal-pressure hydrocephalus. Meningioma involving the sagittal sinus, carcinomatous or lymphomatous meningitis, and mass lesions at the tentorium can all produce the clinical picture of normal-pressure hydrocephalus.

Numerous entities that produce partial or intermittent obstruction to the outflow channel are known to produce a communicating obstructive hydrocephalus. Tumors such as colloid cysts of the third ventricle, cholesteatomas, metastases involving the third or fourth ventricle, and even pituitary adenomas have been reported as causes of NPH (Katzman, 1977). Incomplete mechanical obstruction to the outflow such as aqueductal stenosis (Vanneste and Hyman 1986), cerebellar hematoma, or tumor mass and basilar impression have also been associated with the disorder. Katzman and Pappius (1973) estimate that as many as 20 percent of individuals with the NPH syndrome actually have a partial obstruction of ventricular outflow.

One frequently mentioned but controversial entity, ectatic basilar artery, may be associated with NPH (Breig et al, 1967; Ekbom et al, 1969b; Kak and Taylor, 1967). Atherosclerotic alteration of the wall of the basilar artery can produce an unyielding stiffened and straightened vessel (pipestem artery). With advancing age, the brain has a tendency to settle and the nonelastic basilar artery can project upward into the base of the brain,. affecting the inferior and anterior aspects of the third ventricle. The resultant partial obstruction of the third ventricle can cause an enlargement of the ventricles, leading to a hydrocephalic dementia syndrome. In this situation, the lateral ventricles will show marked enlargement and the third ventricle may or may not be enlarged while the fourth ventricle will be normal in size.

Hydrocephalus *ex Vacuo*

Among the pathologic entities associated with hydrocephalus and dementia must be included those disorders in which atrophy of the brain substance produces compensatory enlargement of the ventricular system. The most common and best recognized are the degenerative brain disorders, DAT and frontal degenerative dementia. Actually, however, the amount of ventricular enlargement in these disorders is relatively limited, particularly when it is compared to the degree of dementia. Focal ventricular enlargement can be noted in some disorders. For instance, progressive supranuclear palsy causes marked atrophy of the mesencephalon and is readily recognized in brain images, which demonstrate a striking decrease in the thickness of the mesencephalic tectum and a widening of the sylvian aqueduct (Bentson and Keesey, 1974). Similarly the dementia of Huntington's disease is almost constantly accompanied by a focal increase of the size of the frontal horns due to caudate atrophy.

More common as causes of ventricular enlargement on an *ex vacuo* basis are the disorders that produce focal or multifocal brain damage. Cerebral infarction is almost invariably associated with enlargement of the neighboring ventricular system. This enlargement is often asymmetric, providing a good clue to the cause of the hydrocephalus. In vascular dementia associated with multiple lacunes or widespread demyelination, the lateral and third ventricles may be fairly uniformly dilated, a pattern that closely imitates obstructive hydrocephalus. Trauma to cerebral tissues sufficient to produce persistent findings often causes a compensatory enlargement of the ventricles, usually asymmetric. Tumor surgery, the removal of a glioma or a meningioma is often associated with considerable damage to brain tissue and compensatory focal enlargement of the ventricular system. Any of the above disorders may be associated with dementia, and when one includes the presence of hydrocephalus, they must be considered in the differential diagnosis of hydrocephalic dementia. Except for the rather even enlargement of the ventricular system noted in the degenerative brain diseases and some types of vascular dementia, most of the *ex vacuo* causes of hydrocephalic dementia will not be diagnostic problems for the investigator.

Cerebral Cysts

Any disorder capable of producing focal ventricular enlargement—vascular infarction, trauma, tumor surgery, and the like—can also damage an area of brain that may become necrotic and cystic. Damaged cerebrum tends to become fibrotic and shrinks. Modern imaging techniques demonstrate situations in which cerebral cysts enlarge over time. Not infrequently one finds a large cyst in the area of previous insult to the brain in the presence of a normal-appearing ventricular system. Several reports (Adams, 1975a; Benson, 1975; Ojemann et al, 1969) suggest that these cysts represent an atypical form of hydrocephalus. It has been postulated that damage to brain tissue produces a space with less viscoelastic resistance of the involved tissues than that around the ventricles. If this space communicates with a CSF-containing structure, the cyst will enlarge with increases in CSF pressure (force) in preference to the ventricles. Isotope cisternographic studies often demonstrate these cysts and, in addition, demonstrate failure of circulation of the isotope in the normal pathways (Front et al, 1972; Silverberg et al, 1969). Such cysts actually represent a continuation of the ventricular (or, less frequently, the subarachnoid) system. The ventricles would have enlarged (obstructive hydrocephalus) if the cyst were not there to compensate for the increased force. This situation can be considered a forme fruste of normal-pressure hydrocephalus. Cerebral cysts can become symptomatic, often producing focal findings and progressive dementia. A few reports suggest improvement in mental state following shunting in individuals with cerebral cysts.

SYMPTOMATOLOGY OF HYDROCEPHALIC DEMENTIA

While a broad spectrum of symptoms can be seen in patients with progressive hydrocephalus reflecting the various areas of brain that may have been damaged, a comparatively specific triad of disturbances characterizes the hydrocephalic dementias; motor disturbance, dementia, and incontinence (Katzman, 1977). There is considerable variation in these features, however, and additional neurologic and neurobehavioral findings secondary to focal damage can produce a wide variety of clinical pictures. Even when partially obscured, the triad is present to some degree in most patients with hydro-cephalic dementia and provides an important diagnostic clue. Any adult with impaired intellectual function who shows both gait disturbance and incontinence deserves consideration for a diagnosis of acquired hydrocephalus.

Motor Disturbance

Gait disturbance is the most characteristic and usually the most prominent feature of hydrocephalic dementia, but the disturbance varies greatly, ranging from a subtle awkwardness to a totally akinetic state (Sudarsky and Simon, 1987). One of the most consistent findings is some degree of spasticity involving the lower extremities most extensively (Katzman, 1977). This pattern mirrors the anatomically relevant pattern described by Yakovlev (1947) in children with developmental hydrocephalus. Spasticity is greater in the lower extremities than it is in the upper because the distended ventricles produce a far greater deviation of the medially arising fibers controlling leg activities than they do of the more laterally originating fibers involved in upper extremity and facial activity (Fig. 8–2). With sufficient hydrocephalus, a total quadriparesis can occur, although a milder disturbance of gait is more common. While spasticity is usual, an appreciable ataxic quality may be present, often with the characteristics of Bruyn's ataxia, ostensibly based on frontal lobe dysfunction (Meyer and Barron, 1960). The

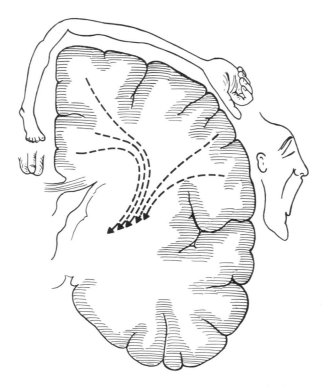

FIGURE 8–2.   The relation of motor fibers distributed to the legs and sphincters to the expanded ventricular system in hydrocephalus. Ataxia and incontinence result from the greater deviation required for those fibers arising from the medial cortex.

patient has difficulty initiating movement, described by Messert and Baker (1966) as though the patient's feet were "glued to the floor" or "held by a magnet." Once engaged in motion the activities become freer, at times returning to near-normal levels. The difficulty in starting bears a resemblance to parkinsonism, but the considerable improvement as activity progresses suggests frontal motor disturbance (Moore, 1969; Sypert et al, 1973).

Exaggerated muscle stretch reflexes and extensor plantar responses are common in hydrocephalic dementia, and when the disorder becomes severe, additional findings such as Hoffmann's sign, hyperactive jaw jerk, snout and grasp reflexes, extrapyramidal motor disturbances, akinetic mutism, or quadriparesis may occur. Neuroophthalmic abnormalities are rare but may occur if distention of the suprapineal recess produces pressure on the upper midbrain (Shallat et al, 1973).

It has been stated that the best results from surgical treatment of hydrocephalus are improvements in the motor disturbances (Benson et al,

1970; Graff-Radford and Godersky, 1986; Katzman, 1974; Messert and Wannamaker, 1974). Movement disorder is certainly a major aspect of hydrocephalic dementia and it is difficult (although not impossible) to make this diagnosis in the absence of some degree of movement abnormality.

Mental Changes

The impairment of mental status associated with hydrocephalus also varies widely. The disorder may be no more than minor intellectual slowing, some decrease in spontaneity, mild inattention, or apathy. In the early stages, intellectual retardation is minimal. With progression, however, greater deterioration occurs so that patients with hydrocephalic dementia show distinct memory disturbance in addition to slowed mental processes. The memory disturbance, disorientation, and mental slowing produce a marked disability (McHugh, 1964; Ojcmann et al, 1969). Impaired abstraction, poor performance on tasks requiring sequential analysis, and difficulty with complex computation are characteristic. The basic features of hydrocephalic dementia correspond closely to those observed in subcortical dementia (slowing, apathy, forgetfulness) but often coexist with signs of cortical dysfunction.

Most patients with hydrocephalic dementia are quiet, withdrawn, and slow to respond, but an occasional patient is anxious, aggressive (Crowell et al, 1973), or paranoid. Only rarely are delusional thinking, hallucinations, or ideas of reference apparent (Dewan and Bick, 1985), and these psychiatric disturbances are thought by some to represent a basic, underlying mental disturbance released by the hydrocephalic process (Rice and Gendelman, 1973). Patients with hydrocephalic dementia often appear depressed (Price and Tucker, 1977), but slowing of mental and physical processes (psychomotor retardation) imitate depression and misdiagnosis is a potential pitfall. Most patients with hydrocephalic dementia do not express depressive thought content.

In more advanced forms of disease, alterations in the state of consciousness may be seen. The patient may become obtunded, show akinetic mutism, or lapse into coma. Some patients with normal-pressure hydrocephalus became comatose following pneumoencephalography (Bannister et al. 1967). Gilbert (1971) suggested that injecting a quantity of air greater than the amount of fluid removed could produce an acutely increased pressure but, in other situations, the presence of an unsuspected mass lesion or an advanced stage of hydrocephalus may have been important factors. Inasmuch as pneumoencephalography is almost never performed now, this has become a pedantic consideration.

Incontinence

The third portion of the triad, urinary incontinence, is frequent in hydro-cephalic dementia but often does not appear until late in the course, and some individuals with hydrocephalic dementia report no incontinence. Fecal incontinence is rare. Like motor fibers concerned with leg function, neurons controlling bladder and bowel sphincters arise medially in the posterior frontal cortex and may be subject to distortion as the ventricular system enlarges. While often considered a pathognomonic symptom, incontinence is of limited diagnostic value as it only occurs late and is not unusual in late stages of DAT and other types of progressive dementia.

DIAGNOSTIC TECHNIQUES

In the face of the variable clinical picture of the hydrocephalic dementias, some laboratory support is necessary for a definitive diagnosis. A review of the diagnostic techniques used to study all dementias is presented in Chapter 12; only those specific for the hydrocephalic dementias are summarized here.

Psychometric testing can be useful, but the dementing process may be too advanced to allow performance of a full neuropsychological battery. At present there is no guaranteed method for differentiating hydrocephalic dementia from other dementing disorders by psychological testing.

The most useful diagnostic procedure is brain imaging by X-ray CT scan or MRI which show not only a considerable enlargement but a ballooned appearance of the ventricles suggestive of an obstructive process (Gado et al, 1976; Haan and Thomeer, 1988; Jacobs and Kinkel, 1976). The frontal and temporal horns often show a disproportionate enlargement compared to the more posterior portions of the lateral ventricles (LeMay and Hochberg, 1979; Sjaastad et al, 1969). In acute cases, transependymal migration of CSF may create identifiable high signal areas surrounding the ventricles (see Fig. 8–3). In sharp contrast, the cortical subarachnoid spaces often appear relatively normal, even in the presence of a considerable hydrocephalus (Fig. 8–4).

Even better than the X-ray CT for definition of a hydrocephalus is air encephalography, but this procedure has both morbidity and mortality and is rarely used. With pneumoencephalography the hydrocephalus is more accurately demarcated and evidence of incisural block, mass lesion obstructing either anterior or posterior third ventricle, or other obstructive process is often obvious. Classic pneumoencephalographic findings in NPH include enlargement of the anterior portion of the lateral ventricle, a corpus callosal angle of 120 degrees or less with the patient in the brow-up position, and obstruction of air flow over the cerebral convexities (LeMay and New, 1970).

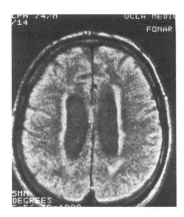

FIGURE 8-3.   MRI of a patient with normal pressure hydrocephalus. Note enlarged lateral ventricles with bright lateral boundaries formed by fluid, probably a
transependymal exudation of CSF.

Isotope cisternography remains useful for identification of some types
of hydrocephalic dementia (Benson et al, 1970). Isotope injected into the
lumbar region in cases of communicating obstructive hydrocephalus rapidly
diffuses into the ventricles (ventricular reflux) but fails to rise into the sagittal
region (subarachnoid block) over the next 48 to 72 hours (Fig. 8–5). Both
of these features are abnormal, and the combination suggests abnormal CSF
circulation with failure of sagittal absorption. Isotope cisternography can
have both false positive and false negative results, however, and does not
reliably predict response to treatment (Wolinsky et al, 1973).

Infusion manometric tests (Coblentz et al, 1973; Katzman and Hussey,
1970) can demonstrate the lack of CSF flow but also have false positive and
false negative results. Because of technical problems manometric infusion
has not gained wide usage but, when it is properly performed, accurately
demonstrates a disturbance of CSF absorption. More popular are techniques
for CSF drainage to evaluate improvement if any. The most formal technique, external lumbar drainage (ELD), connects a tube in the lumbar
subarachnoid space to an external collector and drains CSF for five days
(Haan and Thomeer, 1988). Far more common is a single removal of a large
quantity (30 to 50 cc) of CSF, sometimes called the Fisher Test. With both
techniques the final judgement is based on observed improvement of gait
or mentation. Both have proved successful.

Angiography may be useful in some instances, primarily to demonstrate
vascular abnormalities producing an obstruction. EEG has been used, but
the results are inconsistent. The reports from series with mixed causes of
hydrocephalus prove inconclusive (Brown and Goldensohn, 1973). Studies
of cerebral blood flow using isotopes indicate decreased cerebral blood flow

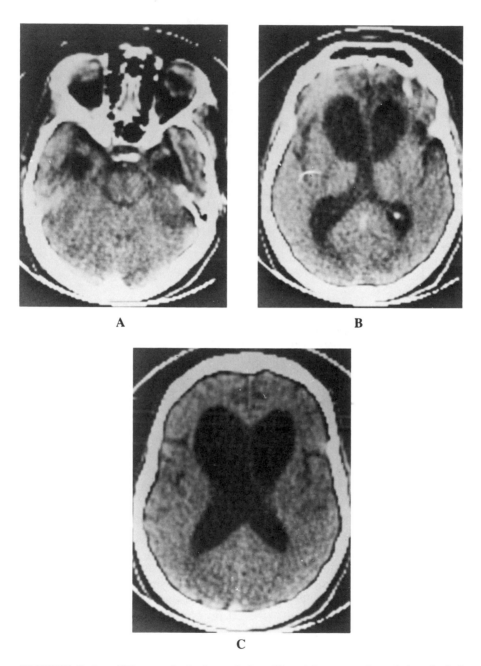

A   B

C

FIGURE 8–4.   CT scans in hydrocephalus. Ventricles are enlarged (particularly the frontal (B and C) and temporal (A) horns) while the cortical sulci are relatively normal.

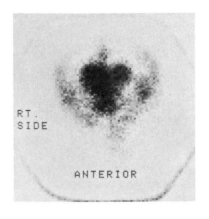
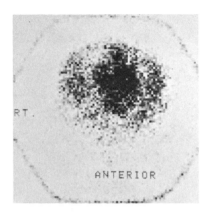
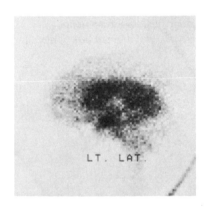
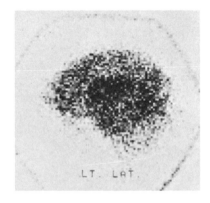

FIGURE 8–5.   Cisternography in normal-pressure hydrocephalus. Ventricular reflux occurs soon after injection of the radionuclide, and flow over the convexities is
obstructed.

in hydrocephalus (particularly frontally) and, in the case of obstructive
hydrocephalus, the cerebral blood flow increases after CSF shunting (Graff-
Radford et al, 1987; Greitz, 1969; Greitz et al, 1969; Mathew at al, 1975).
Unfortunately, an increase in cerebral blood flow does not always coincide
with a decrease in dementia. Some studies suggest that careful monitoring
of intracranial CSF pressure can produce information indicative of potential
for success of shunting in individuals with hydrocephalic dementia (Crockard
et al, 1977; Hartmann and Alberti, 1977; Symon et al, 1972), but again have
not proved consistently accurate (Huckman, 1981). Emission tomography
(PET, SPECT) may reveal ventricular enlargement and only modest decrease in cortical glucose metabolism (Fig. 8–6) or cerebral blood flow.
These tests are not sufficiently specific to be diagnostic.

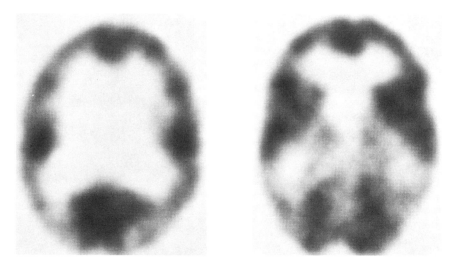

FIGURE 8–6.   PET in normal-pressure hydrocephalus. Notable ventricular enlargement and only modestly decreased cortical glucose metabolism are evident.

In summary, the most successful diagnostic technique remains the neurologic examination with the probable diagnosis confirmed by one of the imaging studies. A CSF drainage study may then be undertaken on those patients being considered for shunt therapy.

PATHOLOGY

Grossly, the brains of patients who die with an obstructive hydrocephalus appear normal except for slight flattening of the gyri. Coronal sections of the hemispheres show widely dilated lateral ventricles, with the dilatation most marked in the frontal and temporal horns (Fig. 8–7). Histologic studies may reveal leptomeningeal or pacchionian fibrosis responsible for the absorption block (in cases of NPH), ventricular ependymal disruption and subependymal gliosis produced by the ventricular dilatation, and periventricular demyelination and spongiosis (Di Rocco et al, 1977). The last changes are manifested clinically in the gait ataxia and incontinence that result from disruption of the periventricular fibers. In addition to these neuropathologic findings associated with the hydrocephalus per se, evidence of the underlying process (trauma, hemorrhage, neoplasm, and so forth) may also be identified.

The gross specimen will not always demonstrate the presence of hydrocephalus even in cases where laboratory studies have shown a considerable enlargement of the ventricles in life. Messert and colleagues (1972)

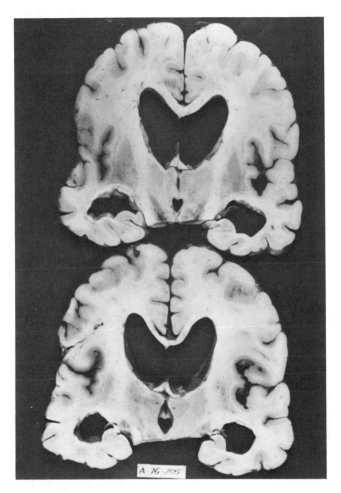

FIGURE 8–7.   Coronal section of brain with hydrocephalus. The lateral ventricles and temporal horns are enormously dilated; the callosal angle between the ventricles is less than 120 degrees; and the cerebral sulci are not enlarged.

have demonstrated that, particularly in cases of acute or subacute hydrocephalus, the elasticity of the periventricular tissues may remain sufficiently intact to allow return of the ventricles to near-normal size when the abnormal force is relaxed. They contend that the ventricles are almost always smaller at postmortem than they are *in vivo*.

The pathophysiology of hydrocephalic dementia remains as much a mystery as do the mechanisms involved in the production of hydrocephalus, and several factors probably contribute to the ultimate intellectual disability. The dilatation of the anterior portions of the ventricular system, compromised function of periventricular tracts and structures, diminished frontal blood flow, increased periventricular parenchymal fluid, and other, as yet unidentified, factors may all play a role in producing the mental status changes.

TREATMENT

There can be little question that the rapid acceptance of hydrocephalic dementia as a distinct entity reflected the concomitant introduction of a rational and frequently successful treatment. In addition to treatment of the underlying etiology (for example, removal of mass lesion), hydrocephalic dementia can be corrected by a shunting procedure to divert CSF from the intracranial spaces to an extracranial site (Scarf, 1963). The original procedures involved shunting from a lateral ventricle to a mastoid space (Foltz and Ward, 1956); later procedures attempted to channel the CSF to the cardiac atrium (ventriculoatrial shunt). Next the peritoneum was used to divert CSF (ventriculoperitoneal shunt), and in some instances, a shunt from the lumbar subarachnoid space to the peritoneum (lumboperitoneal shunt) has been used for communicating types of hydrocephalus. In cases where ventricular outflow is obstructed but subarachnoid channels are normal, the Torkildsen procedure, a shunt from a ventricle into the cisterna magna, can be successful.

Each procedure has certain advantages and certain technical problems; all have serious potential complications. The advantage of the ventricular shunt is that the CSF is removed from the area adversely affected; on the other hand, the lumboperitoneal shunt is safer to perform as it does not demand an intracranial approach or cerebral puncture; however, it can be used only in cases of communicating hydrocephalus and demands precise pressure control gauging.

Maintaining patency of the shunt once it has been inserted has been a persistent technical problem. The intake of the shunt is easily occluded by choroid plexus or, if improperly placed, by brain tissue. The peritoneum has the capability of occluding the outflow orifice, providing yet another potential problem.

Even more difficult is control of residual ventricular pressure. This is particularly true with the lumboperitoneal shunt in which the substantial difference in spinal fluid pressure depends on whether the patient is standing or recumbent and can prove difficult to manage. With all types of ventricular shunting the maintenance of a proper pressure is difficult. One-way valves are available with a variety of pressure gradients, and the ultimate success of a shunting procedure is at least partially dependent on choice of a valve that maintains the correct final pressure. Too high a pressure may result in no alteration in the hydrocephalus while too low a pressure may allow too great a decompression of the intracranial tissues with the danger of subdural hematoma.

There are many complications of the shunt procedures. The most common, but not the most serious, is plugging of the shunt causing recurrence of the hydrocephalic dementia. A small compressible reservoir is often placed in a portion of the tube lying just under the scalp. Manual compression of the reservoir is thought to clear both the intake and output orifices. Unfortunately this procedure has not proved reliable. Not infrequently, compressibility is interpreted as indicating patency although the shunt is eventually proved to be occluded. The only reliable check of patency is through a repeat isotope cisternogram or through injection of the tubing itself with an isotope.

More threatening complications include production of a subdural hematoma (secondary to acute change in CSF dynamics) (McCullough and Fox, 1974) or development of infectious processes that invade the foreign body (shunt). Possible infections include meningitis and abscess formation. When ventriculoatrial shunts were used, the formation of infected emboli within the jugular vein produced bacterial endocarditis.

Other complications have been reported and should be considered in the patient who fails to improve after the surgical intervention. Epileptogenic EEGs and seizures are approximately twice as common in hydrocephalic patients who have been shunted as in those who have not. As many as 50 percent of shunted patients have seizures compared to 20 percent of unshunted hydrocephalics (Graebner and Celesia, 1973; Ines and Markand, 1977). The peritoneal end of the shunt may produce intestinal volvulus, and rare cases of perforation of intestines, pleura, scrotum, gallbladder, vagina, or abdominal wall have occurred (Adeloye, 1973; Portnoy and Croissant, 1973; Ramani, 1974; Sakoda et al, 1971; Sells and Loeser, 1973; Wilson and Bertan, 1966). Most perforations occurred in children and have become less common with use of more flexible tubing. Abdominal catheters may cause inflammatory pseudotumor or loculated abdominal cysts, and on rare occasions, CSF ascites has occurred when the peritoneum was unable to absorb the diverted fluid (Cummings et al, 1976; Fischer and Shillito, 1969; Keen and Weitzner, 1973; Parry et al, 1975). Because of the intravascular location of ventriculojugular and ventriculoatrial shunts, they were subject to more numerous and more serious complications, including infection, hydrothorax, cardiac tamponade, vena caval occlusion, pulmonary emboli, and pleural effusion (Forrest and Cooper, 1968); as a consequence, they are rarely performed at present.

To say the least, the currently available treatments for hydrocephalic dementia are far from perfect. Nonetheless, success is so gratifying and occurs in a sufficient number of cases to warrant continued use of shunts coupled with ongoing attempts to improve both predictors of shunt responsiveness and the surgical procedure.

PROGNOSIS

Many cases of spontaneous improvement have been recorded in individuals with hydrocephalic dementia, particularly normal-pressure hydrocephalus (Hughes et al, 1978). Most often the patients developed hydrocephalus acutely following subarachnoid hemorrhage or trauma, showed the clinical and laboratory presence of a hydrocephalic dementia for several weeks or longer, and then without specific therapy improved clinically, and repeat laboratory studies demonstrated resolution of the hydrocephalus. It seems almost unquestionable that the cortical subarachnoid channels, originally occluded, reopened and once again allowed circulation of CSF to the sagittal region. Spontaneous recovery is not predictable, however, and many patients with hydrocephalic dementia must be treated for the problem. The percentage of patients in whom neurosurgical shunt procedures have led to clearcut improvement is variable, dependent on many factors. A considerable literature has appeared on this subject over the past few years, and when differences in reporting are taken into consideration, most series suggest recovery rates ranging between 40 and 65 percent (Hughes et al, 1978; Shenkin et al, 1973; Udvarhelyi et al, 1975) with an overall frequency of about 55 percent (Katzman, 1977).

One of the most discouraging aspects of treating hydrocephalic-dementia is the inability to predict who will improve following therapy. A number of factors affect prognosis. These include whether an appropriate diagnosis has been made; the presence of underlying brain injury such as cerebral infarction, traumatic degeneration, degenerative brain disease, and others; the technical success of the shunting procedure; and the duration of hydrocephalic symptoms before treatment is instituted. The most important consideration in prognosis concerns etiology. When the hydrocephalus is secondary to a known disturbance, the recovery rate is comparatively high (65 to 80 percent). In contrast, treatment of idiopathic types of hydrocephalic dementia with shunting has a success rate of only about 40 percent (Katzman, 1977; Stein and Langfitt, 1974). The presence of motor abnormalities tends to correlate with clinical improvement following shunting (Graff-Radford and Godersky, 1986; Jacobs et al, 1976; Thomsen et al, 1986); most investigators agree that motor problems have the best chance of improvement following a shunt procedure. No single laboratory test adequately predicts responsiveness; CSF drainage studies are widely used and are often the best currently available predictors of shunt success.

There can be little doubt that long duration of hydrocephalus before treatment decreases the potential for improvement (Wood et al, 1974). Thus the presence of the condition for many years before a diagnosis is made usually means that shunting will not produce a significant improvement. Permanent alteration of brain structures is thought to occur on the basis of longstanding compression.

When the shunting procedure is unsuccessful, many individuals merely need replacement of the shunt. In some cases, replacement of one valve with another of lower or higher pressure has resulted in improvement. The risk of the procedure, however, also affects the prognosis. The mortality rate is reported to be between 6 and 9 percent (Illingsworth et al, 1971; Wood et al, 1974). In addition, epidural and subdural hematomas have been said to occur in over 5 percent of shunted patients (Driesen and Elies, 1974), and the other complications already noted can occur. Finally attempts to shunt individuals with hydrocephalus *ex vacuo* (for example, DAT) invariably lead to failure of the treatment (Ojemann et al, 1969; Salmon and Armitage, 1968).

While successful treatment of hydrocephalic dementia is inconsistent, proper selection of patients and use of appropriate techniques can result in salvage of severely disabled patients. Known etiology, short duration before treatment, presence of motor signs, positive imaging and cisternographic findings, and improvement following CSF drainage are the best indicators of possible surgical success; they do not represent operative criteria, however. Shunting should not be withheld from any patient whose clinical and laboratory evaluation suggests that obstructive hydrocephalus is an important contributing factor to the mental status alterations.

9

Dementia Syndromes Associated with Psychiatric Disorders: The "Pseudodementias"

Apparent intellectual impairment associated with psychiatric disorders has traditionally been considered under the rubric of "pseudodementia." The term is included here because of this precedent, but it should be recognized that the prefix "pseudo" implies there is something false about the mental status changes, a questionable implication. In this volume, "dementia" indicates a clinical syndrome of diverse etiology and variable prognosis: it is incorrect to consider the cognitive and personality alterations occurring in the course of psychiatric disturbances as pseudo-changes. Intellectual compromise often occurs in the course of psychiatric illness, and it is often reversible. The degree to which these processes may mimic dementias associated with degenerative disorders of CNS provides one of the great challenges to clinicians working with intellectually impaired patients.

The word "pseudodementia" has been applied to at least two different groups of patients. The first group includes depressed individuals whose cognitive impairment improves when the depression is successfully treated. In the second group, "pseudodementia" is used as a more inclusive term encompassing all patients with apparent cognitive impairment secondary to psychiatric disturbance. Caine (1981) suggested four criteria necessary to define and diagnose pseudodementia. First there is intellectual impairment in a patient with a primary psychiatric disorder; second the features of the syndrome resemble those induced by the degenerative CNS disorders; third the intellectual compromise is reversible; and fourth the patient has no

TABLE 9–1.   Psychiatric disorders that may be associated with dementia.

Affective disorders	Schizophrenia	Hysterical dementia	Miscellaneous pseudodementias
Depression Mania	Acute psychosis with transient intellectual impairment Buffoonery syndrome Persistent psychosis with neuropsychological disturbance Late deterioration	Conversion hysteria with dementia Ganser's syndrome	Malingering Obsessional-ruminative states Anxiety neurosis

primary identifiable neurologic disease that can account for the cognitive changes. Although depression accounts for a majority of pseudodementias, the syndrome can be produced by a number of psychiatric disturbances including mania, schizophrenia, hysterical conversion reactions, and Ganser's syndrome (Table 9–1). Caine (1981) noted that older patients with pseudodementia nearly always have depression as the underlying etiologic disorder, whereas younger patients may be suffering from any one of a heterogeneous group of psychiatric conditions.

The frequency of pseudodementia varies greatly depending on the methods of ascertainment. Of patients admitted to neurologic or psychiatric services for evaluation of dementia, from 2 to 32 percent will be found to have a pseudodementia (Freemon, 1976: Rabins, 1981). Most studies suggest a prevalence of approximately 10 percent among patients evaluated for a history of progressive intellectual deterioration (Marsden and Harrison, 1972: Seltzer and Sherwin, 1978: Smith and Kiloh, 1981: Smith et al, 1976). Follow-up studies, however, suggest that degenerative dementia is overdiagnosed, and in some studies as many as 20 to 50 percent of patients discharged from the hospital with a diagnosis of dementia may actually be suffering from a primary psychiatric disorder with pseudodementia (Nott and Fleminger, 1975: Ron et al, 1979). The principal psychiatric disturbances associated with pseudodementia are presented below.

MOOD DISORDERS

Mood disorders, particularly depression, account for a majority of cases of pseudodementia. Occasionally mania produces a clinical syndrome with forgetfulness, disinhibited behavior, and altered personality that resembles dementia associated with CNS degeneration.

Depression

Depression is the final diagnosis of from 50 to 100 percent of pseudodementias among patients admitted for evaluation of progressive intellectual decline (Caine, 1981; Freemon, 1976; Good, 1981; Marsden and Harrison, 1972; Ron et al, 1979; Seltzer and Sherwin 1978; Smith and Kiloh, 1981). A dementia syndrome can occur with depression in the course of a biopolar disorder, in major depressions (single episode or recurrent), or with depression with elements of character disorder (Caine, 1981; Folstein and McHugh, 1978; McHugh and Folstein, 1979; Wells, 1979). Depression can also significantly exacerbate the intellectual compromise occurring in poststroke depression and in Parkinson's disease with depression (Rogers et al, 1987; Starkstein et al, 1989). The dementia of depression is an age-related phenomenon, and patients who become severely depressed or psychotic during recurrent depressive episodes in early and midlife may manifest a dementia syndrome when depression recurs at a more advanced age. While depressive dementia can occur in young patients, it is uncommon in early or midlife (Cavenar et al, 1979). The prevalence of depressive dementia varies with the population studied of the diagnostic criteria applied. Many severely depressed patients will manifest cognitive alterations, including poor concentration, abnormal attention and impaired memory (Cohen et al, 1982). In most cases, the cognitive deficits are mild in comparison with the depression, and consideration of a primary dementia is unlikely. Kay and associates (1955) found that 10 percent of patients over age 65 years who have mood disorders manifest prominent memory and intellectual deficits consistent with the diagnosis of dementia, and Rabins et al (1984) found that 30 percent of patients admitted for depression had sufficient intellectual impairment to warrant a diagnosis of dementia.

Patients with the dementia of depression are distinguished from depressed patients without cognitive impairment by more frequent presence of delusions, greater anxiety, and more marked cerebral atrophy on brain imaging studies in addition to intellectual impairment (La Rue et al, 1986; Pearlson et al, 1989; Rabins et al, 1984).

The behavioral characteristics of the dementia syndrome include slowness of responses, forgetfulness, disorientation, impaired attention, and disturbed ability to abstract and grasp the meaning of situations (Caine, 1981; Folstein and McHugh, 1978; Hart and Kwenters, 1987; McHugh and Folstein, 1979; Rogers et al, 1987). Depressed mood and affect is usually apparent and the patient may express guilt, shame, and self-deprecatory feelings. Patients may respond with "I don't know" to direct questions or fail to make or complete a response. If psychosis is present, there may be hallucinations, self-deprecatory nihilistic delusions, or paranoid ideation. Delusions of this type are rarely seen in dementias without depression (McHugh, 1981). Signs of cortical impairment such as aphasia, apraxia and

TABLE 9–2.   Comparison of the clinical features of the dementia syndrome of
depression. Parkinson's disease with dementia, and DAT.

Clinical feature	Dementia syndrome of depression	Parkinson's disease	DAT
Bradykinesia	+	+	−
Stooped posture	+	+	−
Rigidity	+/−	+	−
Tremor	−	+	−
Depressed mood	+	+	+/−
Slowness of response	+	+	−
Memory disturbance	+	+	+
Poor recall	+	+	+
Poor recognition	−	−	+
Aphasia	−	−	+
Agnosia	−	−	+
Apraxia	−	+/−	+

agnosia are not present. The dementia syndrome of depression resembles
Parkinson's disease with dementia and has few similarities to cortical degenerative processes such as DAT (Table 9–2).

The natural history of the dementia syndrome of depression is controversial. Some investigators regard the condition as a common harbinger of
degenerative dementia and report a high frequency of DAT among patients
previously manifesting the disorder (Kral, 1983). Other studies, using standardized diagnostic criteria and comprehensive evaluative techniques, however, find no increased prevalence of degenerative dementia among patients
followed for several years after an episode of "pseudodementia" (La Rue
et al, 1986; Rabins et al, 1984). Moreover the elderly with depressive
disorders as a group are not at increased risk for the development of
degenerative diseases (Kay et al, 1955). Thus, most evidence suggests that
the dementia of depression should be regarded as a unique subtype of
depression and not as an early stage or forerunner of DAT.

Many of the physical characteristics of patients with retarded depression
resemble the clinical features of Parkinson's disease. Facial movement is
diminished, and gross motor slowing with increased muscle tension is present
(Greden and Carroll, 1981; Schwartz et al, 1976). Neurovegetative disturbances include loss of appetite, constipation, impotence, and sleep disturbances. Speech is slowed and hypophonic, and speech pause time (the silent
interval between phonations during automatic speech) is elongated (Greden
et al, 1981; Greden and Carroll, 1980). The striking similarities between the
neuropsychological and somatic manifestations of Parkinson's disease and

those of depression suggest that similar pathophysiological mechanisms may be involved in the two conditions and imply the presence of subcortical dysfunction in depression.

Neuropsychological evaluation of depressed patients reveals deficits in several areas of intellectual function. Memory, attention, concentration, processing speed, spontaneous elaboration of information, and analysis of detail are impaired. Learning new information and recent memory functions appear to suffer most in depression (Cronholm and Otteson, 1961; Friedman, 1964; Sternberg and Jarvik, 1976; Whitehead, 1973). The memory deficits are at least partially related to inattention and distractibility, leading to poor organization and encoding of stimulus materials. If depressed patients are provided with structure and organization, the learning-memory deficits are less apparent (Weingartner et al, 1981). Depressed patients are often acutely aware of their memory problems, and complaints may be out of proportion to the actual degree of impairment (Kahn et al, 1975; Wells, 1979). Unpleasant remote experiences may be recalled more easily than are pleasant memories during a depressive episode (Lloyd and Lishman, 1975). Throughout testing, errors of omission are more evident than are errors of commission, and there may be substantial variations in performance from test to test (Miller and Lewis, 1977; Wells, 1979; Whitehead, 1973). Deficits in recent memory lead to disorientation in time and place, paucity of knowledge of current events, and difficulties learning new ward or domestic routines. Although memory impairment and disorientation are more severe in DAT than is dementia of depression, memory abnormalities are common in both and depressed patients omit details on tests of copying and construction, give concrete interpretation of proverbs, perform poorly on other tests of abstraction, have difficulty maintaining set on trail-making tests, generate inadequate word lists (impaired verbal fluency), and have distorted time perception (Caine, 1981; Miller, 1975). Memory disturbance cannot be used to distinguish degenerative dementias from the dementia syndrome of depression. The poor performance on neuropsychological tests may mislead the clinician into making a diagnosis of dementia with the implication that the poor test results indicate structural brain damage. Such interpretations may lead to abandoning treatment efforts with tragic consequences for the depressed patient whose dementia is reversible with appropriate therapy (Cowdry and Goodwin, 1981).

Until recently, laboratory investigation has not been helpful in evaluation of depression. Routine studies of blood, serum, urine, and CSF are unremarkable. The EEG and CT scan show only the expected age-related alterations (Shagass, 1965; Williams, 1954). Patients with late onset depression have more evidence of deep white matter ischemia on MRI than do nondepressed elderly individuals, suggesting that subclinical ischemic episodes increase the likelihood of mood changes (Coffey et al, 1988, 1989, 1990). PET with fluorodeoxyglucose (FDG) has consistently shown diminished metabolism of the anterolateral dorsal prefrontal cortex during the course of depressive episodes (Baxter et al, 1989). As in other conditions with diminished intellectual activity, cerebral blood flow is decreased in depression, and the flow reduction correlates with the severity of the depression (Mathew et al, 1980). Studies of auditory evoked potentials suggest that patients with bipolar affective disorders may show greater augmentation of response amplitude with increasing stimulus intensity, whereas unipolar depressed patients often show a reduction in response amplitude (Buchsbaum et al, 1971).

Neuroendocrinologic testing has added a new dimension to the evaluation of depression. Failure to suppress levels of endogenous cortisol after the administration of dexamethasone occurs in 50 to 70 percent of patients with endogenous depression (Brown et al, 1970; Carroll et al, 1981; Schlesser et al, 1980). Similarly the majority of patients with major depressive episodes will have less elevation of TSH in response to thyrotropin-releasing hormone (TRH) than will those with healthy controls (Gold et al, 1981; Kirkegaard et al, 1978). Patients with depressive dementia usually have an abnormal dexamethasone suppression test (McAllister et al, 1982), but unfortunately some patients with dementia who have no evidence of coexisting depression also have an abnormal test response (Gierl et al, 1987; Jenike and Albert, 1984; Kafona and Aldridge, 1985; Spar and Gerner, 1982), and this evaluation cannot be relied on to distinguish depressive dementia from other dementing illnesses. A similar lack of specificity and differential diagnostic utility has been established for the TRH test (McAllister and Hays, 1987).

The pathophysiology of depression (and depressive dementia) is not understood. Traditional dynamic explanations suggest that internal distractions and ruminations, poor motivation, and learned helplessness account for the impaired mental function of depressed patients. Studies of the neurobiology of depression suggest alternative explanations. Improvement in depression following administration of drugs that block monoamine reuptake at the synaptic cleft or that prevent metabolism of released amines at the synapse along with the observation that depression can be induced by agents that interfere with monoamine availability (reserpine, alpha-methyldopa), suggest that depression is a manifestation of altered monoamine metabolism (Baldessarini, 1975; Schildkraut, 1969; Schildkraut et al, 1967). Norepinephrine is the neurotransmitter most implicated in depression, but serotonin and dopamine, as well as other neurotransmitters and neuroregulators may also play important roles. Multiple transmitter systems are thought to contribute to expression of the depression syndrome with noradrenergic dysfunction hypothesized to predominate in the production of anhedonia, apathy, hopelessness, and anorexia; altered serotonin and acetylcholine function in the etiology of dysphoria, self-reproach, guilt, low self esteem, and thoughts of suicide and death; and dopamine dysfunction in the causation of retardation, fatigue, diminished initiative, poor concentration, and indecisiveness (Whybrow et al, 1984). Transmitter alterations also impact on neuroendocrincologic function, adding a hormonal dimension to the syndrome.

The monoamine transmitters arise in brainstem nuclei and project by way of ascending tracts to subcortical structures, medial limbic cortex, hippocampus, and neocortex (Anden et al, 1966; Lindvall et al, 1974; Ungerstedt, 1971). In addition to the involvement of nigrostriatal connections in motor activity, the ascending projections to frontal and limbic cortex may function in alertness, attention, activation, and behavioral preparedness (Mandell et al, 1962). Disruption of the function of these connections may provide the physiologic basis for some of the disturbed motor and cognitive function in depression as well as the mood alterations. Conversely, the intimate correlations of mood, cognition, and motor function with subcortical structures may help explain the high frequency of affective disorders in subcortical dementing disorders such as Parkinson's disease and Huntington's disease (see Chapter 4).

Depressive dementia is treated with the same interventions used in any severe depressive illness. The dementia syndrome of depression is one of the dementias that can be completely reversed, and the importance of looking for this syndrome among patients with progressive intellectual deterioration cannot be overemphasized. Specific agents, techniques, and precautions in the treatment of depression and dementia are presented in Chapter 13. The first line of therapy involves the use of non-monoamine oxidase inhibitor antidepressants (Glass et al, 1981; Good, 1981). If these fail, monoamine oxidase inhibitors may be tried and some patients may respond to treatment with lithium (Cowdry and Goodwin, 1981). The occurrence of intolerable side effects or failure to respond with improved mood or cognition are indications for electroconvulsive therapy; improvement in the dementia may occur after only a few treatments (Folstein and McHugh, 1978; McHugh and Folstein, 1979; Malloy et al, 1982).

When one is evaluating the depressed patient with intellectual impairment, several considerations in addition to depressive dementia must be borne in mind. Depression can be a major feature of the mental status changes associated with subcortical disorders. In Parkinson's disease and Huntington's disease among others, depression may occur early and be the initial manifestation of a more pervasive dementing process. When dementia and depression coexist, the cognitive deficits are exaggerated, and the dementia may improve with antidepressant therapy. Although depression is not a common clinical manifestation of the cortical dementing disorders (DAT and Pick's disease), it may be present in the early phases and may exaggerate the intellectual deterioration (Liston, 1977; Shraberg, 1978). Depression is sufficiently common in multi-infarct dementia to be included as a component of the diagnostic ischemia scale (Hachinski et al, 1975). Drugs used to treat patients with dementing illnesses can also produce

TABLE 9–3.   Major characteristics of the dementia syndrome of depression (all characteristics need not be present).

Mental status changes	Motor manifestations
Dysphoria	Bradykinesia
Apathy	Masked facies
Decreased motivation	Stooped posture
Anxiety	Slow, hypophonic speech
Depressed affect	History
Persecutory delusions	Age > 60
Psychomotor retardation	Subacute onset and rapid
Impaired memory retrieval	progression of intellectual decline
Poor wordlist generation	Past history of mood disorder
Dilapidation of cognition	Family history of mood disorder
(calculation, abstraction)	Laboratory
Variable performance	Positive dexamethasone suppression
Awareness of cognitive deficit	test
Neurovegetative signs	Enlarged lateral ventricles
Sleep disturbance	
Loss of appetite and weight	
Constipation	
Impotence	

depression. This is particularly important in vascular dementias where depression may be produced by antihypertensive medications. Reserpine is well known to produce depression in some patients (Schildkraut, 1969), but the agent is seldom used in contemporary antihypertensive regimens. Propranolol, however, has come into wide use for hypertension and other cardiovascular disorders and can induce severe depression (Petrie et al, 1982). Haloperidol, frequently used to calm elderly individuals with dementia, can produce the appearance of depression including psychomotor retardation, stooped posture, apathy, and dysphoria (Benson, 1990).

Specific focal lesions may influence mood and produce depression, particularly strokes involving the left frontal lobe and multi-infarct dementia (Starkstein et al, 1987). Frontal and subcortical lesions are also associated with depression (Robinson and Benson, 1981; Robinson and Szetela, 1981; Starkstein et al, 1987; Trimble and Cummings, 1981). and right hemispheric lesions are reported to modify the clinical manifestations of depression (Ross and Mesulam, 1979; Ross and Rush, 1981).

Table 9–3 summarizes the characteristics of the dementia syndrome of depression. In addition to the usual cognitive alterations and clinical features noted above, neurovegetative signs of depression or a personal or family history of mood disorder should alert the clinician to the possible importance of depression in the etiology of intellectual deterioration. The dementia of depression is typically of shorter duration and progresses more rapidly than do the insidiously developing degenerative dementias.

Mania

Mania is an unusual cause of dementia. Smith and colleagues (Smith et al, 1976; Smith and Kiloh, 1981) and Casey and Fitzgerald (1988) reported manic patients who were diagnosed as demented on the basis of progressive memory impairment, aggressive outbursts, hypersexuality, and disinhibited behavior. After appropriate diagnosis, the patients were treated with lithium and showed dramatic and sustained responses. Mania can be divided into three stages (Carlson and Goodwin, 1973). In the initial stage, there is heightened psychomotor activity with increased initiation, rate of speech, and physical activity. Euphoria and irritability lead to expansiveness, grandiosity, and overconfidence. Increased sexual activity, abundant talking and writing, and racing thoughts occur. In the second stage, psychomotor activity and rate of speech increase. Flight of ideas and delusional thinking occur and cognition becomes more disorganized. In the third stage, the activity increases further and may become bizarre. Hallucinations and idiosyncratic delusions are present, and the mood is dysphoric. Disorientation in time and place may occur in this stage. Verbal output is characteristically abnormal in mania; sentences are rarely completed, and there is a tendency to self-stimulate and free associate, derailing the progression of the spoken response (Andreasen and Pfohl, 1976; Benson, 1989; Durbin and Martin, 1977; Lorenz and Cobb, 1952). Insomnia becomes prominent as the mania progresses. Disorientation in this stage of mania frequently leads to suspicions that the patient may be suffering from a degenerative dementia.

Lithium is the drug of choice for both treatment and prophylaxis of mania; its effect is slow, however, and some patients may require a major tranquilizer to control the acute phase of the manic episode (Baldessarini and Lipinski, 1975). Complications of this therapy that may be considered in the patient with mania and dementia include lithium encephalopathy (Fetzer et al, 1981; Shopsin et al, 1979) and lithium-induced thyroid dysfunction (Fieve and Platman, 1968). Carbamazepine may be an effective antimanic agent in some patients who fail to improve with lithium or develop lithium-induced complications (Ballenger and Post, 1980; Okuma et al, 1973).

Manic dementia must be distinguished from the excited disinhibited behavior occurring in dementias with prominent frontal lobe involvement such as Pick's disease, frontal lobe tumors, and general paresis. Secondary manic behavior also occurs in a variety of neurologic processes including stroke and trauma, postencephalitic syndromes, deep-seated cerebral neoplasms, and in response to treatment with levodopa, steroids, isoniazid, sympathomimetics, and amphetamines (Alpers, 1937; Krauthammer and Klerman, 1978; Oppler, 1950, Starkstein et al, 1987; Steinberg et al, 1972; Stern and Dancey, 1942; Sultzer and Cummings, 1989; Waters and Lapierre, 1981; Weisert and Hendrie, 1977).

SCHIZOPHRENIA

Dementia may occur in several situations during the course of schizophrenia. Intellectual impairment may be seen during an acute psychotic episode, some subtypes have ongoing intellectual impairment, and some patients with chronic schizophrenia experience progressive intellectual deterioration late in the course of the illness.

The course of schizophrenia is characterized by relapses and remissions with psychotic episodes lasting from days to months; between exacerbations, personality and cognition do not return to normal. The duration and frequency of the psychotic periods have been greatly modified by the major tranquilizers. Between episodes, the symptomatology is less flagrant but abnormal affect and unusual beliefs persist. During the psychotic period, the patient's language, thought, and movement may be profoundly disturbed, producing a schizophrenic dementia. Memory impairment, disorientation, difficulties with calculation and abstraction, and poor retrieval of general information may be present along with hallucinations, delusions, or disorders of thought (Bienfeld and Hartford, 1982). Bizarre themes, tangential digressions, and lack of involvement with the listener characterize the language of schizophrenics and reflect their abnormal thought process (Gerson et al, 1977). Thinking is overinclusive and concrete (Cameron, 1939; Hanfmann, 1939). A variety of movement disorders may occur in schizophrenia, including waxy flexibility, grimacing, mannerisms, and stereotypes (Hamilton, 1976; Jones, 1965; Marsden et al, 1975; Stevens, 1974; Trimble, 1981), and ocular movements and blinking may be abnormal (Stevens, 1978).

In addition to the intellectual compromise that may occur in the course of an acute psychotic episode, schizophrenics may rarely manifest a bizarre state known as the buffoonery syndrome, in which they exhibit clowning, excessive jocularity, and facetious replies to questions (Hamilton, 1976). Any attempt to engage the patient in cognitive assessment fails (Lishman, 1978). The syndrome combines elements of schizophrenic and hysterical pseudodementias.

Neuropsychological assessment of schizophrenics suggests that some patients are intellectually impaired and perform poorly on tests of memory, intelligence, and psychomotor skills. Recent studies indicate that the neuropsychological impairment correlates with CT evidence of ventricular dilatation and sulcal enlargement, negative symptoms of schizophrenia, normal platelet monoamine oxidase (MAO) activity, poor premorbid adjustment,

TABLE 9–4.   Comparison of characteristics of schizophrenics with and without neuropsychological impairment.

Schizophrenia with neuropsychological impairment	Schizophrenia without neuropsychological impairment
Abnormal CT with ventricular dilatation and sulcal widening	Normal CT scan
Negative clinical symptoms (flat affect, retardation, poverty of speech, social withdrawal) predominate	Positive clinical symptoms (hallucinations, delusions) predominate
Poor premorbid adjustment	Better premorbid adjustment
Poor response to neuroleptics	Good response to neuroleptics
Normal platelet MAO activity	Low platelet MAO activity
Postulated pathology—cell loss	Postulated pathology—increased dopamine receptors
Poor prognosis	Good prognosis

and poor response to neuroleptics (Table 9–4) (Andreason and Olsen, 1982; Andreason et al, 1982; Crow, 1980; Depue et al, 1975; Golden et al, 1980a, b, 1981; Jeste et al, 1982; Johnstone et al, 1976, 1978). This constellation portends a poor prognosis. In this schizophrenic subtype, neuropsychological impairment is not limited to acute psychotic episodes but is instead continuously present.

Although schizophrenia was originally called dementia praecox, dementia per se usually has not been stressed as a feature of the disorder. Bleuler denied that intellectual deterioration occurred in schizophrenia, whereas Kraepelin maintained that a "terminal dementia" or "general decay of mental efficiency" occurred in the late stages (Johnstone et al, 1978). Based on his large experience with schizophrenia, Arieti (1974) reported that in some cases a terminal stage with oral behaviors, perceptual alterations, and behavioral deterioration may be seen. The proportion of schizophrenic patients who follow this course of late deterioration is unknown, but it may be characteristic of the neuropsychologically impaired group discussed above.

The mechanism of intellectual impairment in schizophrenia has not been determined. Preoccupation with delusions and hallucinations has been suggested as a dynamic explanation for poor test performance, but this is not supported by the poor correlation of dementia with these positive schizophrenic symptoms and good correlation with negative symptoms (Andreason et al, 1982). The success of treating schizophrenic symptoms with dopamine-blocking agents and the fidelity with which catecholaminergic agents such as amphetamines reproduce the schizophrenic syndrome suggest that disordered monoamine function underlies schizophrenia (Baldessarini,

1977b; Snyder et al, 1974), and increased concentrations of monoamine have been found in limbic system structures of the brain in autopsied schizophrenics (Bird et al, 1979; Farley et al, 1978). Weinberger (1986) hypothesized that the schizophrenic syndrome is comprised of limbic hyperactivity and prefrontal hypofunction. In this model, positive symptoms such as delusions and hallucinations reflect exaggerated mesolimbic dopaminergic activity whereas the cognitive impairment and negative symptom complex are produced by the hypofunction of frontal dopaminergic systems.

The differential diagnosis of schizophrenia with intellectual impairment includes a large number of neurologic processes that produce schizophrenia-like illnesses closely mimicking primary schizophrenia (Davison and Bagely, 1969). Schizophrenia-like psychoses appear to be particularly common as presenting manifestations of subcortical-limbic disturbances such as Huntington's disease, idiopathic basal ganglia calcification, bilateral subcortical focal lesions, and temporal lobe epilepsy (Cummings, 1985; Cummings et al, 1983a; Francis 1979; McHugh and Folstein, 1975; Slater et al, 1963; Trimble and Cummings, 1981).

Finally the possible role of a drug-induced encephalopathy must also be considered in the schizophrenic patient with intellectual impairment. Chapter 7 lists the drugs used in schizophrenia that are known to interfere with mentation, and their role should be considered in the schizophrenic with mental impairment.

HYSTERICAL DEMENTIA

"Hysteria" and "hysterical" are much-abused terms that often indicate more about the physician's misunderstanding than they do about the patient's disability. Nevertheless dementia can be a manifestation of a conversion reaction in some patients just as amnesia, mutism, or monoparesis is in others. Hysteria is an infrequent diagnosis, and dementia is an infrequent conversion symptom, making hysterical dementia a rare syndrome. The most striking clinical observation in patients with hysterical dementia is the disparity between the patients' ability to answer questions on mental status tests and their abilities in unstructured situations (Kiloh, 1961; McEvoy and Wells, 1979, Merskey, 1979). Patients give many "I don't know" replies or fail to answer simple questions correctly but may engage in intellectually demanding games with other patients, read the newspaper, or give detailed accounts of their last illnesses and complaints. Secondary gain in terms of resolving psychosocial issues or gaining financial advantage may be apparent, although identification of causative psychological conflicts may mislead the clinician into overlooking alternative explanations (Miller et al, 1986b).

Two problems plague the diagnosis of conversion hysteria in general and of dementia as a conversion reaction in particular. The first is the readiness with which the label "hysterical" is appended to clinical phenomena outside the clinician's experience. In one series, 13 percent of the patients with neurologic disease were regarded initially as suffering from a psychiatric disorder as their primary disturbance (Tissenbaum et al, 1951). Females and male homosexuals are the groups most likely to be labeled as hysterical (Miller et al, 1986). In a few cases, misdiagnosis may continue for years with inestimable harm to the patient's care. The other problem to be borne in mind is the frequency with which symptoms considered hysterical occur as the harbinger of neurologic or major psychiatric disease. Follow-up studies of patients given a diagnosis of hysterical conversion reaction show that between 50 and 70 percent eventually develop an organic CNS disorder (Merskey and Buhrich, 1975; Whitlock, 1967a). Most of the remaining patients suffer from a personality disorder, depression, or schizophrenia (Guze et al, 1971; Stefansson et al, 1976). Conversion reactions are symptom complexes, not the diagnosis, and identification of conversion symptoms demands a careful evaluation for an underlying neurologic or psychiatric disorder. As Slater (1965) stated: "The diagnosis of 'hysteria' is a disguise for ignorance and a fertile source of clinical error. It is in fact not only a delusion but also a snare."

GANSER'S SYNDROME

Ganser's syndrome is considered by many to be a variant of hysterical dementia (Whitlock, 1967b) but is discussed separately because of its unique clinical features and its etiologic implications. Sometimes known as the "syndrome of approximate answers," unusual nearly correct verbal responses are only one portion of a symptom complex that also includes disturbances of consciousness with subsequent amnesia for the episode, hallucinations, and sensory or motor changes similar to those seen in conversion reactions. The episode terminates abruptly with restoration of normal mental function (Enoch and Trethowan, 1979; Whitlock, 1967b). Ganser originally described the syndrome in three prisoners, and in his subsequent critical review of the condition. Wertham commented that the Ganser state was a "hysterical pseudostupidity which occurs almost exclusively in jails and in old-fashioned German textbooks" (quoted by Whitlock, 1967b). This criticism has not been sustained, however; Ganser's syndrome or Ganser's symptoms have been described in a wide variety of neurologic and toxic-metabolic conditions (toxic confusional periods, general paresis, head trauma, alcoholic dementia, and so forth) and in psychotic states (May et al, 1960; Weiner and Braiman, 1955; Whitlock, 1967a). All three of Ganser's original patients had known organic mental problems (Whitlock, 1967b). The clinical features may be hysterical or malingered (Goldin and MacDonald, 1955; Tyndel, 1956), but an underlying disorder should be sought.

The unusual verbal replies are the most emphasized portion of this syndrome and the clinical aspect that brings the condition to diagnostic consideration. Answers to questions are often close but not exactly correct, and paralogia may be manifested by talking past the answer or giving random or absurd answers. In most cases, the nature of the replies suggests an awareness of the correct response (Tyndel, 1956; Whitlock, 1967a).

Ganser-type responses occurring in toxic-metabolic encephalopathies improve with resolution of the underlying disorder. If based on structural brain changes, however, the syndrome may persist for years. The Ganser state warrants careful search for a specific etiology and application of appropriate therapy.

MISCELLANEOUS PSEUDODEMENTIAS

Lishman (1978) points out that on rare occasions, dementia may be a manifestation of malingering. In most cases, the motivation is apparent and the ruse cannot be maintained for any substantial length of time. Two other conditions—obsessional ruminative states and severe anxiety neurosis—may impair concentration and the ability to participate in testing sufficiently to suggest dementia (Lishman, 1978). Treatment of the underlying disorder restores intellectual abilities.

10

Dementias Associated with Trauma, Neoplasms, Enzyme Deficiencies, Multiple Sclerosis, and Other Acquired and Inherited Disorders

This chapter presents the neurobehavioral findings of several acquired and hereditary dementia syndromes that have not been considered in earlier sections. A heterogeneous group of disorders is included, from common causes of dementia such as head trauma to rare dementias associated with infrequent enzyme deficiencies.

ACQUIRED DEMENTIAS

Posttraumatic Dementia

Each year, head injuries produce permanent cognitive and behavioral deficits in a large number of individuals. In the United States, there are 500,000 head injuries sufficiently serious to require hospitalization; 70,000 to 90,000 of those involved in head injuries annually will have a life-long disability (Alexander, 1982; Goldstein, 1990). Automobile accidents account for most

TABLE 10–1.   Dementia syndromes associated with trauma.

Cerebral trauma (direct)
   Multiple contusions and/or lacerations
   Diffuse axonal injury (Strich lesions)
Dementia pugilistica ("punch drunk," "slap happy")
Subdural hematoma
Normal-pressure hydrocephalus
Multi-infarct dementia
   Traumatic cerebrovascular occlusion
   Chest trauma with multiple cerebral emboli
   Multiple fat emboli from fractures of large bones
   Diffuse intravascular coagulation

head trauma sustained in western nations, and head trauma accounts for 70 percent of injuries sustained in motor vehicle accidents (Feiring and Brock, 1974). Fifty percent of patients with significant head trauma die at the scene of the accident or within 48 hours of admission to the hospital; approximately 15 percent of those who survive the trauma require prolonged hospitalization and have temporary or permanent neurologic disability (Alexander, 1982; Lishman, 1978). The incidence of posttraumatic dementia is difficult to estimate, but in patients whose posttraumatic amnesia exceeds three weeks, some degree of measurable deficit is often permanent (Jennett and Teasdale, 1981). In some cases, substantial posttraumatic amnesia and residual intellectual deficits may follow head injuries unaccompanied by loss of consciousness. Traumatic brain injury occurs twice as often in men as it does in women, and between the ages of 15 and 24 years and in cases of motor vehicle accidents, men are involved four times as often as women (Alexander, 1982).

Table 10–1 summarizes the varieties of dementia that occur following trauma. This section concentrates on dementia as a consequence of direct cerebral injury. Hydrocephalic dementias are considered in Chapter 7 and the characteristics of multi-infarct dementia are presented in Chapter 5.

Cerebral Trauma

The type of intellectual impairment observed following traumatic brain injury (TBI) reflects the location and extent of injury. Many serious head injuries produce widespread bilateral abnormalities although specific focal deficits may be superimposed. There are three distinct types of neuropathological alterations that may result from closed head injury: (1) diffuse axonal injury; (2) focal contusions, hemorrhages, and lacerations; and (3) hypoxic-ischemic insults. Diffuse axonal injury arises from shearing forces and affects the subcortical white matter fibers, the mesencephalon, and diencephalon (Strich, 1956, 1961). Focal injuries arise from direct contusion, vascular occlusion with vessel compression, or vessel disruption and hemorrhage. Hypoxic-ischemic injuries result from circulatory collapse or airway obstruction that may occur in conjunction with head trauma. These three types of pathology may be present in any combination producing a complex array of neurobehavioral problems. The most ubiquitous and easily detectable neuropsychological disturbance that follows head trauma is posttraumatic amnesia. The patient will not remember what occurred during any period of unconsciousness or the confusional period that initiates recovery from coma. Even when the confusion subsides, anterograde amnesia characterized by ongoing difficulties in acquiring new information as well as retrograde amnesia, an inability to remember what happened for hours, days, or even months prior to the accident, often persists. Anterograde posttraumatic amnesia gradually improves after which the duration of the retrograde amnesia commonly shows a progressive shrinking to within a few minutes or seconds of the accident (Benson and Geschwind, 1967; Russell, 1971; Whitty and Zangwill, 1977). Recovery is not always complete and some degree of permanent memory disturbance may persist as a component of posttraumatic dementia. Neuropsychological assessment in this chronic phase of posttraumatic amnesia reveals deficits in both encoding and retrieval with relative preservation of procedural memory (Crosson et al, 1988; Levin, 1989).

Aphasia is seen in approximately 30 percent of patients who survive significant TBI. In the study by Jennett and colleagues (Jennett and Teasdale, 1981) aphasia was seen as the only neurologic sign in 7 percent of survivors of severe head injury and occurred in combination with other neurologic deficits in another 21 percent. Fluent aphasias, either the anomic or Wernicke types are the most common patterns of language disturbance (Heilman et al, 1971). The long-term prognosis for language recovery is good (Miller and Stern, 1965).

Additional neurobehavioral changes that characterize posttraumatic dementia include cognitive disorganization, emotional withdrawal, anxiety, depression, psychomotor retardation, impaired ability to abstract, and poor concentration (Jennett and Teasdale, 1981; Kinsella et al, 1988; Levin and Grossman, 1978; Schilder, 1934). Signs of interhemispheric disconnection (left-sided apraxia and agraphia) occur if the corpus callosum is injured (Rubens et al, 1977). Hemiparesis, cranial nerve dysfunction, and ataxia commonly accompany posttraumatic dementia. While few long-term follow-up studies of patients with posttraumatic dementia have been accomplished, some investigations have documented continued recovery over several years with only minimal to moderate permanent disability in many patients (Miller, 1966; Miller and Stern, 1965).

The cognitive deficits observed in posttraumatic dementia reflect the distribution of lesions produced in the brain. Cerebral injury may occur at the point of injury (coup injury) with a more extensive lesion on the opposite side of the brain (contrecoup injury) (Courville, 1950; Lindenberg and Freytag, 1960). Traumatic contusions of brain tissue tend to be concentrated in the anterotemporal lobes and inferofrontal lobes (Adams and Victor, 1977); the lesions are most prominent on the crests of the gyri (Romanul, 1970). Local hemorrhage and considerable cerebral edema accompany the contusions in the acute stages. Edema may lead to secondary herniation, causing vascular occlusion that further complicates the intracranial changes. In some cases, extensive degeneration of white matter is found at autopsy (Adams et al, 1982; Jellinger and Seitelberger, 1970; Strich, 1956, 1961). Contusions of the anterotemporal and inferofrontal regions correlate with the occurrence of posttraumatic amnesia, aphasia, and personality changes, and callosal contusion by the falx accounts for posttraumatic callosal disconnection signs.

X-ray CT with contrast enhancement frequently shows areas of cerebral contusion in the acute phase of severe closed head injury, and cerebral atrophy is evident in the chronic phase (Callum and Bigler, 1986). MRI reveals abnormalities, particularly in the white matter of the frontal and temporal lobes, in many patients with posttraumatic dementia (Gandy et al, 1984; Levin et al, 1985, 1987). Both CT and MRI, however, can appear normal in patients with permanent posttraumatic disabilities. Cerebral blood flow studies and PET with FDG demonstrate focal areas of reduced cerebral perfusion and decreased metabolism (Barclay et al, 1985b; Ruff et al, 1989).

Dementia Pugilistica

Martland introduced the term "punch drunk" into the medical literature in 1928. He took the designation from fans, promoters, and prizefighters who recognized that, after years in the ring and repeated head trauma, some boxers developed a syndrome characterized by progressive ataxia and dementia. The entity has had a variety of names including "slug nutty," "slap happy," traumatic encephalopathy, and dementia pugilistica (Critchley, 1957; Martland, 1928). The syndrome characteristically begins with a gait disturbance and slurring dysarthria and gradually progresses into an extrapyramidal Parkinson-type syndrome variably combined with evidence of pyramidal and cerebellar dysfunction (Corsellis et al, 1973; Critchley, 1957; Jordan, 1987; Mawdsley and Ferguson, 1963; Spillane, 1962). Seizures occur in a minority of patients. Dementia appears later in the clinical course and first becomes evident as a disturbance of memory. Recollection of recent events is more affected than memory for remote information, but old information is not completely spared. Psychomotor retardation is apparent, and personality changes and general intellectual decline also occur. Psychiatric alterations are common but highly variable and include paranoia, euphoria, or depression (Corsellis et al, 1973; Winterstein, 1937).

The motor abnormalities of dementia pugilistica often become evident toward the end of a boxer's career and may contribute to his retirement. The appearance of dementia may be delayed 10 to 20 years, becoming manifest in the fifth to seventh decades of life. The prevalence of dementia pugilistica is estimated at between 10 and 50 percent of professional fighters (Corsellis et al, 1973; Sercl and Jaros, 1962). It occurs in men who begin fighting in their teens and have several hundred bouts during their careers. Nearly all affected boxers have been professionals and most were known for their ability to "take a punch."

The EEG may show slowing of background rhythms or diffuse cerebral slow-wave activity. A CT scan reveals cerebral atrophy with ventricular dilatation, and many patients have a cavum septum pellucidum (Bogdanoff and Natter, 1989; Casson et al, 1982; Jordan, 1987; Ross et al, 1983).

Few detailed neuropathologic studies have been undertaken, but Corsellis and colleagues (1973) performed careful investigation of the brains of 15 boxers, most of whom suffered from dementia pugilistica. Grossly the brains were atrophic and coronal sections demonstrated ventricular dilatation. A cavum septum pellucidum was evident in 80 percent. In many, the fornix was almost completely detached from the undersurface of the corpus callosum and the callosum itself was markedly thinned. Cortical scarring was not prominent although evidence of previous perivascular hemorrhage is common (Adams and Bruton, 1989). The substantia nigra was often grossly depigmented and the midbrain atrophic. Histologically, the most dramatic feature was the presence of neurofibrillary tangles in cortical neurons. The affected neurons were diffusely distributed but were most numerous in the hippocampus and other medial temporal structures. Tangles were also found in small numbers in the basal ganglia, thalamus, substantia nigra, locus ceruleus, and other brainstem structures. Immunocytochemical studies reveal identical staining characteristics of the neurofibrillary tangles of dementia pugilistica and those of DAT (Roberts, 1988). In contrast, senile plaques were either sparse or totally absent. This disparity between the abundance of neurofibrillary tangles and the lack of senile plaques distinguishes the pathologic appearance of dementia pugilistica from DAT. Neuron loss and astrocyte proliferation were also evident in the cerebral cortex, but the white matter was normal or mildly gliotic. The pathogenetic relationship between the trauma and the neurofibrillary tangles remains obscure. In a smaller study by Payne (1968), microscopic cortical scars and perivascular foci of demyelination were noted.

Subdural Hematoma

Subdural hematomas can produce alterations of mental status that are readily misdiagnosed as DAT or multi-infarct dementia (Perlmutter and Gobles, 1961; Stuteville and Welch, 1958). In addition, when brain atrophy occurs with advancing age, bridging veins crossing from the cortical surface to the dural sinuses become more vulnerable to trauma, and subdural hematoma may occur to complicate the course of preexisting dementing illness (Govan and Walsh, 1947). Mental status alterations with fluctuating arousal, poor attention, irritability, and impaired memory are the most common manifestations of subdural hematomas in the elderly (Stuteville and Welch, 1958). Focal signs may mislead the clinician into diagnosing stroke or transient ischemic attacks (Feldman et al, 1963b; Welsh et al, 1979). A history of head trauma may be minimal or entirely absent. Subdural blood collections can also lead to inappropriate secretion of antidiuretic hormone with hyponatremia and metabolic encephalopathy (Maroon and Campbell, 1970).

Studies of CSF frequently reveal elevated protein and mild pleocytosis in the presence of chronic subdural hematomas but can be entirely normal. Similarly, the EEG is almost always abnormal; the findings are nonspecific. Bilateral slowing is usually present and the amplitude may be reduced on the side of the lesion (Jaffe et al, 1968; Kiloh et al, 1972). The CT scan may reveal subdural hematomas. The hematomas tend to become isodense with brain in the chronic state and may be difficult to detect. Shift of midline structures and unilateral ablation of cortical sulci are CT signs indicating a lateralized lesion; bilateral absence of sulci and unusual narrowing of ventricles are indicative of bilateral isodense subdural hematomas (Greenhouse and Barr, 1979; Jacobson and Farmer, 1979). Subdural hematomas are readily visible on MRI scans, and MRI is the technique of choice for demonstrating these lesions.

Surgical drainage of subdural hematomas is recommended when significant disability is being produced by the mass effect. Less symptomatic lesions may resolve spontaneously, and conservative treatment with careful observation is often advised (Ambrosetto, 1962; Gannon et al, 1962).

Posttraumatic subdural hematomas must be distinguished from posttraumatic hydrocephalus (Chapter 8) and from traumatic occlusion of intracranial vessels (Duman and Stephens, 1963; Hughes and Brownell, 1968; Mastaglia et al, 1969).

Dementia with Intracranial Neoplasms

Intracranial neoplasms can disturb cognition through a variety of mechanisms. Local infiltration or compression can give rise to focal syndromes such as aphasia, amnesia, or apraxia; edema and increased intracranial pressure may compromise arousal and attention to produce psychomotor retardation; and tumors strategically located near the ventricular system can cause hydrocephalus and hydrocephalic dementia. Onset is usually insidious and headache may be prominent as the tumor increases in size. Tumors located in the posterofrontal, anteroparietal, or occipital lobes may give rise to weakness, somatosensory disturbances, or visual field disturbances respectively, in addition to mental status alterations. The appearance of these focal disturbances suggests the presence of a localized lesion and usually leads to discovery of the tumor. Some tumors, however, produce few changes beyond intellectual and personality deterioration, and the neoplastic etiology of the dementia syndrome can be overlooked easily. Tumors involving one or both frontal lobes, the midline, and the temporal lobes are particularly likely to present with early and prominent cognitive changes that may be misdiagnosed as degenerative or vascular dementia (Keschner et al, 1938; McIntyre and McIntyre, 1942; Minski, 1933; Selecki, 1965).

Mental status changes occur in 90 percent of patients with frontal lobe tumors and dementia is found in 70 percent (Avery, 1971; Direkze et al, 1971; Frazier, 1936; Hecaen, 1964; Kolodny, 1929; Strauss and Keschner, 1935). Alterations of personality with euphoria and facetiousness or apathy may be early symptoms, followed by poor concentration, impaired memory, and disorientation. Motor and language changes appear later and approximately one-half of patients have seizures. Any type of frontal tumor may produce a dementia syndrome, but this is particularly characteristic of subfrontal meningiomas arising from the olfactory grooves and planum sphenoidale (Avery, 1971; Fisher, 1969; Hunter et al, 1968; Sachs, 1950). Gliomas and metastatic tumors that invade the anterior corpus callosum and spread to involve both frontal lobes also produce a marked dementia (Alpers, 1936; Alpers and Grant, 1931; Nasrallah and McChesney, 1981; Selecki, 1964). Temporal lobe tumors have a tendency to produce personality alterations and cognitive impairment early in the clinical course (Keschner et al, 1936). If the left temporal lobe is involved, language disturbances may predominate. Dementia is also a major manifestation of tumors that involve the cerebral cortex in a diffuse manner such as gliomatosis cerebri (Dickson et al, 1988; Dunn and Kernohan, 1957) or the encephalitic form of metastatic carcinoma (Floeter et al, 1987; Madow and Alpers, 1951).

Tumors originating in subcortical structures can produce dementia syndromes not too dissimilar from those seen with cortical tumors. Deep midline tumors frequently invade commissural structures to produce bilateral hemispheric dysfunction. Brain dysfunction may result from superficial extension of the tumors or from pressure induced by the expanding mass and surrounding edema. Brainstem tumors cause dementia syndromes characterized by personality changes, lethargy, disorientation, memory impairment, and mutism (Cairns, 1950; Wallack et al, 1977). Tumors originating in the thalamus produce confusional states, memory loss, emotional lability, and mental dullness (Cheek and Taveras, 1966; McKissock and Paine, 1958; Smyth and Stern, 1938). Hemiparesis is demonstrable in a majority of patients with thalamic tumor. Tumors of the basal ganglia may present with impairment of attention and concentration, poor memory, personality changes and depression (Whitty, 1956). Tumors in the region of the hypothalamus, pituitary, and third ventricle produce endocrine dysfunction as well as intellectual deterioration and personality changes (White and Cobb, 1955). When the hypothalamus is invaded the symptomatology may include hyperphagia, somnolence, and rage attacks (Beal et al, 1981a; Reeves and Plum, 1969).

Results of studies of the CSF are usually abnormal when an intracranial neoplasm exists. Elevated protein, normal glucose, and mild pleocytosis are the usual findings. Tumors that border on the ventricular system or subarachnoid space may produce the most striking CSF abnormalities. The EEG recordings are abnormal in a majority of cases and radionuclide brain scans usually show increased radioactivity in the region of the tumor. The contrast-enhanced CT scan is excellent in tumor detection as well as in determining the location and size of the lesion. An X-ray CT will also demonstrate the edema surrounding a tumor, lateral shifting of midline structures, and secondary hydrocephalus. Most of these changes are better demonstrated by MRI than by CT.

Corticosteroids are used to reduce the edema surrounding intracranial neoplasms and to decrease intracranial pressure. Anticonvulsants are administered to limit the risk of seizure activity. Depending on their histologic type and location, intracranial tumors are treated with some combination of surgical removal or debulking, chemotherapy, or radiotherapy.

Multiple Sclerosis

Multiple sclerosis is an inflammatory disorder of undetermined etiology that involves the white matter of the cerebral hemispheres, brainstem, optic nerves, cerebellum, and spinal cord. The incidence and prevalence of the disease vary with the geographic latitude of the reported population. It is two to six times more common in the northern United States than in the southern states, and this geographic trend has been confirmed worldwide. Epidemiologic information varies from study to study, but most indicate a prevalence in the northern latitudes of 30 to 60 per 100,000 population compared with 5 to 15 per 100,000 in the southern latitudes (Kurland, 1970). Small geographic areas with clusters of cases of multiple sclerosis producing prevalence rates of 100 to 150 per 100,000 population have been described (Eastman et al, 1973). Individuals migrating between areas of high and low prevalence acquire the risk of the new region only if they migrate before the age of 15 years but retain the risk of the original area if they move after the age of 15 (Poser, 1978).

The disease does not appear to be inherited, but 5 to 10 percent of affected individuals have family members who are also affected, and a genetically determined susceptibility or a common environmental exposure is suspected. Multiple sclerosis begins at any age between childhood and the sixth decade, but 60 to 70 percent of cases have their first symptoms between the ages of 20 and 40. It is more common in females than it is in males by a ratio of 1.4:1 (Poser, 1978; Victor and Adams, 1981). Recurrent episodes of demyelination characteristically produce a relapsing and remitting course. The average duration of the disease is at least 22 years, and the 10-year survival rate has been found to be about 85 percent of the rate for the healthy population. Approximately 50 percent of victims can still walk and work 10 years after the onset of the disease (Kurland, 1970; MacLean and Berkson, 1951; Sibley, 1990).

Clinical Manifestations

Neuropsychological abnormalities are common in multiple sclerosis, and an overt dementia is evident by the late stages in a majority of patients. The profile of deficits resembles that of a subcortical dementia with decreased speed of information processing, impaired memory, and a general dilapidation of cognitive processes (Rao, 1986).

In a study of 108 victims, Surridge (1969) found no intellectual deterioration in 40 percent, slight intellectual compromise in 40 percent, and moderate to severe deficits in the remaining 20 percent. The dementia was characterized by memory disturbances, impairment of conceptual thinking, and naming errors. Aphasia is not common in multiple sclerosis, but articulatory disturbances, paraphasia, and anomia are the usual manifestations when changes of verbal output occur (Beatty et al, 1988; Olmos-Lau et al, 1977). There is a significant association between severity of dementia and increasing physical disability (Kurtze, 1970; Surridge, 1969). In rare cases, dementia is the predominant manifestation, the presenting feature or even less commonly, virtually the only manifestation of the disorder (Kahana et al, 1971; Koenig, 1968; Poser, 1957; Young et al, 1976). Rapidly progressive dementia leading to early death occurs when there is extensive and intense cerebral involvement (Bergin, 1957).

Neuropsychological assessment reveals that deficits in learning and delayed recall of verbal and visual information is present in a majority of patients early in the clinical course or when physical disability is mild (Grant et al, 1984; Lyon-Caen et al, 1986; van den Burg et al, 1987). Later in the disease, memory abnormalities are more evident; deficits in information processing such as wordlist generation, symbol-digit substitution, memory scanning, and problem solving are commonly observed (Beatty and Gange, 1977; Beatty et al, 1988a, 1989; Franklin et al, 1989; Jambor, 1969; Peyser et al, 1980; Rao et al, 1984, 1989b). Some, but not all, studies have demonstrated a correlation between severity of cognitive function and extent of hemispheric pathology as revealed by MRI (Franklin et al, 1988; Rao et al, 1989a).

Personality alterations, mood disturbances, and psychotic episodes may occur during the course of multiple sclerosis. Euphoria has often been commented on and was present at the time of study in 20 percent of the patients investigated by Surridge (1969). Depression is not infrequent, may be the presenting feature of the disorder, and is more common in multiple sclerosis than it is in many other chronic neurologic disorders (Joffe et al, 1987; Goodstein and Ferrell, 1977; Whitlock and Siskind, 1980). Psychosis may be the major manifestation of multiple sclerosis in some cases (Kohler et al, 1988; Mur et al, 1966; Salguero et al, 1969; Schiffer and Babigan, 1984), and a predisposition of these patients to conversion reactions has been suggested (Aring, 1965; Caplan and Nadelson, 1980) but is difficult to confirm.

Sensory and motor disturbances are usually prominent in the clinical presentation and course of multiple sclerosis. Neuroophthalmic abnormalities are often among the earliest signs of multiple sclerosis and remain an important indicator of the disease throughout its course. Internuclear ophthalmoplegia is characteristic, and other varieties of ophthalmoparesis, nystagmus, pupillary abnormalities, and optic neuritis occur in some patients (Percy et al, 1972). Spastic paraparesis, cerebellar ataxia, exaggerated muscle stretch reflexes, and extensor plantar responses are common motor disturbances. Typical sensory findings include loss of vibration and position sense particularly in the lower extremities (Kurtze, 1970; Poser, 1978). Incontinence of urine is frequent, and impotence occurs early. Seizures occur in approximately 4 percent of patients (Drake and Macrae, 1961). The symptoms and signs wax and wane over time, but permanent deficits gradually accumulate as the disease progresses.

Laboratory Evaluation

The diagnosis of multiple sclerosis is aided by studies of CSF and electrophysiologic and radiologic procedures. Results of routine blood, serum, and urine examinations are normal. Blood tests based on lymphocyte abnormalities are being developed, but their sensitivity and specificity are not yet determined (Levy et al, 1976; Offner et al, 1977). Abnormalities of the CSF are present in 60 to 80 percent of multiple sclerosis patients. Thirty percent have CSF pleocytosis, usually in the range of 5 to 10 mononuclear cells, and 30 to 50 percent have an elevated protein content (rarely exceeding 100 mg per 100 ml) (Poser, 1978). Elevated CSF gamma globulin, particularly immunoglobin G (IgG), is more specific for the diagnosis of multiple sclerosis but is not pathognomonic (Table 10–2). Levels of IgG in excess of 13 percent of the total protein content occur in 60 to 70 percent of patients (Lamoureux et al, 1975; Poser, 1978; Swanson, 1989; Tourtellotte, 1970). Elevation of IgG also occurs in neurosyphilis, subacute sclerosing panencephalitis, in conditions with elevated serum IgG, and rarely in other diseases (Lisak and Keshgegian, 1980; Yahr et al, 1954). In multiple sclerosis the CSF gamma globulin is concentrated in discrete oligoclonal bands rather than occurring in the normal diffuse pattern (Hart and Sherman, 1982).

TABLE 10–2.   Conditions that may elevate CSF gamma globulin content.

Multiple sclerosis
Inflammatory CNS diseases
   Subacute sclerosing panencephalitis
   Progressive rubella encephalitis
   Inflammatory neuropathies
   Neurosyphilis
   Viral encephalitis
   Meningitis
Conditions with elevated serum gamma globulin
   Behçet disease
   Rheumatoid arthritis
   Sarcoidosis
   Leprosy
   Cirrhosis
Miscellaneous disorders (rare)
   Degenerative CNS diseases
   CNS tumors
   Vascular disturbances
   Adrenoleukodystrophy

Adapted from RP Lisak and AA Keshgegian, Oligoclonal immunoglobins in cerebrospinal fluid in multiple sclerosis, Clin Chem 1980;26:1340–1345 and MD Yahr et al, Further studies on the gamma globulin content of cerebrospinal fluid in multiple sclerosis and other neurological diseases, Ann NY Acad Sci 1954;58:613 614.

A majority of patients with multiple sclerosis will have diffuse or focal abnormalities on their EEGs, but these changes are nonspecific (Ashworth and Emery, 1963). If demyelinating lesions affect the visual pathways, visual evoked responses will be delayed (Halliday et al, 1972). Visual evoked potentials, brain stem auditory evoked potentials, and somatosensory evoked potentials are frequently abnormal in multiple sclerosis even when no symptoms relating to these sensory systems have been elicited (Geisser et al, 1987; Swanson, 1989).

CT scan can contribute to the diagnosis of multiple sclerosis. Acute lesions appear as low-density areas in the cerebral white matter and enhance with contrast infusion or after delayed-infusion scans (Aita et al, 1978; Morariu et al, 1980; Warren et al, 1976). In approximately one-third of well-established cases, low-density areas will be seen in the periventricular regions (Gyldensted, 1976; Hershey et al, 1979; Swanson, 1989).

MRI is substantially more sensitive than CT for the detection of abnormalities in multiple sclerosis (Jacobs et al, 1986; Stewart et al, 1987). Demyelinating lesions are most evident in the periventricular border, cerebral and cerebellar white matter, and brain stem (Fazekas et al, 1988; Kirshner et al, 1985; Stewart et al, 1987).

Pathology and Pathogenesis

Grossly, the brain and spinal cord of the patient with multiple sclerosis appear normal or slightly to moderately atrophic. Coronal sections of the cerebral hemispheres reveal a characteristic topographic distribution of the multiple sclerosis plaques. The sclerotic lesions occur most frequently in the superolateral corners of the lateral ventricles. A smaller number of lesions is distributed throughout the cerebral white matter with a tendency to spare the subcortical U fibers, cortex, and deep gray-matter structures (Oppenheimer, 1976a, Zimmerman and Netsky, 1950). In the spinal cord, the plaques concentrate in the center of the posterior columns, in the center and posterior two-thirds of the lateral columns, and symmetrically on both sides of the anterior median fissure in the ventral columns (Fog, 1950).

Acute lesions have bubbly expansions of the myelin, microglial proliferation, astrocytic hyperplasia, and lymphocytic perivascular cuffing. Extracellular myelin fragments and sudanophilic lipids may be visible, and oligodendrocytes partially or completely disappear. Neurons and axons occurring within the lesions are usually preserved. In chronic plaques, fibrillary gliosis becomes prominent, lipid phagocytes congregate around blood vessels, and sudanophilic lipid material is absent (Oppenheimer, 1976a; Zimmerman and Netsky, 1950). Although perivascular lymphocytic infiltration is common, the blood vessels themselves are usually unaffected in multiple sclerosis. A rare dementing disorder with demyelinating lesions and clinical course similar to multiple sclerosis but associated with cerebrovascular amyloid angiopathy has been reported (Heffner et al, 1976).

A specific type of demyelinating lesion, Balo's concentric sclerosis, consists of alternating bands of intact myelin and zones of myelin loss (Balo, 1928; Grcevic, 1960). These lesions may represent an intermediate stage in the development of a more typical mature plaque (Moore et al, 1985).

The etiology and pathogenesis of multiple sclerosis is undetermined. Environmental toxins, viral agents, and autoimmune reactions have been implicated as etiologically significant (Rodriguez, 1989). Cellular hypersensitivity to myelin basic protein, loss of peripheral suppressor T cells, antibodies to oligodendroglia, and other abnormalities of the immune system have been demonstrated (Abramsky et al, 1977; Reinherz et al, 1980; Sheremata et al, 1974). Immunologic mechanisms appear to play an important but probably secondary role in the pathogenesis of the disorder; the inciting agent, event, or substance has not been discovered.

Treatment

Until the etiology and pathogenesis of multiple sclerosis are more fully understood, treatment attempts must be directed at the secondary and symptomatic aspects of the disease. Treatment with intravenous ACTH or oral steroid agents to limit the inflammatory reaction is popular. Controlled study of the use of these agents suggests that they have little impact on the overall course of the disorder but may shorten the duration of individual exacerbations (Cooperative Study Report, 1970). Aminopyridine, a potassium channel-blocking agent that restores conduction in demyelinated nerves, has been reported to be beneficial to multiple sclerosis patients (Davis et al, 1990). Spasticity, a major problem limiting the mobility of these patients, may be improved through the use of contraction-blocking agents such as baclofen (Feldman et al, 1978; Sachais et al, 1977), and the neuropathic pain that occasionally occurs responds well to carbamazepine (Albert, 1969). Amantadine hydrochloride may ameliorate the chronic fatigue experienced by many multiple sclerosis patients (Cohen and Fisher, 1989). Amitriptyline decreases the pathological displays of affect occurring with pseudobulbar palsy (Schiffer et al, 1985). Rehabilitation regimens aid in maximizing function and minimizing disability and substantially benefit disabled patients (Erickson et al, 1989).

Differential Diagnosis

Any disorder producing multiple relapsing and remitting lesions in the CNS can mimic the clinical course of multiple sclerosis, and other demyelinating disorders can produce similar clinical, radiologic, and laboratory findings. The principal waxing and waning diseases that may simulate multiple sclerosis clinically are the inflammatory collagen-vascular disorders, particularly SLE (Fulford et al, 1972). Lupus occurs in the same age group as multiple sclerosis and may produce elevations of CSF gamma globulin levels. It can usually be identified by its involvement of non-CNS organs and by specific blood tests.

There are several demyelinating diseases that produce dementia and must be differentiated from multiple sclerosis (Table 10–3) (Poser, 1978). Most of these can be distinguished by their course, identifiable inciting event, or family history. Inherited disorders of myelin are discussed below.

Superficial Hemosiderosis of the CNS

Superficial hemosiderosis of the CNS could be discussed among vascular, hydrocephalic, or neoplastic dementias and can be considered in the differential diagnosis of all these conditions. The disorder occurs following repeated episodes of subarachnoid hemorrhage. The bleeding episodes may be asymptomatic or signaled by recurrent symptoms and neurologic findings. Gradually, a fairly uniform clinical syndrome evolves composed of progressive dementia, nerve deafness, pyramidal signs, and cerebellar ataxia (Adams and Victor, 1981; Tomlinson and Walton, 1964). The dementia includes memory impairment, disorientation, poor attention, apathy, and lethargy

TABLE 10–3.   Diseases of myelin that can produce dementia in adults.

Demyelinating disorders (acquired disorders of myelin)
    Idiopathic
        Multiple sclerosis
    Secondary
        Hyperergic
            Postinfectious encephalomyelopathy
            Postvaccinal encephalomyelopathy
        Vascular
            Binswanger's disease
        Infectious
            Subacute sclerosing panencephalitis
            Progressive multifocal leukoencephalopathy
            Progressive rubella panencephalitis
            Lyme disease
            HIV encephalopathy
        Toxic–metabolic
            Vitamin B_{12} deficiency
            Carbon monoxide encephalopathy
            Toluene exposure
            Mercury intoxication
            Marchiafava-Bignami disease
            Lead encephalopathy
            Ergotamine encephalopathy
            Arsenic intoxication
            Radio/chemotherapy (delayed demyelination)
            Anoxic encephalopathy (delayed demyelination)
            Central pontine myelinolysis with hemispheric demyelination
Dysmyelinating disorders (inherited disorders of myelin)
    Adrenoleukodystrophy
    Metachromatic leukodystrophy
    Membranous lipodystrophy
    Cerebrotendinous xanthomatosis
    Hereditary adult-onset leukodystrophy

(McGee et al, 1962; Tomlinson and Walton, 1964). Pathologically, an iron-containing pigment is widely distributed in outer layers of the brain, cerebellum, and spinal cord. The outer layers of the cortex are damaged with marked proliferation of astrocytes, loss of neurons, and injury to myelin sheaths. Pigment-containing macrophages are abundant and numerous hyaline bodies are present in involved areas (Lewey and Govons, 1942; McGee et al, 1962; Neumann, 1948; Tomlinson and Walton, 1964). The recurrent subarachnoid hemorrhage may be produced by a variety of conditions including carcinomatosis of the meninges, aneurysms, arteriovenous malformations, and a variety of intracranial tumors. In addition to the hemosiderosis

TABLE 10–4.   Differential diagnosis of dementia with seizures.

Generalized or focal seizure disorder (epilepsy)
    Brain damage associated with epilepsy
    Frequent, recurrent, or prolonged seizures
    Anticonvulsant-related intellectual decline
        Anticonvulsant toxicity
        Folate deficiency
    Epilepsy-associated psychiatric disorder
        Schizophrenia-like psychosis
        Depression
Seizures with associated neurologic disease
    DAT
    Pick's disease
    Multi-infarct dementia
    Jakob-Creutzfeldt disease
    Posttraumatic dementia
    Myoclonic epilepsy with dementia
    Neuronal storage disorders

---

and the direct effects of the underlying etiologic process, hydrocephalus is frequently present and contributes to the dementia syndrome. Treatment is directed toward identifying the etiology of the recurrent bleeding. Hemosiderosis does not affect other organs, and the CNS is spared in generalized hemochromatosis.

Epilepsy

In the past, epilepsy was regarded as a degenerative condition with inevitable intellectual deterioration. Few reliable treatments were available and epileptics were sequestered in colonies where they were socially isolated and subject to repeated uncontrolled seizures. The outlook has improved considerably and there is little evidence that epilepsy per se is associated with dementia (Brown and Reynolds, 1981). Nevertheless, there are circumstances in which intellectual deterioration occurs in the epileptic patient (Table 10–4). A major contributing factor is the amount and location of any associated underlying brain injury. Patients with inherited forms of epilepsy may have no identifiable cerebral pathology, but those with acquired generalized or focal seizure disorders have associated brain lesions that cause the seizures and may also limit intellectual performance (Glowinski, 1973; Quadfasel and Pruyser, 1955). These injuries may be congenital, giving rise to mental retardation, or acquired later in life, producing posttraumatic, postinfectious, or poststroke symptoms with cognitive impairment.

Prolonged, frequent, and recurrent seizures can lead to progressive intellectual disability (Dikman and Matthews, 1977; Dodrill and Troupin, 1976). Increasing epileptiform activity on the EEG also correlates with intellectual impairment compared to matched patients with fewer paroxysmal EEG abnormalities (Bornstein et al, 1988; Dodrill and Wilkus, 1976a, b).

Currently, the most common cause of intellectual impairment in epileptics is inadvertent chronic anticonvulsant intoxication. Phenytoin, mesantoin, phenobarbital, and ethosuximide have all been reported to produce changes in mental status that reverse when the drug is discontinued or the dosage lowered (Giordani et al, 1983) (Chapter 7). Folate metabolism may also be impaired by anticonvulsants and lead to a chronic folate-deficiency dementia (Chapter 7).

Epilepsy has been associated with a schizophrenia-like psychosis and with an unusual propensity to develop affective disorders (Betts, 1981; Slater and Beard, 1963; Toone, 1981). The neuropsychiatric disorders predispose the epileptic patient to the dementias associated with psychiatric disorders presented in Chapter 9.

Finally, the intellectual compromise occurring in some patients with epilepsy must be distinguished from progressive dementing illnesses that have seizures as one potential manifestation of the CNS disorder. These include DAT, Pick's disease, multi-infarct dementia, Jakob-Creutzfeldt disease, lipid storage diseases, and so on. Seizures are far more common with cortical than they are with subcortical dementias.

INHERITED DISORDERS WITH DEMENTIA

Most inherited biochemical defects are recessively inherited disorders that become manifest in infancy or early childhood. The child fails to develop skills at the expected age or may lose previously mastered abilities. Deficits in motor and intellectual development are present. In some cases, however, biochemical deficiencies do not become apparent until adolescence or adulthood. Table 10–5 lists the inherited adult-onset biochemical disorders that produce dementia as a main feature of their clinical symptomatology.

Leukodystrophies

There are three inherited diseases of the white matter that first appear in adult life; metachromatic leukodystrophy (MLD), adrenoleukodystrophy (ALD), and membranous lipodystrophy. Acquired mental impairment is characteristic of each.

Metachromatic Leukodystrophy (MLD)

MLD is a lipid storage disease in which sulfatides accumulate in central and peripheral nervous system tissues producing progressive dementia, py-

TABLE 10–5.   Inherited adult-onset biochemical disorders that produce dementia.

Leukoencephalopathies
  Metachromatic leukodystrophy
  Adrenoleukodystrophy
  Membranous lipodystrophy
  Cerebrotendinous xanthomatosis
  Hereditary adult-onset leukodystrophy
Polioencephalopathies
  Adult GM, gangliosidosis
  Adult GM_2 gangliosidosis (adult Tay-Sach's disease)
  Adult Gaucher's disease (type III)
  Fabry's disease
  Adult cerebral lipidosis (including ceroid lipofuscinosis)
  Adult polyglucosan body disease
Miscellaneous biochemical disorders
  Mitochondrial encephalomyopathies
  Leigh's disease
  Homocystinuria
  Wilson's disease
  Porphyria

ramidal and extrapyramidal motor abnormalities, seizures, and peripheral neuropathy (Austin et al, 1968; Muller et al, 1969; Sourander and Svennerholm, 1962). It is an autosomal recessive disorder with infantile, juvenile, and adult forms. The adult form is arbitrarily defined by onset of symptoms after the age of 21 years (Hirose and Bass, 1972). One patient whose disease began at age 63 has been reported, and several patients have survived into the seventh decade (Bosch and Hart, 1978). The infantile and juvenile forms characteristically begin with motor disturbances whereas the adult variety most commonly presents with insidious mental status alterations. The course of the disease is widely variable, lasting 1 to 44 years with an average duration of 15 years (Ettinger, 1965; Muller et al, 1969).

Several adults with MLD had initial manifestations simulating a psychiatric disorder. Some were thought to be suffering from schizophrenia (Betts et al, 1968; Manowitz et al, 1978; Sourander and Svennerholm, 1962; Waltz et al, 1987) whereas others presented with delusions of grandeur and self-importance suggestive of mania (Muller et al, 1969; Van Bogaert and DeWulf, 1939). All reports of adult-onset MLD describe a dementia early in the course of the illness. The dementia has prominent features suggesting subcortical dysfunction with outstanding characteristics of apathy, progressive memory impairment with disorientation, and loss of insight (Bosch and Hart, 1978). Visuospatial functions may be compromised more than language skills are (Manowitz et al, 1978). Motor disturbances—rigidity, ataxia, athetosis, or tremor—usually appear within a few months of onset. Dysarthria and pseudobulbar palsy become prominent as the disease advances, and peripheral neuropathy is consistently present. The latter is often asymptomatic but occasionally causes dysesthesia and can be demonstrated with nerve conduction studies. Seizures are typically a late feature but may occur in the early phases of disease.

EEGs of patients with MLD show diffuse slowing, and CT findings have been variable. Bosch and Hart (1978) reported that the CT scan in their patient showed slightly enlarged ventricles, prominent cortical sulci, and normal density of white matter. Lane and co-workers (1978) described a case of MLD in which the CT scan revealed symmetric areas of low density in the deep white matter of both hemispheres. MRI studies reveal abnormal high signal areas on T_2-weighted images in the periventricular regions (Fisher et al, 1987; Waltz et al, 1987). Visual and somatosensory evoked potentials are delayed and nerve conduction velocities are slowed (Wulff and Trojaborg, 1985). Nonopacification of the gallbladder by cholecystography and elevation of the CSF protein provide supportive evidence for the diagnosis but are less reliable in adult than in infantile disease (Bosch and Hart, 1978). The presence of a peripheral neuropathy is an important finding as few diseases affect both the central and peripheral nervous systems (Bosch and Hart, 1978). Once MLD is suspected, the diagnosis can usually be confirmed by demonstration of diminished arylsulfatase A in urine, leukocytes, or skin fibroblasts (Percy and Kaback, 1971) or by doing a biopsy of peripheral nerve tissue and showing the accumulation of metachromatic material in Schwann cells and macrophages (Olsson and Sourander, 1969).

Pathologically, MLD is characterized by symmetric demyelination of all lobes of the cerebral hemispheres with variable myelin loss in the cerebellum, brainstem, and spinal cord. The subcortical U fibers are uniformly spared. With appropriate stains, metachromatic material is demonstrated in the glial cells of the cerebral white matter and occasionally in the cortical neurons. Metachromatic inclusions are also present in the neurons of the lower brainstem and dentate nucleus of the cerebellum (Austin et al, 1968; Guseo et al, 1975; Sourander and Svennerholm, 1962). In some cases, metachromatic products have been observed in the liver, gallbladder, kidney, hypophysis, and/or testis (Sourander and Svennerholm, 1962). The peripheral nerves in MLD show accumulation of copious amounts of a yellow-brown staining substance in Schwann cells and perivascular and subperineurial phagocytes, and there is segmental interruption of the myelin sheaths (Olsson and Sourander, 1969). Electron microscopic investigation reveals myelin fragments in phagocytes, homogeneous granular material in neurons, and lamellated structures in oligodendrocytes and astrocytes (Guseo et al, 1975; Joosten et al, 1975). Neurochemical assays of brain tissues show a relative increase in the sulfatide content of both gray and white matter (Sourander and Svennerholm, 1962).

The pathophysiologic basis of MLD has been delineated in recent years. The accumulation of sulfatide in the body suggested a deficit in catabolism of this lipid, and arylsulfatase A, the enzyme necessary for degrading intracellular sulfatide, was shown to be decreased or absent in the urine, leukocytes, and skin fibroblasts of affected patients (Bosch and Hart, 1978; Hirose and Bass, 1972; Percy and Kaback, 1971). Myelin is synthesized normally but the inherited enzyme deficiency results in insufficient catabolism of sulfatides by oligodendrocytes and Schwann cells. Intermediate products in the metabolic pathway accumulate in the cells, resulting in disruption of myelin maintenance and eventual breakdown of the myelin sheaths (Muller et al, 1969). The delineation of the mechanism of myelin destruction in MLD has not led to the development of effective intervention, and all attempts to halt progression of the disease have met with failure.

Adrenoleukodystrophy (ALD)

ALD is an X-linked disorder of white matter with progressive neurologic deterioration leading to dementia, blindness, quadriparesis, and death. There is variable evidence of adrenal insufficiency. The condition has been known by a variety of names during its confusing history, including diffuse sclerosis, melanodermic leukodystrophy, sudanophilic leukodystrophy, and Schilder's disease. Typically its onset is between ages 3 and 12, but several patients have been reported with onset in the third and fourth decades and a few as late as the sixth decade (Powell et al, 1975; Schaumburg et al, 1974, 1975). A change in behavior followed soon after by evidence of intellectual deterioration initiates the disorder. Gait disturbances are an early feature, and visual failure and seizures may occur at any time in the course. The initial findings may be asymmetric with hemiparesis preceding quadriparesis and hemianopia antedating blindness. Death occurs one to nine years after onset. Occasionally adrenal failure is the first manifestation of the disorder. Fatigue, hypotension, and hyperpigmentation of the skin and gums are then evident. As a rule the CNS disturbances appear first and the adrenal dysfunction is asymptomatic, but an impaired adrenal response to adrenocorticotropic hormone stimulation is demonstrable in most cases (Gray, 1969; Powell et al, 1975; Schaumburg et al, 1975). Steroid replacement therapy relieves the addisonian symptoms but has no effect on the course of neurologic deterioration.

Peripheral neuropathy is not part of ALD, but a variant of the disorder known as adrenomyeloneuropathy presents with a peripheral neuropathy and spastic paraparesis. Dementia is a late feature of this related illness, which sometimes occurs among family members of patients with typical ALD (Griffin et al, 1977).

The characteristics of the dementia in ALD have not been fully described. The patient reported by Valenstein and colleagues (1971) was inattentive, had impaired memory and poor calculation, and showed little concern about his progressive visual failure. Gray (1969) emphasized disinhibited, distractable behavior, and social irresponsibility. Impaired speech and paraphasia were observed in one patient (Bresnan and Richardson, 1979), and psychotic symptoms including hallucinations and delusions have occurred in others (Powell et al, 1974; Weiss et al, 1980).

The EEGs reveal generalized slowing, and auditory evoked responses may be abnormal (Black et al, 1979). In some cases radionuclide brain scans show abnormal uptake of isotope in the posterior hemispheric areas (Sanchez and Lopez, 1976; Valenstein et al, 1971). CT scans demonstrate low-density confluent areas in the white matter of the posterotemporal, parietal, and occipital regions. The ventricles may be enlarged in the area of the trigone and occipital horns, and there is marked contrast enhancement at the edges of the lesions (Greenberg et al, 1977; Lane et al, 1978). MRI demonstrates regions of increased signal intensity on T_2-weighted images. The abnormalities are most evident in the motor tracts, and visual radiations and abnormalities may be apparent prior to the occurrence of overt neurologic symptoms (Auborg et al, 1989). Cultured skin fibroblasts from patients with ALD have elevated levels of C26 fatty acid (Moser et al, 1980, 1984a; O'Neill et al, 1982). Demonstration of adrenal insufficiency in a patient with the appropriate clinical and radiologic findings supports the diagnosis. Biopsy of adrenal tissue has been suggested as the most reliable method of histologic verification (Schaumburg et al, 1975; Weiss et al, 1980) although some authors have championed the use of less invasive biopsies of skin or conjunctiva (Martin et al, 1977b, 1980). Studies of CSF may reveal a lymphocytosis or increased protein but are usually normal. The CSF immunoelectrophoresis demonstrates a nonspecific increase in IgG (Sanchez and Lopez, 1976).

Pathologically, there are large confluent areas of demyelination in the posterotemporal, parietal, and occipital areas of the brain. The frontal regions are relatively spared or may be involved asymmetrically. There is extensive gliosis, loss of axons, and a prominent inflammatory response in the demyelinated areas with subcortical U fibers spared. The inflammatory cells are primarily T lymphocytes, suggesting an immunologically mediated component to the illness (Griffen et al, 1985). The optic nerves are severely involved, and the cerebellum shows variable demyelination. Examination of the adrenal glands reveals ballooned cortical cells with striated cytoplasm and macrovacuoles in the zona fasciculata and zona reticularis. Electron microscopy shows that the striations are curvilinear or twisted lamellar accumulations consisting of leaflets separated by clear spaces (Powers and Schaumburg, 1974). Similar inclusions have been demonstrated in Schwann cells, testis, skin, conjunctiva, CNS macrophages, and microglial cells and appear to be specific for ALD (Martin et al, 1977b; Powell et al, 1975; Schaumburg et al, 1975).

The genetic abnormality of ALD has been mapped to chromosome Xq28 (Moser et al, 1984a). The inherited defect results in the failure to degrade and hence the accumulation of very long chain fatty acids; all affected persons show increased levels of these compounds, particularly hexocosanoate (C26:0). There is abnormal storage of abnormal gangliosides and cholesterol esters in the cerebral white matter, adrenal cortex, and other tissues (Griffin et al, 1985). Metabolism of these substances normally takes place in a subcellular organelle, the peroxisome, and ALD is properly considered a peroxisomal disorder (Moser et al, 1984a). The adrenal insufficiency can be managed successfully with cortisol replacement therapy but no treatment is available for the neurologic deterioration. High-dose prednisone therapy and immunosuppression fail to halt progression of the disease (Stumpf et al, 1981). Use of diets with restricted amounts of very long chain fatty acids and bone marrow transplantation result in lowered levels of plasma fatty acids but have not altered the neurological status or progression of the patients (Moser et al,1984b; Suzuki et al, 1986). Erucic acid therapy also lowers long chain fatty acid levels and may slow progression of symptoms in mild cases of ALD (Rizzo et al, 1989).

Membranous Lipodystrophy

Membranous lipodystrophy (lipomembranous polycystic osteodysplasia; Nasu-Hakola disease; brain, bone, and fat disease) is an uncommon autosomal recessive disorder manifested by the onset of bone pain at age 20 years followed by a tendency to fracture bones easily by age 30 years; neuropsychiatric symptoms appear when the patient is in the thirties; and death usually occurs in the late thirties or early forties (Hakola, 1972). The X-rays reveal cystic lesions of the bone. Neurologic abnormalities include rigidity, exaggerated muscle stretch reflexes, and extensor plantar responses. Optic atrophy is apparent in some cases and seizures are not uncommon. Perseveration in spontaneous speech, monotonous verbal output, and abnormalities of word stress occur. Memory impairment, disorientation, and dilapidation of intellectual functions are combined with euphoria, mania, and disinhibition. The EEG reveals nonspecific slowing of the background rhythms, and skull X-rays and X-ray CT scans may demonstrate calcification of the basal ganglia (Bird et al, 1983; Hakola, 1972). Autopsy studies reveal that the most marked changes occur in the hemispheric white matter where dense fibrillary gliosis is noted. Axonal spheroids are common (Matushita et al, 1981; Nasu et al, 1973). Light and electron microscopy of the bone cysts shows invaginated and corrugated fat cell membranes without lipid storage (Bird et al, 1983; Nasu et al, 1973). No treatment for the disorder is currently available.

Cerebrotendinous Xanthomatosis

Cerebrotendinous xanthomatosis is a rare familial disorder presenting with dementia or organic psychosis, slowly progressive cerebellar dysfunction, and myoclonus (Crome and Stern, 1976). Juvenile cataracts and mild peripheral neuropathy may be present. Most patients have xanthomata of the tendons and lungs with xanthelasma of the eyelids although occasional patients have no peripheral manifestations of the disease (Neumann, 1971). The CT scans show diffuse hypodensity of the hemispheric white matter (Beringer et al, 1981). MRI demonstrates diffuse areas of increased signal in the hemispheric white matter on T_2-weighted images (Swanson and Cromwell, 1986). Cholestanol, a degradation product of cholesterol, is increased in the brain, lungs, bones, and tendons. Within the brain, the most extensive changes are evident in the basal ganglia, cerebellum, and inferior olives, and there is widespread demyelination of the white matter. Serum cholesterol levels are normal in most cases but cholestanol levels increase. An enzymatic defect has not been identified.

Hereditary Adult-Onset Leukodystrophy

One large kindred with an autosomal dominant adult-onset leukodystrophy has been described (Eldridge et al, 1984). Symptoms begin in the fourth or fifth decade and include autonomic dysfunction as well as cerebellar and pyramidal stem abnormalities. Patients commonly survive 20 years following onset. CT reveals hypodensity of the hemispheric white matter, and T_2-weighted MRI scans show regions of increased signal intensity in the frontoparietal white matter, brain stem, and cerebellar white matter (Schwankhaus et al, 1988).

Polioencephalopathies (Neuronal Storage Diseases)

Many infantile lipidoses and mucoploysaccharidoses have been characterized biochemically, but only a few of the adult neuronal storage diseases have been extensively studied. Adult neuronal storage diseases are rare disorders that typically produce a wide variety of neurologic disturbances including dementia, myoclonus, seizures, ataxia, and spasticity.

GM_1 gangliosidosis has early- and late-onset forms. In adults it produces a dementia, parkinsonism, myoclonus, ataxia, or pyramidal system dysfunction (Mutoh et al, 1986; Ohta et al, 1985). The underlying abnormality is a deficiency in beta-galactosidase resulting in the accumulation of GM_1 ganglioside in brain. The disorder is inherited in an autosomal recessive manner.

Several cases of adult GM_2 gangliosidosis have been reported (Miyatake et al, 1979; Navon et al, 1981; O'Neill et al, 1978; Rapin et al, 1976;

Specola et al, 1990). The ganglioside accumulation results from hexosaminidase A deficiency. In some cases, neurologic abnormalities became evident in childhood and progressed as the patient aged. In others, no neurologic disturbances were evident prior to the third or fourth decade of life. The dementia includes memory impairment and behavioral changes. Seizures, cranial nerve palsies, spasticity, and ataxia are also present. At autopsy, the neurons are ballooned and periodic acid-Schiff-positive granules are present in both neurons and glial cells. Intracellular membranous cytoplasmic bodies are shown by electron microscopy.

Gaucher's disease usually affects children, but the uncommon type III variant produces dementia, myoclonus, and generalized seizures in adults. The disease has its onset in adolescence and leads to death within 10 years. It results from acid beta-glucosidase deficiency (Kolodny and Cable, 1982; Nishimura and Barranger, 1980).

Fabry's disease (angiokeratoma corporis diffusum, hereditary dystrophic lipidosis) is anther disorder of sphingolipid metabolism that may not become manifest until adulthood. It is an X-linked disorder, but female carriers may show partial involvement. Alpha-galactosidase is the deficient enzyme and ceramide trihexoside accumulates in many body organs, CNS, autonomic nervous system, and blood vessels (Crome and Stern, 1976; Kaye et al, 1988; Rahman and Lindenberg, 1963). Ballooned neurons may be found in central autonomic and deep gray structures, but most of the neurologic abnormalities are secondary to vascular occlusion. Symptoms include a multi-infarct type of dementia combined with limb pain, impaired renal function, focal neurologic signs, and autonomic dysfunction (Cable et al, 1982). Keratotic macules and papules on the lower trunk and limbs and corneal opacities are characteristic of the disease (Lou and Reske-Neilsen, 1971; Wise et al, 1962).

Kuf's disease is an adult-onset autosomal recessive cerebral lipidosis that presents with an insidious dementia, myclonus, seizures, spasticity, and cerebellar dysfunction (Crome and Stern, 1976; Dekaban and Herman, 1974; Greenwood and Nelson, 1978; Tobo et al, 1984). Classically, the disorder is considered a form of neuronal ceroid lipofuscinosis. Lipofuscin is visible by light microscopy in many of the cortical neurons, and electron microscopy reveals neuronal inclusion bodies consisting of membrane fragments and amorphous granular material.

Adult polyglucosan body disease is a disorder of polysaccharide metabolism presenting with dementia (Gray et al, 1988). Deterioration usually begins in the sixth or seventh decade of life and progresses to death in 3 to 8 years, but rare cases have had chronic courses lasting 20 years or more. The disorder is characterized by progressive dementia, marked sensory loss, and upper and lower motor neuron dysfunction (Peress et al, 1979; Robitaille et al, 1980; Suzuki et al, 1971). Pathologically, intraneuronal inclusion bodies identical to Lafora bodies are found throughout the CNS. Histochemical investigation demonstrates the polysaccharide nature of the inclusions, but no specific enzyme defect has been identified. Unlike myoclonic epilepsy with Lafora bodies (discussed below) the patients do not have myoclonus, and the inclusion bodies are concentrated in the neuronal processes rather than in the cell body.

Miscellaneous Inherited Dementing Disorders

Leigh's Disease

Leigh's disease (subacute necrotizing encephalomyelopathy) usually appears in infancy or childhood but occasionally presents in late adolescence or adulthood (Hardman et al, 1968; Kalimo et al, 1979; Sipe, 1973). Deficiencies of pyruvate dehydrogenase and cytochrome c oxidase have been demonstrated (Miranda et al, 1989). Some patients have been mildly intellectually retarded from birth, and cognitive impairment advances as the other manifestations of the disease become evident. The disease is characterized by bilateral optic atrophy, progressive brainstem dysfunction, ataxia, seizures, and a peripheral neuropathy. CT may reveal radiolucent lesions involving the basal ganglia, brain stem, and cerebellum. MRI is more sensitive than CT in the demonstration of abnormalities (Koch et al, 1986). At autopsy there is mild demyelination plus capillary and glial proliferation involving periventricular areas that pathologically resembles Wernicke's encephalopathy but affects the optic nerves, basal ganglia, substantia nigra, tectum of the midbrain, cerebellar cortex, dentate nucleus, and inferior olives.

Progressive Myoclonus Epilepsy

In 1891 Unverricht described the occurrence of myoclonus and epilepsy in a family of 11 siblings. In 1903 and 1912 Lundborg described several more families with the same syndrome and used the term progressive myoclonus epilepsy. He noted that in addition to myoclonic jerks and seizures, rigidity, hyperactive reflexes, and dementia were constant features (Dam and Moller, 1968).

Two variants of progressive myoclonus epilepsy (Unverricht-Lundborg disease) have been identified. Both syndromes present with myoclonus, epilepsy, and dementia. Lafora bodies are found in the cell bodies of one variant (Lafora type) whereas the other has neuron loss and gliosis without distinctive inclusions (Harriman and Miller, 1955). Progressive myoclonic epilepsy is rare outside of Scandinavia where its prevalence is estimated at 1 in 140,000 (Harenko and Toivakka, 1961; Koskiniemi et al, 1974a, b). The disorder is inherited in an autosomal recessive manner, has its onset between 6 and 15 years of age, and leads to death in 3 to 22 years. The initial symptoms include myoclonus or generalized seizures and as the disease advances bulbar dysfunction, dysarthria, extrapyramidal disorders, cerebellar symptoms, and profound dementia become apparent (Grinker et al, 1938). The dementia is of the subcortical type and is characterized by psychomotor retardation, poor concentration, memory impairment, and personality alterations. Visual hallucinations, aberrant sexual behavior, depression, and outbursts of rage were seen in some cases (Grinker et al, 1938; Harenko and Toivakka, 1961; Harriman and Miller, 1955; Janeway et al, 1967; Koskiniemi et al, 1974a; Schwarz and Yanoff, 1965). The EEG changes include slowing of background rhythms, paroxysmal spike and wave activity, and photosensitive myoclonus (Janeway et al, 1967; Koskiniemi et al, 1974b; Wada et al, 1960). Pathologic examination reveals cerebellar, olivary, and spinal degeneration. Mesencephalic and substantia nigra involvement is apparent in some cases and changes have sometimes been noted in the cerebral cortex (Haltia et al, 1969; Koskinicmi et al, 1974a; Matthews et al, 1969; Yokoi et al, 1965). In the Lafora body type of progressive myoclonic epilepsy, Lafora bodies are found throughout the CNS but are most abundant in the substantia nigra, dentate nuclei, thalami, and globus pallidus (Schwarz and Yanoff, 1965). Lafora inclusions are concentric rounded bodies of varying size occurring in the neuronal cytoplasm (Corsellis and Meldrum, 1976). Chemically they are composed of acid mucopolysaccharides and glycoproteins (Janeway et at, 1967; Schwarz and Yanoff, 1965).

The disease is inexorably progressive, and the course, unalterable. Seizure activity and myoclonic jerking respond at least partially to a variety of anticonvulsants including sodium valproate, phenobarbital, phenylacetylurea, and clonazepam (Grinker et al, 1938; Iivanainen and Himberg, 1982; Koskiniemi et al, 1974b, Peterson and Hambert, 1966).

The differential diagnosis of progressive myoclonus epilepsy includes a large number of syndromes that combine myoclonus and progressive dementia (Table 10–6). Watson and Denny-Brown (1953) noted that the combination of dementia and myoclonic jerking occurs in many disorders that affect the CNS diffusely, particularly neuronal storage diseases and subacute sclerosing panencephalitis. Noad and Lance (1960) pointed out that myoclonus epilepsy and progressive spinocerebellar degenerations share many clinical and pathologic features. Other disorders that produce myoclonus and dementia include Jakob-Creutzfeldt disease, metabolic encephalopathies, postanoxic brain injury, and degenerative disorders (Aigner and Mulder, 1969; Lance and Adams, 1963; Swanson et al, 1962).

Mitochondrial Encephalomyopathies

Mitochondrial encephalomyopathies are a diverse group of illnesses resulting from abnormal mitochondrial function (Pavlakis et al, 1988). Three

TABLE 10–6.   Differential diagnosis of principal syndromes manifesting
dementia and myoclonus.

Chronic viral encephalitis
    Jakob-Creutzfeldt disease
    Subacute sclerosing panencephalitis
Metabolic encephalopathies
    Uremic encephalopathy
    Pulmonary encephalopathy
    Postanoxic dementia with intention myoclonus
Inherited metabolic disorders
    Neuronal storage diseases
Degenerative disorders
    Spinocerebellar degenerations
    Progressive myoclonus epilepsy
    DAT

Myoclonus has been reported as a symptom in rare examples of almost every disorder that produces dementia.

mitochondrial syndromes may manifest dementia—Kearns-Sayre syndrome; myoclonus epilepsy with ragged red fibers (MERRF); and mitochondrial myopathy, encephalopathy, lactic acidosis, and strokeline episodes (ME-LAS). Kearns-Sayre syndrome is a disorder of children characterized by progressive external opthalmoplegia, pigmentary retinopathy, and cardiac conduction defects. Mental retardation occurs in some cases and progressive dementia in others. The MERRF syndrome patients typically exhibit ataxia, dementia, myoclonus, and hearing loss (Lombes et al, 1989; Pavlakis et al, 1988). The MELAS syndrome patients manifest dementia, seizures, short stature, elevated serum lactic acid levels, and multiple focal neurologic signs (Pavlakis et al, 1988; Talley and Faber, 1989). Basal ganglia calcification may be evident in MELAS patients. All the mitochondrial encephalopathies share maternal transmission as the characteristic hereditary pattern.

Mast Syndrome

Mast syndrome (not to be confused with mast cell disease) is an autosomal recessive disease of the nervous system that occurs primarily in Amish communities of Ohio, Indiana, and Pennsylvania in the United States (Cross and McKusick, 1967). The syndrome initially becomes manifest as a gait disorder appearing in the second decade. Over the next three to four decades, dysarthria, cerebellar disturbances, increased tone, athetosis, and dementia become evident. The dementia is characterized by apathy, poor concentration, impaired memory, disturbed comprehension, and emotional lability.

Sensory Radicular Neuropathy (Denny-Brown Disease)

Geschwind and Segarra (1969) reported a patient with hereditary sensory neuropathy, sensorineural deafness, ataxia, seizures, and progressive dementia. The disorder began at age 18, and the patient died at age 35. Pathologically there was widespread neuron loss and glial proliferation in the cerebral cortex. Astrocytic proliferation was evident in the white matter. Neuron loss was evident in the cerebellum, putamen, caudate, and inferior olives. The posterior roots of the spinal cord showed marked fiber loss with intense neurilemmal proliferation. Dementia was an early feature of this case, appearing at age 18 with hearing impairment and progressing steadily to severe intellectual deficiency at the time of death.

Myotonic Dystrophy

Myotonic dystrophy (dystrophia myotonica, myotonia atrophica) is an autosomal dominant systemic disorder manifested by myopathy, cataracts, frontal baldness (in males), gonadal atrophy, heart disease, impaired pulmonary ventilation, endocrine abnormalities, bone changes, and abnormalities of serum immunoglobulins (Adams, 1975b, Walton and Gardner-Medwin, 1974). Congenital mental retardation occurs in some patients and a progressive dementia is seen in others. Onset of symptoms is normally between ages 20 and 50, with ptosis, facial weakness, dysarthria, and weakness of the distal limb muscles. Muscle wasting becomes evident, and myotonia, the abnormal persistence of muscle contraction, becomes evident in the hands and tongue. The course is steadily progressive and death occurs after 20 to 25 years from aspiration pneumonia or cardiac failure.

The dementia that sometimes accompanies myotonic dystrophy has been studied little, but progressive impairment of attention, memory, abstraction, calculation, and initiation have been noted, and cognitive slowing is evident (Culebras et al, 1973; Woodward et al, 1982). Huber et al (1989c) identified abnormalities in attention, effortful memory, and visuospatial reasoning. Aphasia, agnosia, and/or apraxia have not been reported. Dementia secondary to impaired pulmonary or cardiac function or to endocrine disturbances must be excluded, however, before the dementia of myotonic dystrophy is attributed to a primary CNS process. MRI reveals cerebral cortical atrophy, increased skull thickness, focal abnormalities in the cerebral white matter, and linear areas of high signal in the anterior medial temporal lobes (Huber et al, 1989c). Culebras and colleagues (1973) found that patients with myotic dystrophy with dementia had abundant eosinophilic intracytoplasmic bodies in the thalamus, particularly the dorsomedial and anterior thalamic nuclei. Such bodies occur in up to 1 percent of neurons in normal elderly individuals but were present in 10 to 30 percent of patients with myotonic dystrophy and dementia.

A number of inherited disorders with biochemical defects has been presented in earlier chapters. Homocystinuria, Wilson's disease, and porphyria all have inherited metabolic abnormalitites and may lead to progressive intellectual deterioration. Many diseases that are currently classified as degenerative will no doubt eventually be found to have enzymatic defects that account for their progressive course.

11
Aging and Senility

One difficult problem facing the clinician who is attempting to diagnose dementia concerns the alterations in mental activity (usually described as some degree of mental impairment) that occur during the course of "normal" aging. While epidemiologists estimate that between 5 and 20 percent of the population over 65 years of age suffer from mild to severe dementia (see Chapter 1), many, in fact most, of the remaining members of the geriatric population also show some degree of mental alteration. This process has been discussed under a variety of terms such as senescence, senility, or primary senile dementia. Current research suggests that the problem may be at least partially artificial, a product of extracerebral physical and/or social factors (Rowe and Kahn, 1987). Differences in usual versus successful aging, young-old (under 70 years) versus old-old (over 70), and other divisions demonstrate that not all elderly show mental decline to the same degree. Nonetheless many elderly do show mental impairment of some degree.

A number of explanations for cognitive decline have been offered and in recent years some suggest that all mental impairment seen in the aging individual represents the effect of greater or lesser degrees of Alzheimer-type cortical neuropathologic changes. While it is conveniently inclusive, this approach has shortcomings and appears incorrect.

Do these elderly individuals have a milder degree of cortical dementia or is the mental change part of the normal aging process? The term *senes-*

cence has been used to indicate the changes of normal aging and *senility* for those of abnormal aging, but the boundary is obscure. For the purposes of this chapter *senility* will be used to indicate the milder degrees of mental alteration that occur in nondemented elderly people. Determining the boundary between the normal and the dementing population is fraught with pitfalls for the clinician; some of these problems will be outlined.

CLINICAL ALTERATIONS IN SENILITY

Slowness

One of the most consistent changes noted with aging is a general slowing of intellectual and physical performance (Katzman, 1982). This is obviously true of motor activity. For instance, the fastest time for a marathon distance run increases linearly with age so that the best time ever recorded for a person over 75 is approximately twice that of the 21-year-old recordholders (Clark, 1979). Other motor activities such as finger tapping, rates of moving the arms or the legs, and all types of reaction time tests also show progressive slowing with advancing age (Birren, 1974; Welford, 1965). These changes are not absolute, however, and many younger individuals have slow reaction times while some elderly people perform rapidly. Observation suggests an association between continued involvement in physical activities throughout life and the maintenance of motor speed. Nonetheless the slowing down of motor activities is pervasive and is clearly present in the majority of the elderly; it must be accepted as a factor of consequence in normal aging.

Just as there is a decrease in motor speed (bradykinesia), there is also slowing of the processing of sensory information as demonstrated by visual, auditory, and somatosensory reaction times (Birren, 1974; Salthouse, 1976). Numerous studies suggest that the most profound slowing occurs in central processing and can be called bradyphrenia (Welford, 1965; Fozard et al, 1976), but peripheral alterations affect visual, auditory, and tactile senses and add to the delay of the elderly individual's response to sensory stimulation. The slowing of sensorimotor processing appears to involve all three aspects of the reflex arc—the sensory pathways, the central processing of the sensory information, and the motor response mechanism. Decreased speed of processing correlates well with advancing age (Van Gorp et al, 1990).

Forgetfulness

Many elderly individuals complain about their memory and, when they are questioned, admit to forgetfulness. Formal testing, however, demonstrates normal capability in immediate recall (digit span, and so forth), normal retrieval from long-term storage and retained ability to learn long lists of unrelated words. It takes elderly subjects somewhat longer to learn the lists, but when they are retested, they retain as much of the newly learned information as do younger subjects (Craik, 1977). Recall of nonverbal material is affected more than verbal recall is (Eslinger et al, 1988). Incidental learning, the remembering of events during testing that were not the primary material to be learned, is less successful in older individuals when compared to the young (Katzman, 1982). Also the elderly improve on memory tests if offered semantic clues, whereas younger subjects require fewer aids for recall (Smith, 1977). The greatest change in memory in the aged appears to be decreased retrieval of learned information, not ability to learn. Literally, the elderly forget to remember. Nonetheless, the learning process in the elderly is affected by slowness and is less efficient than it is in the young (Crook et al, 1986). In the past decade two terms, *benign senescent forgetfulness* and *age-associated memory impairment,* have been introduced to characterize the alterations in memory function that appear with advancing age.

Language

Verbal intelligence test responses, as a whole, tend to be preserved until the seventh decade and then decline only gradually (Dopplet and Wallace, 1955); ability on the vocabulary subtests of the Wechsler Adult Intelligence Scale is remarkably preserved (Riegel, 1968). Nonetheless, older subjects regularly complain of difficulty in finding words and may perform relatively poorly on confrontation naming tests (Goodglass, 1980). This is particularly noticeable with proper names. Elderly individuals often recognize a long-time acquaintance but cannot recollect the person's name, a form of forgetfulness, not a language impairment. Anomic language disturbance may be one of the earliest signs of senility, however, and, as it develops, the language disturbance can resemble a mild form of Wernicke aphasia with compromised comprehension of language in addition to the naming difficulties (Albert, 1981). Much of the indistinctness in reports of the language changes with aging stem from failure to separate varieties of dementia from senility. Most studies still treat dementia as a single disease process. Recent studies, however, posit a subcortical-frontal problem that affects language processing (Albert and Kaplan, 1980; Van Gorp et al, 1988). More and better research is needed, but it is abundantly clear that linguistic alterations are mild and language disability is not a major problem of senility. In fact, some language-related functions such as narrative style may actually show increasing complexity with advancing years and become more complex during the aging process (Obler, 1979).

Visuospatial Discrimination

Visuospatial competence also changes with aging. While tests such as the Raven Matrices and the Block Design Subtest of the Wechsler Adult Intelligence Scale are performed normally, or nearly so, by healthy elderly subjects (Katzman, 1982), formal, timed, spatial tests are performed poorly in comparison to young control subjects (Gaylord and Marsh, 1975). Again slowness is a factor of key significance in the mental processes of the elderly (Salthouse, 1985).

Careful analysis of some specific aspects of two- and three-dimensional drawing skills suggests greater involvement of frontal than of parietal functions (Albert and Kaplan, 1980). Among the more prominent abnormalities in drawing by the elderly are segmentation (poor integration of individual elements of a production) and perseveration (Veroff, 1980). Age-related deficits have been reported in block construction, stick design, clock setting, and the Hooper Visual Organization Test (Farver, 1975). These alterations may be interpreted as manifestations of either frontal or parietal compromise.

Cognition

The ability to manipulate knowledge is also fairly well maintained by the normal elderly. Thus while Botwinick (1977) found a general decline in intelligence test results after age 60 years, the worst declines were in tests demanding speed. Verbal test score levels were maintained for almost two additional decades, and the level of general intellectual function was maintained well into old age.

More recent studies (Ernst, 1987) suggest that the elderly have problems in concept formation and problem-solving tasks. In particular, tests sensitive to frontal dysfunction such as the Stroop (1935) and verbal fluency tasks are performed less well by the elderly (Veroff, 1980; Whelihan and Lesher, 1985). Reese and Rodeheaver (1985) concluded that elderly individuals perform more poorly because of persevervations and the use of more primitive strategies.

Personality and Mood

While basic traits remain, personal styles tend to change as the individual gets older. Most changes center around the slowing of a person's lifestyle; fewer new challenges are sought, and fewer goals are accomplished. Most elderly seem to accept this alteration, entering a somewhat apathetic state. Drive appears decreased even though desire may remain; the elderly come to accept that they can accomplish less in a given amount of time. There is a trend toward decreased ability to concentrate and to maintain selective attention over prolonged periods of time, a disturbance that creates problems in judgment and other higher cognitive functions. With advancing years, most individuals show decreased desire for novelty, accepting and actually coveting the security of a routine. This trait appears early in many and is well defined in a sizeable majority by age 60. Such a tendency for self-protection appears to be a normal personality style of advancing years, but the age at which it commences varies considerably.

The most serious mood disturbance of advancing age is a tendency for depression. In some ways, depression should be expected in the elderly. For instance, many elderly must attempt to maintain their standard of living on an inadequate, fixed income in the face of increasing costs—an automatic pathway to failure. Immediate family members (particularly children) grow away, and most social companions tend to be elderly, have few new interests, tend to become ill, and eventually die. The spouse is often chronically ill, demanding considerable care before eventually dying; this produces a constricting demand, replaced by a major void in established life patterns. Such factors greatly curtail the social environment of an elderly individual. Ill health represents an additional problem for many (over half of individuals over age 65 have at least one major physical disability). Both exercise and diet are often inadequate, leading to decreased strength and a generally unhealthy state. Any or all of these factors should be sufficient to produce a significant degree of reactive depression. This is not the picture, however. Many elderly are amazingly resilient and combat their adversities with optimism. Severe depression in the elderly is a physical disturbance, an illness correctable by physical methods such as medication or electroconvulsive therapy. As noted in Chapter 9, depression and depressive dementia can produce significant alterations in mental capacity; milder degrees of depression may be a pertinent factor in the apparent mental impairment that has been called senility.

Physical Changes

In addition to the mental changes, a number of physical alterations occur with advancing age. For instance, hearing is diminished in most aged persons, and decreased ability to perceive high-frequency sounds begins at about age 50 in most individuals. The acoustic trauma of a lifetime has been suggested as the basis for this change (Weiss, 1959), but relative deafness is present in such a sizeable number of the elderly that others consider it a product of physiologic aging.

Vision is generally altered. Most elderly individuals show impaired accommodation for near objects, so-called presbyopia. Changes in distant vision also occur although they often start at a later age. The tendency for cataract formation increases with advancing age and, once begun, inexorably increases in density to produce significant visual problems. Corrective surgery for cataracts often leaves residual visual inadequacies. The elderly usually need greater illumination to see accurately. Impaired color vision is common, most often on the basis of lens opacities. Even ocular motility is slowed, and many elderly develop difficulty with upward gaze (Jenkyn and Reeves, 1981).

Changes in the motor system occur with advancing age. The gait becomes hesitant and slightly broad-based with somewhat shorter steps. Many of the characteristics of early Parkinson's disease such as stooped posture, diminished arm swing, and a tendency to make movements or turns en bloc are seen. Almost all individuals above age 75 demonstrate some abnormality of station and gait. Increased muscle tone produces a mild axial and/or appendicular rigidity and tendency for tremor (Jenkyn and Reeves, 1981). The latter is said to be overemphasized in that fewer than 2 percent of the elderly have a significant tremor (Larsen and Sjøgren, 1960). Some degree of hesitation and tremulousness (uncertainty) is present in many elderly persons, however.

Gait problems are often exaggerated by dizziness. Maintenance of awareness of position and movement in space demands accurate visual, vestibular, proprioceptive, tactile, and auditory perceptions. The slowing of both peripheral and central processing of all sensory modalities leads to a feeling of uncertainty. The elderly tend to walk closer to a wall, they appreciate being able to lean on the arm of someone else, and many use a stick to aid balance. Even when they do not complain of objective dizziness, many show unsteadiness of their movements (Drachman, 1979).

Another important problem for the elderly concerns altered sleep patterns. The most common complaint is of insomnia. Formal sleep studies suggest that the total time per night spent sleeping does not change or diminishes modestly with aging, but the elderly tend to awaken more frequently during the night, spend more time lying awake than do young adults, and show a decrease in the amount of stage 4 deep sleep (Feinberg, 1978). The use of sleep medications often complicates rather than corrects the naturally occurring change.

Individually or in combination, a number of physical difficulties seen more frequently in the elderly add to the actual physical disease states to produce the altered mental state called senility.

LABORATORY CHANGES IN SENILITY

Several laboratory studies reflect the functional changes that occur during normal aging. For instance, the EEG characteristically shows some slowing of the background rhythm. There is a shift of the average alpha frequency from 11 to 12 Hz in the young to 8 to 9 Hz in the aged. By age 65 some degree of slowing of alpha rhythms is present in more than half of otherwise healthy subjects (Drachman and Hughes, 1971), and slowing becomes more prevalent with advancing years. A similar degree of EEG slowing is present in the early stages of dementia of the Alzheimer type but, in later stages of this disorder, the slowing goes beyond the range of age-matched normal subjects. Visual, auditory, and somatosensory evoked responses in the elderly show an increased latency in the late components (Goodin et al, 1978), possibly reflecting the slowing of central processing.

X-ray CT scan and MRI clearly demonstrate alterations in the skull: brain ratio with advancing age. Mild enlargement of the ventricular system appears and increases steadily with with advancing age, concomitant with widening of the cortical sulci. The same changes are more prevalent and noteworthy in the demented population; in one study 60 percent of demented patients showed atrophy while only 15 percent of age-matched healthy controls showed the same degree of change (Huckman et al, 1975). There is far too much overlap, however, for DAT to be diagnosed merely from the presence of atrophy on the X-ray CT scan. MRI produces an even more confusing picture with advancing years. Over one-third of individuals over 65 years of age will show some areas of increased signal intensity in the deep white matter. While termed deep white-matter lesions (DWMLs), Binswanger's disease, leukoaraiosis and/or subcortical arteriosclerotic encephalopathy, these MRI findings often have no clinical correlates. That they represent subtle but meaningful brain changes appears possible.

POSTULATED CAUSES OF SENILITY

Many theories have been offered as to the cause of altered mental performance with advancing age; each remains speculative. Despite considerable evidence of ongoing mental alteration and some ability to correlate this change with physical, social, and biologic factors, none of the theories accounts for all observed changes.

One of the more obvious potential causes of changed function concerns bodily health. If over 50 percent of all individuals over age 65 suffer from at least one major health disturbance such as cardiac disease, pulmonary insufficiency, osteoporosis, and so on, all bodily functions can be expected to be detrimentally affected including those of the brain. In addition to these major dysfunctions, many lesser but nonetheless significant health problems occur in the elderly. For instance, decreased visual competency together with the similar deterioration in hearing increase the isolation of elderly persons, leading to slowed mentation and depression. Dizziness is common, and peripheral neuropathy and ataxia are other frequent disturbances that interfere with normal function. In addition, most elderly tend to be in poor general health. In part, this reflects normal wear and tear, the breakdown of muscle fibers, ligaments, and the like over the years, but some deterioration comes from decreased exercise, poor nutrition, lowered resistance to infectious diseases, slowed recovery from comparatively minor illnesses, and many related factors, all of which contribute to the apparent impairment of mental function in the elderly.

Health factors are aggravated by the many psychological problems already noted. Specifically, many elderly suffer depression. Both psychological and physical factors can act as the source of the depression that produces a neurophysiologic process that impairs both the general health and the mentation of the elderly.

A number of investigators now suggest that subcortical or frontal systems dysfunction (the two are often used interchangeably) is a paramount factor in the cognitive decline of aging (Albert and Kaplan, 1980; Hicks and Birren, 1970; Van Gorp and Mahler, 1990; Veroff, 1980). Most evidence for this conjecture is based on psychological test results and Goldberg (1986) has noted that diffusely spread brain damage first involves the frontal-executive tasks and the focal nature of neurobiologic changes in the elderly remains to be determined.

Regardless of the many factors known to alter mental activity, natural body changes appear crucial to this problem. In fact, the process of aging appears to begin in youth and continues inexorably. Sight and hearing are said to be at their zenith at about age 10 years, intellect at age 21, and motor strength and coordination reach their peaks at about age 25. Cerebral blood flow decreases by 20 percent between the ages of 30 and 75, and the brain weight actually decreases by 10 percent between these ages (Cohen, 1982). Certain brain cells age and disappear much faster than others; thus the cerebellum loses 40 percent of its cells between the fourth and the eighth decades, and Betz cells (the unique giant pyramidal cells of the primary motor cortex) become distorted and then disappear completely with advancing age (Scheibel, 1977).

Aging affects many cells, including those of the brain. In fact, observations from many different species suggest that genetic programming allows the individual cell only a limited life span (Hayflick, 1976). Thus the life span of a single species (for example, dog, rat) while somewhat variable among individuals of the species is relatively stable and quite different from that of another species (for example, man, turtle). Work with tissue culture has demonstrated a relatively consistent limit to the number of reproductions a cell will undergo before the cell line is discontinued (Hayflick, 1965). Whether this is also true of cells in the living human remains unknown, but experience with cell cultures suggests a temporal limitation for living tissues.

In addition to a genetic program for aging, other factors that may limit cell longevity have been suggested such as loss of an essential trophic factor

(Appel, 1981), death of neurons due to autoimmune reaction, and cellular response to chronic exposure to endogenous or exogenous toxins; it has even been suggested that certain viruses may specifically involve aging neurons. The possibility of an alteration (degeneration) of one or more neurotransmitter systems in a manner analogous to the disturbance of dopamine that produces parkinsonian motor dysfunction has also been postulated (McGeer and McGeer, 1976). Each consideration is speculative with little firm supporting evidence, but each is plausible, and one or several may be correct.

Despite many intriguing theories concerning the apparent inevitability of aging and death, no definite causes are known to underlie the alterations in mind and body that occur with advancing age. The changes can be described but the cause remains obscure. Most would agree on a combination of cellularly based (genetic) alterations leading to aging and death that can be hastened by a number of extrinsic factors. It is the physician's responsibility to identify and if possible correct as many of the latter as possible.

DIFFERENTIAL PROBLEMS

Mental alterations do occur in most individuals as they advance in age. The process called senility is different and must be separated from senile dementia of the Alzheimer type. The statement that senile dementia of the Alzheimer type represents a disease process and not a normal biologic alteration (Katzman and Karasu, 1975) is strongly supported. The clinical differences between senility and senile dementia are not negligible, and they carry a crucial difference in prognosis.

For the clinician, the most difficult differential problem is the separation of senility from early stages of dementia of the Alzheimer type in the elderly individual. The use of positive diagnostic criteria for DAT can be helpful, and serial evaluations over a period of months eventually identify individuals with DAT whose mentation progressively deteriorates although their physical state remains good. Differentiation of a subcortical problem that is producing a dementia state from normal mental slowing is far more difficult but even more rewarding. Many causes of subcortical dementia can be treated. At present, only careful clinical evaluation and a high degree of suspicion can provide the answer. Demonstration of a treatable, possibly even curable, cause of dementia makes this effort worthwhile.

TREATMENT OF SENILITY

Most successful treatments currently suggested for the mental impairment of advancing age are preventive. Maintenance of good health through good nutrition, healthy living, and considerable physical and mental activity are essential. Active individuals, particularly those who engage in physically vigorous activities such as racket sports, swimming, hiking, and so on, will lead a longer life and maintain better mentation (Rowe and Kahn, 1987). The tendency of the aging individual to eat less, and particularly to consume less healthful foods, can lead to a generalized deterioration in all functions including mentation; sustaining good nutrition is important for the aging individual. Depression is a treatable cause of cognitive impairment in the elderly (Chapter 9), and antidepressant therapy should be initiated if significant depression is detected.

Whether ongoing high-level mental activity (vigorous in the athletic sense) can help an individual maintain better levels of mental function with advancing age is more controversial. While many anecdotal demonstrations of the value of ongoing mental challenges are offered, convincing proof that mental exercising effectively slows mental aging remains to be presented. Animal experimentation does show that the more stimulating the environment, the greater the thickness of the cortical mantle (Diamond, 1978). Such demonstrations certainly suggest that increased mental activity could be a valuable antidote for some of the cognitive alterations of senility.

The possibility that some medication can be developed that would combat the effects of aging, including mental impairment, is eternally alluring. The fountain of youth remains a coveted dream. Many scientists are currently engaged in projects that will hopefully lead to pharmacologic agents or biologic programs allowing longer life, including maintenance of youthful bodily and mental functions. The possibility of a replacement neurotransmitter program for the aging nervous system based on the model of levodopa therapy for parkinsonism, is enticing. To date there is no evidence that such changes can be effected in the living human, but it is certainly possible that some day we will have a better understanding of senility and therefore a better chance for appropriate intervention.

12

Laboratory Aids in the Diagnosis of Dementia

Despite the necessity for and basic accuracy of clinical observations, it is almost always wise to perform some type of laboratory testing to confirm and help specify the etiology of a dementing process. The laboratory can be extremely valuable but is almost only used to confirm, not to diagnose the cause of dementia.

Many laboratory studies are used to study dementia, including many studies developed recently. Several laboratory techniques appeared to have value and were promoted strongly before serious weaknesses were found and they dwindled in popularity. No single technique completely dominates the diagnostic approach, but many have value for specified problems.

Dementia cannot be evaluated adequately by using a single dementia battery. Rather clinicians must select appropriate diagnostic techniques from the multitude of available tests based on the individual patient's problem. Unfortunately many physicians still rely on a preselected set of tests and, if no diagnostic result is forthcoming, discontinue the search for a specific diagnosis. This approach is seriously flawed. Physicians who conclude from negative results of a series of laboratory studies (for example, CT scan, EEG, B_{12}, thyroid and other blood studies) that patients must be suffering from an irreversible degenerative process are not only being lulled into a false interpretation but quite possibly are sentencing the patients to a lifetime of unnecessary mental impairment. While physicians who deal with dementia should be aware of available laboratory techniques, they must rely on their own clinical competence above that of the laboratory. Laboratory tests are easily misinterpreted and can lead to incorrect explanations of dementia. For example, an abnormal glucose tolerance curve in an elderly individual with mental impairment is significant and demands specific management but may have nothing to do with the dementing process. On the other hand, laboratory testing may provide significant findings that were not anticipated. Any lead that can help determine the cause of dementia is valuable. Many laboratory procedures can provide useful information in some cases; only a select group of primary tools will be presented here.

CLINICAL LABORATORY AND PATHOLOGIC STUDIES

The clinical laboratory may provide information that pinpoints a treatable, sometimes curable condition. This poses problems for the clinician, however. Almost all of the pertinent laboratory tests are disorder-specific, not general; with few exceptions, clinical laboratory studies are not good screening tools. The clinician must select the appropriate test based on diagnostic clues or educated curiosity that will confirm or discover the cause of the dementia. Unfortunately the number of causes and the corresponding number of laboratory tests is so vast that no clinician can truly master the field. To present even an outline of all these tests, an artificial subdivision must be made and only a limited overview can be provided. Table 12–1 gives the principal diagnostic tests and their roles in evaluation of dementia.

Blood and Serum Studies

Many blood tests are crucially important for the diagnosis of dementia. Patients being evaluated for mental impairment deserve a full battery of routine tests including complete blood count, differential count, red cell indices, erythrocyte sedimentation rate (ESR), and so on. Additional routine studies include electrolyte and blood chemistry tests. Electrolyte abnormalities such as low sodium (associated with inappropriate antidiuretic hormone syndrome), while they are uncommon, are of obvious diagnostic significance. More specific studies such as liver and renal function tests can be of diagnostic importance when organ failure is known or suspected. Serologic studies are also valuable. While neurosyphilis is now rare, its incidence is again on the rise, and it is a well known cause of progressive dementia. HIV antibody tests are positive in most individuals carrying the HIV virus and in all patients with HIV encephalopathy. Serum HIV testing should be pursued in any individual with appropriate risk factors (homosexual or bisexual behavior, repeated exposure to blood products) or in anyone who has laboratory or clinical findings suggestive of AIDS (see Chapter 6 for

TABLE 12–1. Laboratory tests in the diagnosis of dementia.

Dementing condition	Laboratory test
Pulmonary dysfunction	Arterial blood gases, pulmonary function tests, EEG
Cardiac conditions	EKG, chest X-ray, Holter monitor, echocardiography, cardiac angiography, EEG
Anemic anoxia	Hematocrit, hemoglobin, studies of red cell morphology, bone marrow studies, EEG
Renal failure	Blood urea nitrogen, serum creatinine, urinalysis, intravenous pyelography, renal biopsy, EEG
Hepatic encephalopathy	Serum ammonia, liver function tests, liver biopsy, EEG
Pancreatic encephalopathy	Serum amylase, blood sugar, EEG
Vitamin deficiencies	Serum B_{12} and folate levels; hematocrit and hemoglobin; red cell indices; bone marrow studies
Endocrinopathies	Thyroid function tests, serum cortisol levels, serum calcium and phosphorus
Systemic illnesses	
Inflammatory illnesses	Erythrocyte sedimentation rate, antinuclear factor, lupus erythematosus cell preparation, EEG, CT, angiography
CNS infections	White blood cell count; CSF cell count, protein, glucose, antibody levels; culture of CSF, blood urine, sputum; EEG; HIV serum antibody
CNS syphilis	Serum VDRL and FTS-ABS; CSF VDRL, cell count, gamma globulin
Toxic dementias	
Drug intoxication	Serum drug levels, EEG
Heavy metal intoxication	Serum and urine metal levels (hair or nail studies appropriate in some cases), EEG
Vascular dementia	EKG, chest X-ray, Holter monitor, echocardiography, cardiac angiography, carotid angiography, EEG, CT, technetium brain scan
Hydrocephalus	EEG, CT, isotope cisternography, (pneumoencephalography or ventriculography as indicated)
Intracranial tumor	EEG, CT, technetium brain scan, cerebral arteriography
Subdural hematoma	EEG, CT, technetium brain scan, arteriography
Depression	Dexamethasone suppression test, thyrotropin-releasing factor test
Wilson's disease	Serum copper and ceruloplasmin, 24-hour urinary copper excretion, CT, EEG
Adrenoleukodystrophy	Adrenal stimulation test, CT, EEG
Metachromatic leukodystrophy	Urinary arylsulfatase A assay, CT, EEG, nerve conduction studies
Multiple sclerosis	CSF gamma globulin, CSF cell count, CT, EEG, oligoclonal bands in CSF

additional details). Vitamin deficiencies, particularly of vitamin B_{12} and folate, can underlie dementia (Strachan and Henderson, 1965) and should be assayed if poor nutrition is suspected or if neuropathy, myelopathy, or anemia is present. Other tests to be used in selected instances would include hormonal assays, tests of endocrine function (particularly thyroid tests including TSH) or screening determinations for heavy metals. The typical heavy metal screen includes lead, mercury, and arsenic, but in selected cases, particularly those with a history of exposure to a specific metal, special assays may indicate the etiology of dementia. Tests of immunologic abnormality, tests for the inflammatory disorders (antinuclear antibody, lupus erythematosus cell preparations, and so forth), blood cultures, blood gas determinations, pH determination, and many other investigations may provide useful information in selected instances.

So many tests can be performed that no predetermined battery can possibly provide the correct information for all or even a majority of individuals with dementia. Thus intelligent selection by the clinician is crucial in using the laboratory for diagnostic purposes. The preceding chapters have suggested laboratory studies of particular value in specific disease states and Table 12–1 provides an overview of laboratory studies of significance for major categories of dementia-producing disorders.

Urinalysis

Routine urinalysis rarely provides diagnostic information concerning dementia, although renal disease as a cause of mental impairment can occur. Of more importance are assays of hormonal function and heavy metal excretion performed with 24-hour urine specimens. In selected cases (Wilson's disease, metachromatic leukodystrophy, metal intoxication), these tests may provide the definitive answer for the cause of a dementing illness.

Cerebrospinal Fluid (CSF) Tests

CSF dynamics and constituents may be of importance in the evaluation of dementia. The routine study of a CSF sample should include opening and closing pressures, the appearance of the fluid, the presence and number of both red and white blood cells, and chemical determinations of protein and glucose. If malignancy is suspected, sufficient fluid should be removed for cytology studies. Similarly, CSF can be studied for the presence of organisms by appropriate stains and additional fluid should be taken for culture when an infectious etiology is suspected. In some types of fungal disorder, careful study of CSF provides one of the few positive diagnostic clues. Levels of immunoglobulin may provide specific information in some inflammatory and demyelinating disorders.

A number of special tests of CSF pressure dynamics have been discussed in Chapter 8. While they are potentially useful, many causes of false negative and false positive results continue to plague their interpretation (Benson, 1985).

Tissue Samples

In some instances study of tissue samples may provide diagnostic information. For instance, excessive arsenic may be demonstrated by chemical assay of hair samples. Leprosy, amyloidosis, and some of the vasculitides may be diagnosed from samples of peripheral nerve or study of small blood vessels. Skin tests for fungi and other pathogens may provide critical information. In each instance, choice of the specific test is dependent on the clinician's recognition that an uncommon disorder may be the cause of the dementia. One method of tissue sampling, brain biopsy, deserves separate consideration.

Brain Biopsy

Relatively few morbid pathologic studies have proved valuable for the diagnosis of dementia in the living patient. Samples of brain tissue have been taken for biopsy, but the value of this procedure for the diagnosis of dementia remains at best controversial (Parr, 1955). The presence of an Alzheimer plaque in cortical biopsy material was at one time accepted as a positive marker of the presence of DAT (Sim et al, 1966), and brain biopsy was performed with fair frequency. The occurrence of both false positive and false negative results was discouraging, and few now recommend this test to diagnose DAT (Glen and Christie, 1979). More recent studies suggest that some valuable information may be derived through study of enzyme activity in biopsy material (Bowen et al, 1982). Great caution must be taken in correlating data from these specialized studies with a specific dementia diagnosis, however, and at present there appear to be few indications for brain biopsy in the diagnostic work-up of dementia.

Biopsy of cortical tissue remains an enticing possibility, however, particularly for the diagnosis of disorders such as DAT or Pick's disease that preferentially involve cortical tissue or infections or vascular inflammatory disorders centered in the meninges. Improved laboratory techniques may eventually provide a process through which small pieces of cortical or meningeal tissue will yield diagnostically important information.

Autopsy

The definitive determination of the cause of dementia has traditionally rested with the autopsy, results of which provide important, sometimes essential, information. Even autopsy material, however, is not without problems of interpretation. Alzheimer neuropathologic changes are present in the brains of most older people (Tomlinson, 1977), and the mere presence of neuritic plaques, neurofibrillary tangles, or even granulovacuolar degeneration is no longer considered diagnostic (Ball et al, 1988; Khachaturian, 1985). Only when the quantity of these tissue abnormalities is exceptionally high can they be considered diagnostic; good quantitative studies are almost prohibitively difficult and are rarely performed. Like all laboratory tests, autopsy is most valuable when correlated with the clinical evaluation. No matter what the quantity of Alzheimer neuropathologic changes present at postmortem, if the individual was not demented in life DAT is not a likely diagnosis. Dependent upon the number of plaques and tangles demanded, many neuropathologic specimens are compatible with a diagnosis of DAT but the diagnosis can be made only if correlated with an appropriate clinical picture (McKhann et al, 1984).

One problem hindering the current pathologic investigations of dementia is the diminishing availability of postmortem studies. Autopsy rates have decreased while the number of elderly has greatly increased; a large number (probably a majority) of demented patients die in nursing homes, and pathologic determinations helpful for understanding the dementia are not performed. Even when demented subjects come to postmortem, the study is most often performed by a local pathologist who lacks the training and facilities necessary to carry out a definitive determination of the cause of the dementia. Incorrect autopsy diagnoses of the cause of dementia (most often DAT based on the presence of a few plaques and/or tangles) complicates the current diagnostic difficulty (Wisniewski et al, 1989). With the many specialized studies of autopsy material now available (such as transfer to animals of the causative virus, biochemical and tissue enzyme determinations, electron microscopic studies, and so on), it can be anticipated that future autopsy studies will provide information for more intelligent determinations of the causes of dementia.

In summary, the clinical laboratory often demonstrates a specific cause of dementia but the results are almost always dependent on the clinician's selection of the appropriate test. No single battery will adequately cover the many possible causes. Nonetheless some laboratory studies are abnormal with sufficient frequency that their use is warranted in the diagnostic work-up of all patients with dementia.

RADIOLOGIC EXAMINATIONS

Routine X-rays of Chest, Skull, and Spine

In most instances, routine X-ray studies of the skull, cervical spine, chest, and so on do not provide useful information in the differential diagnosis of dementia. There are exceptions, however, that deserve consideration.

On rare occasions, X-rays of the skull may provide a diagnostic clue. For instance, the multiple osteolytic areas of Paget's disease of the skull may be the first indication of the condition. Most often, however, many other symptoms are present, and the diagnosis is made without the films. Similarly, plain skull films indicating bony metastases or bone changes indicative of a meningioma may prove diagnostic. Evidence of an old skull fracture, either a linear fracture of the convexity or a basilar skull fracture, may be of significance. In some instances, particularly in youngsters with chronic increased intracranial pressure, a characteristic mottling of the inner surface of the skull, the so-called beaten-silver appearance, may be noted. Inasmuch as this bony abnormality may remain for many years, its presence on the plain film suggests abnormally increased intracranial pressure during development, a possible factor in the mental impairment of later life.

The most common clue from a plain film of the skull in a patient with dementia is abnormality of the sella turcica. Bony erosion of the clinoid processes or enlargement of the sella suggests intrasellar or suprasellar pathology, often associated with hormonal alterations or ventricular outflow problems, both capable of causing dementia. The empty-sella syndrome, while often demanding broader radiologic investigation or actual surgical intervention for diagnostic confirmation, may be associated with progressive mental impairment (Kaufman et al, 1973). Similarly tumors in the perisellar area such as clivus chordoma, meningioma, and the like are routinely slow growing, produce few focal findings, are known to present as a progressive dementia, and may be suspected from bony alterations in the region of the sella.

While X-rays of the cervical spine rarely indicate the specific cause of dementia, they deserve comment. One important abnormality that can be demonstrated is basilar impression (Spillane, 1960). Alterations in the junction of the upper cervical spine and skull may jam cerebral tissues into the cisterna magna, producing altered CSF circulation and subsequent dementia (Chapter 8). Less common abnormalities such as the Klippel-Feil and Arnold-Chiari syndromes (Spillane, 1960) may be the source of mental impairment and have suggestive radiographic abnormalities.

X-rays of the nasal sinuses may produce information not readily available through other tests. Chronic infectious disorders and low-grade malignancies including granulomas frequently begin in the nasal pharynx or sinus passages and can produce vague neurologic symptomatology including mental impairment.

None of the above abnormalities is common and, in general, plain films are not of diagnostic value in the evaluation of dementia; they are, however, simple, safe procedures and may prove valuable in selected cases of mental impairment.

X-ray Computed Tomography (CT)

X-ray CT of the brain has become a major tool in neurologic diagnosis, largely replacing plain films of the skull, and occupies an important place in the laboratory evaluation of dementia. At present, almost every individual who presents with acquired mental impairment deserves some form of brain image study. Like plain X-rays, X-ray CT is simple and comparatively safe, and with the more technically advanced equipment now available, sophisticated evaluations can be obtained (Oldendorf, 1980). While they are expensive, when the cost of laboratory tests no longer necessary are considered, they are actually cost efficient (Baker et al, 1974). There are two areas in which X-ray CT is particularly valuable for the study of dementia: the presence of focal abnormalities and the presence of generalized structural changes affecting the ventricular system or cerebral mantle. These are discussed separately.

In evaluation of dementia, the X-ray CT scan achieves its greatest success demonstrating underlying focal disorders. Many of these have been discussed in earlier chapters and need only be listed here. The presence of intracranial mass lesions such as primary neoplasm (glioblastoma, astrocytoma, ependymoma, oligodendroglioma, and the like) and primary extracerebral tumors such as meningioma, chordoma, craniopharyngioma, and so on is usually demonstrated readily by X-ray CT, as are most metastatic tumors to the brain. While it is not absolute, differentiation of metastatic from primary intracranial tumors is often suggested by X-ray CT appearance. Other nonmalignant intracranial space-occupying lesions such as abscesses and calcific lesions (for example, cysticercosis) can be demonstrated and diagnosed by this procedure. Most tumors are demonstrated to best advantage after intravenous administration of radiopaque dye. The contrast agent makes vascularized lesions more apparent and demonstrates blood-brain barrier disruption. Contrast enhancement improves the diagnostic yield of the scan in all but degenerative and static (old stroke, old trauma) conditions.

One valuable use of X-ray CT is demonstration of blood collections within the cranium. Both intracerebral hematomas and the various extracerebral blood collections such as subdural and epidural hematomas can usually be defined precisely. Establishing the presence of a hematoma in an individual with impaired mental capability can be valuable; the problem is often treatable. Bilateral isodense hematomas may produce a hypernormal

CT image (small ventricles, obliteration of cerebral sulci) (Jacobson and Farmer, 1979) and are capable of causing serious mental impairment.

X-ray CT can demonstrate vascular infarctions if several considerations are carefully observed. First the procedure often fails to demonstrate altered cerebral density for a few days following infarction. The tissues remain isodense initially, and it may be 10 days or more before sufficient alteration results to allow demonstration of the infarction. This deficiency can be overcome with use of contrast enhancement (Ambrose, 1973), but even this may sometimes fail (Oldendorf, 1980). Best results are obtained several (usually three or more) weeks after infarction when a distinct alteration in tissue density accurately demarcates the area of destroyed cerebral tissue. A second consideration concerns the size of the infarction. Occlusion of a major vessel with destruction of a considerable area of tissue can be demonstrated routinely, but smaller infarctions (lacunes) such as those that may occur with hypertension or embolic disease (Chapter 5) are often too small to be visualized. In general, the cerebral lesion must be a half-centimeter or greater in size to be noted with most currently available equipment. Inasmuch as the quality of many X-ray CT machines in use is less than optimal, many of the small lacunes that underlie cases of vascular dementia are not visualized. Absence of scan evidence of infarction cannot be equated with absence of significant cerebrovascular disease.

Several generalized alterations demonstrated by X-ray CT are of clinical significance. Cerebral edema is often evident at least if it is severe. A diagnosis of pseudotumor cerebri can often be confirmed based on the widespread edema and decreased ventricular size in the presence of increased intracranial pressure. Hydrocephalus is often clearly demonstrated by X-ray CT although cautious interpretation of the pattern of ventricular enlargement is necessary to distinguish among its various causes and degrees (Chapter 8). When the hydrocephalus is associated with increased sulcal markings, the scan is often interpreted as showing cerebral atrophy (Gado, 1981; Naeser et al, 1982). In most cases of obstructive hydrocephalus, the degree of ventricular dilatation is out of proportion to the size of the cerebral sulci, and the frontal and temporal horns are more dilated than are the posterior aspects of the ventricular system (Jacobs and Kinkel, 1976). Unfortunately both false negative and false positive interpretations occur even when strict criteria are applied, and isotope cisternography (discussed below) is often indicated to help determine the cause of ventricular enlargement. In addition to obstructive hydrocephalus, enlarged ventricles may be present in metabolic alterations, particularly in chronic alcoholism, in a variety of progressive dementia conditions and in normal aging (Gumasekera and Richardson, 1977). Both the presence and the underlying cause of hydrocephalus may be difficult to determine from X-ray CT, but the procedure is safe and easily performed and offers excellent information in the initial work-up for hydrocephalus.

The more generalized changes that can occur in the brain in some types of dementia are far more difficult to interpret from X-ray CT and have been overinterpreted in the past. The original tendency to diagnose "cerebral atrophy" on the basis of X-ray CT appearance is being corrected; widening of sulci and ventricular dilatation on X-ray CT cannot be equated with dementia (Gado, 1981; Naeser et al, 1980).

In the degenerative dementias, uncertainty about the value of X-ray CT remains. In Pick's disease, considerable atrophy may be present in the anterior portion of the frontal or temporal lobes bilaterally (Cummings and Duchen, 1981). When it is associated with the appropriate clinical picture (Chapter 3), a diagnosis of Pick's disease or frontal lobe degeneration is probable. Atrophy of anterior temporal lobe is not an early finding, however, and in some well-established cases it may not be present.

DAT has proved difficult to characterize by X-ray CT. The enlarged ventricles and increased sulcal markings seen on X-ray CT are similar to findings demonstrated by pneumoencephalography in DAT. Many patients with these findings on CT examination do not have the clinical findings of DAT, however, and a euphemism, "cerebral atrophy," is commonly used in the readings. This usage appears questionable since metabolic changes as well as normal aging can produce the appearance of atrophy (ventricular dilatation and enlarged sulcal markings) without detectable structural abnormalities. Numerous reports (Ceade et al, 1976; Gawler et al, 1976; Hachinski et al, 1975; Roberts et al, 1976) indicate that definite changes of ventricular and sulcal markings occur in patients with DAT and that these abnormalities increase as the disease progresses. The reciprocal statement, that individuals with increasing dilatation of ventricles and sulci on X-ray CT must have DAT, appears incorrect. Gado (1981), Naeser and colleagues (1982), and others have demonstrated that the alterations in both the ventricular size and sulcal markings of DAT are not significantly different from those of advancing age. Naeser and co-workers (1980) suggest that white-matter density decreases in DAT, but this has not proved reliable for differential diagnosis. There is no single alteration of the X-ray CT diagnostic of DAT. Figure 12–1 graphically illustrates the problem. The individual in Figure 12–1A was referred to the hospital because of the marked alterations on X-ray CT, and a diagnosis of Pick's disease had been suggested by the referring neurologist. Clinical evaluation showed no dementia (IQ was 137 at the time the scan was done), but a history of alcohol abuse was obtained. In contrast, the individual in Figure 12–1B had a well-advanced DAT on clinical examination, but X-ray CT of this individual was interpreted as within normal limits for his age.

In summary despite some limitations, the X-ray CT scan remains the single most widely useful laboratory test currently available in the evaluation of dementia, but overinterpretation must be avoided. Most specifically, DAT can neither be diagnosed nor excluded from the appearance of the scan alone; appropriate clinical findings must be the determining factor.

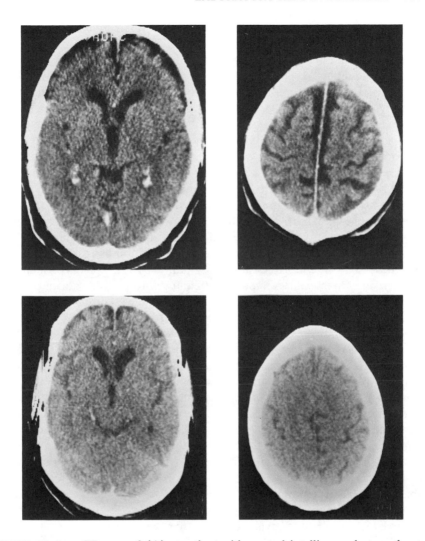

FIGURE 12–1.   CT scan of (A) a patient with normal intelligence but moderate ventricular enlargement and marked widening of sulci suggestive of "cerebral atrophy" and (B) a patient with advanced DAT and normal CT scan. (Reprinted by permission of the publisher from Benson DF, Treatable dementias, in Benson and Blumer, Psychiatric aspects of neurologic disease, vol. 2. New York: Grune & Stratton, 1982b.)

Magnetic Resonance Imaging (MRI)

Although it does not use radiation, the technique of brain imaging by use of magnetic fields (MRI) is most often conducted in radiology departments, and the scans are interpreted by radiologists. The ultrahigh-intensity magnetism temporarily alters polarity of selected cellular elements; appropriate measurements and interpretations of the electrical currents produced by the return of these elements to normal polarity can be converted into a visual display (Oldendorf, 1980). Like CT, MRI produces a tomographic image of the brain. Dependent upon the timing of the relaxation phase, fluids, particularly water, will be visualized as black or white in contrast to the intermediate tones of brain structures, yielding a sharply resolved image. MRI is expensive and not yet widely available but has already proved superior to any other brain imaging method because of better resolution and greater sensitivity to white-matter pathology.

MR scans are valuable in the evaluation of dementia, particularly in their ability to delineate mass lesions, hydrocephalus, hematomas, and cerebral infarctions—both old and recent. In these tasks, MRI is as good as, or superior to, CT scanning. MRI does not show intracranial calcification as well and is not as sensitive to subarachnoid blood as is CT.

Intriguing in the evaluation of dementia is the presence of MRI hyperintensities, particularly in periventricular white matter. Variously termed white-matter hyperintensities (WMH), Binswanger's disease, white-matter lesions or abnormalities, or just unidentified bright objects (UBOs), MRI white-matter changes are common in the elderly. They have been reported in as many as 30 percent of normal elderly (Bradley et al, 1984) and up to 80 percent or more of stroke patients (Dewitt et al, 1984). Attempts to correlate WMH with dementia produce mixed results (Hunt et al, 1989; Kertesz et al, 1990). Most vascular dementia cases show white matter lesions of some type, but they are also seen to a limited extent in DAT patients (Brun and England, 1986; Rezek et al, 1987). Neither the source nor the significance of white-matter lesions is settled.

The limitations of diagnostic competency outlined for X-ray CT scanning are also true for MRI. While atrophy can be interpreted, specific labeling of various degenerative dementias is usually not possible. Like all laboratory studies, MRI is most valuable to support or confirm a clinical diagnosis. As such, it is a valuable resource.

Pneumoencephalography and Ventriculography

For many years, studies of the ventricular system using air as a contrast material ranked among the most important of diagnostic tools for dementia. With the advent of the X-ray CT, this use of ventriculography and pneumoencephalography has almost disappeared, being reserved only for specialized cases. Air studies can offer information of value; they can outline mass lesions and demonstrate hydrocephalus. Delineation of the ventricular boundaries and cerebral structures surrounding the ventricles is considerably sharper with air studies than it is with X-ray CT. In selected cases of normal-pressure hydrocephalus and cerebral cysts (Chapter 8), air studies provide specific findings that, if not absolutely diagnostic, are strongly suggestive of underlying etiology. Because of consistent morbidity (headache) and occasional mortality, air studies are indicated only when less dangerous procedures fail to provide definite answers.

Angiography

Angiographic studies are rarely indicated in the evaluation of an individual with dementia. They can offer valuable information, however, particularly in the study of cerebral circulation and are still used in selected cases. Angiography remains the best technique to locate vascular lesions, both vascular abnormalities (hemangioma, aneurysm, and so on) and the occlusions that produce infarction. In selected cases, angiography may help define a cerebral vasculitis (Chapter 5). Again as with air studies, angiography has a definite morbidity and is to be considered in the evaluation of dementia only in special circumstances.

ELECTROPHYSIOLOGIC STUDIES

The electroencephalogram (EEG) has been recognized as a tool for the diagnosis of acute confusional states (delirium) (Strub and Black, 1981), but many consider it of limited usefulness in the diagnosis of dementia. Harner (1975) and others (Wilson et al, 1977) have demonstrated that the electroencephalogram offers useful information in the diagnosis of dementia and a modification of electroencephalography using stimulus-evoked and event-related responses has proved useful in the study of dementia.

Electroencephalography (EEG)

Although EEG is a well-established and widely practiced diagnostic process, its usefulness in dementia has always been questionable. The test is of greatest value in the demonstration of epilepsy and has become recognized as an important means of indicating neurophysiologic changes of delirium and other acute confusional processes. Early reports of EEG in patients with dementia suggested severe abnormality with widespread, irregular slow-wave activity (Letemendia and Pampiglione 1958; Liddell, 1958). Most of these early studies emanated from institutions for the mentally disabled and reported only patients with severe, end-stage disease. Earlier in the course of dementia such gross alterations of cortical electrical activity are not consistently demonstrable (Sim, 1979). Some demented patients do have severely disordered EEG patterns, but others, even those with striking dementia, show only mild degrees of slowing. The degree of abnormality is not consistently correlated with the severity of mental deterioration, and the test was considered unreliable for differential diagnosis in dementia (Glen and Christie, 1979). Harner (1975) correlated the varieties of EEG abnormality with the underlying cerebral disorder causing the dementia and demonstrated that the procedure had considerable value in the diagnostic work-up. Three findings have diagnostic significance for dementia: (1) normal EEG in the face of severe dementia, (2) very abnormal EEG in the face of mild dementia, and (3) seizure activity. The abnormal EEG with diffuse changes in an individual with severe dementia is not so helpful. The first of the three findings has produced most consternation and disagreement concerning the test's usefulness in dementia. As noted, most early reports of EEG in DAT and other advanced dementias indicated striking abnormality whereas more recent studies often report little or no abnormality in the early stages. Slowing of the EEG does not appear to reflect the severity of mental abnormality until the late stages of disease when a marked disturbance of cerebral function correlates with wide-spread EEG abnormality. This can be a valuable diagnostic clue. A patient with a marked degree of dementia who shows only minimal slowing—in other words, one whose EEG appears considerably closer to normal than the mental state—is a likely candidate for diagnosis of one of the progressive degenerative dementias such as DAT or Pick's disease. Exceptions to this rule exist, however, and demand careful attention. For instance, depression (and depressive dementia) produce little effect on the EEG, a state that is not concordant with the severe abnormality of mental function noted clinically. The practitioner must depend also on clinical and laboratory information. Nonetheless, if the history, physical examination, and mental status findings are suggestive of the early stages of a dementia of the Alzheimer's or Pick's type, a normal or near-normal EEG can act as supportive evidence.

In contrast, many disorders that produce dementia also cause severe alterations of the EEG pattern. Some are classic, with almost pathognomonic patterns. In Jakob-Creutzfeldt disease (Chapter 6), paroxysmal sharp waves on a slow background are usually accepted as confirmation of the diagnosis if the clinical picture is appropriate (Fisher, 1969; Goto et al, 1976). Some heavy metal poisonings, hepatic encephalopathy, and subacute encephalitides produce triphasic waves typically in a less paroxysmal manner than are the sharp waves of Jakob-Creutzfeldt disease (Lesse et al, 1958; May, 1968). The presence of triphasic waves in the EEG of a patient with dementia indicates one of only a few disorders; in most instances, the history and/or physical examination provide the information necessary.

Even more distinctive are the focal slow waves seen with intracranial masses such as tumors, hematomas, abscesses, and the like (Fischer-Williams et al, 1962; Friedman and Odom, 1972). The presence of focal slowing of the EEG in a patient with a clinical picture of dementia is a strong indication of a treatable condition and a thorough diagnostic effort is indicated.

The most common EEG abnormality in individuals with dementia is diffuse slow-wave activity. This may be pronounced, with slow waves of 2 to 3 Hz in all leads. While most characteristic of acute delirium, slow-wave activity also characterizes chronic confusional disorders with dementia, including metabolic disorders, nutritional disorders, intoxications, and so on. While not diagnostic, the presence of widespread slow-wave activity in an EEG of a patient with acquired mental impairment should suggest the possibility of a metabolic or toxic factor; appropriate investigation may demonstrate the culprit and lead to appropriate treatment. The most common cause of slow-wave activity in a demented patient is an iatrogenic pharmacologic poisoning that can produce both seriously impaired mental capacity and a significant slowing of the EEG pattern. Barbiturates, phenothiazines, opiates, anticonvulsants, and many other drugs used in excess can produce such a change.

A more common finding is a lesser degree of EEG slow activity. With a theta rhythm frequency between 4 and 7 Hz, a multitude of abnormalities must be considered. Even so, this pattern in a patient with dementia suggests certain broad outlines for diagnostic work-up. For instance if the dementia is longstanding and severe with the clinical features of DAT, this pattern could be anticipated. On the other hand if the dementia is of comparatively recent onset or less severe, an extrinsic factor (metabolic, toxic, inflammatory, or systemic) is probably present and must be sought. Many patients with a generalized slow EEG pattern have correctable disorders.

The presence and characteristics of EEG abnormality in hydrocephalus are debated. Some studies of normal-pressure hydrocephalus suggest that there is no consistent abnormality of the EEG (Brown and Goldensohn, 1973); others suggest that a specific abnormality is seen (Jacobs et al, 1976). The difference of opinion may reflect the etiologic process associated with the hydrocephalus. DAT can produce sizeable ventricular dilatation in individuals with a near-normal EEG pattern, and it seems probable that some studies have intermixed DAT patients with other cases of hydrocephalus. A considerable improvement in the EEG pattern following shunting of normal-pressure hydrocephalus has been suggested (Benson, 1974) but has not been reported consistently. In general, obstructive hydrocephalus, whether communicating or noncommunicating, will be associated with an abnormal EEG pattern; in contrast, hydrocephalus ex vacuo will more often be associated with a normal or only mildly slowed pattern.

Finally, the presence of spike or sharp-wave activity suggestive of seizure may be of considerable importance in the evaluation of a patient with dementia. The presence of a seizure disorder, particularly an occult seizure problem, may be overlooked, and a seizure disorder producing a decrease in mental capacity is treatable. More common, however, epileptogenic focus is based on focal cerebral abnormality (trauma, tumor, or infarction), again an important finding with treatment implications.

In general, the investigation of dementia should include a screening EEG. For interpretation, a simple basic rule suggests that, if the mental state looks worse than the EEG (an admittedly unwieldy comparison), the patient is likely to have a degenerative dementing disorder or a depressive dementia. On the other hand if the EEG pattern looks worse than the patient's mental state, some other cause is probable, quite possibly a treatable disorder. While it is often not diagnostic, the EEG may provide helpful leads toward the diagnosis of dementia.

Refinements in EEG techniques and analysis may be useful in the identification and differential diagnosis of dementia syndromes and the application of EEG studies to dementia patients. EEG data obtained from scalp electrodes can be subjected to spectral analysis and used to create topographic maps of brain electrical activity, typically portraying the spatial distribution of delta, theta, alpha, and beta activity. Differences in the quantity and distribution of slow-wave activity have been demonstrated between dementia and normal aging and between dementia and depression (Brenner et al, 1986; Duffy et al, 1984). Preliminary differences in synchronization of EEG activity from different brain regions have been shown between DAT and vascular dementia (Leuchter et al, 1987). The information available from brain mapping is the same as that from routine EEG tracings; no superiority of brain mapping technique over conventional EEG techniques has been demonstrated.

Evoked Response Studies

Stimulus-evoked and event-related responses have been widely used in the study of brain activity. Simple somesthetic, visual, or auditory stimuli are repetitively presented while EEG tracings with specifically located leads are performed. Through computerized analysis, the background EEG activity can be subtracted, leaving a pattern reflecting cerebral responses to the stimuli. Evoked response studies have value in demonstrating abnormalities in the peripheral nervous system (Allison et al, 1978; Desmedt and Noel, 1973) and brainstem (Chiappa, 1980; Starr and Achor, 1975). With the use of more complex stimuli and advanced computer analysis techniques, alterations referable to cortical activity can be demonstrated (Gevins et al, 1981), and some investigators have suggested that appropriate evoked response studies can be useful in the diagnosis of dementia (Goodin et al, 1978). Original reports suggested a delay of late evoked responses (P300) in dementia, but did not separate varieties of dementia. Attempts to replicate and refine these studies produced conflicting results (Drake et al, 1982; Laurian et al, 1982; Hendrickson et al, 1979; Syndulko et al, 1982). Evoked potential information can also be mapped topographically onto brain templates similar to the brain activity mapping of spectral EEG data (Duffy, 1979; Gevins et al, 1981). The utility of these studies in dementia evaluation is under study. Sensory evoked response testing, particularly responses correlating with higher cortical functions, may be useful in the future, but routine EEG readings remain more accurate and easier to interpret (Visser et al, 1985).

NUCLEAR MEDICINE INVESTIGATIONS

A variety of nuclear medicine techniques have been developed for intracranial testing; some of these have proved useful for dementia evaluation.

Isotope Cisternography

Following the pioneering work of DiChiro and co-workers (1964), a technique for demonstrating CSF circulation by use of radioactive materials came into general use. This procedure, now called isotope cisternography, remains available in most nuclear medicine laboratories but is not widely used. The technique is comparatively simple but the different flow patterns require knowledgeable interpretation (Table 12–2). Radioactive material is injected into the CSF by means of a lumbar puncture. The isotope rapidly diffuses through the CSF but, because of the one-way flow from the ventricles, rarely enters the ventricular system; if there is hydrocephalus, however, the isotope will enter and outline the ventricular system (ventricular reflux). The radioactive material circulates as the CSF circulates, collecting in the sagittal sinus region in about 24 hours, where it is absorbed and largely disappears within 48 to 72 hours.

In the presence of hydrocephalus ex vacuo (for example, DAT) the CSF circulation is slow; isotope refluxes into the ventricles and only slowly circulates to the parasagittal region. Scans taken in the first 24 hours show concentration of isotope in the ventricles with little midline sagittal activity; later scans (particularly 48 to 72 hours after injection) reveal that most of the radioactivity is concentrated in the sagittal area.

When there is obstruction to CSF flow, several different patterns can occur. If the ventricular outflow channels are obstructed, all isotope will flow over the cerebral convexities and be reabsorbed in a normal manner. The isotope cisternogram will appear normal despite evidence of enlarged ventricles on X-ray CT or MRI. If the obstruction is over the convexities, however, the isotope will reflux into the ventricles and remain there for the life of the radioactive substance (see Chapter 8 for additional descriptions of isotope cisternography in normal-pressure hydrocephalus). Isotope cis-

TABLE 12–2.   CT findings and results of isotope cisternography in dementing disorders.

Condition	CT findings	Cisternography
Normal	Normal sulci and ventricles	Tracer ascends in cisterns and is absorbed over cerebral convexities without ventricular reflux
Hydrocephalus ex vacuo (DAT, Pick's disease, vascular dementia, and so on)	Enlarged ventricles and dilated cerebral sulci	Tracer ascends in cisterns, refluxes into ventricles, then is absorbed over cerebral convexities
Communicating obstructive hydrocephalus (normal-pressure hydrocephalus)	Enlarged ventricles, normal cerebral sulci	Tracer ascends in cisterns, refluxes into ventricles; there is no absorption over the cerebral convexities
Noncommunicating obstructive hydrocephalus (aqueductal stenosis, midbrain tumors, and so on)	Enlarged ventricles, normal cerebral sulci	Tracer ascends in cisterns and is absorbed over cerebral convexities without ventricular reflux (normal flow pattern despite enlarged ventricles)

ternography can clearly demonstrate NPH (Benson et al, 1970), but both false positive and false negative results occur and the procedure is infrequently used. In combination with X-ray CT or MRI, it remains a valuable tool, however, offering information on the dynamic activity of CSF circulation that is not available from static imaging studies.

Single Photon Emission Computed Tomography (SPECT)

SPECT has become a widely used diagnostic tool in the evaluation of dementia in the past few years. The technique uses relatively stable, inexpensive isotopes and can be performed in most nuclear medicine laboratories; the major deficiency of the procedure is limited spatial resolution. Relative values for cortical areas can be obtained, and the technique has proved useful in dementia evaluation (Gemell et al, 1984; Jagust et al, 1987).

While a number of different isotopes have been reported and the scanning equipment varies considerably, all techniques tend to show decreased cerebral blood flow in the temporal-parietal area in DAT (Mueller et al, 1986; Sharp et al, 1986). Frontal hypoperfusion has been demonstrated in frontal lobe degenerative disorder (Chapter 3) (Giombetti et al, 1989) and in progressive supranuclear palsy (Terta et al, 1988). Dementia based on multiple infarctions, Huntington's disease, and alcoholic encephalopathy present different SPECT patterns (Jagust et al, 1987; Sharp et al, 1986; Smith, et al, 1988) but are not sufficiently distinctive to be diagnostic. Posterior cortex hypoperfusion has been reported in posterior cortical atrophy (Benson et al, 1988), and focal left cortical hypoperfusion has been seen in cases of progressive aphasia (Kempler et al, 1990). False positive results, particularly bilateral temporal-parietal hypoperfusion, are not infrequent, however; at best, SPECT can be used as a confirmatory finding, not as a standard for diagnosis.

Because of its easy availability, safety, and relatively modest cost, SPECT will remain a popular diagnostic technique in dementia evaluation. Future improvements in radiopharmaceuticals and scanning equipment should enhance its diagnostic potential but relatively poor resolution will continue to limit the value of SPECT.

Positron Emission Tomography (PET)

A second, more sophisticated radioisotope diagnostic tool, PET (Kuhl et al, 1973; Phelps et al, 1979), has been used for assessment of dementia in the past few years. Radioactive materials are tagged to selected chemicals and, following intravenous injection, counts of radioactivity can be performed and reconstructed as tomographic slices. The most useful isotopes produce positrons (Phelps, 1977) but, unfortunately, production of positron-emitting ions demands use of a cyclotron so that only a limited number of centers currently perform this procedure. Most studies still use either oxygen 15 (for cerebral blood flow and oxygen utilization) or fluorine 18–labeled deoxyglucose (metabolism of glucose) (Frackowiak et al, 1981; Phelps et al, 1979). Early studies demonstrated abnormal metabolism in vascular disease (Kuhl et al, 1980b), tumor, epilepsy (Kuhl et al, 1980a) and dementia (Benson et al, 1983; Ferris et al, 1980; Frackowiak et al, 1981). Both isotopes demonstrate decreased use of these basic metabolites in individuals with dementia when compared to age-matched healthy subjects. Studies by Frackowiak and colleagues (1981) and Benson and associates (1983) demonstrated pattern differences of abnormal metabolism between individuals with DAT or Pick's disease and those with other causes of dementia such as normal-pressure hydrocephalus, vascular dementia, and Huntington's disease. A considerable decrease of glucose or oxygen metabolism was noted in the association cortex of patients with DAT or Pick's disease, whereas cortical metabolic rates were close to normal in many other types of dementing diseases. For instance, in Huntington's disease, despite the presence of considerable dementia, cortical glucose metabolic rates appeared within the range of normal controls, whereas there was a severe decrease in glucose metabolism in the area of the caudate nucleus (Kuhl et al, 1982).

Following the early reports that established the use of PET metabolic and blood-flow studies as valuable diagnostic aids in dementia assessment, many laboratories replicated the findings (Duara et al, 1986; Foster et al, 1983; Friedland et al, 1983). DAT, the most thoroughly studied condition, is characterized by bilateral temporal-parietal hypometabolism/hypoperfusion in the early stages with bifrontal decreases appearing in the later stages. Considerable variation is reported, particularly lateral asymmetry (Foster et al, 1983; Koss et al, 1985). Vascular dementia tends to show a variable PET picture with irregularly scattered areas of cortical and subcortical hypometabolism (Kuhl et al, 1983). A number of other dementia-producing conditions are also said to present distinctive PET metabolism pictures. Normal-pressure hydrocephalus (Jagust et al, 1985), Pick's disease (Friedland et al, 1986), Huntington's disease (Kuhl et al, 1982), Wilson's disease (Hawkins et al, 1983), Jakob-Creutzfeldt disease (Friedland et al, 1986; Horowitz et al, 1982), posterior cortical atrophy (Benson et al, 1988), and progressive aphasia (Kempler et al, 1990) have distinguishing features on PET studies. Others, particularly Parkinsonian dementia, the dementia of depression, and the many systemic disorders that produce mental impairment, do not have diagnostic characteristics on PET study. Just as with SPECT, the results of PET scanning are not sufficiently robust to provide a positive diagnosis from the laboratory study alone, but they do offer substantial confirmatory data.

To date, most published studies of PET abnormalities in DAT have studied metabolism or cerebral blood flow of the brain in a quiet, restful state. It appears probable that more information could be gained by investigating brain activity under conditions demanding cognitive function. "Activation" studies have proved fruitful in schizophrenia research (Buchsbaum et al, 1982; Ingvar and Franzen, 1974) and show promise for demonstrating areas of cerebral dysfunction in DAT (Ingvar et al, 1975; Marc-Vergenes et al, 1985).

13

Treatment, Long-Term Management, and Working with Caregivers

Many dementing illnesses are progressive or remain stable after substantial irreversible impairment has occurred. Survival after onset of dementia often spans a decade during which the patient undergoes progressive loss of function and requires constantly changing types of medical, family, and community support. Pharmacotherapy may be required for treatment of agitation, delusions, or depression; nonpharmacologic interventions and residential and domestic resources such as day care, respite care, and nursing-home care may ameliorate patient distress and family burden; and medical surveillance of the demented patient is necessary to prevent excess disability stemming from overmedication, pneumonia, dehydration, malnutrition, decubiti, and other complications of extended incapacity. Family members must respond to the changing needs of the patient while simultaneously striving to attain psychological accommodation to the gradual loss of the spouse, parent, or sibling. Financial and legal counseling is needed to preserve income and capital for the surviving spouse and facilitate decision making for the impaired patient. Substantial unresolved ethical issues encumber long-term management, including decisions regarding life extension, vital function support, and research participation.

Disease-specific treatment of each dementia has been addressed in previous chapters. Nonspecific aspects of long-term management, pharmacologic treatment, nonpharmacologic interventions, community resources, and caregiving issues will be discussed in this chapter.

MEDICAL ISSUES IN LONG-TERM CARE

Dementia patients must be carefully monitored for co-occurring medical illnesses, drug toxicity, delirium, and seizures. In addition, dementia-related behaviors such as incontinence and wandering may require medical evaluation and treatment.

Co-Occurring Medical Disorders

Dementia patients are subject to all the ailments of their age group plus any additional medical risks that stem from the presence of the brain disease. Dementia patients rarely die as a direct consequence of dementing disease but succumb to aspiration pneumonia, dehydration, malnutrition, sepsis from urinary tract or decubitus infection, or incidental age-related diseases such as cardiac disorders or cancer. The most common chronic illnesses of those over age 65 are arthritis, hypertension, hearing loss, ischemic heart disease, diabetes, cataracts, stroke, malignant neoplasms, varicose veins, and lower extremity orthopedic involvement (Cassel and Brody, 1990). Dementia patients may suffer from any of these common disorders of the elderly, and several may be present simultaneously. The presence of dementia makes it likely that concurrent medical illnesses will be underreported and underrecognized. Larson et al (1984), for example, found that 48 dementia patients harbored 88 previously unrecognized conditions that potentially exacerbated their dementia; the disorders included depression, Parkinson's disease, congestive heart failure, urinary tract infection, arthritis, dermatitis, low folate levels, iron deficiency anemia, drug toxicity, and chronic lung disease. Thus, careful surveillance of dementia patients for co-occurring medical illnesses, particularly infections, neoplasms, cardiovascular disorders, pulmonary disease, diabetes, and drug intoxication, is crucial. Effects of visual and hearing loss in contributing to poor social engagement and limited comprehension in dementia patients should also be assessed.

In the late phases of dementia, patients are bedbound, incontinent, and unable to feed themselves. Nutrition and hydration must be maintained, and the patient must be turned in bed sufficiently often to avoid decubitus ulcerations. In addition, seizures are not uncommon in the late stages of DAT and other dementing illnesses. They require treatment with antiepileptic drugs, but sedating medications such as barbiturates should be avoided; the agents of choice are phenytoin or carbamazepine. Metabolic disturbances must be excluded as the cause of the seizures.

Finally, oral and dental disorders can be the cause of pain and may contribute to poor nutrition. They may easily go unnoticed in the demented patient, and regular examinations of the patient's mouth, gums, and teeth should be carried out (Jones et al, 1988).

Delirium

Delirium is common in geriatric patients and can prove difficult to detect in the demented individual. Dementia patients are more likely than are those without cognitive compromise to develop an acute confusional state in response to toxic or metabolic alterations (Giombetti and Miller, 1990). Estimates of the prevalence of delirium in hospitalized dementia patients vary but reported rates indicate that between 25 and 40 percent of hospitalized dementia victims manifest a delirious episode (Lipowski, 1980a). Delirium should be suspected when demented patients have any acute change in behavior, sleep disturbance, increased inattentiveness or distractibility, or motor restlessness. Visual hallucinations are more prominent in delirium than they are in dementia, and a marked increase in hallucinosis may signal the occurrence of a superimposed encephalopathy (Cummings et al, 1987).

Incontinence

Urinary incontinence is present in 40 to 60 percent of ambulatory dementia patients and eventually occurs in nearly all. Fecal incontinence is common among those with frequent urinary incontinence (Ouslander, 1990). Loss of continence is a major cause of distress to caregivers and often figures prominently in the decision to institutionalize the patient. The principal causes of incontinence are delirium, restricted mobility, infection, retention with overflow, inflammation, fecal impaction, polyuria, and pharmaceuticals (Ouslander, 1990). A careful review of these factors along with appropriate laboratory tests and physical examination procedures are necessary before assuming that incontinence is an irreversible aspect of the dementia syndrome.

Incontinence in dementia may be minimized by developing routine toileting habits, increasing the availability and ease of use of toilet facilities, wearing incontinence undergarments and pads, avoiding fluid intake in the evening, and using external collection devices, particularly at night. Indwelling catheters should be avoided.

Wandering

Although not strictly a medical condition, wandering, like incontinence, is a frequent problem in the long-term care of the dementia patient. Wandering refers to aimless or purposeful motor activity that leads to getting lost, leaving a safe environment, or intruding in inappropriate places (Morishita, 1990). Approximately 10 percent of nursing home residents exhibit wandering behavior. Three options exist to combat wandering: medication, restraint, and behavioral and environmental modification. The last has the fewest adverse consequences and should be exercised whenever possible. Several types of interventions may be helpful: identify and eliminate precipitants of wandering, withdraw neuroleptic agents and sedative hypnotics that may exacerbate wandering, initiate alternating periods of exercise and rest, and repeatedly instruct the patient to stay away from doors (Morishita, 1990). In the nursing-home setting, the concept of "sheltered freedom" is being adopted in response to the challenge posed by the wandering patient. Areas that optimally include the patient's room, adjoining corridors, recreational space, and an outdoor exposure are rendered safe and contained. The patient may wander, pace, explore, and remain active in an uninhibited but safe environment. Such institutional programs help minimize the use of medications and restraints. Dementia patients should have medical-alert wrist bands with identification and diagnostic information, and relatives should have a recent photograph of the patient readily available in case the patient wanders away and a search is necessary.

BEHAVIORAL MANAGEMENT IN LONG-TERM CARE

Troublesome and disruptive behaviors are common in dementia and represent a source of considerable anguish for family members and professional caregivers. In DAT, for example, agitation has been described in from 24 to 61 percent of patients, assaultive behavior in 21 percent, wandering in 26 percent, delusions in 30 to 50 percent, and sleep disturbances in at least 50 percent (Cummings et al, 1987; Merriam et al, 1988; Reisberg et al, 1987; Swearer et al, 1988; Teri et al, 1988; Wragg and Jeste, 1989). These behaviors are among the most distressing to caregivers and are often the determinants of the need for institutionalization or the administration of sedating tranquilizing medications. Rabins and colleagues (1982) found that violence, accusatory behavior, and catastrophic reactions were as disturbing to families as was the memory impairment exhibited by the dementia patient. Effective management of these behaviors may include pharmacotherapy, psychotherapy, and environmental manipulations.

Pharmacotherapy

Drug usage should be minimized in the dementia patient. Adverse consequences are common and well-intentioned drug treatment may lead to increased disability and exacerbation of the suffering of patient and family. Psychotropic drug use has been associated with an increased risk of hip fracture and confusion, and extrapyramidal side effects are common in elderly demented individuals treated with neuroleptic agents (Devanand et al, 1989; Ray et al, 1987). Studies of prescribing practices in nursing homes indicate that psychotropic medications are overprescribed and that potentially toxic combinations of medications are not uncommon (Avorn et al, 1989; Blazer et al, 1983, Ray et al, 1980).

The majority of dementia patients are elderly, and prescribing habits must be altered to account for changes in pharmacodynamics and pharmacokinetics in this age group. Absorption, distribution, metabolism, excretion, and organ/receptor sensitivity are often altered in the aged patient (Ouslander, 1981). Absorption is relatively stable across the life span but may be affected to a small extent by alterations in absorptive surface, decreased splanchnic blood flow, increased gastric pH, or altered gastrointestinal motility. Distribution of ingested medication is affected by the decreased lean body mass of the elderly, decreased total body water, decreased serum albumin, increased body fat, and altered protein binding. Metabolism may be changed through reductions in liver mass, decreased liver blood flow, and diminished oxidative enzyme activity. Excretion is altered by reduced renal blood flow, decreased glomerular filtration rate, and diminished tubular secretory function. End organ responsiveness may be affected by a reduced number of receptors or diminished receptor affinity, reduced second messenger function, and reduced magnitude of cellular responses (Greenblatt et al, 1982; Ouslander, 1981; Thompson et al. 1983). These age-related changes make it more difficult to predict the response to any administered dosage of drug, and in most cases, the changes increase the likelihood of toxicity ensuing from a given dose in the elderly compared to the young.

Guidelines that help avoid pharmacotoxicity in the elderly have been developed; those that apply to the use of drugs in the aged demented patient are summarized in Table 13–1 (Jenike, 1985; Montamat et al, 1989; Thompson et al, 1983). The most prudent approach is to avoid the use of drugs and seek nonpharmacologic alternatives (described below) whenever possible. A careful medication history including review of over-the-counter agents, beneficial or adverse responses to previous medications, and treatment adherence should be obtained. Establish an accurate diagnosis of the dementing condition plus any concurrent illnesses, and choose specific target symptoms for treatment. Introduce drugs at one-half to one-third the doses suggested for younger adults, increase the dose in small increments, and use the minimal dose required to achieve the desired response. In some cases, partial responses may have to be accepted. Avoid multiple drug regimens whenever possible. Provide written as well as verbal medication instructions to the patient and the caregiver; review medication schedules regularly; and delete medications whenever possible. Monitor serum drug levels where they may help guide treatment decisions. While exercising caution in medication administration, do not avoid treating the elderly because of age or presence of dementia; the patient may benefit substantially from effective drug therapy. Similarly do not avoid doses recommended for younger patients if the patient fails to respond to smaller dosages and does not exhibit side effects

TABLE 13–1.   Guidelines for pharmacotherapy in dementia.

Minimize the use of medications and seek nonpharmacologic alternatives where possible.

Take a careful medication history including over-the-counter drugs and responses to previously administered agents.

Evaluate adherence to treatment instructions.

Establish the most accurate possible diagnosis of the dementing disorder as well as any concurrent illnesses.

Choose specific target symptoms for treatment, and carefully monitor the response to therapy.

Provide easily read and easily understood written, as well as verbal, instructions to both the patient and the caregiver.

Introduce pharmacotherapy at one-third to one-half the dose recommended for younger adults.

Increase the drug dosage in small increments.

Minimize the total dose administered.

Accept partial responses if more complete target responses are associated with unacceptable side effects.

Know the pharmacology, side-effect profile, and potential drug interactions of each agent administered to the patient.

Avoid multiple drug regimens whenever possible, and beware of potential additive toxicity.

Review drug regimens frequently, discontinuing unnecessary medications and simplifying dosage schedules in concert with changes in the patient's condition.

Obtain serum drug levels when they may help guide dosage decisions.

Monitor side effects regularly.

Do not avoid pharmacotherapy just because of the age of the patient or the presence of a dementing disorder.

Do not avoid dosages recommended for younger adults if the patient fails to respond to lower doses and does not manifest adverse side effects at higher doses.

with higher doses. The pharmacology, side-effect profile and drug interactions of administered agents must be understood by the prescribing clinician and side effects must be monitored frequently.

The agents most frequently prescribed for behavior problems in demented patients are neuroleptics, antidepressants, and sedative hypnotics. Table 13–2 lists the agents, usual dosage ranges, and target symptoms used in constructing a psychopharmacologic regimen for a dementia patient. No specific neuroleptic agent has been demonstrated to be superior to others in controlling delusions and agitation in dementia, and drug choice depends on the patient's response and the side effects produced by the drug (Gottlieb and Piotrowski, 1990; Helms, 1985; Risse and Barnes, 1986; Steele et al, 1986). High potency agents such as haloperidol or fluphenazine have a

TABLE 13–2.   Commonly used agents and dosage ranges to control specific target symptoms in dementia patients.

Symptom	Available agents	Usual daily dose (P.O.: range)
Agitation	Haloperidol	1 mg (0.5–3 mg)
	Fluphenazine	1 mg (1–5 mg)
	Thiothixene	2 mg (1–10 mg)
	Thioridazine	75 mg (30–150 mg)
	Molindone	75 mg (5–125 mg)
	Propranolol	120 mg (80–240 mg)
	Trazodone	300 mg (200–500 mg)
	Fluoxetine	40 mg (20–80 mg)
	Buspirone	15 mg (15–30 mg)
	Carbamazepine	1000 mg (800–1200 mg)
Delusions	Haloperidol	1 mg (0.5–3 mg)
	Fluphenazine	1 mg (1–5 mg)
	Thiothixene	2 mg (1–10 mg)
	Thioridazine	75 mg (30–150 mg)
Depression	Nortriptyline	50 mg (50–100 mg)
	Desipramine	50 mg (50–150 mg)
	Doxepin	50 mg (50–150 mg)
	Trazodone	100 mg (100–400 mg)
	Fluoxetine	40 mg (20–80 mg)
Anxiety	Oxazepam	30 mg (20–60 mg)
	Lorazepam	1 mg (0.5–6 mg)
Insomnia	Thioridazine	25 mg (25–75 mg)
	Temazepam	15 mg (15–30 mg)
	Lorazepam	1 mg (0.2–4 mg)
	Nortriptyline	45 mg (20–75 mg)
Sexual aggression (males)	Medroxyprogesterone	300 mg/wk IM

greater tendency to produce extrapyramidal symptoms but are less likely to cause sedation and hypotension. The opposite side-effect profile character-ized low-potency agents such as thioridazine. Thiothixene occupies an in-termediate position with regard to these effects. Non-neuroleptic agents reported to be useful in the control of agitation include propranolol, tra-zodone, fluoxetine, buspirone, and carbamazepine (Risse and Barnes, 1986). Benzodiazepines tend to increase confusion in aged individuals and should not be used as the drugs of choice for treatment of agitation. If neuroleptics fail to relieve agitation, however, benzodiazepines may be used as an alternative.

Depression is common in many forms of dementia, particularly vascular dementia and dementia in Parkinson's disease (Cummings, 1988; Mayeux et al, 1981b). A wide variety of antidepressant agents are now available, and none has been shown to be superior to others in relieving depression associated with dementia. Many antidepressant agents have anticholinergic effects potentially deleterious to the cognitively impaired patient while others tend to produce postural hypotension or adversely affect cardiac function (Thompson et al, 1983). Agents commonly used in the treatment of depression in dementia are listed in Table 13–2; they include nortriptyline, desipramine, doxepin, trazodone, and fluoxetine.

Anxiety may complicate dementia syndromes and is not uncommon in the early stages of DAT. Some benzodiazepines such as diazepam, frequently prescribed for anxiety states, undergo marked changes in metabolism in the elderly, have very extended half lives, and should not be used in aged individuals. Other agents such as oxazepam and lorazepam undergo relatively little change in metabolism and can safely be used in this age group (Thompson et al, 1983).

Insomnia and nocturnal wandering are common disruptive behavioral changes in dementia, exhausting the caregiver and endangering the patient. Sedative hypnotics often increase daytime confusion and should be used with caution. Short-acting benzodiazepines (Table 13–2) (Thompson et al. 1983) may be used for brief periods in an attempt to reentrain diurnal rhythms in the patient and provide relief for the caregiver. Sedating neuroleptic agents (for example, thioridazine) are the agents of choice for persistent insomnia, and nortriptyline has also been used successfully (Reynolds et al, 1988). Antihistamines such as diphenhydramine have substantial anticholinergic activity, increase the risk of delirium in the demented elderly individual, and should be avoided.

Sexual aggression is uncommon in dementia but may occasionally occur as a major behavioral problem. Exhibitionism, frequent masturbation, indiscriminant sexual advances, and attempted forced intercourse have been reported. Sexually aggressive males may be treated with medroxyprogresterone acetate given as a daily oral dose or a weekly or monthly injection (Cooper, 1987).

Psychotherapy

Psychotherapy can be broadly construed to include any nonpharmacologic treatment intended to modify the behavior of the dementia patient. Modalities potentially available for use with the dementia patient include conventional psychotherapy and behavior/operant, group, family, supportive, reminiscence, directive, reality, and cognitive therapies (Maletta, 1988). The mode of therapy chosen is determined by the patient's level of intellectual function, the specific problems to be addressed, and the availability of knowledgeable therapists. The most appropriate type of therapy will change over time in patients with progressive conditions. Early in a progressive illness, insight-oriented, group, and/or family therapies may be recommended.

Early loss of introspection and self-insight limit traditional psychodynamic psychotherapy to the initial phases of the illness, but during this time, alleviation of anxiety, increasing the sense of control, addressing feelings of shame and embarrassment, discussing fear of becoming a burden on one's family, improving communication with others, and alleviating distress to forestall maladaptive behaviors are reasonable treatment goals (Miller, 1989; Verwoerdt, 1981). Cognitive therapies depend on memory function, and their usefulness is also limited to the early phases of the disease when sufficient memory skills remain. In some instances, group therapy may provide a safe, nonjudgmental environment where emotional, social, economic, and legal issues common to dementia patients may be discussed. Family therapy, with or without the patient present, may facilitate the open exchange of information and emotional exchange necessary to optimize the carc of the dementia patient in the family setting.

Supportive psychotherapy may be useful in many stages of dementia. Goals are to provide guidance, offer reassurance, modulate anxiety and insecurity, provide an empathic listener, and assist in obtaining community resources (Maletta, 1988). This may be effectively combined with reminiscence therapy, using the more intact remote memories of the demented patient to maintain a connection with the past. Photographs and family albums as well as discussions that include family members and long-term friends aid this process. As the disease worsens, reality therapy focusing on appropriate eating, toileting, and socialization behavior as well as directive therapy providing advice to the patient are most relevant (Maletta, 1988).

Behavior modification and operant techniques become useful later in the disease course when maladaptive and destructive behaviors may emerge. These techniques depend on identifying the environmental events that precipitate, encourage, or maintain aberrant behaviors and then manipulating the environmental contingencies to extinguish destructive behaviors and reinforce constructive responses (Eisdorfer et al, 1981). Operant techniques have been used successfully to increase personal care, improve socialization, increase exercise, and decrease aggressive incidents in dementia patients (McEvoy, 1990; Pinkston et al, 1988).

COMMUNITY RESOURCES

Many dementia patients have progressive illnesses that require constant changes in community and family support. The continuum of required care may be arranged by a case manager, nurse, or social worker familiar with local resources or may be identified and arranged by family members. The Alzheimer's Association provides services to dementia patients and their families and maintains directories of community resources. In addition to home care supports, day care, respite care, and nursing home care, dementia patients may also benefit from services available to other senior citizens such as senior centers, congregate meals, meals on wheels, escort services, and transportation programs.

Home Care

The most important community resource is the patient's home, and efforts to keep patients in their familiar environments should be pursued whenever it is feasible for the patient and the family. Programs that may help the patient stay at home include home care support, day care, and respite care. Approximately 80 percent of all dementia care is delivered by family members. In most cases, the caregiver is the spouse (approximately 50 percent of caregivers) or an adult daughter or daughter-in-law (one-quarter to one-third of caregivers) (Office of Technology Assessment Task Force, 1988). As dementia becomes evident, the caregiver gradually assumes household duties such as shopping, meal preparation, check writing, and driving. As the disease progresses, they provide help with dressing, eating, bathing, and toileting. A spectrum of help providers—untrained domestic workers, home health aides, and nurses—may be employed to provide services in the home or relieve the caregiver. In-home respite care allows the caregiver to leave the home for a few hours to pursue recreational activities, shopping, or other duties. Home visits by specialized practitioners lead to recommendations regarding behavioral changes in the patient, safety, caregiver well being, and social issues based on problems often not evident in the course of office-based assessments (Ramsdell et al, 1989). If no family support is available, dementia patients may stay in board-and-care homes or foster homes that serve, at least temporarily, as surrogate family settings.

Family members should be involved in educational programs that allow them to be more effective in communicating and interacting with dementia patients. Table 13–3 lists techniques for improving communications with dementia patients (Ostuni and Pietro, 1986). The basic tenets emphasize simple vocabulary and frequent repetition. In advanced stages, dementia patients may respond to a soothing, familiar voice; gentle touch; or soft music (Hoffman et al, 1985; Norberg et al, 1986).

Family members should be taught behavioral management techniques to improve patient behavior, decrease caregiver stress, and delay institutionalizing the patient (Green et al, 1986; Pinkston et al, 1988). Zarit and co-workers (1985) have shown the utility of a multistep process whereby family members are encouraged to focus on individual problem behaviors

TABLE 13–3.   Techniques to improve communication with dementia patients (adapted from Ostuni and Pietro, 1986).

Conversation
    Maintain topic by asking relevant questions.
    Remind patient of topic and summarize conversation frequently.
    Avoid frustrating and potentially embarrassing situations including strangers or multiple participants.
    Encourage interactions with friends and family members within the bounds of the patient's memory and language skills.
    Orient the patient to situations ahead of time and repeat frequently.
    Adopt a reassuring, respectful, and affectionate but not demeaning style.
    Do not avoid conversation even if it is not reciprocated.
    Maintain social rituals (greetings, farewells, etc).
    Avoid asking open questions; offer a few limited responses ("Do you want coffee or tea?" rather than "Do you want something to drink?").
    Do not correct, hurry, or interrupt the patient's conversation.
    Guess what is meant when word-finding difficulties occur.
    Avoid abstract or metaphorical words and phrases.
    Do not respond to angry or incoherent utterances; temporarily stop or redirect the conversation.
Instructions
    Repeat messages frequently.
    Paraphrase messages and use synonyms.
    Use short sentences with simple structures.
    Break messages into components, and allow individual tasks to be completed before proceeding to another task.
    Give instructions close to the time the act is to be done.
    Avoid competing conversations with television, radio, other conversations, and so on.
    Speak slowly.
    Use a simple vocabulary, and avoid abstract words.
    Enhance message with gestures, appropriate inflections, objects, and pictures.
    Written messages and reminders may aid in some circumstances.
    Use a calm, soothing tone, but do not belittle or infantilize the patient.

exhibited by the patient, generate alternative means of responding, consider the pros and cons of each potential solution, choose the solution that seems best, rehearse the intervention before applying it with the patient, carry out the plan, evaluate the outcome, and continue with the chosen solution if it proves promising or choose an alternate if the results are unsatisfactory.

    Adjustments in the home environment are usually necessary. The principal aim is to facilitate basic living activities and create a safe living space that is maximally free (Carroll, 1989). Residential adjustments should not make the home unfamiliar to the patient or unacceptable to the caregiver.

Hot surfaces such as radiators and light bulbs should be protected; sharp objects and small items that can be placed in the mouth should be removed; loose rugs should be removed or secured in place. Lighting should be ample in all areas, and electric cords should be safely placed. In the bathroom and kitchen, toxic substances should be securely stored, and antiscald measures should be taken (remove hot water faucet handles or turn down temperature of the water heater). If the patient is physically disabled, grab bars will be required in the bathroom, and railings will be needed in walkways. The kitchen stove is a major source of problems and should be secured with a gas turn-off valve or electric switch. Locks will be needed to secure wandering patients and prevent them from leaving the home without appropriate supervision. Double bolt locks, one of which turns clockwise and one counterclockwise, or more sophisticated electronic devices may be installed. The yard must also be secured and most advanced patients will require supervision while outside to avoid elopement or ingestion of foreign material.

Decisions regarding driving invariably arise in the course of progressive dementing illnesses. Loss of driving privileges is an affront to the autonomy of the patient and may threaten the independence of the spouse if the patient has been the principal driver. Dementia, however, is a definite risk factor for motor vehicle accidents: 30 percent of driving dementia patients have accidents after disease onset and crashes are several times more common among dementia patients than among age-matched controls (Friedland et al, 1988; Lucas-Blaustein et al, 1988). Some states now require that patients with dementing illnesses be reported to the Department of Motor Vehicles. Patients then retake the driving test, and licensing is suspended if they fail. Until such measures are widely enacted, families and physicians must take responsibility for prohibiting driving as soon as impairment is evident.

Day Care

Day care programs are facilities located in the community or operated in conjunction with medical centers that provide daily programs to elderly patients. Lunch is usually included, and the programs provide structured activities including games, crafts, music, exercise, and recreation. Patients spend several hours per day one to five days per week in the program, and most dementia patients will stay in day care for one to three years (Bergmann et al, 1978). Programs commonly include 10 to 20 patients and may consist exclusively of dementia patients or of a mix of intellectually impaired and cognitively intact individuals. Transition from home care to day care can be difficult, and it may take patients several weeks to successfully adjust to program routines. Day care programs are cost-effective alternatives to nursing home care and delay institutionalization of patients that cannot be managed at home on a full-time basis. Day programs allow caregivers to continue employment and to be relieved of full-time caregiving responsibilities (Chodosh et al, 1986; Panella et al, 1984).

Respite Care

Community respite care usually involves admitting the patient for a brief period of time (from a few days to a few weeks) to an extended-care institution. Admission of the patient provides the caregiver more prolonged relief than is possible with in-home respite or day-care-based respite. These longer respite periods allow the caregiver to spend time with family members, take care of personal health needs, or simply to relax for longer periods of time. Respite renews the caregiver's vigor and is likely to delay permanent nursing home placement. Respite may also allow the patient's physician to introduce new medications under supervised conditions. Patients, however, often have temporary difficulty adjusting to the new environment and may exhibit transient exacerbations of behavioral abnormalities, disruption of sleep patterns, or loss of continence.

NURSING HOME CARE

Nursing homes have become an integral component of the continuum of care needed by dementia patients. Their number has expanded rapidly in recent years, increasing from 25,000 beds in 1200 homes in 1939 to 1.5 million beds in 15,000 homes by 1988 (Office of Technology Assessment Task Force, 1988; Read, 1990). This rate of expansion will continue as the size of the aged population expands, and a nursing home census of 3 million is expected by the year 2030 (Stotsky and Stotsky, 1983). Five percent of the U.S. population over the age of 65 lives in nursing homes and 40 to 70 percent of nursing home residents are demented (Office of Technology Assessment Task Force, 1988; Rovner et al, 1986). Dementia patients account for approximately 50 percent of the $40 billion spent annually on nursing-home care. A majority of dementia patients spend the terminal phases of their illness in a nursing home.

Several levels of care are available in nursing homes, and complex and changing terminologies complicate referral of the dementia patient to the proper residential facility. Approximately half of all nursing homes are certified by Medicare or Medicaid as skilled nursing facilities (SNFs). These facilities provide 24-hour services by licensed practical nurses and have at least one registered nurse on the day shift, seven days per week. Intermediate care facilities (ICFs) are less intensively staffed and have at least one licensed practical nurse on duty during the day shift, seven days per week.

The decision to place one's family member in a nursing home is usually the most daunting issue faced by the caregiver. It is rarely made without personal anguish, considerable guilt, and recurrent misgiving and self-doubt. It is often the focal point of family disagreement. Some families have little tolerance for even the most limited aberrant behavior and pursue nursing home placement early in the patient's clinical course, others maintain the patient at home until death. Most families will decide that nursing home residence is superior to home care at some point between these extremes.

Caregiver characteristics and circumstances, not patient characteristics or disease status, are the principal determinants of institutionalization (Colerick and George, 1986). Male caregivers are more likely to institutionalize female patients than vice versa. Patients are more likely to be institutionalized if they are cared for by an adult child than if their caregiver is a spouse. Employed caregivers are more likely to use nursing homes than are unemployed or retired caregivers. High stress, better income level, and relative youth of caregiver also increase the chance of institutionalization (Colerick and George, 1986).

Costs of nursing homes vary widely but currently average $18,500 to $26,500 per person per annum, a prohibitive financial burden for most families. Half of the costs of nursing-home care are borne by the patients and their families (Office of Technology Assessment Task Force, 1988). Options such as long-term care insurance, health maintenance programs for the elderly, life-care communities, and religious organizations with nursing facilities currently account for only a small portion of the expense of extended care. In the past, state mental hospitals provided long-term care to the mentally disabled elderly, but this practice has been drastically curtailed since the deinstitutionalization movement of the 1960s.

Department of Veterans Affairs (formerly Veterans Administration [VA]) Medical Centers have affiliated nursing homes that are regularly inspected for standards of health care provided. Families bear most of the costs of placement in these homes. A few VAs also have their own nursing homes that provide extended care to eligible veterans at no cost to the family, but most residents must have a service-connected disability to be eligible for admission.

Nursing homes vary drastically in quality from poorly staffed human warehouses with custodial philosophies to pleasant residences with a wide variety of programmatic options to enrich the lives of clients. A few nursing homes have established specialized units for the care of dementia patients, whereas others encourage a mix of those with and without cognitive impairment: Neither option has been demonstrated to be clearly superior (Rabins, 1986). Choosing a nursing home should include consideration of many elements: cost, proximity to family members, physical environment and cleanliness, staffing, staff knowledge of dementia, quality of nursing care, availability of medical care, range of programs for the residents, food services, management and care philosophy, availability of dental and podiatry services, and participation in a quality assurance program (Cohen and Eisdorfer, 1986). Family members may continue to visit the resident frequently and often play a major role in feeding, dressing, and toileting the patient even after nursing-home residence has been initiated.

Every effort must be made to maintain the dignity of the nursing-home patient. They should be treated according to their actual age; diminutive names or "cute" ribbons are rarely appropriate. Clothes are less anonymous than pajamas, and soiled clothing should be changed quickly. Nurses and aides should be acquainted with the patient's biography, so they see him or her as a former athlete, nurse, truck driver, or engineer rather than simply as a confused aged individual.

The transition from home to nursing home is difficult for most patients; increased confusion and worsened behavior can be anticipated for the first one to two weeks following the move. Once admitted to a nursing home, most patients will not return home for more than brief periods if at all and nearly all eventually die in the nursing home or shortly after transfer from the home to an acute-care facility. After admission, the caregiver, with medical and nursing-home staff collaboration, should develop a plan for responding to any life-threatening illness that develops for the patient—transfer to a hospital, initiation of life-saving procedures, provision of pain-relief only, and so forth. The need for funeral arrangements and a means of facilitating patient autopsy should also be anticipated.

CAREGIVERS

As experience has grown with the care of dementia patients, it has become obvious that one cannot simply treat the patient; the needs of both the patient and the family must be addressed. "Burden" refers to the extent to which caregivers perceive their emotional or physical health, social life, and financial status as suffering as a result of caring for their demented relative. The concept of burden has proven a useful means of communicating the extent of caregiver stress, and an inventory has been developed that assists in its assessment (Scott et al, 1986; Zarit et al, 1980, 1986). Burden is ameliorated when other family members provide support, share in the caregiving, visit the patient and caregiver, and facilitate brief respite periods for the primary caregiver (Scott et al, 1986). Higher burden scores indicate greater distress and correlate with an increased likelihood of nursing-home placement of patients.

Depression, symptoms of psychological distress, use of psychotropic drugs, and physical illness are all increased among dementia caregivers (Pruchno and Potashnik, 1989). Cohen and Eisdorfer (1988) found that 55 percent of caregivers had symptoms of depression, and those with depressive symptoms were more likely to perceive a lack of control over their situation than were those without such symptoms. Depression may be ameliorated through participation in support groups or group therapy; in some cases, individual therapy or medications may be required.

Education regarding the diagnosis, nature, and prognosis of the specific dementia syndrome is an essential first step in aiding the caregiver to understand the patient's disease and changing behavior. Several books are also available to help family members understand dementias and the challenges of caregiving; among the best are *The 36-Hour Day* (Mace and Rabins, 1981) and *Understanding Alzheimer's Disease* (Aronson, 1988).

Family therapy can help alleviate the distress of caregivers and improve their sense of control (Kahan et al, 1985; Rabins, 1990). Problems common to caregivers include disappointment about lost life goals, frustration with the patient's limitations, guilt about nursing-home placement, anxiety about role reversals, and mourning the slow death of the dementia patient. Conflict among family members regarding caregiving responsibilities and nursing home placement are also common. These themes can be discussed in a therapeutic setting where problems can be identified, open communication encouraged, and solutions derived.

Support groups where caregivers can exchange information and share emotional distress can be of substantial benefit. Groups serve to impart information, provide imitative learning of positive behaviors, allow catharsis, and enhance cohesiveness among members that may generalize beyond the group setting (Zarit et al, 1985). Groups can be arranged through the local chapter of the Alzheimer's Association or with mental health professionals.

Sexual relationships are a frequent source of concern for the spouse-caregiver. The problems are not uniform: some patients experience loss of libido, some have no change, and a minority exhibit increased sexual drive or sexual disinhibition. Spouses may find continuing sexual activities with the patient distasteful because of the changes in their relationship, or they may be frustrated that this area of interpersonal gratification has also been lost. Frank discussion of these problems with suggestions for redirecting unwanted sexual attention or encouraging desirable affection may be helpful.

LEGAL COUNSELING

Family members almost invariably require legal counsel when a spouse, a parent, or a sibling is identified as suffering from a dementing illness. Financial planning and protection of assets, conservatorship/mental competence issues, and decisions to withhold resuscitation measures may require advice from an attorney. As long as Medicaid restrictions require the patient to be pauperized before being eligible for support, the transfer of resources to children may be expedient. Currently this must be done at least 30 months prior to request for aid, however, and so must be anticipated early in the disease course before a crisis arises (Overman and Stoudemire, 1988). The taxation consequences of these financial shifts must be calculated; new laws currently being formulated are likely to increase the complexity of these considerations.

Early in the course of the illness, the dementia patient may be competent to make decisions but will eventually be unable to do so if the mental disorder progresses. A surrogate decision maker should be designated. The best means of legally formalizing this relationship is to obtain a durable power of attorney. This document differs from other forms of power of attorney in that it is not abrogated when the patient becomes physically or mentally incapacitated (Overman and Stoudemire, 1988).

Optimally, the patient will consider a living will while he or she is still able to make decisions. This allows the patient to make explicit his or her wishes regarding life support and the scope of medical care to be pursued in the terminal phases of illness. Early discussions of this issue will save the family the pain of making the decision later under more emotionally trying circumstances.

ETHICAL ISSUES

Many ethical issues arise in the course of dementing illnesses. Most prominent are the decision to provide sustenance or to treat infections in the terminally ill state, the decision to resuscitate, and the decision to participate in research projects. Such decisions are easiest when the patient has made his or her wishes known at a time when mental competence was not in question; even this is not infallible, however, since both demented and nondemented patients should have the right to change their minds as unanticipated situations arise. Early discussions of these problems are the exception since almost no patient or family is emotionally prepared to comprehend the full ramifications of the diagnosis of a progressive dementing illness. In the absence of guidance from the victim, family members must make painful decisions regarding the vigor of intervention and support measures. In some cases, this is made easier by encouraging family members to ask "What would he want for himself if he were cognizant of his circumstances?" rather than "Should I continue his life?" No decisions applicable to all patients in these circumstances are possible, and individualized choices must be made for each patient and with each family. The decision-making process should include defining the goals of the intervention under consideration, seeking input from all involved family members as well as representatives of disciplines involved in the care of the patient, observing the patient for clues as to quality of life (groans, smiles, and so on), discussion of the social and psychological consequences of the proposed intervention, and review of the possible adverse or beneficial outcomes of pursuing a particular course (Alexander, 1988; Lo and Dornbrand, 1984; Wanzer et al, 1984). Advice may be solicited from institutional ethics panels, clergy, or other qualified individuals, but the burden of the final decision falls on the family.

The ethics of research using dementia patients may also emerge as an issue, particularly in research intensive university environments. An unresolvable conflict exists between the inability of the demented patient to give informed consent on the one hand and the clear need for dementia-related research on the other (Cassel, 1985). Currently, research participation is allowed provided full disclosure of potential risks and benefits is given to the spouse or guardian as well as the patient and an informed consent agreement has been explained and signed. In the absence of full comprehension by the patient, the investigator must accept additional responsibility to insure that no unnecessary suffering is experienced as a consequence of research participation.

The clinician-investigator must recognize that his or her two roles—patient care and research—provide a potential conflict of interest and must insure that presentation of the research to the patient and the family has been made in an unbiased fashion. Having performed research involving a vulnerable human subject, the investigator is obligated to report the results to the scientific community as quickly as is feasible in order to spare other patients the need for similar jeopardy.

14

Conclusions and Directions

GENERALIZATIONS CONCERNING THE DEMENTIAS

Dementia is a clinical syndrome, etiologically nonspecific, and can be reversible as well as irreversible. Determination of the cause of dementia is essential for proper treatment and management. Both identification and characterization of the intellectual changes of dementia are dependent on careful testing of mental status; this examination is crucial for establishing etiology and diagnosis.

Dementia is not a part of normal aging, and the existence of a dementia syndrome implies the presence of a specific medical condition adversely affecting intellectual function. Every demented individual, regardless of age, deserves thorough evaluation in search of a reversible cause of mental status impairment. Intellectual functions, however, change with age and among the commonly observed alterations are psychomotor slowing, forgetfulness, garrulousness, and a decrease in active vocabulary. Called senescence, these changes do not represent a dementia syndrome in the healthy elderly individual.

The incidence of dementia increases with advancing age until it affects 20 to 40 percent of the population over 80 years of age. The higher prevalence among the elderly reflects the increased frequency of degenerative disorders, as well as the increased occurrence of systemic illnesses and the correspondingly greater use of pharmacologic agents that combine to produce intellectual impairment.

Two broad but clinically distinct patterns of mental status change are readily identified. Dementias associated with primary dysfunction of the cerebral cortex produce aphasia, amnesia, acalculia, apraxia, and/or agnosia; judgment and insight are impaired. Personality may be relatively preserved in the cortical dementias although disinterest, unconcern, or disinhibition may occur and suspiciousness and paranoid ideation are common. Dementias occurring with disorders affecting the basal ganglia, thalamus, rostral brainstem, and their frontal lobe projections tend to be characterized by slow intellectual processing, forgetfulness, dilapidation of cognition, and the occurrence of affective disorders. The subcortical dementias often include prominent neuropsychiatric disorders including depression, mania, and schizophrenia-like illnesses. Movement disorders—tremor, rigidity, chorea, bradykinesia, ataxia, and dysarthria—frequently accompany the dementias produced by involvement of subcortical structures. In contrast, patients with the cortical dementias routinely remain free of motor involvement until late in the disease.

Dementia based on metabolic or toxic disorders shares many features of the acute confusional state but may last for weeks and months and must be considered among the common causes of acquired chronic intellectual impairment. The pattern of intellectual impairment in the toxic-metabolic conditions resembles that observed with degenerative disorders of the subcortical structures. The cardinal features of cortical involvement—aphasia, amnesia, agnosia, apraxia—are not seen, whereas slowing and dilapidation of intellect occur and disorders of movement such as rigidity, asterixis, tremor, and myoclonus are often prominent. Peripheral neuropathy is common in metabolic and toxic diseases but rare in degenerative disorders.

A dementia syndrome may occur as part of a variety of psychiatric disturbances, including depression, schizophrenia, and hysterical conversion reactions such as the Ganser syndrome. The mental impairments of these disorders are broadly variable in their characteristics but rarely show the clinical features associated with cortical dementias.

The laboratory evaluation of all demented patients should include a brain image (CT or MRI) and standard laboratory tests of blood, serum, and urine. Additional studies such as EEG, evoked responses, brain mapping, SPECT or PET scans, CSF studies, heavy metal and drug levels, and other laboratory assays should be selected on the basis of clinical hypotheses. Given the large number of causes of dementia, it is impossible to construct a single battery that can detect all possible etiologies. Specific laboratory tests needed are selected based on history, general physical and neurologic examinations, mental status testing, and basic laboratory studies.

Many dementias are reversible or curable (Table 14–1). Toxic dementias, including iatrogenic ones, frequently reverse when exposure to the

TABLE 14–1.   Reversible dementias and the appropriate intervention.

Reversible dementia	Intervention
Toxic dementias (including pharmaceutical abuse)	Limitation of exposure to toxic substance
Metabolic dementias	Treatment of underlying illness
Heavy metal poisoning	Chelation, removal of source
Infectious dementias	Administration of appropriate antibiotic agents
Inflammatory disorders	Therapy with antiinflammatory drugs
Multi-infarct dementia	Identification of source of emboli or treatment of hypertension/hypotension; aspirin therapy
Wilson's disease	Penicillamine
Parkinson's disease	Levodopa
Hydrocephalic dementia	Shunt
Neoplastic dementia	Removal or decompression of intracranial tumor, appropriate chemo- or radiation therapy
Subdural hematoma	Surgical removal
Dementia of depression	Antidepressant agents, ECT

noxious agent is limited, and treatment of the underlying illness will cure many metabolic dementias. Identification of an embolic source will halt the progression of multi-infarct dementia and considerable spontaneous recovery may follow. Total or partial reversal of subcortical dementia in Wilson's disease may occur with institution of appropriate treatment, and the dementia of Parkinson's disease may be improved by levodopa administration. Some hydrocephalic dementias are curable with appropriate shunting procedures, and neoplastic dementias may be cured or greatly alleviated by removal of the offending neoplasm and/or appropriate medical oncology therapy. The dementia syndrome of depression may remit spontaneously, but it can be actively treated pharmacologically or with electroconvulsive therapy. Essentially all reversible and curable dementias have features of subcortical dysfunction; identification of the specific characteristics that identify subcortical dementia indicates the need for a thorough search for reversible etiologies.

Treatment of patients with advanced degenerative dementing illnesses is based on health maintenance and includes guarding against decubitus ulceration, aspiration pneumonia, and urinary tract infections. This, plus prevention of contractures and the maintenance of good nutritional status, facilitates the management of patients with late-stage dementias of all types. Family counseling and support can prepare family members for the expected course of disease and is an essential part of good management.

Effective management depends on using all available clinical information to establish an etiology. In most cases, it is possible to arrive at a clinical diagnosis if a thorough evaluation is pursued. History, general physical and neurologic examinations, mental status testing, and laboratory information all provide important data leading to a diagnosis and appropriate disease-specific management.

CHANGING CONCEPTS OF DAT

With the documented increase in the frequency of dementia over the past few decades, a broader awareness and a paradoxically increased confusion concerning the problem has affected the lay public as well as many physicians and scientists. Much of the confusion stems from the greatly expanded publicity given to one specific type of dementia, DAT. For many, Alzheimer's disease (as DAT is popularly called) has become a generic term encompassing all causes of progressive dementia. This looseness of definition has produced significant changes in the concept of DAT and exemplifies the current confusion that characterizes dementia.

For over a half century after it was first described, DAT was considered a relatively rare disorder. It was strictly linked to the presenile onset of a progressive dementia and carefully separated from a less clearly defined entity called "senile dementia." The age at which an individual changed from presenile to senile provoked controversy, no identifiable neuropathologic distinctions between the two disorders could be found, and in the 1960s the two disorders were amalgamated into one. The combination was called senile dementia of the Alzheimer type, dementia of the Alzheimer type (DAT), or simply Alzheimer's disease. Concomitant with the change in terminology, two additional factors were occurring. First the number of elderly citizens increased markedly; second Blessed and colleagues (1968) demonstrated that elderly individuals who became demented had many cortical plaques and tangles. It was accepted that plaques and tangles were the neuropathologic base of DAT, and it was then suggested that the mental impairment of the elderly was based on plaque and tangle disease (Plum, 1979). Not only was dementia made interchangeable with DAT, but both were made interchangeable with the presence of plaques and tangles in the brain.

A correlation of dementia/DAT/plaques and tangles was often correct, but studies published in the 1970s (Tomlinson, 1977) had already demonstrated that some individuals, considered demented on a clinical basis, did not have significant numbers of plaques or tangles. Not all dementia was based on Alzheimer-type pathology. Improved diagnostic criteria for DAT were produced, first as *primary degenerative dementia* (PDD) in the *Diagnostic and Statistical Manual of Mental Disorders, Third Edition* (DSM-III) (American Psychiatric Association, 1980) and later as *possible, probable, or definite Alzheimer's disease* by the National Institute of Neurologic and Communicative Disorders and Stroke/Alzheimer's Disease and Related Disorders Association (McKhann et al, 1984). At the same time, it was noted that some patients with sizeable numbers of plaques and tangles at histologic study had not shown evidence of dementia during life (Tomlinson, 1977); criteria for the minimum number of plaques and/or tangles located in specific brain areas to warrant the diagnosis of DAT were established by neuro-pathologists (Ball, 1988; Khachaturian, 1985; Tomlinson, 1977). Despite improvements in clinical and pathological criteria, individuals with non-Alzheimer-type behavioral changes who show multiple plaques and tangles at postmortem and the opposite, those with the accepted clinical features of DAT who have no plaques or tangles, continue to be reported.

In the past decade, many alternate approaches to the diagnosis of DAT have been suggested; most stress pathognomonic findings on laboratory tests. Neuropsychological batteries, EEGs including brain mapping and evoked potential studies, nuclear medicine studies, brain imaging, and specific chemical markers (for example, choline acetyltransferase) plus numerous additional laboratory studies have been suggested. At best, these techniques provide only nonspecific correlations. Most are reasonably accurate in supporting a clinical impression of DAT (about 60 to 70 percent correlation in selected DAT series) but suffer high false positive levels and have proved almost useless in cases in which the diagnosis is in question. To date, no laboratory studies have provided unequivocal evidence for demarcating DAT.

A different approach that became popular in the 1980s featured search for a basic defect in DAT. Individual investigators have championed the importance of viral infection or prion abnormality, of circulating amyloid proteins, of inherent abnormalities of neural membranes, of autoimmune problems, of aluminum as a brain toxin, of genetic factors including search for the abnormal chromosomes and/or genes of DAT, and many more. Again none of these approaches has presented sufficiently reliable data to aid in recognition of DAT as a specific entity.

In fact, the more DAT is studied and the more frequently the term appears in lay and medical literature, the less distinct it becomes as a specific entity. *Clinical Alzheimer's disease* may define a population that overlaps but does not precisely coincide with *neuropathological Alzheimer's disease*. At present, it must be accepted that more than one type of DAT exists based on the methodology and definition in use.

The problem is not a mere nosological conundrum. The current use of DAT as a synonym for dementia poses a serious trap for both the physician and the patient. No specific treatment for DAT exists, but there are treatments for many other causes of dementia; it would be safer if the term DAT was reserved to identify a specific segment of the dementia population.

FUTURE TRENDS

Despite the confusion in nomenclature, dementia is a medical problem of major consequence, a status that will persist and in all probability increase significantly in future years. Ongoing improvements in the treatment of systemic illness will add to human longevity, creating an increasing number of individuals susceptible to late-life dementing problems. Barring global war, nuclear catastrophe, or environmental disaster dementia will be the most formidable medical problem of the early twenty-first century.

As the number of demented individuals increases, the modalities of treatment, the means of care and management, and the facilities available for these functions must expand. This process has already started and will grow exponentially in future years. Sheltered freedom for the seriously demented individual will become a mainstay of medical management. At the same time, the number of social support structures available for the mildly demented, allowing them to remain in the community, will increase. Retirement villages, currently mostly warm-weather, semiresort arenas for the affluent, will be established in all portions of the country. Governmental participation in defraying the cost of long-term care will be obligatory and the evolution of federal and state as well as private insurance mechanisms for financing extended care can be anticipated.

To cope with this large population of demented individuals, additional specialization within the medical profession will be necessary. The number of physicians who specialize in the problems of aging and dementia will increase in step with the increase in the aged patient population. These specialists will combine knowledge of the medical problems of the aged with particular expertise in the diagnosis and management of dementing disorders.

Expertise in the management of dementia patients is necessarily transdisciplinary, requiring knowledge of geriatric medicine, neurology, psychiatry, and pharmacology. The practice of arrogating dementia by a particular medical specialty does a disservice to the complex needs of the patient and the caregiver. Moreover, multidisciplinary input is usually required with the services of experts in psychology, nursing, social work, gerontology, and rehabilitation medicine complementing the diagnostic and management skills of the physician.

Improvements in diagnostic accuracy of the dementias can be expected. Neuroimaging promises to offer greater specificity in diagnosis of individual disease states. Magnetic resonance spectroscopy will allow *in vitro* characterization of aspects of brain neurochemistry and diagnostic biochemical profiles will likely be developed. Radiolabeling of additional biochemical substrates that can be visualized with PET may allow improved diagnostic utility and facilitate study of metabolic function in dementing disorders. Assay of CSF metabolites and breakdown products may assume increasing diagnostic importance. Molecular biology and molecular genetics are rapidly gaining ascendance as the dominant approach to the study of neurobiological illnesses and advances can be anticipated in understanding the molecular events that lead to plaque, tangle, and amyloid production in DAT. Genetic diagnosis of DAT, including prenatal recognition of the individual who will develop the illness 60 or 70 years later, may be possible. Animal models of portions of the DAT process—such as amyloid production by cells harvested from trisomy-16 mice—will accelerate the pace of unraveling the molecular mechanisms of DAT.

In addition to being tragic illnesses that inflict inestimable suffering, DAT and related disorders are also valuable teachers and can serve as model disorders whose study can reveal important aspects of normal aging as well as providing information applicable to other disease states. Careful neuropsychological investigation of memory disturbances in cortical and subcortical dementias, for example, has provided validation of the cortical/subcortical classificatory approach and has produced insights into the mechanisms of normal and abnormal learning and memory. The failure of storage or very rapid loss from storage of information in DAT can be distinguished from the recall disturbances of patients with Huntington's and other subcortical diseases. These observations have confirmed the importance of the hippocampus in new learning and storage and directed attention to frontal-subcortical structures as the anatomical system mediating access to stored material. Study of psychosis in DAT and of depression in vascular dementia and Parkinson's disease may provide valuable information relevant to understanding schizophrenia and major mood disorders.

Treatment breakthroughs may substantially affect the course of DAT and other dementing illnesses. Until recently, treatment of degenerative diseases has been exclusively symptomatic, unable to affect the underlying disease process. Contemporary investigations of the use of selegiline in Parkinson's disease, however, suggest that this agent may intervene in the basic degenerative process. By inhibiting monoamine oxidase, selegiline decreases the production of hydroxyl radicals that destroy phospholipid membranes including those of neurons. Prevention of cellular death and rescue of failing neurons is a revolutionary therapeutic option; selegiline will serve as a prototype of other such agents. Antiamyloid agents could be considered as another approach to DAT therapy. While amyloid production is likely to result from other more basic changes, amyloid may be neurotoxic and elimination or reduction of the brain amyloid burden may stabilize or slow the disease. Progress in understanding the molecular biological aspects of DAT may lead to new therapies such as preemptive intervention in the processes leading to plaque and tangle formation. Transmitter replacement strategies are expected to be of limited utility given the degree of neuronal loss and dysfunction in degenerative disorders such as DAT, but there may be an as yet undefined window of therapeutic opportunity when optimization of the multiple transmitters involved in DAT would provide clinically meaningful improvement in function. Syphilis, tuberculosis, and polio have all appeared to be invincible foes of humanity in the past, and each has given way to the march of science. No less is expected for DAT and other dementing diseases.

References

Aaron AM, Freeman JM, Carter S. The natural history of Sydenham's chorea. Am J Med 1965;38:83–95.

Abd el Naby S, Hassanein. Neuropsychiatric manifestations of chronic manganese poisoning. J Neurol Neurosurg Psychiatry 1965;28:282–288.

Abend WK, Tyler HR. Thyroid disease and the nervous system. In: Aminoff MJ, ed. Neurology and general medicine. Churchill Livingstone, New York, 1989: 257–271.

Abramsky O. Common and uncommon neurological manifestations as presenting symptoms of vitamin B_{12} deficiency. J Am Geriatr Soc 1972;20:93–96.

Abramsky O, Lisak RP, Silberberg DH, Pleasure DE. Antibodies to oligodendroglia in patients with multiple sclerosis. N Engl J Med 1977;297:1207–1211.

Adachi M, Wellmann KF, Volk BW. Histochemical studies on the pathogenesis of idiopathic non-arteriosclerotic cerebral calcification. J Neuropathol Exp Neurol 1968;27:483–499.

Adam J, Crow TJ, Duchen LW, Scaravilli F, Spokes E. Familial cerebral amyloidosis and spongiform encephalopathy. J Neurol Neurosurg Psychiatry 1982;45:37–45.

Adams CWM, Bruton CJ. The cerebral vasculature in dementia pugilistica. J Neurol Neurosurg Psychiatry 1989;52:600–604.

Adams JH. Virus diseases of the nervous system. In: Blackwood W, Corsellis JAN, eds. Greenfield's neuropathology. Year Book Medical Publishers, Chicago, 1976:292–326.

Adams JH, Brierley JB, Connor RCR, Treip CS. The effects of systemic hypotension upon the human brain. Clinical and neuropathological observations on 11 cases. Brain 1966;89:235–267.

Adams JH, Graham DI, Murray LS, Scott G. Diffuse axonal injury due to nonmissile head injury in humans: An analysis of 45 cases. Ann Neurol 1982;12:557–563.

Adams M, Rhyner PA, Day J, De Armond S, Smuckler EA. Whipple's disease confined to the central nervous system. Ann Neurol 1987;21:104–108.

Adams RD. Diverticulation of the cerebral ventricles: a cause of progressive focal encephalopathy. Dev Med Child Neurol 1975a;17(suppl 35):135–137.

Adams RD. Diseases of muscle. 3rd ed. Harper & Row, New York, 1975b.

Adams RD, Fisher CM, Hakim S, Ojemann R, Sweet W. Symptomatic occult hydrocephalus with "normal" cerebrospinal fluid pressure: a treatable syndrome. N Engl J Med 1965;273:117–126.

Adams RD, Kubik CS. Subacute degeneration of the brain in pernicious anemia. N Engl J Med 1944;231:1–9.

Adams RD, Van Bogaert L, Vander Eecken H. Striato-nigral degeneration. J Neuropathol Exp Neurol 1964;23:584–608.

Adams RD, Victor M. Principles of neurology. McGraw-Hill, New York, 1977.

Adams RD, Victor M. Principles of neurology, 2nd ed. McGraw-Hill Book Company, New York, 1981.

Adams RD, Victor M. Principles of neurology, 4th ed. McGraw-Hill, New York, 1989.

Adams RD, Victor M, Mancall EL. Central pontine myelinolysis. Arch Neurol Psychiatry 1959;81:154–172.

Adeloye A. Spontaneous extrusion of the abdominal tube through the umbilicus complicating peritoneal shunt for hydrocephalus. J Neurosurg 1973;38:758–760.

Adler S. Methyldopa-induced decrease in mental activity. JAMA 1974;230:1428–1429.

Affleck DC, Treptow KR, Herrick HD. The effects of isoxsuprine hydrochloride (Vasodilan) on chronic cerebral arteriosclerosis. J Nerv Ment Dis 1961;132:335–338.

Agamanolis DP, Tan JS, Parker DL. Immunosuppressive measles encephalitis in a patient with a renal transplant. Arch Neurol 1979;36:686–690.

Aigner BR, Mulder DW. Myoclonus. Arch Neurol 1960;2:600–615.

Aisen AM, Martel W, Gabrielsen TO, Glazer GM, Brewer G, Young AB, Hill G. Wilson disease of the brain: MR imaging. Radiology 1985;157:137–141.

Aita JF, Bennett DR, Anderson RE, Ziter F. Cranial CT appearance of acute multiple sclerosis. Neurology 1978;28:251–255.

de Ajuriaguerra J, Tissot R. Some aspects of language in various forms of senile dementia (comparisons with language in childhood). In: Lenneberg EH, Lenneberg H, eds. Foundations of language development. A multidisciplinary approach, Vol 1. Academic Press, New York, 1975:323–339.

Akelaitis AJ. Hereditary form of primary parenchymatous atrophy of the cerebellar cortex associated with mental deficiency. Am J Psychiatry 1937–1938;94:1115–1140.

Akelaitis AJ. Lead encephalopathy in children and adults. J Nerv Ment Dis 1941; 93:313–332.

Akelaitis AJ. Atrophy of the basal ganglia in Pick's disease. Arch Neurol Psychiatry 1944;51:27–34.

Alberca R, Rafel E. Chinchon I, Vadillo J, Navarro A. Late onset parkinsonism in Hallervorden-Spatz disease. J Neurol Neurosurg Psychiatry 1987;50:1665–1668.

Albert ML. Treatment of pain in multiple sclerosis—preliminary report. N Engl J Med 1969;280:1395.

Albert ML. Subcortical dementia. In: Katzman R, Terry RD, Bick KL, eds. Alzheimer's disease, senile dementia and related disorders. Raven Press, New York, 1978:173–180.

Albert ML. Language in normal and dementing elderly. In: Obler LK, Albert ML, eds. Language and communication in the elderly. Lexington Books, Lexington, Mass.; 1980:145–150.

Albert ML, Changes in language with aging. Semin Neurol 1981;1(1):43–46.

Albert ML, Feldman RG, Willis AL. The "subcortical dementia" of progressive supranuclear palsy. J Neurol Neurosurg Psychiatry 1974;37:121–130.

Albert ML, Soffer D, Silverberg R, Reches A. The anatomic basis of visual agnosia. Neurology 1979;29:876–879.

Albert MS, Butters N, Brandt J. Patterns of remote memory in amnestic and demented patients. Arch Neurol 1981;38:495–500.

Albert MS, Butters N, Levin J. Temporal gradients in the retrograde amnesia of patients with alcoholic Korsakoff's disease. Arch Neurol 1979;36:211–216.

Albert MS, Kaplan E. Organic implications of neuropsychological deficits in the elderly. In: Poon LW, Fozard JL, Cermak LS, Erenberg D. Thompson LW, eds., New Directions in memory and aging: proceedings of the George A. Talland Memorial Conference. Lawrence Erlbaum Associates, New Jersey, 1980, pp 430–432.

Al Deeb SM, Yaqub BA, Sharif HS, Phadke JG. Neurobrucellosis: Clinical characteristics, diagnosis, and outcome. Neurology 1989;39:498–501.

Alexander FG, Selesnick ST. The history of psychiatry. New American Library, New York, 1966.

Alexander GE, DeLong MR, Strik PL. Parallel organization of functionally segregated circuits linking basal ganglia and cortex. Ann Rev Neurosci 1986;9:357–381.

Alexander MP. Traumatic brain injury. In: Benson DF, Blumer D, eds. Psychiatric aspects of neurologic disease, Vol 2. Grune & Stratton, New York, 1982:219–248.

Alexander MP. Clinical determination of mental competence—a theory and a retrospective study. Arch Neurol 1988;45:23–26.

Alexander MP, Schmitt MA. The aphasia syndrome of stroke in the left anterior cerebral artery territory. Arch Neurol 1980;37:97–100.

Alfrey AC, Legendre CR, Kaehny WD. The dialysis encephalopathy syndrome. Possible aluminum intoxication. N Engl J Med 1976;294:184–188.

Alfrey AC, Mishell JM, Burks J, et al. Syndrome of dyspraxia and multifocal seizures associated with chronic hemodialysis. Trans Am Soc Artif Intern Organs 1972;18:257–261.

Allen EM, Singer FR, Melamed D. Electroencephalographic abnormalities in hypercalcemia. Neurology 1970;20:15–22.

Allen N. Solvents and other industrial organic compounds. In: Vinken PJ, Bruyn GW, eds. Intoxications of the nervous system. Part I, vol. 36. Handbook of clinical neurology. North-Holland, New York, 1979:361–389.

Allen RM, Flemenbaum A. Delirium associated with combined fluphenazine-clonidine therapy. J Clin Psychiatry 1979;40:236–237.

Allen W. Inheritance of the shaking palsy. Arch Intern Med 1937;60:424–436.

Allison RS, Bedford PD, Meyer A. Discussion on the clinical consequences of cerebral anoxia. Proc R Soc Med 1956;49:609–622.

Allison T, Goff WR. Wood CC. Auditory, somatosensory and visual evoked potentials in the diagnosis of neuropathology. In: Lehman D, Calloway E, eds. Human evoked potentials: applications and problems. Plenum Press, New York, 1978:1–16.

Alpers BJ. A note on the mental syndrome of corpus callosum tumors. J Nerv Ment Dis 1936;84:621–627.

Alpers BJ. Relation of the hypothalamus to disorders of personality. Arch Neurol Psychiatry 1937;38:291–303.

Alpers BJ, Grant FC. The clinical syndrome of the corpus callosum. Arch Neurol Psychiatry 1931;25:67–86.

Alvord EC Jr. The pathology of Parkinsonism. Part II. An interpretation with special reference to other changes in the aging brain. In: McDowell FH, Markham CH, eds. Recent advances in Parkinson's disease. FA Davis, Philadelphia, 1971:131–161.

Alvord EC Jr, Forno LS, Kusske JA, Kauffman RJ, Rhodes JS, Goetowski CR. The pathology of parkinsonism: a comparison of degenerations in cerebral cortex and brainstem. Adv Neurol 1974;5:175–193.

Ambrose J. Computerized transverse axial scanning (tomography). Part 2. Clinical application. Br J Radiol 1973;46:1023–1047.

Ambrosetto C. Post-traumatic subdural hematoma. Arch Neurol 1962;6:287–292.

Ambrosetto G, Tassinari CA, Baruzzi A, Lugaresi E. Phenytoin encephalopathy as probable idiosyncratic reaction: case report. Epilepsia 1977;18:405–408.

Ambrosetto P, Kim, M. Progressive supranuclear palsy. Arch Neurol 1981;38:672.

American Psychiatric Association. Diagnostic and statistical manual of mental disorders. 3rd ed. American Psychiatric Press, Washington, D.C., 1980.

American Psychiatric Association. Diagnostic and statistical manual of mental disorders, revised 3rd edition. American Psychiatric Press, Washington, D.C. 1987.

Aminoff MJ, Marshall J, Smith EM, Wyke MA. Pattern of intellectual impairment in Huntington's chorea. Psychol Med 1975;5:169–172.

Anden N-E, Dalstrom A, Fuxe K, Larsson K, Olson L, Ungerstedt U. Ascending monoamine neurons to the telencephalon and diencephalon. Acta Physiol Scand 1966;67:313–326.

Andreason NJC, Olsen SA. Negative v positive schizophrenia. Arch Gen Psychiatry 1982;39:789–794.

Andreasen NJC, Olsen SA, Dennert JW, Smith MR. Ventricular enlargement in schizophrenia: relationship to positive and negative symptoms. Am J Psychiatry 1982;139:297–302.

Andreasen NJC, Pfohl B. Linguistic analysis of speech in affective disorders. Arch Gen Psychiatry 1976;33:1361–1367.

Anzil AP, Herrlinger H, Blinzinger K, Heldrich A. Ultrastructure of brain and nerve biopsy tissue in Wilson disease. Arch Neurol 1974;31:94–100.

Appell J, Kertesz A, Fishman M. A study of language functioning in Alzheimer patients. Brain Lang 1982;17:73–91.

Appel SH. A unifying hypothesis for the cause of amyotrophic lateral sclerosis, Parkinsonism and Alzheimer disease. Ann Neurol 1981;10:499–505.

Aquilonius S-M, Eckernas S-A. Choline therapy in Huntington chorea. Neurology 1977;27:887–889.

Aquilonius S-M, Sjostrom R. Cholinergic and dopaminergic mechanisms in Huntington's chorea. Life Sci 1971;10:405–414.

Arai H, Emson PC, Carrasco LH. Huntington's disease: changes in tachykinin content in postmortem brains. Ann Neurol 1987;22:587–594.

Arieff AI, Cooper JD, Armstrong D, Lazarowitz VC. Dementia, renal failure, and brain aluminum. Ann Intern Med 1979;90:741–747.

Arieff AI, Llach F, Massry SG. Neurological manifestations of hyponatremia: correlation with brain water and electrolytes. Medicine 1976;55:121–129.

Arieti S. Interpretation of schizophrenia. Basic Books, New York, 1974.

Arimitsu T, Jabbari B, Buckler RE, DiChiro G. Computed tomography in a verified case of tuberculous meningitis. Neurology 1979;29:384–386.

Aring CD. Observations on multiple sclerosis and conversion hysteria. Brain 1965;88:663–674.

Arlien-Soborg P, Bruhn P, Gyldensted C, Melgaard B. Chronic painter's syndrome. Acta Neurol Scand 1979;60:149–156.

Arnold BM, Casal G, Higgins HP. Apathetic thyrotoxicosis. Can Med Assoc J 1974;3:957–958.

Aronson MK, ed. Understanding Alzheimer's disease. Charles Scribners' Sons, New York, 1988.

Aronson SM, Aronson BE. Clinical neuropathological conference. Dis Nerv Syst 1973;34:124–130.

Arregui A, Bennett JP Jr, Bird ED, Yamamura HI, Iversen LL, Snyder SS. Huntington's chorea: selective depletion of activity of angiotensin converting enzyme in the corpus striatum. Ann Neurol 1977;2:294–298.

Arseni C, Nereantiu F, Horvath L. Ciurea V. Inclusion encephalitis evolving concomitantly with a cerebellar tumor in a child. Eur Neurol 1978;17:188–192.

Asher R. Myxoedematous madness. Br Med J 1949;2:555–562.

Asher SW, Aminoff MJ. Tetrabenazine and movement disorders. Neurology 1981; 31:1051–1054.

Ashworth B, Emery V. Cerebral dysrhythmia in disseminated sclerosis. Brain 1963;86:173–188.

Asken MJ, Hobson RW II. Intellectual change and carotid endarterectomy, subjective speculation or objective reality: a review. J Surg Res 1977;23:367–375.

Asnis G. Parkinson's disease, depression, and ECT: a review and case report. Am J Psychiatry 1977;134:191–195.

Asso D. WAIS scores in a group of parkinson patients. Br J Psychiatry 1969;115:555–556.

Atack JR, May C. Kaye JA, Kay AD, Rapoport SI. Cerebrospinal fluid cholinesterases in aging and in dementia of the Alzheimer type. Ann Neurol 1988;23:161–167.

Au WJ, Gabor AJ, Vijayan N, Markand O. Periodic lateralized epileptiform complexes (PLEDs) in Creutzfeldt-Jakob disease. Neurology 1980;30:611–617.

Auborg P, Sellier N, Chaussain JL, Kalifa G. MRI detects cerebral involvement in neurologically asymptomatic patients with adrenoleukodystrophy. Neurology 1989;39:1619–1621.

Aurbach GD. Parathyroid. In: Beeson PB, McDermott W, eds. Cecil-Loeb: textbook of medicine. 13th ed. WB Saunders, Philadelphia, 1971:1846–1855.

Austen FK, Carmichael MW, Adams RD. Neurologic manifestations of chronic pulmonary insufficiency. N. Engl J Med 1957;257:579–590.

Austin J, Armstrong D, Fouch S, et al. Metachromatic leukodystophy (MLD). Arch Neurol 1968;18:225–240.

Avery TL. Seven cases of frontal tumour with psychiatric presentation. Br J Psychiatry 1971;119:19–23.

Avorn J, Dreyer P, Connelly K, Soumerai SB. Use of psychoactive medication and the quality of care in rest homes. N Engl J Med 1989;320:227–232.

Avram MM, Feinfeld DA, Huatuco AH. Search for the uremic toxin. N Engl J Med 1978;298:1000–1003.

Babbitt DP, Tang T, Dobbs J, Berk R. Idiopathic familial cerebrovascular ferrocalcinosis (Fahr's disease) and review of differential diagnosis of intracranial calcification in children. Am J Roentgenol 1969;105:352–358.

Babior BM, Bunn HF. Megaloblastic anemias. In: Braunwald E, Isselbacher KJ, Petersdorf RG, Wilson JD, Martin JB, Fauci AS, eds. Harrison's principles of internal medicine, 11th ed. McGraw-Hill Book Company, New York, 1987;1498–1504.

Bacchus M. Encephalopathy in pulmonary disease. Arch Intern Med 1958;102:194–198.

Bailey P, Baker AB, eds. Sequelae of the arthropod-borne encephalitides. Neurology 1958;8:878–896.

Baker HL, Campbell JK, Houser DW. Computer-assisted tomography of the head. Mayo Clin Proc 1974;49:17–27.

Bala Manyam NV, Hare TA, Katz L, Glaeser BS. Huntington's disease. Cerebrospinal fluid GABA levels in at-risk individuals. Arch Neurol 1978;35:728–730.

Balajthy B. Symptomatology of the temporal lobe in Pick's convolutional atrophy. Acta Med Acad Sci Hung 1964;20:310–316.

Baldessarini RJ. The basis for amine hypotheses in affective disorders. Arch Gen Psychiatry 1975;32:1087–1093.

Baldessarini RJ. Chemotherapy in psychiatry. Harvard University Press, Cambridge, Mass., 1977a.

Baldessarini RJ. Schizophrenia. N Engl J Med 1977b;297:988–995.

Baldessarini RJ, Lipinski JF. Lithium salts: 1970–1975. Ann Intern Med 1975;83:527–533.

Baldwin JN, Dalessio DJ. Folic acid therapy and spinal-cord degeneration in pernicious anemia. N Engl J Med 1961;164:1339–1342.

Ball JAC, Taylor AR. Effect of cyclandelate on mental function and cerebral blood flow in elderly patients. Br Med J 1967;3:525–528.

Ball MJ. Topography of Pick inclusion bodies in hippocampi of demented patients. J Neuropathol Exp Neurol 1979;38:614–620.

Ball MJ, Griffin-Brooks S, MacGregor J, Nagy B, Ojalvo-Rose E, Fewster PH.

Neuropathological definition of Alzheimer's disease: multivariate analyses in the morphometric distinction between Alzheimer dementia and normal aging. Alzheimer Disease and Associated Disorders 1988; 2(1):29–37.

Ball MJ, Nuttall K. Neurofibrillary tangles, granulovacuolar degeneration, and neuron loss in Down syndrome: quantitative comparison with Alzheimer dementia. Ann Neurol 1980;7:462–465.

Ballard PA, Tetrud JW, Langston JW. Permanent human parkinsonism due to 1-methyl-4-phenyl-1,2,3,6-tetrahydropyridine (MPTP): seven cases. Neurology 1985;35:949–956.

Ballenger JC, Post RM. Carbamazepine in manic-depressive illness: a new treatment. Am J Psychiatry 1980;137:782–790.

Balo J. Encephalitis periaxialis concentrica. Arch Neurol Psychiatry 1928;19:242–264.

Baloh RW, Yee RD, Boder E. Eye movements in ataxia-telangiectasia. Neurology 1978;28:1099–1104.

Bamford KA, Caine ED, Kido DK, Plassche WM, Shoulson I. Clinical-pathologic correlation in Huntington's disease: a neuropsychological and computed tomography study. Neurology 1989;39:796–801.

Banerji NK, Millar JHD. Chiari malformations presenting in adult life. Brain 1974;97:157–168.

Bank WJ, Pleasure DE, Suzuki K, Nigro M, Katz R. Thallium poisoning. Arch Neurol 1972;26:456–464.

Bannister R, Gilford E, Kocen R. Isotope encephalography in the diagnosis of dementia due to communicating hydrocephalus. Lancet 1967;2:1014–1017.

Bannister R, Oppenheimer DR. Degenerative diseases of the nervous system associated with autonomic failure. Brain 1972;95:457–474.

Baratz R, Herzog AG. The communication disorder in dialysis dementia: a case report. Brain Lang 1980;10:378–389.

Barbeau A. L-dopa in juvenile Huntington's disease. Lancet 1969;2:1066.

Barbeau A, Friesen H. Treatment of Wilson's disease with L-dopa after failure with penicillamine. Lancet 1970;1:1180–1181.

Barclay L, Zemcov A, Blass JP, McDowell F. Rates of decrease of cerebral blood flow in progressive dementias. Neurology 1984;34:1555–1560.

Barclay L, Zemcov A, Blass JP, Sansone J. Survival in Alzheimer's disease and vascular dementia. Neurology 1985a;35:834–840.

Barclay L, Zemcov A, Reichert W, Blass JP. Cerebral blood flow decrements in chronic head injury syndrome. Biol Psychiatry 1985b;20:146–157.

Bareggi SR, Franceschi M, Bonini L, Zecca L, Smirne S. Decreased CSF concentrations of homovanillic acid and gamma-aminobutyric acid in Alzheimer's disease. Arch Neurol 1982;39:709–712.

Baringer JR, Gajdusek C, Gibbs CS Jr. Masters CL, Stern WE, Terry RD. Transmissible dementias: current problems in tissue handling. Neurology 1980;30:302–303.

Barker MG, Lawson JS. Nominal aphasia in dementia. Br J Psychiatry 1968;114:1351–1356.

Barkley DS, Hardiwidjaja S, Menkes JH. Abnormalities in growth of skin fibroblasts of patients with Huntington's disease. Ann Neurol 1977;1:426–430.

Barr AN, Fischer JH, Koller WC, Spunt AL, Singhal A. Serum haloperidol concentration and choreiform movements in Huntington's disease. Neurology 1988;38:84–88.

Barr AN, Heinze WJ, Dobben GD, Valvassori GE, Sugar O. Bicaudate index in computerized tomography in Huntington disease and cerebral atrophy. Neurology 1978a;28:1196–1200.

Barr AN, Heinze W, Mendoza JE, Perlik S. Long term treatment of Huntington disease with L-glutamate and pyridoxine. Neurology 1978b;28:1280–1282.

Barrett AM. A case of Alzheimer's disease with unusual neurological disturbances. J Nerv Ment Dis 1913;40:361–374.

Barron KD, Siguerra E, Hirano A. Cerebral embolism caused by nonbacterial thrombotic endocarditis. Neurology 1960;10:391–397.

Barry PP, Moskowitz MA. The diagnosis of reversible dementia in the elderly. Arch Intern Med 1988;148:1914–1918.

Bass NH, Hess HH, Pope A. Altered cell membranes in Creutzfeldt-Jakob disease. Arch Neurol 1974;31:174–182.

Bauer WR, Turel AP Jr, Johnson KP. Progressive multifocal leukoencephalopathy and cytarabine. JAMA 1973;226:174–176.

Baxter LR Jr, Schwartz JM, Phelps ME, Mazziotta JC, Guze BH, Selin CE, Gerner RH, Sumida RM. Reduction of prefrontal cortex glucose metabolism common to three types of depression. Arch Gen Psychiatry 1989;46:243–250.

Bayles KA, Tomoeda CK. Confrontation naming impairment in dementia. Brain Lang 1983;19:98–114.

Bayles KA, Tomoeda CK, Kaszniak AW, Stern LZ, Eagans KK. Verbal perseveration of dementia patients. Brain Lang 1985;25:102–116.

Beal MF, Kleinman GM, Ojemann RG, Hochberg FH. Gangliocytoma of the third ventricle: hyperphagia, somnolence, and dementia. Neurology 1981a;31:1224–1228.

Beal MF, Mazurek MF. Substance P-like immunoreactivity is reduced in Alzheimer's disease cerebral cortex. Neurology 1987;37:1205–1209.

Beal MF, Mazurek MF, Ellison DW, Swartz KJ, McGarvey U, Bird ED, Martin JB. Somatostatin and neuropeptide Y concentrations in pathologically graded cases of Huntington's disease. Ann Neurol 1988;23:562–569.

Beal MF, Mazurek MF, Svendsen CN, Bird ED, Martin JB. Widespread reduction of somatostatin-like immunoreactivity in the cerebral cortex in Alzheimer's disease. Ann Neurol 1986;20:489–495.

Beal MF, Williams RS, Richardson EP Jr, Fisher CM. Cholesterol embolism as a cause of transient ischemic attacks and cerebral infarction. Neurology 1981b; 31:860–865.

Beard AW. The association of hepatolenticular degeneration with schizophrenia. Acta Psychiatr Neurol 1959;34:411–428.

Beatty PA, Gange JJ. Neuropsychological aspects of multiple sclerosis. J Nerv Ment Dis 1977;164:42–50.

Beatty WW, Goodkin DE, Monson N, Beatty PA. Cognitive disturbances in patients with relapsing remitting multiple sclerosis. Arch Neurol 1989;46:1113–1119.

Beatty WW, Goodkin DE, Monson N, Beatty PA, Hertsgaard D. Anterograde and retrograde amnesia in patients with chronic progressive multiple sclerosis. Arch Neurol 1988a;45:611–619.

Beatty WW, Salmon DP, Butters N, Heindel WC, Granholm EL. Retrograde amnesia in patients with Alzheimer's disease or Huntington's disease. Neurobiol Aging 1988b;9:181–186.

Bebb GL. A study of memory deterioration in encephalitis lethargica. J Nerv Ment Dis 1925;61:356–365.

Bechar M, Lakke JPWF, van der Hem GK, Beks JWF, Penning L. Subdural hematoma during long-term hemodialysis. Arch Neurol 1972;26:513–516.

Beck AT. Thinking and depression: idiosyncratic content and cognitive disorders. Arch Gen Psychiatry 1963;9:324–333.

Begeer JH, Haaxma R, Snoek JW, Boonstra S, le Coultre R. Signs of focal posterior cerebral abnormality in early subacute sclerosing panencephalitis. Ann Neurol 1986;19:200–202.

Behan PO, Behan WMH. Possible immunological factors in Alzheimer's disease. In: Glen AIM, Whalley LJ, eds. Alzheimer's disease. Early recognition of potentially reversible deficits. Churchill Livingstone, London, 1979:33–35.

Behan PO, Feldman RG. Serum proteins, amyloid, and Alzheimer's disease. J Am Geriatr Soc 1970;18:792–797.

Behrman S, Carroll JD, Janota I, Matthews WB. Progressive supranuclear palsy. Brain 1969;92:663–678.

Bell JA, Hodgson HJF. Coma after cardiac arrest. Brain 1974;97:361–372.

Bell WE, McCormick WF. Increased intracranial pressure in children. WB Saunders, Philadelphia, 1972.

Bellin EL, Silva M, Lawyer T Jr. Central nervous system histoplasmosis in a Puerto Rican. Neurology 1962;12:148–152.

Belloni G, di Rocco C, Focacci C, Galli G, Maira G, Rossi GF. Surgical indications in normotensive hydrocephalus. A retrospective analysis of the relations of some diagnostic findings to the results of surgical treatment. Acta Neurochir 1976;33:1–21.

Belman AL, Lantos G, Horoupian D, Novick BE, Ultman MH, Dickson DW, Rubinstein A. AIDS: calcification of the basal ganglia in infants and children. Neurology 1986;36:1192–1199.

Benedek S, McGovern VJ. A case of Alzheimer's disease with amyloidosis of the vessels of the cerebral cortex. Med J Aust 1949;2:429–430.

Bennett AE, Mowery GL, Fort JT. Brain damage from chronic alcoholism: the diagnosis of intermediate stage of alcoholic brain disease. Am J Psychiatry 1960;116:705–711.

Bennett JC, Maffly RH, Steinbach HL. The significance of bilateral basal ganglia calcification. Radiology 1959;72:368–377.

Bennett JE. Chemotherapy of systemic mycoses. N Engl J Med 1974;290:320–322.

Bennett JE, Dismukes WE, Duma RJ, et al. A comparison of amphotericin B alone and combined with flucytosine in the treatment of cryptococcal meningitis. N Engl J Med 1979;301:126–131.

Benson DF. Fluency in aphasia: correlation with radioactive scan localization. Cortex 1967;3:373–394.

Benson DF: Normal pressure hydrocephalus: a controversial entity. Geriatrics 1974;29:126–132.

Benson DF. The hydrocephalic dementias. In: Benson DF, Blumer D, eds. Psychiatric aspects of neurologic disease. Grune & Stratton, New York, 1975:83–97.

Benson DF. Amnesia. South Med J 1978;71:1221–1228.

Benson DF. Aphasia, alexia, and agraphia. Churchill Livingstone, New York, 1979a.

Benson DF. Neurologic correlates of anomia. In: Whitaker H, Whitaker HA, eds. Studies in neurolinguistics. Vol. 4. Academic Press, New York, 1979b:298–328.

Benson DF. The use of positron emission scanning techniques in the diagnosis of Alzheimer's disease. In: Corkin S, Davis KL, Growdon JH, Usdin E, Wurtman RJ. eds. Alzheimer's disease: a report of progress in research. Raven Press, New York, 1982a:79–82.

Benson DF. The treatable dementias. In: Benson DF. Blumer D, eds. Psychiatric aspects of neurologic disease, Vol. 2. Grune & Stratton, New York, 1982b:123–148.

Benson DF. Parkinsonian dementia. Cortical or subcortical? In: Hassler RG, Christ JF, eds. Advances in neurology, vol. 40: Parkinsonian-specific motor and mental disorders. Raven Press, New York, 1984:235–240.

Benson DF. Hydrocephalic dementia. In: Frederiks JAM, ed. Handbook of clinical neurology, 2nd ed., Vol. 46: Neurobehavioral disorders. Elsevier Science Publishers, Amsterdam, 1985:323–333.

Benson DF. Disorders of verbal expression in neuropsychiatry. In: Reynolds EH, Trimble M, eds. The bridge between neurology and psychiatry. Churchill Livingstone, London, 1989:88–105.

Benson DF. Psychomotor retardation. Neuropsychiatry, Neuropsychol, Behav Neurol 1990;3:36–47.

Benson DF, Barton MI. Disturbances in constructional ability. Cortex 1970;6:19–46.

Benson DF, Blumer D. Amnesia: A clinical approach to memory. In: Benson DF, Blumer D, eds. Psychiatric aspects of neurologic disease. Vol. 2. Grune and Stratton, New York, 1982:251–277.

Benson DF, Cummings JL, Kuhl DE. Dementia: cortical-subcortical. Neurology 1981a;31:101.

Benson DF, Cummings JL, Tsai SY. Angular gyrus syndrome simulating Alzheimer disease. Arch Neurol 1982;39:616–620.

Benson DF, Davis RJ, Snyder BD. Posterior cortical atrophy. Arch Neurol 1988; 45:789–793.

Benson DF, Geschwind N. Shrinking retrograde amnesia. J. Neurol Neurosurg Psychiatry 1967;30:539–544.

Benson DF, Geschwind N. Psychiatric conditions associated with focal lesions of the central nervous system. In: Arieti S, Reiser M, eds. American handbook of psychiatry, Vol. 4 Basic Books, New York, 1975:208–243.

Benson DF, Geschwind N. The aphasias and related disturbances. In: Baker AB, Baker LH, eds. Clinical neurology, Vol. 1. Harper and Row, New York, 1976:1–28.

Benson DF, Kuhl DE, Hawkins RA, Phelps ME, Cummings JL, Tsai SY. Positron computed tomography in the diagnosis of dementia. Ann Neurol 1981b;10:76.

Benson DF, Kuhl DE, Hawkins RA, Phelps ME, Cummings JL, Tsai SY. The fluorodeoxyglucose 18F scan in Alzheimer's disease and multi-infarct dementia. Arch Neurol 1983;40:711–714.

Benson DF, LeMay M, Patten DH, Rubens AB. Diagnosis of normal-pressure hydrocephalus. N Engl J Med 1970;283:609-615.

Benson DF, Marsden CD, Meadows JC. The amnestic syndrome of posterior cerebral artery occlusion. Acta Neutrol Scand 1974a;50:133–145.

Benson DF, Segarra J, Albert ML. Visual agnosia-prosopagnosia. A clinicopathologic correlation. Arch Neurol 1974b;30:307–310.

Benson DF, Stuss DT. Motor abilities after frontal leukotomy. Neurology 1982; 32:1353–1357.

Benson DF, Tomlinson EB. Hemiplegic syndrome of the posterior cerebral artery. Stroke 1971;2:559–564.

Bentson JR, Keesey JC. Pneumoencephalography of progressive supranuclear palsy. Radiology 1974;113:89–94.

Berciano J. Olivopontocerebellar atrophy. a review of 117 cases. J Neurol Sci 1982;53:253–272.

Berent S, Giordani B, Lehtinen S, Markel D, Penney JB, Buchtel HA, Starosta-Rubinstein S, Hichwa R, Young AB, Positron emission tomographic scan investigations of Huntington's disease: cerebral metabolic correlates of cognitive function. Ann Neurol 1988;23:541–546.

Beresin EV. Delirium in the elderly. J Geriatr Psychiatry Neurol 1988;1:127–143.

Berg L, Hughes CP, Cuben LA, Danziger WL, Martin RL, Knesevich J. Mild senile dementia of Alzheimer type: research diagnostic criteria, recruitment, and description of a study population. J Neurol Neurosurg Psychiatry 1982;45:926–968.

Berger JR, Ayyar R. Neurological complications of ethylene glycol intoxications. Arch Neurol 1981;38:724–726.

Berger JR, Ross DB. Reversible Parkinson syndrome complicating postoperative hypoparathyroidism. Neurology 1981;31:881–882.

Bergin JD. Rapidly progressing dementia in disseminated sclerosis. J Neurol Neurosurg Psychiatry 1957;20:285–292.

Bergmann K, Foster EM, Justice AW, Matthews V. Management of the demented elderly patient in the community. Br J Psychiatry 1978;132:441–449.

Bergvall V, Galera R. Time relationship between subarachnoid hemorrhage, arterial spasm, changes in circulation and posthemorrhagic hydrocephalus. Acta Radiol (Diagn) (Stockh) 1969;9:229–237.

Beringer VM, Beringer J, Salen G, Shefer S, Zimmerman RD. Computed tomography in cerebrotendinous xanthomatosis. Neurology 1981;31:1463–1465.

Berl T, Anderson RJ, McDonald KM, Schrier RW. Clinical disorders of water metabolism. Kidney Int 1976;10:117–132.

Berlin L. Presenile sclerosis (Alzheimer's disease) with features resembling Pick's disease. Arch Neurol Psychiatry 1949;61:369–384.

Berlyne N. Confabulation. Brit J Psychiatry 1972;120:31–39.

Bernoulli C, Siegfried J, Baumgartner G, et al. Danger of accidental person-to-person transmission of Creutzfeldt-Jakob disease by surgery. Lancet 1977;1:478–479.

Bes A, Guell A, Fabre N, Dupui Ph, Victor G, Geraud G. Cerebral blood flow studied by xenon-133 inhalation technique in parkinsonism: loss of hyperfrontal pattern. J Cereb Blood Flow Metab 1983;3:33–37.

Betts TA. Depression, anxiety, and epilepsy. In: Reynolds EH, Trimble MR, eds. Epilepsy and psychiatry. Churchill Livingstone, New York, 1981;60–71.

Betts TA, Smith WT, Kelly RE. Adult metachromatic leukodystrophy (sulphatide lipidosis) simulating acute schizophrenia. Neurology 1968;18:1140–1142.

Bharucha NE, Bharucha EP, Bhabha SK. Machado-Joseph-Azorean disease in India. Arch Neurol 1986;43:142–144.

Bianchine JR. Drug therapy of parkinsonism. N Engl J Med 1976;295:814–818.

Bickel H, Neale FC, Hall G. A clinical and biochemical study of hepatolenticular degeneration (Wilson's disease). Q J Med 1957;26:527–558.

Bicknell JM, Holland JV. Neurologic manifestations of Cogan syndrome. Neurology 1978;28:278–281.

Biemond A. On Binswanger's subcortical arteriosclerotic encephalopathy and the possibility of its clinical recognition. Psychiatr Neurol Neurochir 1970;73:413–417.

Bienfeld D, Hartford JT. Pseudodementia in an elderly woman with schizophrenia. Am J Psychiatry 1982;139:114–115.

Binns JK, Robertson EE. Pick's disease in old age. J Ment Sci 1962;108:804–810.

Bird ED, Mackay AVP, Rayner CN, Iversen LL. Reduced glutamic-acid-decarboxylase activity of post-mortem brain in Huntington's chorea. Lancet 1973;1:1090–1092.

Bird ED, Spokes EGS, Iversen LL. Increased dopamine concentration in limbic areas of brain from patients dying with schizophrenia. Brain 1979;102:347–360.

Bird MT, Paulson GW. The rigid form of Huntington's chorea. Neurology 1971;21:271–276.

Bird TD, Cederbaum S, Valpey RW, Stahl WL. Familial degeneration of the basal ganglia with acanthocytosis: a clinical neuropathological and neurochemical study. Ann Neurol 1978;3:253–258.

Bird TD, Koerker RM, Leaird BT, Vleck BW, Thorning DR. Lipomembranous polycystic osteodysplasia (brain, bone, and fat disease): A genetic cause of presenile dementia. Neurology 1983;33:81–86.

Birren JE. Translation in gerontology—from lab to life: psychophysiology and speed of response. Am Psychol 1974;29:808–815.

Bittenbender JB, Quadfasel FA. Rigid and akinetic forms of Huntington's chorea. Arch Neurol 1962;7:275–288.

Black JA, Fariello RG, Chun RW. Brainstem auditory evoked response in adrenoleukodystrophy. Ann Neurol 1979;6:269–270.

Blass JP, Gibson GE. Abnormality of thiamine-requiring enzyme in patients with Wernicke-Korsakoff syndrome. N Engl J Med 1977;297:1367–1370.

Blass JP, Kark RAP, Menon NK. Low activities of the pyruvate and oxoglutarate dehydrogenase complexes in five patients with Friedreich's ataxia. N Engl J Med 1976;295:62–67.

Blazer DG II, Federspiel CF, Ray WA, Schaffner W. The risk of anticholinergic toxicity in the elderly: a study of prescribing practices in two populations. J Gerontol 1983;38:31–35.

Blessed G, Tomlinson BE, Roth M. The association between quantitative measures of dementia and of senile change in the cerebral grey matter of elderly subjects. Br J Psychiatry 1968;114:797–811.

Bleuler M. Acute mental concomitants of physical diseases. In: Benson DF, Blumer

D, eds. Psychiatric Aspects of Neurologic Disease. Grune & Stratton, New York, 1975;37–61.

Blumbergs P, Beran R, Hicks P. Myoclonus in Down's syndrome. Arch Neurol 1981;38:453–544.

Blumenthal H, Miller C. Motor nuclear involvement in progressive supranuclear palsy. Arch Neurol 1969;20:362–367.

Blusewicz MJ, Dustman RE, Schenkenberg T, Beck EC. Neuropsychological correlates of chronic alcoholism and aging. J Nerv Ment Dis 1977;165:348–355.

Bockner S, Coltart N. New cases of GPI. Br Med J 1961;1:18–20.

Bodensteiner JB, Goldblum RM, Goldman AS. Progressive dystonia masking ataxia in ataxia-telangiectasia. Arch Neurol 1980;37:464–465.

Bodis-Wollner I, Yahr MD. Measurements of visual evoked potentials in Parkinson's disease. Brain 1978;101:661–671.

Bogdanoff B, Natter HM. Incidence of cavum septum pellucidum in adults: a sign of boxer's encephalopathy. Neurology 1989;39:991–992.

Bokobza B, Ruberg M, Scatton B, Javoy-Agid F, Agid Y. [3H]Spiperone binding, dopamine and HVA concentrations in Parkinson's disease and supranuclear palsy. Eur J Pharmacol 1984;99:167–175.

Boller F. Mental status of patients with Parkinson's disease. J Clin Neuropsychol 1980;2:157–172.

Boller F, Boller M, Denes G, Timberlake WH, Zieper I, Albert ML. Familial palilalia. Neurology 1973;23:1117–1125.

Boller F, Lopez OL, Moossy J. Diagnosis of dementia: clinicopathologic correlations. Neurology 1989;39:76–79.

Boller F, Mizutani T, Roessmann V, Gambetti P. Parkinson disease, dementia, and Alzheimer disease: clinicopathological correlations. Ann Neurol 1980;7:329–335.

Boller F, Passafiume D, Keefe NC, Rogers K, Morrow L, Kim Y. Visuospatial impairment in Parkinson's disease. Role of perceptual and motor factors. Arch Neurol 1984;41:485–490.

Bondareff W, Baldy R, Levy R. Quantitative computed tomography in senile dementia. Arch Gen Psychiatry 1981;38:1365–1368.

Bondareff W, Mountjoy CQ, Roth M. Loss of neurons of origin of the adrenergic projection to cerebral cortex (nucleus locus ceruleus) in senile dementia. Neurology 1982;32:164–168.

Bondareff W, Mountjoy CQ, Roth M, Rossor MN, Iversen LL, Reynolds GP. Age and histopathologic heterogeneity in Alzheimer's disease. Arch Gen Psychiatry 1987;44:412–417.

Bondy PK. Hypoglycemic states. In: Beeson PB, McDermont W, eds. Cecil-Loeb: textbook of medicine. 13th ed. WB Saunders, Philadelphia, 1971:1656–1659.

Bornstein RA, Pakainis A, Drake ME, Suga LJ. Effects of seizure type and waveform abnormality on memory and attention. Arch Neurol 1988;45:884–887.

Bosch EP, Hart MN. Late adult-onset metachromatic leukodystrophy. Arch Neurol 1978;35:475–477.

Botez MI, Botez T, Maag U. The Wechsler subtests in mild organic brain damage associated with folate deficiency. Psychol Med 1984;14:431–437.

Botwinick J. Intellectual abilities. In: Birren JE, Schaie KW, eds. Handbook of the psychology of aging. Van Nostrand, New York, 1977:580–605.

Bouchard JP, Barbeau A, Bouchard R, Bouchard RW. Autosomal recessive spastic ataxia of Charlevoix-Saquenay. Can J Neurol Sci 1978;5:61–69.

Bouton SM Jr. Pick's disease: clinicopathologic case reports. J Nerv Ment Dis 1940;91:9–30.

Bowen DL, Lane HC, Fauci AS. Immunopathogenesis of the acquired immunodeficiency syndrome. Ann Int Med 1985;103:704–709.

Bowen DM, Davison AN. Changes in brain lysosomal activity, neurotransmitter-related enzymes and other proteins in senile dementia. In: Katzman R, Terry RD, Bick KL, eds. Alzheimer's disease, senile dementia and related disorders. Raven Press, New York, 1978:421–426.

Bowen DM, Sims NR, Benton S, et al. Biochemical changes in cortical brain biopsies from demented patients in relation to morphological findings and pathogenesis. In: Corkin S, Davis KL, Growdon JH et al. Alzheimer's disease: A report of progress in research. Raven Press, New York, 1982:1–8.

Bowen DM, Smith CB, White P, Davison AN. Neurotransmitter-related enzymes and indices of hypoxia in senile dementia and other abiotrophies. Brain 1976;99:459–496.

Bowen FP, Kamienny RS, Burns MM, Yahr MD. Parkinsonism: effects of levodopa treatment on concept formation. Neurology 1975;25:701–704.

Boyd DA. A contribution to the psychopathology of Alzheimer's disease. Am J Psychiatry 1936–1937;93:155–175.

Boyd PR, Walker G, Henderson IN. The treatment of tetraethyl lead poisoning. Lancet 1957;1:181–185.

Boyd WD, Graham-White J, Blackwood J, Glen I, McQueen J. Clinical effects of choline in Alzheimer presenile dementia. Lancet 1977;2:711.

Boyer SH IV, Chisholm AW, McKusick VA. Cardiac aspects of Friedreich's ataxia. Circulation 1962;25:493–505.

Bradley WG Jr, Waluch V, Brant-Zawadzki M, Yadley RA, Wycoff RR. Patchy, periventricular white matter lesions in the elderly: A common observation during NMR imaging. Noninvasive Medical Imaging 1984;1:35–41.

Braham J. Jakob-Creutzfeldt disease: treatment by amantadine. Br Med J 1971;4:212–213.

Brain L. The neurological complications of neoplasms. Lancet 1963;1:179–184.

Brain L, Walton JN. Brain's diseases of the nervous system, 7th ed. Oxford University Press, London, 1969.

Brain L, Wilkinson M. Subacute cerebellar degeneration associated with neoplasms. Brain 1965;88:465–478.

Brain WR, Daniel PM, Greenfield JG. Subacute cortical cerebellar degeneration and its relation to carcinoma. J Neurol Neurosurg Psychiatry 1951;14:59–75.

Branconnier RJ, Cole JD. Effects of chronic papaverine administration on mild senile organic brain syndrome. J Am Geriatr Soc 1977;25:458–462.

Brandt J, Butters N, Ryan C, Bayog R. Cognitive loss and recovery in long-term alcohol abusers. Arch Gen Psychiatry 1983;40:435–442.

Brandt J, Folstein ME, Folstein MF. Differential cognitive impairment in Alzheimer's disease and Huntington's disease. Ann Neurol 1988;23:555–561.

Brandt KD, Lessell S, Cohen AS. Cerebral disorders of vision in systemic lupus erythematosus. Ann Intern Med 1975;83:163–169.

Brant-Zawadzki M, Fein G, Van Dyke C, Kiernan R, Davenport L, de Groot J. MR imaging of the aging brain: patchy white-matter lesions and dementia. Am J Neuroradiol 1985;6:675–682.

Breig A, Ekbom K, Greitz T, Kugelberg E. Hydrocephalus due to elongated basilar artery. Lancet 1967;1:874–875.

Breitner JCS, Folstein MF. Familial Alzheimer dementia: a prevalent disorder with specific clinical features. Psychol Med 1984;14:63–80.

Breitner JCS, Silverman JM, Mohs RC, Davis KL. Familial aggregation in Alzheimer's disease: comparison of risk among relatives of early- and late-onset cases, and among male and female relatives in successive generations. Neurology 1988;38:207–212.

Brenner RP, Snyder RD. Late EEG findings and clinical status after organic mercurial poisoning. Arch Neurol 1980;37:282–284.

Brenner RP, Ulrich RF, Spiker DG, Sclabassi RJ, Reynolds CF III, Marin RS, Boller F. Computerized EEG spectral analysis in elderly normal, demented, and depressed subjects. EEG Clin Neurophysiol 1986;64:483–492.

Bresnan MJ, Richardson EP Jr. Case 18-1979. N Engl J Med 1979;300:1037–1045.

Brewer C, Perrett L. Brain damage due to alcohol consumption: an air-encephalographic, psychometric and electroencephalographic study. Br J Addict 1971;66:170–182.

Brewer GJ, Terry CA, Aisen AM, Hill GM. Worsening of neurologic syndrome in patients with Wilson's disease with initial penicillamine therapy. Arch Neurol 1987;44:490–493.

Brierley JB. Cerebral hypoxia. In: Blackwood W, Corsellis JAN, eds. Greenfield's neuropathology. Year Book Medical Publishers, Chicago, 1976:43–85.

Brierley JB, Corsellis JAN, Hierons R, Nevin S. Subacute encephalitis of later adult life mainly affecting the limbic areas. Brain 1960;83:357–368.

Brierley JB, Graham DI, Adams JH, Simpson JA. Neocortical death after cardiac arrest. Lancet 1971;2:560–565.

Briley DP, Coull BM, Goodnight SH Jr. Neurological disease associated with antiphospholipid antibodies. Ann Neurol 1989;25:221–227.

Brinkman SD, Largen JW Jr. Changes in brain ventricular size with repeated CAT scans in suspected Alzheimer's disease. Am J Psychiatry 1984;141:81–83.

British Medical Journal. Editorial: Dangerous antihypertensive treatment. Br Med J 1979;2:228–229.

Brody IA, Chase TN, Gordon EK. Depressed monoamine catabolite levels in cerebrospinal fluid of patients with parkinsonism dementia of Guam. N Engl J Med 1970;282:947–950.

Brody JA, Wilkins RH. Wernicke's encephalopathy. Arch Neurol 1968;19:228–232.

Broe GA, Caird FI. Levodopa for parkinsonism in elderly and demented patients. Med J Aust 1973;1:630–635.

Bronsky D, Kushner DS, Dubin A, Snapper I. Idiopathic hypoparathyroidism and pseudohypoparathyroidism: case reports and review of the literature. Medicine 1958;37:317–352.

Brouwers P, Cox C, Martin A, Chase T, Fedio P. Differential perceptual-spatial impairment in Huntington's and Alzheimer's dementias. Arch Neurol 1984; 41:1073–1076.

Brown DG, Goldensohn ES. The electroencephalogram in normal pressure hydrocephalus. Arch Neurol 1973;29:70–71.

Brown GLaV, Wilson WP. Parkinsonism and depression. South Med J 1972;65:540–545.

Brown JJ, Hesselink JR, Rothrock JF. MR and CT of lacunar infarcts. Am J Radiol 1988;151:367–372.

Brown JR. Diseases of the cerebellum. In: Baker AB, Baker LH, eds. Clinical neurology. Harper & Row, New York, 1971;1–38.

Brown P, Cathala F, Castaigne P, Gajdusek DC. Creutzfeldt-Jakob disease: Clinical analysis of a consecutive series of 230 neuropathologically verified cases. Ann Neurol 1986;20:597–602.

Brown P, Cathala F, Gajdusek DC. Creutzfeldt-Jakob disease in France. III. Epidemiological study of 170 patients dying during the decade. Ann Neurol 1979;38–46.

Brown P, Rodgers-Johnson P, Cathala F, Gibbs CJ Jr, Gajdusek DC. Creutzfeldt-Jakob disease of long duration: clinicopathological characteristics, transmissibility, and differential diagnosis. Ann Neurol 1984;16:295–304.

Brown RG, Marsden CD. An investigation of the phenomenon of "set" in Parkinson's disease. Movement Disorders 1988;3:152–161.

Brown SW, Reynolds EH. Cognitive impairment in epileptic patients. In: Reynolds EH, Trimble MR, eds. Epilepsy and psychiatry. Churchill Livingstone, London, 1981:147–164.

Brownell B, Oppenheimer DR. An ataxic form of subacute presenile polioencephalopathy (Jakob-Creutzfeldt disease). J Neurol Neurosurg Psychiatry 1965;28:350–361.

Bruetsch WL. Neurosyphilitic conditions. In: Arieti S, ed. American handbook of psychiatry. Basic Books, New York, 1959:1003–1020.

Brun A. Frontal lobe degeneration of the non-Alzheimer type. I. Neuropathology. Arch Gerontol Geriatr 1987;6:193–208.

Brun A, Englund E. A white matter disorder in dementia of the Alzheimer type: A pathoanatomical study. Ann Neurol 1986;19:253–262.

Brun A, Gustafson L. Limbic lobe involvement in presenile dementia. Arch Psychiat Nervenkr 1978;226:79–93.

Bruyn GW. Huntington's chorea. Historical, clinical, and laboratory synopsis. In: Vinken PJ, Bruyn GW, eds. Handbook of clinical neurology. Vol. 6: Diseases of the basal ganglia. American Elsevier, New York, 1968;298–378.

Bruyn GW, Bots GThA, Staal A. Familial bilateral vascular calcifications in the central nervous system. Psychiatr Neurol Neurochir 1964;67:342–376.

Buchsbaum M, Goodwin F, Murphy D, Borge G. AER in affective disorders. Am J Psychiatry 1971;128:19–25.

Buchsbaum MS, Ingvar DH, Kessler R, Waters RN, Cappelletti J, van Kammen DP, King C, Johnson JL, Manning RG, Flynn RW, Mann LS, Bunney WE Jr., Sokoloff L. Cerebral glucography with positron tomography-use in normal subjects and patients with schizophrenia. Arch Gen Psychiat 1982;39:251–259.

Bucht G, Adolfsson R, Winblad B. Dementia of the Alzheimer type and multi-infarct dementia: a clinical description and diagnostic problems. J Am Geriatr Soc 1984;32:491–498.

Bucy PC, Klüver H. An anatomic investigation of the temporal lobe in monkey (*Macaca mulatta*). J Comp Neurol 1955;103:151–252.

Bucy PC, Weaver TA, Camp EH. Bromide intoxication of unusual severity and chronicity resulting from self-medication with Bromo-Seltzer. JAMA 1941; 117:1256–1258.

Budinger T. Nuclear magnetic resonance: prospects for brain tissue characterization, flow measurements, and non-invasive metabolic studies. Presentation at 106th Annual Meeting of the American Neurological Association, San Francisco, Calif., September 14–16, 1981.

Buge A, Supino-Viterbo V, Rancurel G, Pontes C. Epileptic phenomena in bismuth toxic encephalopathy. J Neurol Neurosurg Psychiatry 1981;44:62–67.

Bulger RJ, Schrier RW, Arend WP, Swanson AG. Spinal-fluid acidosis and the diagnosis of pulmonary encephalopathy. N Engl J Med 1966;274:433–437.

Buonanno FS, Brady TJ, Pykett IL, et al. Proton NMR imaging in experimental ischemic cerebral infarction. Presented at 106th Annual Meeting of the American Neurological Association, San Francisco, Calif., September 14–16, 1981.

de la Burde B, Choate MS. Early asymptomatic lead exposure and development at school age. J Pediatr 1975;87:638–642.

van den Burg W, van Zomeren AH, Minderhoud JM, Prange AJA, Meijer NSA. Cognitive impairment in patients with multiple sclerosis and mild physical disability. Arch Neurol 1987;44:494–501.

Burger LJ, Rowan AJ, Goldensohn ES. Creutzfeldt-Jakob disease. An electroencephalographic study. Arch Neurol 1972;26:428–433.

Burger PC, Burch JG, Kunze U. Subcortical arteriosclerotic encephalopathy. Stroke 1976;7:626–631.

Burger PC, Vogel FS. The development of the pathologic changes of Alzheimer's disease and senile dementia in patients with Down's syndrome. Am J Pathol 1973;73:457–468.

Burke DS, Brundage JF, Redfield RR, Damato JJ, Schable CA, Putman P, Visintine R, Kim HI. Measurement of the false positive rate in a screening program for human immunodeficiency virus infections. N Engl J Med 1988;319:961–964.

Burks JS, Huddlestone J, Alfrey AC, Norenberg MD, Lewin E. A fatal encephalopathy in chronic haemodialysis patients. Lancet 1976;1:764–768.

Burks TF. Autonomic agents. In: Levenson AJ, ed. Neuropsychiatric side effects of drugs in the elderly. Raven Press, New York, 1979:69–78.

Bursten B. Psychoses associated with thyrotoxicosis. Arch Gen Psychiatry 1961;4:267–273.

Burston J, Blackwood W. A case of aspergillus infection of the brain. J Pathol Bacteriol 1963;86:225–228.

Burton RA, Raskin NH. Alimentary (postgastrectomy) hypoglycemia. Arch Neurol 1970;23:14–17.

Burvill PW, Jackson JM, Smith WG. Psychiatric symptoms due to vitamin B_{12} deficiency without anaemia. Med J Aust 1969;2:388–390.

Butters N, Albert MS, Sax D. Investigations of the memory disorders of patients with Huntington's disease. Adv Neurol 1979;23:203–213.

Butters N, Albert MS, Sax DS, Miliotis P, Nagode J, Sterste A. The effect of verbal mediators on the pictorial memory of brain-damaged patients. Neuropsychologia 1983;21:307–323.

Butters N, Cermak LS. Alcoholic Korsakoff's syndrome. Academic Press, New York, 1980.

Butters N, Sax D, Montgomery K, Tarlow S. Comparison of the neuropsychological deficits associated with early and advanced Huntington's disease. Arch Neurol 1978;35:585–589.

Butters N, Wolfe J, Granholm E, Martone M. An assessment of verbal recall, recognition and fluency abilities in patients with Huntington's disease. Cortex 1986;22:11–32.

Byers RK, Gilles FH, Fung C. Huntington's disease in children. Neurology 1973;23:561–569.

Cable WJL, Kolodny EH, Adams RD. Fabry disease: impaired autonomic function. Neurology 1982;32:498–502.

Cadilhac J, Ribstein M. The EEG in metabolic disorders. World Neurol 1961;2:296–308.

Caine ED. Pseudodementia. Current concepts and future directions. Arch Gen Psychiatry 1981;38:1359–1364.

Caine ED, Ebert MH, Weingartner H. An outline for the analysis of dementia. The memory disorder of Huntington's disease. Neurology 1977;27:1087–1092.

Caine ED, Hunt RD, Weingartner H, Ebert MH. Huntington's dementia. Clinical and neuropsychological features. Arch Neurol 1978;35:377–384.

Caine ED, Shoulson I. Psychiatric syndromes in Huntington's disease. Am J Psychiatry 1983;140:728–733.

Cairns H. Mental disorders with tumours of the pons. Folia Psychiatr Neurol Jpn 1950;53:193–203.

Cala LA, Jones B, Mastaglia FL, Wiley B. Brain atrophy and intellectual impairment in heavy drinkers—a clinical, psychometric and computerized tomography study. Aust NZ J Med 1978;8:147–153.

Callum CM, Bigler ED. Ventricle size, cortical atrophy and the relationship with neuropsychological status in closed head injury: a quantitative analysis. J Clin Exp Neuropsychol 1986;8:437–452.

Cameron KR, Birchal SM, Mose MA. Isolation of foamy virus from patient with dialysis encephalopathy. Lancet 1978;2:796.

Cameron N. Deterioration and regression in schizophrenic thinking. J Abnorm Soc Psychol 1939;34:265–270.

Caplan LR, Nadelson T. Multiple sclerosis and hysteria. JAMA 1980;243:2418–2421.

Caplan LR, Schoene WC. Clinical features of subcortical arteriosclerotic encephalopathy (Binswanger disease). Neurology 1978;28:1206–1215.

Cares RM, Gordon BS, Kreuger E. Boeck's sarcoid in chronic meningoencephalitis. J Neuropathol Exp Neurol 1957;16:544–554.

Carlen PL, Wilkinson A, Wortzman G, et al. Cerebral atrophy and functional deficits in alcoholics without clinically apparent liver disease. Neurology 1981;31:377–385.

Carlen PL, Wortzman G, Holgate RC, Wilkinson DA, Rankin JG. Reversible atrophy in recently abstinent chronic alcoholics measured by computed tomography scans. Science 1978;200:1076–1078.

Carlson GA, Goodwin FK. The stages of mania. Arch Gen Psychiatry 1973;28:221–228.

Carney MWP. Five cases of bromism. Lancet 1971;2:523–524.

Carpenter PC. Cushing's syndrome: Update of diagnosis and management. Mayo Clin Proc 1986;61:49–58.

Carroll BJ, Feinberg M, Greden JF, et al. A specific laboratory test for the diagnosis of melancholia. Arch Gen Psychiatry 1981;38:15–22.

Carroll DL. When your loved one has Alzheimer's. Harper and Row, Philadelphia, 1989.

Carter CC, Fuller TJ. Increased intracranial pressure in chronic lung disease. Neurology 1957;7:169–174.

Carter HR, Sukavajuna C. Familial cerebello-olivary degeneration with late development of rigidity and dementia. Neurology 1956;6:876–884.

Cartwright GE. Diagnosis of treatable Wilson's disease. N Engl J Med 1978;298:1347–1350.

Cascino GD, Jensen JM, Nelson LA, Schutta HS. Periodic hyperammonemic encephalopathy associated with a ureterosigmoidostomy. Mayo Clin Proc 1989;64:653–656.

Caselli RJ. Giant cell (temporal) arteritis: a treatable cause of multi-infarct dementia. Neurology 1990;40:753–755.

Casey DA, Fitzgerald BA. Mania and pseudodementia. J Clin Psychiatry 1988;49:73–74.

Cassel C. Research on senile dementia of the Alzheimer's type: ethical issues involving informed consent. In: Melnick VL, Dubler NN, eds. Alzheimer's dementia. Dilemmas in clinical research. Humana Press, Clifton, N.J., 1985:99–108.

Cassel CK, Brody JA. Demography, epidemiology, and aging. In: Cassel CK, Riesenberg DE, Sorensen LB, Walsh JR, eds. Geriatric medicine, 2nd ed. Springer-Verlag, New York, 1990:16–27.

Casson IR, Sham R, Campbell EA, Tarlau M, Didomenico A. Neurological and CT evaluation of knocked-out boxers. J Neurol Neurosurg Psychiatry 1982;45:170–174.

Caudill RG, Smith CE, Reinarz JA. Coccidioidal meningitis. Am J Med 1970;49:360–364.

Cavenar JO, Maltbie AA, Austin L. Depression simulating organic brain disease. Am J Psychiatry 1979;136:521–523.

Ceade MH, Coleman RE, Lee LS, Mickhael MA, Alderson PO, Archer CR. Correlation between computerized transaxial tomography and radionuclide cisternography in dementia. Neurology 1976;26:555–560.

Celesia GG. Pathophysiology of periodic EEG complexes in subacute sclerosing panencephalitis (SSPE). Electroencephalogr Clin Neurophysiol 1973;35:293–300.

Celesia GG, Barr AN. Psychosis and other psychiatric manifestations of levedopa therapy. Arch Neurol 1970;33:193–200.

Celesia GG, Wanamaker WM. Psychiatric disturbances in Parkinson's disease. Dis Nerv Syst 1972;33:577–583.

Centers for Disease Control. Syphilis: recommended treatment schedules, 1976. Ann Intern Med 1976;85:94–96.

Centers for Disease Control. CDC classification system for human T-lymphocytes virus Type III/lymphadenopathy associated virus infection. Mortal Morbid Weekly Report 1987a;36(Suppl):1–9.

Centers for Disease Control. Revision of the CDC surveillance case definition for acquired immunodeficiency syndrome. Morbid Mortal Weekly Report 1987b; 36(Suppl)3S–14S.

Chaffin DS. Phenothiazine-induced acute psychotic reaction: the "psychotoxicity" of a drug. Am J Psychiatry 1964;121:26–32.

Chalupa B, Synkova J, Sevcik M. The assessment of electroencephalographic changes and memory disturbances in acute intoxications with industrial poisons. Br J Ind Med 1960;17:238–241.

Chandler JH, Bebin J. Hereditary cerebellar ataxia. Neurology 1956;6:187–195.

Charness ME, DeLaPaz RL. Mamillary body atrophy in Wernicke's encephalopathy: antemortem identification using magnetic resonance imaging. Ann Neurol 1987;22:595–600.

Charness ME, Simon RP, Greenberg DA. Ethanol and the nervous system. N Engl J Med 1989;321:442–454.

Chawluk JB, Mesulam M-M, Hurtig H, Kusher M, Weintraub S, Saykin A, Rubin N, Alavi A, Reivich M. Slowly progressive aphasia without generalized dementia: Studies with positron emission tomography. Ann Neurol 1986;19:68–74.

Chedru F, Geschwind N. Disorders of higher cortical functions in acute confusional states. Cortex 1972;8:395–411.

Chedru F, Geschwind N. Writing disturbances in acute confusional states. Neuropsychology 1972;10:343–353.

Cheek WR, Taveras JM. Thalamic tumors. J Neurosurg 1966;24:505–513.

Chen K-M, Yase Y. Parkinsonism-dementia, neurofibrillary tangles, and trace elements in the Western Pacific. In: Hutton JT, Kenny AD, eds. Senile dementia of the Alzheimer type. Alan R Liss, New York, 1985:153–173.

Chen L. Neurofibrillary change on Guam. Arch Neurol 1981;38:16–18.

Cherington M. Parkinsonism, L-dopa, and mental depression. J Am Geriatr Soc 1970;18:513–516.

Chernik NL, Armstrong D, Posner JB. Central nervous system infections in patients with cancer. Medicine 1973;52:563–581.

Chhuttani PN, Chopra JS. Arsenic poisoning. In: Vinken PJ, Bruyn GW, eds. Intoxications of the nervous system. Part I, vol. 36. Handbook of clinical neurology. North-Holland, New York, 1979:199–216.

Chiappa K. Pattern shift visual, brainstem auditory and short latency somatosensory evoked potentials in multiple sclerosis. Neurology 1980;30:110–123.

Ch'ien LT, Boehm RM, Robinson H, Lin C, Frenkel LD. Characteristic early electroencephalographic changes in herpes simplex encephalitis. Arch Neurol 1977;34:361–364.

Chiofalo N, Fuentes A, Galvez S. Serial EEG findings in 27 cases of Creutzfeldt-Jakob disease. Arch Neurol 1980;37:143–145.

Chodosh HL, Zeffert B, Muro ES. Treatment of dementia in a medical day care program. J Am Geriatr Soc 1986;34:881–886.

Chokroverty S, Breutman ME, Berger V, Reyes MG. Progressive dialytic encephalopathy. J Neurol Neurosurg Psychiatry 1976;39:411–419.

Chokroverty S, Duvoisin RC, Sachdeo R, Sage J, Lepore F, Nicklas W. Neurophysiological study of olivopontocerebellar atrophy with or without glutamate dehydrogenase deficiency. Neurology 1985;35:652–659.

Chokroverty S, Khedekar R, Derby B, Sachdeo R, Yook C, Lepore F, Nicklas W, Duvoisin RC. Pathology of olivopontocerebellar atrophy with glutamate dehydrogenase deficiency. Neurology 1984;34:1451–1455.

Christensen A. Luria's neuropsychological investigation. Spectrum, New York. 1975.

Christensen E, Brun A. Subacute spongiform encephalopathy. Neurology 1963;13:455–463.

Christie AB. Changing patterns in mental illness in the elderly. Br J Psychiatry 1982;140:154–159.

Christie JE, Glen AIM, Yates CM, et al. Choline and lecithin effects on CSF choline levels and on cognitive function in Alzheimer pre-senile dementia. In: Glen AIM, Whalley LJ, eds. Alzheimer's disease. Early recognition of potentially reversible deficits. Churchill Livingstone, London, 1979:163–168.

Christie JE, Shering A, Ferguson J, Glen AIM. Physostigmine and arecoline: effects of intravenous infusions in Alzheimer presenile dementia. Br J Psychiatry 1981;138:46–50.

Christy NP. Anterior pituitary. In: Beeson PB, McDermott W, eds. Cecil-Loeb: textbook of medicine, 13th ed. WB Saunders, Philadelphia, 1971:1728–1748.

Chu N-S. Tuberculous meningitis. Arch Neurol 1980;37:458–460.

Chui HC, Teng EL, Henderson VW, Moy AC. Clinical subtypes of dementia of the Alzheimer type. Neurology 1985;35:1544–1550.

Chun RWM, Daly RF, Mansheim BJ Jr. Wolcott GJ. Benign familial chorea with onset in childhood. JAMA 1973;225:1603–1607.

Citron BP, Halpern M, McCarron M, et al. Necrotizing angiitis associated with drug abuse. N Engl J Med 1970;283:1003–1011.

Claisse P, Levy C. Etude histologique d'un cas d'hydrocephalie interne. Bull Soc Anat Paris 1897;11:264–266.

Clarfield AM. The reversible dementias: do they reverse? Ann Intern Med 1988;109:476–486.

Clark T. The masters movement: age conquers some but it doesn't conquer all. Runner's World 1979:80–95.

Cleghorn RA. Adrenal cortical insufficiency: psychological and neurological observations. Can Med Assoc J 1951;65:449–454.

Cobb W. The periodic events of subacute sclerosing leucoencephalitis. Electroencephalogr Clin Neurophysiol 1966;21:278–294.

Coblentz JM, Mattis S, Zungesser LH, Kasoff SS, Wisniewski HM, Katzman R. Presenile dementia. Arch Neurol 1973;29:299–308.

Cochran JW, Fox JH, Kelly MP. Reversible mental symptoms in temporal arteritis. J Nerv Ment Dis 1978;166:446–447.

Coffey CE, Figiel GS, Djang WT, Cress M, Saunders WB, Weiner RD. Leukoencephalopathy in elderly depressed patients referred for ECT. Biol Psychiatry 1988;24:143–161.

Coffey CE, Figiel GS, Djang WT, Saunders WB, Weiner RD. White matter hyperintensity on magnetic resonance imaging: neuroanatomical correlates in the depressed elderly. J Neuropsychiatry Clin Neurosci 1989;1:135–144.

Coffey CE, Figiel GS, Djang WT, Weiner RD. Subcortical hyperintensity on magnetic resonance imaging: a comparison of normal and depressed elderly subjects. Am J Psychiatry 1990;147:187–189.

Cohen CR, Duchesneau PM, Weinstein MA. Calcification of the basal ganglia as visualized by computed tomography. Radiology 1980;134:97–99.

Cohen D, Eisdorfer C. The loss of the self. WW Norton, New York, 1986.

Cohen D, Eisdorfer C. Depression in family members caring for a relative with Alzheimer's disease. J Am Geriatr Soc 1988;36:885–889.

Cohen N. Aging and neurobiology. Presented at a conference on Geriatric Medicine at the Eisenhower Medical Center, Palm Springs, Calif., February 11, 1982.

Cohen RA, Fisher M. Amantadine treatment of fatigue associated with multiple sclerosis. Arch Neurol 1989;46:676–680.

Cohen RM, Weingartner H, Smallberg SA, Pickar D, Murphy DL. Effort and cognition in depression. Arch Gen Psychiatry 1982;39:593–597.

Cohen WJ, Cohen NH. Lithium carbonate, haloperidol, and irreversible brain damage. JAMA 1974;230:1283–1287.

Cohn R, Sode J. The EEG in hypercalcemia. Neurology 1971;21:154–161.

Colerick EJ, George LK. Predictors of institutionalization among caregivers of patients with Alzheimer's disease. J Am Geriatr Soc 1986;34:493–498.

Colgan J, Naguib M, Levy R. Computed tomographic density numbers. A comparative study of patients with senile dementia and normal elderly controls. Br J Psychiatry 1986;149:716–719.

Collins RC, Al-Mondhiry H, Chernik NL, Posner JB. Neurologic manifestations of intravascular coagulation in patients with cancer. Neurology 1975;25:795–806.

Condon JV, Backa DR, Gibbs FA. Electroencephalographic abnormalities in hyperthyroidism. J Clin Endocrinol Metabol 1954;14:1511–1518.

Conn HO. Asterixis. Its occurrence in chronic pulmonary disease, with a commentary on its general mechanism. N Engl J Med 1958;259:564–569.

Conn HO. A rational program for the management of hepatic coma. Gastroenterology 1969;57:715–723.

Conomy JP, Beard NS, Matsumoto H, Roessmann U. Cytarabine treatment of progressive multifocal leukoencephalopathy. JAMA 1974;229:1313–1316.

Constantinidis J. Is Alzheimer's disease a major form of senile dementia? Clinical, anatomical, and genetic data. In: Katzman R, Terry RD, Bick KL, eds. Alzheimer's disease, senile dementia and related disorders. Raven Press, New York; 1978:15–25.

Constantinidis J. Zinc metabolism in presenile dementia. In: Glen AIM, Whalley LJ, eds. Alzheimer's disease. Early recognition of potentially reversible deficits. Churchill Livingstone, London, 1979:48–49.

Constantinidis J, Richard J, Tissot R. Pick's disease. Histological and clinical correlations. Eur Neurol 1974;11:208–217.

Constantinidis J, Tissot R. Role of glutamate and zinc in the hippocampal lesions of Pick's disease. Adv Biochem Psychopharm 1981;27:413–422.

Cook DG, Fahn S, Brait KA. Chronic manganese intoxication. Arch Neurol 1974;30:59–64.

Cook P, James I. Cerebral vasodilators. N Engl J Med 1981;305:1508–1513, 1560–1564.

Cook RH, Austin JH. Precautions in familial transmissible dementia. Arch Neurol 1978;35:697–698.

Cook RH, Bard BE, Austin JH. Studies in aging of the brain. IV. Familial Alzheimer disease: relation to transmissible dementia, aneuploidy, and microtubular defects. Neurology 1979;29:1402–1412.

Cook RH, Schneck SA, Clark DB. Twins with Alzheimer's disease. Arch Neurol 1981;38:300–301.

Cools AR, Van Den Bercken JHL, Horstink MWI, Van Spaendonck KPM, Berger HJC. Cognitive and motor shifting aptitude disorder in Parkinson's disease. J Neurol Neurosurg Psychiatry 1984;47:443–453.

Cooper AJ. Medroxyprogesterone acetate (MPA) treatment of sexual acting out in men suffering from dementia. J Clin Psychiatry 1987;48:368–370.

Cooperative Study Report. Cooperative study in the evaluation of therapy in multiple sclerosis. Neurology 1970;20(2):1–59.

Cordingly G, Navarro C, Brust JCM, Healton EB. Sarcoidosis presenting as senile dementia. Neurology 1981;31:1148–1151.

Corin MS, Elizan TS, Bender MB. Oculomotor function in patients with Parkinson's disease. J Neurol Sci 1972;15:251–265.

Corsellis JAN. The limbic areas in Alzheimer's disease and in other conditions associated with dementia. In: Wolstenholme GEW, O'Connor M, eds. Alzheimer's disease and related conditions. J & A Churchill, London, 1970:37–45.

Corsellis JAN. Ageing and the dementias. In: Blackwood W, Corsellis JAN, eds. Greenfield's neuropathology. Year Book Medical Publishers, Chicago, 1976:796–848.

Corsellis, JAN, Brierley JB. An unusual type of presenile dementia (atypical Alzheimer's disease with amyloid vascular change). Brain 1954;77:571–587.

Corsellis JAN, Bruton CJ, Freeman-Browne D. The aftermath of boxing. Psychol Med 1973;3:270–303.

Corsellis JAN, Goldberg GJ, Norton AR. "Limbic encephalitis" and its association with carcinoma. Brain 1968;91:481–496.

Corsellis JAN, Meldrum BS. Epilepsy. In: Blackwood W, Corsellis JAN, eds. Greenfield's neuropathology. Year Book Medical Publishers, Chicago, 1976:771–795.

Corser CM, Baikie E, Brown E. Effect of lecithin in senile dementia: a report of four cases. In: Glen AIM, Whalley LJ, eds. Alzheimer's disease. Early recognition of potentially reversible deficits. Churchill Livingstone, London, 1979:169–172.

Costa DC, Ell PJ, Burns A, Philpot M, Levy R. CBF tomograms with 99m-Tc-HM-PAO in patients with dementia (Alzheimer type and HIV) and Parkinson's disease—initial results. J Cereb Blood Flow Metab 1988;8:S109–S115.

Courville CB. The mechanism of coup-countrecoup injuries of the brain. Bull Los Angeles Neurol Soc 1950;15:72–86.

Coutinho P, Andrade C. Autosomal dominant system degeneration in Portuguese families of the Azores islands. Neurology 1978;28:703–709.

Cowan RJ, Maynard CD, Lassiter KR. Technetium 99m pertechnetate brain scans in the detection of subdural hematomas: a study of the age of the lesion as related to the development of a positive scan. J Neurosurg 1970;32:30–34.

Cowdry RW, Goodwin FK. Dementia of bipolar illness: diagnosis and response to lithium. Am J Psychiatry 1981;138:1118–1119.

Coyle PK, Wolinsky JS. Characterization of immune complexes in progressive rubella panencephalitis. Ann Neurol 1981;9:557–562.

Craik FIM. Age differences in human memory. In: Birren JE, Schaie KW, eds. Handbook of the psychology of aging. Van Nostrand Reinhold, New York, 1977:384–420.

Crapper DR, Dalton AJ, Skopitz M, Eng P, Scott JW, Hachinski VC. Alzheimer degeneration in Down syndrome. Arch Neurol 1975;32:618–623.

Crapper DR, Krishnan SS, Quittkat S. Aluminum, neurofibrillary degeneration and Alzheimer's disease. Brain 1976;99:67–80.

Crapper DR, Quittkat S, DeBoni U. Altered chromatin conformation in Alzheimer's disease. Brain 1979;102:483–495.

Cravioto H, Korein J, Silberman J. Wernicke's encephalopathy. Arch Neurol 1961;4:510–519.

Cremer NE, Oshiro LS, Weil ML, Lennette EH, Itabashi HH, Carnay L. Isolation of rubella virus from brain in chronic progressive panencephalitis. J Gen Virol 1975;29:143–153.

Creutzfeldt HG. On a peculiar focal disease of the central nervous system (preliminary communication). EP Richardson Jr, trans. In: Rottenberg DA, Hochberg FH, eds. Neurological classics in modern translation. Hafner Press, New York, 1977:97–112.

Critchley EMR. Speech disorders in parkinsonism: a review. J Neurol Neurosurg Psychiatry 1981;44:751–758.

Critchley M. Medical aspects of boxing, particularly from a neurological standpoint. Br Med J 1957;1:357–362.

Critchley M. The neurology of old age. Lancet 1931;1:1119–1127, 1221–1230, 1331–1336.

Critchley M, Greenfield JG. Olivoponto-cerebellar atrophy. Brain 1948;71:343–364.

Crockard HA, Hanlon K, Duda EE, Mullan JF. Hydrocephalus as a cause of dementia: evaluation of computerized tomography and intracranial pressure monitoring. J Neurol Neurosurg Psychiatry 1977;40:736–740.

Crome L, Stern J. Inborn lysosomal enzyme deficiencies. In: Blackwood W, Corsellis JAN, eds. Greenfield's neuropathology. Year Book Medical Publishers, Chicago, 1976:500–580.

Cronholm B, Otteson J. Memory functions in endogenous depression. Arch Gen Psychiatry 1961;5:101-107.

Crook T, Bartus RT, Ferris SH, Whitehouse P, Cohen GD, Gershon S. Age associated memory impairment: proposed diagnostic criteria and measures of clinical change—National Institute of Mental Health Work Group. Develop Psychol 1986;2261–2276.

Cross HE, McKusick VA. The mast syndrome. Arch Neurol 1967;16:1–13.

Crosson B, Novack TA, Trenerry MR, Craig PL. California Verbal Learning Test (CVLT) performance in severely head-injured and neurologically normal adult males. J Clin Exp Neuropsychol 1988;10:754–768.

Crow TJ. Molecular pathology of schizophrenia: more than one disease process? Br Med J 1980;280:66–68.

Crowell RM, Tew JM, Mark VH. Aggressive dementia associated with normal pressure hydrocephalus. Neurology 1973;23:461–464.

Crystal HA, Schaumburg HH, Grober E, Fuld PA, Lipton RB. Cognitive impairment and sensory loss associated with chronic low-level ethylene oxide exposure. Neurology 1988;38:567–569.

Crystal RG. Sarcoidosis. In: Braunwald E, Isselbacher KJ, Petersdorf RG, Wilson JD, Martin JB, Fauci AS, eds. Harrison's principles of internal medicine, 11th edition. McGraw-Hill, New York, 1987:1445–1450.

Culebras A, Feldman RG, Fager CA. Hydrocephalus and dementia in Paget's disease of the skull. J Neurol Sci 1974;23:307–321.

Culebras A, Feldman RG, Merk FB. Cytoplasmic inclusion bodies within neurons of the thalamus in myotonic dystrophy. J Neurol Sci 1973;19:319–329.

Cummings J, Sonntag VKH, Scott RM. Ascites complicating ventriculo-peritoneal shunting in an adult. Surg Neurol 1976;6:135–136.

Cummings JL. Introduction. Subcortical dementia. Cummings JL, ed. Oxford University Press, New York, 1990:1–15.

Cummings JL. Intellectual impairment in Parkinson's disease: clinical, pathologic, and biochemical correlates. J Geriatr Psychiatry Neurol 1988;1:24–36.

Cummings JL. Subcortical dementia. Brit J Psychiatry 1986;149:682–697.

Cummings JL. Clinical neuropsychiatry. Grune & Stratton, New York, 1985.

Cummings JL. Cortical dementias. In: Benson DF, Blumer D, eds. Psychiatric aspects of neurologic disease, Vol 2. Grune & Stratton, New York, 1982:93–120.

Cummings JL, Benson DF. The role of the nucleus basalis of Meynert in dementia: review and reconsideration. Alz Dis Assoc Disor 1987;1:128–145.

Cummings JL, Benson DF. Dementia of the Alzheimer type: an inventory of diagnostic clinical features. J Am Gertiatr Soc 1986;34:12–19.

Cummings JL, Benson DF. Subcortical dementia. Arch Neurol 1984;41:874–879.

Cummings JL, Benson DF, Hill MA, Read S. Aphasia in dementia of the Alzheimer type. Neurology 1985;35:394–397.

Cummings JL, Benson DF, LoVerme S Jr. Reversible dementia. JAMA 1980a; 243:2434–2439.

Cummings JL, Darkins A, Mendez M, Hill MA, Benson DF. Alzheimer's disease and Parkinson's disease: comparison of speech and language alterations. Neurology 1988;38:680–684.

Cummings JL, Duchen LW. The Klüver-Bucy syndrome in Pick disease. Neurology 1981;31:1415–1422.

Cummings JL, Gosenfeld L, Houlihan J, McCaffrey T. Neuropsychiatric manifestations of idiopathic calcification of the basal ganglia: case report and review. Biol Psychiatry 1983a;18:591–601.

Cummings JL, Hebben NA, Obler L, Leonard P. Nonphasic misnaming and other neurobehavior features of an unusual toxic encephalopathy: case study. Cortex 1980b:16:315–323.

Cummings JL, Houlihan JP, Hill MA. The pattern of reading deterioration in dementia of the Alzheimer type: observations and implications. Brain Lang 1986;29:315–323.

Cummings JL, Landis T, Benson DF. Environmental disorientation: clinical and radiologic findings. American Academy of Neurology, San Diego, 1983b.

Cummings JL, Miller B, Hill MA, Neshkes R. Neuropsychiatric aspects of multi-infarct dementia and dementia of the Alzheimer type. Arch Neurol 1987;44:389–393.

Cummings JL, Victoroff JI. Noncognitive neuropsychiatric syndromes of Alzheimer's disease. Neuropsychiatry, Neuropsychol, Behav Neurol 1990;3:140–158.

Cummings JL, Wirshing WC. Recognition and differential diagnosis of tardive dyskinesia. Int'l J Psychiatr Med 1989;19:133–144.

Cummings JN. Biochemistry of the basal ganglia. In: Vinken PJ, Bruyn GW, eds. Diseases of the basal ganglia. Vol 6. Handbook of clinical neurology. American Elsevier, New York, 1968:116–132.

Cunningham J, Graus F, Anderson N, Posner JB. Partial characterization of the Purkinje cell antigens in paraneoplastic cerebellar degeneration. Neurology 1986;36:1163–1168.

Curran D. Huntington's chorea without choreiform movements. J Neurol Psychopathol 1930;10:305–310.

Currie S, Henson RA, Morgan HG, Poole AJ. The incidence of non-metastatic neurological syndromes of obscure origin in the reticuloses. Brain 1970;93:629–640.

Currier RD. A classification for ataxia. In: Duvoisin RC, Plaitakis A, eds. The olivopontocerebellar atrophies. Raven Press, New York, 1984:1–4.

Cutler NR, Brown PW, Narayan T, Parisi JE, Janotta F, Baron H. Creutzfeldt-Jakob disease: a case of 16 years' duration. Ann Neurol 1984;15:107–110.

Cutler NR, Haxby JV, Duara R, Grady CL, Kay AD, Kessler RM, Sundaram M, Rapoport Sl. Clinical history, brain metabolism, and neuropsychological function in Alzheimer's disease. Ann Neurol 1985;18:298–309.

Cutler RWP, Watters GV, Hammerstad JP, Merler E. Origin of cerebrospinal fluid gamma globulin in subacute sclerosing leukoencephalitis. Arch Neurol 1967; 17:620–628.

Cutting J. Study of anosognosia. J Neurol Neurosurg Psychiatry 1978a;41:548–555.

Cutting J. The relationship between Korsakov's syndrome and alcoholic dementia. Br J Psychiatry 1978b;132:240–251.

Cutting J. Specific psychological deficits in alcoholism. Br J Psychiatry 1978c;133:119–122.

Cutting J. Alcoholic dementia. In: Benson DF, Blumer D, eds. Psychiatric aspects of neurologic disease, Vol 2. Grune & Stratton, New York, 1982:149–164.

Czlonkowska A, Rodo M. Late onset of Wilson's disease. Arch Neurol 1981;38:729–730.

Dalessio DJ, Benchimol A, Dimond EG. Chronic encephalopathy related to heart block. Neurology 1965;15:499–503.

Dam M, Moller JE. Myoclonus epilepsy. Acta Neurol Scand 1968;44:596–611.

Damasio AR, Lobo-Antunes J, Macedo C. Psychiatric aspects in parkinsonism treated with L-dopa. J Neurol Neurosurg Psychiatry 1971;34:502–507.

Damasio AR, Yamada T, Damasio H, Corbett J, McKee J. Central achromatopsia: behavioral, anatomic, and physiologic aspects. Neurology 1980;30:1064–1071.

Damasio H, Antunes L, Damasio AR. Familial nonprogressive involuntary movements of childhood. Ann Neurol 1977;1:602–603.

D'Amato RJ, Zweig RM, Whitehouse PJ, Wenk GL, Singer HS, Mayeux R, Price DL, Snyder SH. Aminergic systems in Alzheimer's disease and Parkinson's disease. Ann Neurol 1987;22:229–236.

D'Antona R, Baron JC, Samson Y, Serdaru M, Viader F, Agid Y, Cambier J. Subcortical dementia. Frontal cortex hypometabolism detected by positron tomography in patients with progressive supranuclear palsy. Brain 1985;108:785–799.

Dandy WE. Experimental hydrocephalus. Ann Surg 1919;70:129–142.

Dandy WE, Blackfan KD. An experimental and clinical study of internal hydrocephalus. JAMA 1913;61:2216–2217.

Daniels AC, Chokroverty S, Barron KD. Thalamic degeneration, dementia, and seizures. Arch Neurol 1969;21:15–24.

Danta G, Hilton RC. Judgment of the visual vertical and horizontal in patients with parkinsonism. Neurology 1975;25:43–47.

Darkins AW, Fromkin VA, Benson DF. A characterization of the prosodic loss in Parkinson's disease. Brain Lang 1988;34:315–327.

Darley FL, Aronson AE, Brown JR. Motor speech disorders. WB Saunders, Philadelphia, 1975.

Daroff R, Deller JJ Jr, Kastl AJ Jr, Blocker WW Jr. Cerebral malaria. JAMA 1967;202:119–122.

Davanipour Z, Alter M, Sobel E, Asher D, Gajdusek DC. Creutzfeldt-Jakob disease: Possible medical risk factors. Neurology 1985;35:1483–1486.

David NJ, Mackey EA, Smith JL. Further observations in progressive supranuclear palsy. Neurology 1968;18:349–356.

Davidson EA, Robertson EE. Alzheimer's disease with acne rosacea in one of identical twins. J Neurol Neurosurg Psychiatry 1955;18:72–77.

Davies DL. The intelligence of patients with Friedreich's ataxia. J Neurol Neurosurg Psychiatry 1949a;12:34–38.

Davies DL. Psychiatric changes associated with Friedreich's ataxia. J Neurol Neurosurg Psychiatry 1949b;12:246–250.

Davies P. Studies on the neurochemistry of central cholinergic systems in Alzheimer's disease. In: Katzman R, Terry RD, Bick KL, eds. Alzheimer's disease, senile dementia and related disorders. Raven Press, New York, 1978:453–468.

Davies P. Neurotransmitter-related enzymes in senile dementia of the Alzheimer type. Brain Res 1979;171:319–327.

Davies P, Katz DA, Crystal HA. Choline acetyltransferase, somatostatin, and substance P in selected cases of Alzheimer's disease. In: Corkin S, Davies KL, Growdon JH, Usdin E, Wurtman RJ. Alzheimer's disease: a report of progress in research. Raven Press, New York, 1982:9–14.

Davies P, Maloney AJF. Selective loss of central cholinergic neurons in Alzheimer's disease. Lancet 1976;2:1403.

Davies P, Verth AH. Regional distribution of muscarinic acetylcholine receptor in normal and Alzheimer's-type dementia brains. Brain Res 1978;138:385–392.

Davis FA, Stefoski D, Rush J. Orally administered 4-aminopyridine improves clinical signs in multiple sclerosis. Ann Neurol 1990;27:186–192.

Davis KL, Mohs RC, Tinklenberg JR. Enhancement of memory by physostigmine. N Engl J Med 1979;301:946.

Davis KL, Yesavage JA, Berger PA. Possible organophosphate-induced parkinsonism. J Nerv Ment Dis 1978;166:222–225.

Davis LE. A physio-pathologic study of the choroid plexus with the report of a case of villous hypertrophy. J Med Res 1924;44:521–534.

Davis LE, Wands JR, Weiss SA, Price DL, Girling EF. Central nervous system intoxication from mercurous chloride laxatives. Arch Neurol 1974;30:428–431.

Davis PE, Mumford SJ. Cued recall and the nature of the memory disorder in dementia. Brit J Psychiatry 1984;144:383–386.

Davison C. Spastic pseudosclerosis (cortico-pallido-spinal degeneration). Brain 1932;55:247–264.

Davison C. Circumscribed cortical atrophy in the presenile psychoses—Pick's disease. Am J Psychiatry 1938;94:801–818.

Davison C. Progressive subcortical encephalopathy (Binswanger's disease). J Neuropathol Exp Neurol 1942;1:42–48.

Davison C, Brill NQ. Essential hypertension and chronic hypertensive encephalopathy. Ann Intern Med 1939;12:1766–1781.

Davison C, Rabiner AM. Spastic pseudosclerosis (disseminated encephalomyelopathy; corticopallidospinal degeneration). Arch Neurol Psychiatry 1940;44:578–595.

Davison K, Bagely CR. Schizophrenia-like psychoses associated with organic disorders of the central nervous system: a review of the literature. Br J Psychiatry 1969(special issue no. 4): 113–184.

Davous P, Roudier ML, Abramowitz C, Lamous Y. Pharamcological modulation of cortisol secretion and dexamethasone suppression in Alzheimer's disease. Biol Psychiatry 1988;23:13–24.

Dayan AD. Quantitative histological studies on the aged human brain. II. Senile plaques and neurofibrillary tangles in senile dementia. Acta Neuropathol 1970;16:95–102.

Dayan AD, Bhatti I, Gostling JVT. Encephalitis due to herpes simplex in a patient with treated carcinoma of the uterus. Neurology 1967;17:609–613.

De Boni U, Crapper DR. Paired helical filaments of the Alzheimer type in cultured neurons. Nature 1978;271:566–568.

DeGroot LJ. Diseases of the thyroid. In: Beeson PB, McDermott W, eds. Cecil-Loeb: textbook of medicine, 13th ed. WB Saunders, Philadelphia, 1971:1753–1780.

Dehaene I, Bogaerts M. L-dopa in progressive supranuclear palsy. Lancet 1970;2:470.

Deiss A, Lynch RE, Lee GR, Cartwright GE. Long-term therapy of Wilson's disease. Ann Intern Med 1971;75:57–65.

Dekaban AS, Herman MM. Childhood, juvenile, and adult cerebral lipidases. Arch Pathol 1974;97:65–73.

Delaney JF. Spinal fluid aluminum levels in patients with Alzheimer disease. Ann Neurol 1979;5:580–581.

De La Paz R, Enzmann D. Neuroradiology of acquired immunodeficiency syndrome. In: Rosenblum ML, Levy RM, Bredesen DE, eds. AIDS and the nervous system. Raven Press, New York, 1988:121–153.

Della Sala S, Lucchelli F, Spinnler H. Ideomotor apraxia in patients with dementia of Alzheimer type. J Neurol 1987;2324:91–93.

Den Hartog Jager WA, Bethlem J. The distribution of Lewy bodies in the central and autonomic nervous systems in idiopathic paralysis agitans. J Neurol Neurosurg Psychiatry 1960;23:283–290.

Dening TR. Psychiatric aspects of Wilson's disease. Br J Psychiatry 1985;147:677–682.

Dening TR, Berrios GE. Wilson's disease. Psychiatric symptoms in 195 cases. Arch Gen Psychiatry 1989;46:1126–1134.

Denny-Brown D. The basal ganglia. Oxford University Press, London, 1962.

Denny-Brown D. Hepatolenticular degeneration (Wilson's disease). N Engl J Med 1964;270:1149–1156.

Denny-Brown D. Handbook of neurological examination and case recording. Harvard University Press, Cambridge, Mass., 1957.

Depue RA, Dubicki MD, McCarthy T. Differential recovery of intellectual, associational, and psychophysiological functioning in withdrawn and acute schizophrenics. J Abnor Psychol 1975;84:325–330.

DeRenzi E, Scotti G, Spinnler H. Perceptual and associative disorders of visual recognition. Neurology 1969;19:634–642.

DeRenzi E, Spinnler H. Facial recognition in brain-damaged patients. Neurology 1966;16:145–152.

DeRenzi E, Vignolo LA. L-dopa for progressive supranuclear palsy. Lancet 1969; 2:1360.

DeReuck J. The cortico-subcortical arterial angio-architecture in the human brain. Acta Neurol Belg 1972;72:323–329.

DeReuck J, Crevits L, De Coster W, Sieben G, Vander Eecken H. Pathogenesis of Binswanger chronic progressive subcortical encephalopathy. Neurology 1980;30:920–928.

DeReuck J, Vander Eecken H. The arterial angioarchitecture in lacunar state. Acta Neurol Belg 1976;76:142–149.

Desmedt JE, Noel P. Average cerebral evoked potentials in the evaluation of lesions of the sensory nerves and of the central somatosensory pathway. In: Desmedt JE, ed. New developments in electromyography and clinical neurophysiology. Vol. 1. Karger, Basel, 1973:352–371.

De Smet Y, Ruberg M, Serdaru M, Dubois B, Lhermitte F, Agid Y. Confusion, dementia and anticholinergics in Parkinson's disease. J Neurol Neurosurg Psychiatry 1982;45:1161–1164.

Deutsch G, Tweedy JR. Cerebral blood flow in severity-matched Alzheimer and multi-infarct patients. Neurology 1987;37:431–438.

Devanand DP, Sackeim HA, Brown RP, Mayeux R. A pilot study of haloperidol treatment of psychosis and behavioral disturbance in Alzheimer's disease. Arch Neurol 1989;46:854–857.

Devinsky O, Petito CK, Alonso DR. Clinical and neuropathological findings in systemic lupus erythematosus: the role of vasculitis, heart emboli, and thrombotic thrombocytopenic purpura. Ann Neurol 1988;23:380–384.

De Vita VT, Utz JP, Williams T, Carbone PP. Candida meningitis. Arch Intern Med 1966;117:527–535.

Dewan MJ, Bick A. Normal pressure hydrocephalus and psychiatric patients. Biol Psychiat 1985;20:1127–1131.

De Wardener HE, Lennox B. Cerebral beri beri (Wernicke's encephalopathy). Lancet 1947;1:11–17.

Dewhurst K, Oliver JE, McKnight AL. Socio-psychiatric consequences of Huntington's disease. Br J Psychiatry 1970;116:255–258.

Dewhurst K, Oliver J, Trick KLK, McKnight AL. Neuro-psychiatric aspects of Huntington's disease. Confin Neurol 1969;31:258–268.

DeWitt LD, Buonanno FS, Kistler JD, Brady TJ, Pykett IL, Goldman MR, Davies KR. Nuclear magnetic resonance imaging in evaluation of clinical stroke syndromes. Ann Neurol 1984;16:535–545.

Dhib-Jalbut S, Jacobson S, McFarlin DE, McFarland HF. Impaired human leukocyte antigen-restricted measles virus-specific cytotoxic T-cell response in subacute sclerosing panencephalitis. Ann Neurol 1989;25:272–280.

Diamond MC. The aging brain: some enlightening and optimistic results. Am Sci 1978;66:66–71.

Dian L, Cummings JL, Petry S, Hill MA. Personality changes in multi-infarct dementia. Psychosomatics 1990;31:1–6.

DiChiro G, Reames PM, Matthews WB Jr. RISA-ventriculography and RISA-cisternography. Neurology 1964;14:185–191.

Dick MB, Dean M-L, Sands D. Memory for action events in Alzheimer-type dementia: further evidence of an encoding failure. Brain Cognit 1989a;9:71–87.

Dick MB, Kean M-L, Sands D. Memory for internally generated words in Alzheimer-type dementia: breakdown in encoding and semantic memory. Brain Cognit 1989b;9:88–108.

Dickson DW, Horoupian DS, Thal LJ, Davies P, Walkley S, Terry RD. Klüver-Bucy syndrome and amyotrophic lateral sclerosis: a case report with biochemistry, morphometrics, and Golgi study. Neurology 1986;36:1323–1329.

Dickson DW, Horoupian DS, Thal LJ, Lantos G. Gliomatosis cerebri presenting with hydrocephalus and dementia. Am J Neuroradiol 1988;9:200–202.

Dikman S, Matthews CG. Effect of major motor seizure frequency upon cognitive-intellectual functions in adults. Epilepsia 1977;18:21–29.

Diller L, Riklan M. Psychosocial factors in Parkinson's disease. J Am Geriatr Soc 1953;4:1291–1300.

Direkze M, Bayliss SG, Cutting JC. Primary tumours of the frontal lobe. Br J Clin Pract 1971;25:207–213.

Di Rocco C, Di Trapani G, Maira G, Bentivoglio M, Macchi G, Rossi GF. Anatomo-clinical correlations in normotensive hydrocephalus. J Neurol Sci 1977;33:437–452.

Dix RD, Bredesen DE. Opportunistic viral infections in acquired immunodeficiency syndrome. In: Rosenblum ML, Levy RM, Bredesen DE, eds. AIDS and the nervous system. Raven Press, New York, 1988:221–261.

Dix MR, Harrison MJG, Lewis PD. Progressive supranuclear palsy (the Steele-Richardson-Olszewski syndrome). J Neurol Sci 1971;13:237–256.

Dobyns WB, Goldstein NP, Gordon H. Clinical spectrum of Wilson's disease (hepatolenticular degeneration). Mayo Clin Proc 1979;54:35–42.

Dodge PR. Syphilitic infections of the central nervous system. In: Beeson PB, McDermott W, eds. Cecil-Loeb: textbook of medicine, 13th ed. WB Saunders, Philadelphia, 1971:235–240.

Dodrill CB, Troupin AS. Seizures and adaptive abilities. Arch Neurol 1976;33:604–607.

Dodrill CB, Wilkus RJ. Relationships between intelligence and electroencephalographic epileptiform activity in adult epileptics. Neurology 1976a;26:525–531.

Dodrill CB, Wilkus RJ. Neuropsychological correlates of the electroencephalogram in epileptics. I. Topographic distribution and average rate of epileptiform activity. Epilepsia 1976b;17:89–100.

Dolman CL, Sweeney VP, Magil A. Neoplastic angioendotheliosis. Arch Neurol 1979;36:5–7.

Dom R, Malfroid M, Baro F. Neuropathology of Huntington's chorea. Studies of the ventrobasal complex of the thalamus. Neurology 1976;26:64–68.

Domnitz J. Thallium poisoning. A report of six cases. South Med J 1960;53:590–593.

Donaldson AA. CT scan in Alzheimer pre-senile dementia. In: Glen AIM, Whalley LJ, eds. Alzheimer's disease. Early recognition of potentially reversible deficits. Churchill Livingstone, New York, 1979:97–101.

Donaldson I MacG. The treatment of progressive supranuclear palsy with L-dopa. Aust N Z J Med 1973;3:413–416.

Donnan GA, Tress BM, Bladin PF. A prospective study of lacunar infarction using computerized tomography. Neurology 1982;32:49–56.

Dooling EC, Richardson EP Jr. Delayed encephalopathy after strangling. Arch Neurol 1976;33:196–199.

Dooling EC, Richardson EP Jr, Davis KR. Computed tomography in Hallervorden-Spatz disease. Neurology 1980;30:1128–1130.

Dooling EC, Schoene WC, Richardson EP Jr. Hallervorden-Spatz syndrome. Arch Neurol 1974:30:70–83.

Dopplet JE, Wallace WL. Standardization of the Wechsler Adult Intelligence Scale for older persons. J Abnor Soc Psychol 1955;51:312–330.

Dorfman LJ, Forno LS. Paraneoplastic encephalomyelitis. Acta Neurol Scand 1972;48:556–574.

Dorsey FG. Overview of aging and risk of susceptibility to pharmacologic iatrogenic problems in the elderly. In: Levenson AJ, ed. Neuropsychiatric side effects of drugs in the elderly. Raven Press, New York, 1979:1–3.

Dougherty JH Jr, Rawlinson DG, Levy DE, Plum F. Hypoxic-ischemic brain injury and the vegetative state: clinical and neuropathologic correlation. Neurology 1981;31:991–997.

Douglas AC, Maloney AFJ. Sarcoidosis of the central nervous system. J Neurol Neurosurg Psychiatry 1973;36:1024–1033.

Dournon E, Matheron S, Rozenbaum W, Gharakhanian S, Michon C, Girard PM, Perronne C, Salmon D, De Truchis P, Leport C, Bouvet E, Dazza MC, Levacher M, Regnier B, and the Claude Bernard Hospital AZT Study Group. Effects of zidovudine in 365 consecutive patients with AIDS or AIDS-related complex. Lancet 1988;2:1297–1302.

Dowson JH. Neuronal lipofuscin accumulation in ageing and Alzheimer dementia: a pathogenic mechanism? Br J Psychiatry 1982;140:142–148.

Drachman DA. Neurological complications of Wegener's granulomatosis. Arch Neurol 1963;8:145–155.

Drachman DA, Adams RD. Herpes simplex and acute inclusion-body encephalitis. Arch Neurol 1962;7:45–63.

Drachman DA. Dizziness and vertigo. In: Beeson P, McDermott W, Wyngaarden T, eds. Textbook of medicine, 15th ed. WB Saunders, Philadelphia, 1979:737–742.

Drachman DA, Hughes TR. Memory and the hippocampal complexes. III. aging and temporal EEG abnormalities. Neurology 1971;21:1–6.

Drachman DA, Leavitt J. Human memory and the cholinergic system. Arch Neurol 1974;30:113–121.

Drachman DA, Richardson EP Jr. Aqueductal narrowing, congenital and acquired. Arch Neurol 1961;5:552–559.

Drachman DA, Sahakian BJ. Memory and cognitive function in the elderly. Arch Neurol 1980;37:674–675.

Drake ME Jr, Erwin CW, Simpson DW, Heyman A. Early-latency brainstem auditory evoked potentials in Alzheimer disease. Neurology 1982;32:A146.

Drake ME Jr, Macrae D. Epilepsy in multiple sclerosis. Neurology 1961;11:810–816.

Dreese MJ, Netsky MG. Degenerative disorders of the basal ganglia. In: Minckler J, ed. Pathology of the nervous system. McGraw-Hill, New York, 1968:1185–1204.

Dreyfus PM, Geel SE. Vitamin and nutritional deficiencies. In: Siegel GJ, Albers RW, Katzman R, Agranoff BW, eds. Basic neurochemistry, 2nd ed. Little, Brown, Boston, 1976:605–626.

Driesen W, Elies W. Epidural and subdural hematomas as complication of internal drainage of cerebrospinal fluid in hydrocephalus. Acta Neurochir (Wien) 1974;30:85–93.

Duara R, Grady C, Haxby J, Sundaram M, Cutler NR, Heston L, Moore A, Schlageter N, Larson S, Rapoport SI. Positron emission tomography in Alzheimer's disease. Neurology 1986;36:879–887.

Dubinsky RM, Hallett M, Levey R, Di Chiro G. Regional brain glucose metabolism in neuroacanthocytosis. Neurology 1989;39:1253–1255.

Dubinsky RM, Jankovic J. Progressive supranuclear palsy and a multi-infarct state. Neurology 1987;37:570–576.

Dubois B, Pillon B, Legault F, Agid Y, Lhermitte F. Slowing of cognitive processing in progressive supranuclear palsy. Arch Neurol 1988;45:1194–1199.

Dubois-Dalcq M, Coblentz JM, Plect AB. Subacute sclerosing panencephalitis. Unusual nuclear inclusions and lengthy clinical course. Arch Neurol 1974;31:355–363.

Dubovsky SL, Grabon S, Berl T, Schrier RW. Syndrome of inappropriate secretion of antidiuretic hormone with exacerbated psychosis. Ann Intern Med 1973;79:551–554.

Ducas J, Robson HG. Cerebrospinal fluid penicillin levels during therapy for latent syphilis. JAMA 1981;246:2583–2584.

Duffy FH, Albert MS, McAnulty G. Brain electrical activity in patients with presenile and senile dementia of the Alzheimer type. Ann Neurol 1984;16:439–448.

Duffy FH, Birchfield JL, Lombroso CT. Brain electrical activity mapping (BEAM): a method for extending the clinical utility of EEG and evoked potential data. Ann Neurol 1979;5:309–321.

Duffy P, Wolf J, Collins G, DeVoe AG, Streeten B, Cowen D. Possible person-to-person transmission of Creutzfeldt-Jakob disease. N Engl J Med 1974;290:692.

Duguid JR, De La Paz R, DeGroot J. Magnetic resonance imaging of the midbrain in Parkinson's disease. Ann Neurol 1986;20:744–747.

Duman S, Stephens JW. Post-traumatic middle cerebral artery occlusion. Neurology 1963;13:613–616.

Dunea G, Mahurkar SD, Mamdani B, Smith EC. Role of aluminum in dialysis dementia. Ann Intern Med 1978;88:502–504.

Dunn J, Kernohan JW. Gliomatosis cerebri. Arch Pathol 1957;64:82–91.

Durbin M, Martin RL. Speech in mania: syntactic analysis. Brain Lang 1977;4:208–218.

Durso R, Fedio P, Brouwers P, et al. Lysine vasopressin in Alzheimer disease. Neurology 1982;32:674–677.

Duvoisin RC, Yahr MD. Encephalitis and parkinsonism. Arch Neurol 1965;12:227–239.

Duvoisin RC, Yahr MD, Schweitzer MD, Merritt HH. Parkinsonism before and since the epidemic of encephalitis lethargica. Arch Neurol 1963;9:232–236.

Dyck PJ, Johnson WJ, Lambert EH, O'Brien PC. Segmental demyelination secondary to axonal degeneration in uremic neuropathy. Mayo Clin Proc 1971;46:400–431.

Dyck PJ, Ohta J. Neuronal atrophy and degeneration predominantly affecting peripheral sensory neurons. In: Dyck PJ, Thomas PK, Lambert EH, eds. Peripheral neuropathy. WB Saunders, Philadelphia, 1975:791–824.

Dyken PR, Swift A, DuRant RH. Long-term follow-up of patients with subacute sclerosing panencephalitis treated with inosiplex. Ann Neurol 1982;11:359–364.

Eadie MJ, Sutherland JM. Arteriosclerosis in parkinsonism. J Neurol Neurosurg Psychiatry 1964;27:237–240.

Eastman R, Sheridan J, Poskanzer DC. Multiple sclerosis clustering in a small Massachusetts community with possible common exposure 23 years before onset. N Engl J Med 1973;289:793–794.

Ehle AL. Johnson PC. Rapidly evolving EEG changes in a case of Alzheimer disease. Ann Neurol 1977;1:593–595.

Ehmann WD, Alauddin M, Hossain TIM, Markesberry WR. Brain trace elements in Pick's disease. Ann Neurol 1984;15:102–104.

Eisdorfer C, Cohen D, Buckley CE III. Serum immunoglobulins and cognition in the impaired elderly. In: Katzman R, Terry RD, Bick KL, eds. Alzheimer's disease, senile dementia and related disorders. Raven Press, New York, 1978:401–407.

Eisdorfer C, Cohen D, Preston C. Behavioral and psychological therapies for the older patient with cognitive impairment. In: Miller NE, Cohen GD, eds. Clinical aspects of Alzheimer's disease and senile dementia. Raven Press, New York, 1981:209–224.

Ekbom K, Greitz T, Kalmer M, Lopez J, Ottoson S. Cerebrospinal fluid pulsations in occult hydrocephalus due to ectasia of basilar artery. Acta Neurochir 1969a;20:1–8.

Ekbom K, Greitz T, Kugleberg E. Hydrocephalus due to ectasia of the basilar artery. J Neurol Sci 1969b;8:465–477.

Ekholm S, Simon JH. Magnetic resonance imaging and the acquired immunodeficiency syndrome dementia complex. Acta Radiol 1988;29:227–230.

Eldridge R, Anayiotos CP, Schlesinger S, Cowen D, Bever C, Patonas N, McFarland H. Hereditary adult-onset leukodystrophy simulating chronic progressive multiple sclerosis. N Engl J Med 1984;311:948–953.

Elizan TS, Chen K-M, Mathai KV, Dunn D, Kurland LT. Amyotrophic lateral sclerosis and Parkinsonism-dementia complex. Arch Neurol 1966a;14:347–355.

Elizan TS, Hirano A, Abrams BM, Need RL, Van Nuis C, Kurland LT. Amyotrophic lateral sclerosis and Parkinsonism-dementia complex of Guam. Arch Neurol 1966b;14:356–368.

Ellenberger C Jr, Petro DJ, Ziegler SB. The visually evoked potential in Huntington disease. Neurology 1978;28:95–97.

Ellie E, Julien J, Ferrer X. Familial idiopathic striopallidodentate calcifications. Neurology 1989;39:381–385.

Ellington E, Margolis G. Block of arachnoid villus by subarachnoid hemorrhage. J Neurosurg 1969;30:651–657.

Ellis WG, McCulloch JR, Corley CL. Presenile dementia in Down's syndrome. Neurology 1974;24:101–106.

Ellison DW, Beal MF, Mazurek MF, Bird ED, Martin JB. A postmortem study of amino acid neurotransmitters in Alzheimer's disease. Ann Neurol 1986;20:616–621.

Ellner JJ, Bennett JE. Chronic meningitis. Medicine 1976;55:341–369.

Elovaara I, Iivanainen M, Valle S-L, Suni J, Tervo T, Lahdevirta J. CSF protein and cellular profiles in various stages of HIV infection related to neurological manifestations. J Neurol Sci 1987;78:331–342.

Emson PC, Rehfeld JF, Langevin H, Rossor M. Reduction in cholecystokinin-like immunoreactivity in the basal ganglia in Huntington's disease. Brain Res 1980;198:497–500.

Engel GL, Romano J. Delirium, a syndrome of cerebral insufficiency. J Chron Dis 1959;9:260–277.

English WH. Alzheimer's disease. Psychiatr Q 1942;16:91–106.

Englund E, Brun A. Frontal lobe degeneration of the non-Alzheimer type. IV. White matter changes. Arch Gerontol Geriatr 1987;6:235–243.

Enlow RW. Epidemiology and immunology of acquired immune deficiency syndrome. In: Nichols SE, Ostrow DG, eds., Acquired immune deficiency syndrome. American Psychiatric Press, Washington, D.C., 1984;3–16.

Enna SJ, Bird ED, Bennett JP Jr, et al. Huntington's chorea. Changes in neurotransmitter receptors in the brain. N Engl J Med 1976;294:1305–1309.

Enna SJ, Stern LZ, Wastek GJ, Yamamura HI. Cerebrospinal fluid γ-aminobutyric acid variations in neurological disorders. Arch Neurol 1977;34:683–685.

Enoch MD, Trethowan WH. Uncommon psychiatric syndromes. 2nd ed. John Wright & Sons, Bristol, Eng., 1979.

Epstein FH, Levitin H, Glaser G, Lavietes P. Cerebral hyponatremia. N Engl J Med 1961;265:513–518.

Epstein L G and Shaver LR. Neurology of human immunodeficiency virus infection in children. In: Rosenblun ML, Levy RM, Bredesen DE, eds, AIDS and the nervous system, Raven Press, New York, 1988:79–101.

Eraut D. Idiopathic hypoparathyroidism presenting as dementia. Br Med J 1974;1:429–430.

Erickson RP, Lie MR, Wineinger MA. Rehabilitation in multiple sclerosis. Mayo Clin Proc 1989;64:818–828.

Erkinjuntti T. Types of multi-infarct dementia. Acta Neurol Scand 1987;75:391–399.

Erkinjuntti T, Haltia M, Palo J, Sulkava R, Paetau A. Accuracy of the clinical diagnosis of vascular dementia: a prospective clinical and post-mortem neuropathological study. J Neurol Neurosurg Psychiatry 1988;51:1037–1044.

Erkinjuntti T, Ketonen L, Sulkava R, Sipponen J, Vuorialho M, Iivanainen M. Do white matter changes on MRI and CT differentiate vascular dementia from Alzheimer's disease? J Neurol Neurosurg Psychiatry 1987;50:37–42.

Erkinjuntti T, Laaksonen R, Sulkava R, Syrjalainen R, Palo J. Neuropsychological differentiation between normal aging, Alzheimer's disease, and vascular dementia. Acta Neurol Scand 1986;74:393–403.

Erkinjuntti T, Sipponen JT, Iivanainen M, Ketonen L, Sulkava R, Sepponen RE. Cerebral NMR and CT imaging in dementia. J Comp Assist Tomog 1984;8:614–618.

Erkinjuntti T, Sulkava R, Kovanen J, Palo J. Suspected dementia: evaluation of 323 consecutive referrals. Acta Neurol Scand 1987;76:359–364.

Ernst J. Neuropsychological problem-solving skills in the elderly. Psychology and Aging 1987;2:363–365.

Esiri MM, Wilcock GK. Cerebral amyloid angiopathy in dementia and old age. J Neurol Neurosurg Psychiatry 1986;49:1221–1226.

Eslinger PJ, Damasio AR. Preserved motor learning in Alzheimer's disease: Implications for anatomy and behavior. J Neurosci 1986;6:3006–3009.

Eslinger PJ, Pepin L, Benton AL. Different patterns of visual memory errors occur with aging and dementia. J Clin Exper Neuropsychol 1988; 10:60–61 (Abstr.).

Espir MLE, Spalding JMK. Three recent cases of encephalitis lethargica. Br Med J 1956;1:1141–1144.

Essa M. Carbamazepine in dementia. J Clin Psychopharmacol 1986;6:234–236.

Essen-Moller E. A family with Alzheimer's disease. Acta Psychiatr Neurol Scand 1946;21:233–244.

Esteban A, Mateo D, Gimenez-Roldan S. Early detection of Huntington's disease. Blink reflex and levodopa load in presymptomatic and incipient subjects. J Neurol Neurosurg Psychiatry 1981;44:43–48.

Estrin WJ, Cavalieri SA, Wald P, Becker CE, Jones JR, Cone JE. Evidence of neurologic dysfunction related to long-term ethylene oxide exposure. Arch Neurol 1987;44:1283–1286.

Estey E, Lieberman A, Pinto R, Meltzer M, Ransohoff J. Cerebral arteritis in scleroderma. Stroke 1979;10:595–597.

Etienne P, Dastoor D, Gauthier S, Ludwick R, Collier B. Alzheimer disease: lack of effect of lecithin treatment for three months. Neurology 1981;31:1552–4.

Etienne P, Gauthier S, Dastoor D, Collier B, Ratner J. Alzheimer's disease: clinical effect of lecithin treatment. In: Glen AIM, Whalley LJ, eds. Alzheimer's disease. Early recognition of potentially reversible deficits. Churchill Livingstone, London, 1979:173–178.

Etienne P, Gauthier S, Johnson G, et al. Clinical effects of choline in Alzheimer's disease. Lancet 1978;2:508–509.

Ettigi PG, Brown GM. Brain disorders associated with endocrine dysfunction. Psychiatr Clin North Am 1978;1:117–136.

Ettinger A. Adult form of leucodystrophy of type Scholz-Bielschowsky-Henneberg, with metachromatic breakdown products, in a 55-year-old male. Psychiatr Neurol (Basel) 1965;149:225–239.

Evans BM. Cyclic EEG changes in subacute spongiform and anoxic encephalopathy. Electroencephalogr Clin Neurophysiol 1975;39:587–598.

Evans HL, Laties VG, Weiss B. Behavioral effects of mercury and methyl-mercury. Fed Proc 1975;34:1858–1867.

Faber-Langendoen K, Morris JC, Knesevich JW, LaBarge E, Miller JP, Berg L. Aphasia in senile dementia of the Alzheimer type. Ann Neurol 1988;23:365–370.

Faden AI, Townsend JJ. Myoclonus in Alzheimer disease. Arch Neurol 1976;33:278–280.

Fairweather DS. Psychiatric aspects of the post-encephalitic syndrome. J Ment Sci 1947;93:201–254.

Falk RE, Cederbaum SD, Blass JP, Gibson GE, Kark RAP, Carrel RE. Ketonic diet in the management of pyruvate dehydrogenase deficiency. Pediatrics 1976;58:713–721.

Famuyiwa OO, Eccleston D, Donaldson AA, Garside RF. Tardive dyskinesia and dementia. Br J Psychiatry 1979;135:500–504.

Faris AA. Wernicke's encephalopathy in uremia. Neurology 1972;22:1293–1297.

Farley IJ, Price KS, McCullough E, Deck JHN, Hordynski W, Hornykiewicz O. Norepinephrine in chronic paranoid schizophrenia: above normal levels in limbic forebrain. Science 1978;200:456–458.

Farlow MR, Yee RD, Dlouhy SR, Conneally PM, Azzarelli B, Ghetti B. Gerstmann-Straussler-Scheinker disease. I. Extending the clinical spectrum. Neurology 1989;39:1446–1452.

Farnell FJ, Globus JH. Chronic progressive vascular subcortical encephalopathy. Arch Neurol Psychiatry 1932;27:593–604.

Farrell DF. The EEG in progressive multifocal leukoencephalopathy. Electroencephalogr Clin Neurophysiol 1969;26:200–205.

Farrer LA, O'Sullivan DM, Cupples A, Growdon JH, Myers RH. Assessment of genetic risk for Alzheimer's disease among first-degree relatives. Ann Neurol 1989;25:485–493.

Farver P. Performance of older adults on a test battery designed to measure parietal lobe functions. Unpublished master's degree thesis, Boston University, Boston, College of Allied Health Professions, 1975.

Fauci AS, Lane HC. The acquired immunodeficiency syndrome (AIDS). In: Braunwald E, Isselbacher KJ, Petersdorf RG, Wilson JD, Martin JB, Fauci AS, eds. Harrison's principles of internal medicine, 11th ed. McGraw-Hill, New York, 1987;1392–1396.

Fazekas F, Offenbacher H, Fuchs S, Schmidt R, Niederkorn K, Horner S, Lechner H. Criteria for an increased specificity of MRI interpretation in elderly subjects with suspected multiple sclerosis. Neurology 1988;38:1822–1825.

Fehling C, Jagerstad M, Lindstrand K, Elmqvist D. Folate deficiency and neurological disease. Arch Neurol 1974;30:263–265.

Fehrenbach RA, Wallesch C-W, Claus D. Neuropsychological findings in Friedreich's ataxia. Arch Neurol 1984;41:306–308.

Feinberg I. Sleep patterns in dementia: evidence, issues, and strategies. In: Nandy K, ed. Senile dementia: a biomedical approach. North-Holland, New York, 1978.

Feinglass EJ, Arnett FC, Dorsch CA, Zizic TM, Stevens MB. Neuropsychiatric manifestations of systemic lupus erythematosus: diagnosis, clinical spectrum, and relationship to other features of the disease. Medicine 1976;55:323–339.

Feiring EH, Brock S. General considerations in injuries of the brain and spinal cord and their coverings. In: Feiring EH, ed. Brock's injuries of the brain and spinal cord. Springer, New York, 1974:1–41.

Feldman RG. Trichlorethylene. In: Vinken PJ, Bruyn GW, eds. Intoxications of the nervous system. Part I, vol. 36. Handbook of clinical neurology. North-Holland, New York; 1979:457–464.

Feldman RG, Chandler KA, Levy LL, Glaser GH. Familial Alzheimer's disease. Neurology 1963a;13:811–824.

Feldman RG, Cummings. JL. Treatable dementias. In: Slade WR Jr, ed. Geriatric neurology. Futura, New York, 1981:173–197.

Feldman RG, Kelly-Hayes M, Conomy JP, Foley JM. Baclofen for spasticity in multiple sclerosis. Neurology 1978;28:1094–1098.

Feldman RG, Pincus JH, McEntee WJ. Cerebrovascular accident or subdural fluid collection? Arch Intern Med 1963b;112:966–976.

Fernandez F, Adams F, Levy JK, Holmes VF, Neidhart M, Mansell PWA. Cognitive impairment due to AIDS-related complex and its response to psychostimulants. Psychosomatics 1988;29:38–46.

Ferraro A, Jervis GA. Pick's disease. Clinico-pathologic study and report of two cases. Arch Neurol Psychiatry 1936;36:739–767.

Ferraro A, Jervis GA. Alzheimer's disease (an attempt at establishing the adult type of the disease). Psychiatr Q 1941;15:3–16.

Ferrier IN, Johnson JA,Roberts GW, Crow TJ, Corsellis JAN, Lee YC, O'Shaughnessy D, Adrian TE, McGregor GP, Baracese-Hamilton AJ, Bloom SR. Neuropeptides in Alzheimer type dementia. J Neurol Sci 1983;62:159–170.

Ferris EJ. Arteristis. In: Newton TH, Potts DG, eds. Radiology of the skull and brain. Vol 2. St. CV Mosby, Louis, 1974:2566–2597.

Ferris EJ, Levine HL. Cerebral arteritis: a classification, Radiology 1973;109:327–341.

Ferris SH, de Leon MJ, Wolf AP, et al. Positron emission tomography in the study of aging and senile dementia. Neurobiol Aging 1980;1:127–131.

Fetzer J, Kader G, Danahy S. Lithium encephalopathy: a clinical, psychiatric, and EEG evaluation. Am J Psychiatry 1981;138:1622–1623.

Feurle GE, Volk B, Waldherr R. Cerebral Whipple's disease with negative jejunal histology. N Engl J Med 1979;300:907–908.

Fields SD, MacKenzie R, Charlson ME, Perry SW. Reversibility of cognitive impairment in medical inpatients. Arch Intern Med 1986;146:1593–1596.

Fieve RR, Platman S. Lithium and thyroid function in manic-depressive psychosis. Am J Psychiatry 1968;125:527–530.

Filley CM, Heaton RK, Nelson LM, Burks JS, Franklin GM. A comparison of dementia in Alzheimer's disease and multiple sclerosis. Arch Neurol 1989;46:157–161.

Filley CM, Kelly J, Heaton RK. Neurospychologic features of early- and late-onset Alzheimer's disease. Arch Neurol 1986;43:574–576.

Fine EW, Lewis D, Villa-Lauda I, Blakemore CB. The effect of cyclandelate on mental function in patients with arteriosclerotic brain disease. Br J Psychiatry 1970;117:157–161.

Finelli PF, McEntee WJ, Lessell S, Morgan TF, Copetto J. Whipple's disease with predominantly neuro-ophthalmic manifestations. Ann Neurol 1977;1:247–252.

Finlayson MH, Guberman A, Martin JB. Cerebral lesions in familial amyotrophic lateral sclerosis with dementia. Acta Neuropath 1973;26:237–246.

Finlayson RE, Hurt RD, Davis LJ Jr, Morse RM. Alcoholism in elderly persons: a study of the psychiatric and psychosocial features of 216 inpatients. Mayo Clin Proc 1988;63:761–768.

Finlayson MH, Superville B. Distribution of cerebral lesions in acquired hepatocerebral degeneration. Brain 1981;104:79–95.

Fischer EG, Shillito J Jr. Large abdominal cysts: a complication of peritoneal shunts. J Neurosurg 1969;31:441–444.

Fischer P-A, Enzensberger W. Neurological complications of AIDS. J Neurol 1987;234:269–279.

Fischer-Williams M, Bosanquet FD, Daniel PM. Carcinomatosis of the meninges: a report of three cases. Brain 1955;78:42–58.

Fischer-Williams M, Last SL, Lyberi G, Northfield DWC. Clinico-EEG study of 128 gliomas and 50 intracranial metastatic tumors. Brain 1962;85:1–46.

Fisher A. On meningioma presenting with dementia. Proc Aust Assoc Neurol 1969;6:29–38.

Fisher CM. The clinical picture in Creutzfeldt-Jakob disease. Trans Am Neurol Assoc 1960;85:147–150.

Fisher CM. Lacunes: small, deep cerebral infarcts. Neurology 1965a;15:774–784.

Fisher CM. Pure sensory stroke involving face, arm, and leg. Neurology 1965b;15:76–80.

Fisher CM. A lacunar stroke. The dysarthria-clumsy hand syndrome. Neurology 1967;17:614–617.

Fisher CM. The arterial lesions underlying lacunes. Acta Neuropathol 1969;12:1–15.

Fisher CM, Cole M. Homolateral ataxia and crural paresis: a vascular syndrome. J Neurol Neurosurg Psychiatry 1965;28:48–55.

Fisher CM, Curry HB. Pure motor hemiplegia of vascular origin. Arch Neurol 1965;13:30–44.

Fisher CM, Williams HW, Wing ES Jr. Combined encephalopathy and neuropathy with carcinoma. J Neuropathol Exp Neurol 1961;20:535–547.

Fisher M. Senile dementia—a new explanation of its causation. Can Med Assoc J 1951;65:1–7.

Fisher NR, Cope SJ, Lishman WA. Metachromatic leukodystrophy: conduct disorder progressing to dementia. J Neurol, Neurosurg, Psychiatry 1987;50:488–489.

Fishman RA. Occult hydrocephalus. N Engl J Med 1966;274:466–467.

Fitch N, Becker R, Heller A. The inheritance of Alzheimer's disease: a new interpretation. Ann Neurol 1988;23:14–19.

Fitz TE, Hallman BL. Mental changes associated with hyperparathyroidism. Arch Intern Med 1952;89:547–551.

Fitzhugh LC, Fitzhugh KB, Reitan RM. Adaptive abilities and intellectual functioning of hospitalized alcoholics: further considerations. Q J Stud Alcohol 1965;26:402–411.

Fitzsimons JM. Tuberculous meningitis. Tubercle 1963;44:87–102.

Fleming JL, Wiesner RH, Shorter RG. Whipple's disease: clinical, biochemical, and histopathologic features and assessment of treatment in 29 patients. Mayo Clin Proc 1988;63:539–551.

Flendrig JA, Kruis H, Das HA. Aluminum and dialysis dementia. Lancet 1976;1:1235.

Fletcher WA, Sharpe JA. Saccadic eye movement dysfunction in Alzheimer's disease. Ann Neurol 1986;20:464–471.

Fletcher WA, Sharpe JA. Smooth pursuit dysfunction in Alzheimer's disease. Neurology 1988;38:272–277.

Flicker C, Ferris SH, Crook T, Bartus R. Implications of memory and language dysfunction in the naming deficit of senile dementia. Brain Lang 1987;31:187–200.

Floeter MK, So YT, Ross DA, Greenberg D. Miliary metastases to the brain: clinical and radiologic features. Neurology 1987;37:1817–1818.

Flowers KA, Pearce I, Pearce JMS. Recognition memory in Parkinson's disease. J Neurol Neurosurg Psychiatry 1984;47:1174–1181.

Flowers KA, Robertson C. The effect of Parkinson's disease on the ability to maintain a mental set. J Neurol Neurosurg Psychiatry 1985;48:517–529.

Fog T. Topographic distribution of plaques in the spinal cord in multiple sclerosis. Arch Neurol Psychiatry 1950;63:382–414.

Folstein MF, Breitner JCS. Language disorder predicts familial Alzheimer's disease. Johns Hopkins Med J 1981;149:145–147.

Folstein MF, Folstein SE, McHugh PR. "Mini-mental state": a practical method for grading the mental state of patients for the clinician. J Psychiatr Res 1975;12:189–198.

Folstein SE, Folstein MF, McHugh PR. Psychiatric syndromes in Huntington's disease. Adv Neurol 1979;23:281–289.

Folstein MF, Luria RE. Reliability, validity and clinical application of the visual analogue mood scale. Psychol Med 1973;3:479–486.

Folstein MF, McHugh PR. Dementia syndrome of depression. In: Katzman R, Terry RD, Bick KL, eds. Alzheimer's disease, senile dementia and related disorders. Raven Press, New York, 1978:87–93.

Folstein SE, Brandt J, Folstein MF. Huntington's disease. In: Cummings JL, ed. Subcortical dementia. Oxford University Press, New York, 1990:87–107.

Foltz EL. The first seven years of a hydrocephalus project. In: Shulman K, ed. Workshop in hydrocephalus. The Children's Hospital of Philadelphia, Philadelphia, 1966.

Foltz EL, Shurtleff DB. Five-year comparative study of hydrocephalus in children with and without operation (113 cases). J Neurosurg 1963;20:1064–1079.

Foltz EL, Ward AA. Communicating hydrocephalus from subarachnoid bleeding. J Neurosurg 1956;13:546–566.

Foncin JF, Gruner JE. Tin neurotoxicity. In: Vinken PJ, Bruyn GW, eds. Intoxications of the nervous system. Part I, vol. 36. Handbook of clinical neurology. North-Holland, New York, 1979:279–290.

Ford RG, Siekert RG. Central nervous system manifestations of periarteritis nodosa. Neurology 1965;15:114–122.

Forno LS, Barbour PJ, Norville RL. Presenile dementia with Lewy bodies and neurofibrillary tangles. Arch Neurol 1978;35:818–22.

Forno LS, Norville RL. Ultrastructure of the neostriatum in Huntington's and Parkinson's disease. Adv Neurol 1979;23:123–135.

Forrest DM, Cooper DGW. Complications of ventriculo-atrial shunts. J Neurosurg 1968;29:506–512.

Forster W, Schultz S, Henderson AL. Combined hydrogenated alkaloids of ergot in senile and arteriosclerotic psychoses. Geriatrics 1955;10:26–30.

Foster NL, Chase TN, Fedio P, Patronas NJ, Brooks RA, Di Chiro G. Alzheimer's disease: focal cortical changes shown by positron emission tomography. Neurology 1983;33:961–965.

Foster NL, Gilman S, Berent S, Morin EM, Brown MB, Koeppe RA. Cerebral hypometabolism in progressive supranuclear palsy studied with positron emission tomography. Ann Neurol 1988;24:399–406.

Fowler CJ, Harrison MJG. EEG changes in subcortical dementia: a study of 22 patients with Steele-Richardson-Olszweski (SRO) syndrome. EEG Clin Neurophysiol 1986;64:301–303.

Fowler HL. Machado-Joseph-Azorean disease. A ten-year study. Arch Neurol 1984;41:921–925.

Fox IS, Spence AM, Wheelis RF, Healey LA. Cerebral embolism in Libman-Sacks endocarditis. Neurology 1980;30:487–491.

Fox JH, Ramsey RG, Huckman MS, Proske AE. Cerebral ventricular enlargement. Chronic alcoholics examined by computerized tomography. JAMA 1976; 236:365–368.

Fox JH, Topel JL, Huckman MS. Use of computerized tomography in senile dementia. J Neurol Neurosurg Psychiatry 1975;38:948–953.

Fozard JL, Thomas JC, Waugh NC. Effects of age and frequency of stimulus repetitions on two choice reaction times. J Gerontol 1976;31:556–563.

Frackowiak RSJ, Pozzilli C, Legg NJ, et al. Regional cerebral oxygen supply and utilization in dementia. Brain 1981;104:753–758.

Francis AF. Familial basal ganglia calcification and schizophreniform psychosis. Br J Psychiatry 1979;135:360–362.

Frank RA, Shalen PR, Harvey DG, Berg L, Ferguson TB, Schwartz HG. Artrial myxoma with intellectual decline and cerebral growths on CT scan. Ann Neurol 1979;5:396–400.

Franklin GM, Heaton RK, Nelson LM, Filley CM, Seibert C. Correlation of neuropsychological and MRI findings in chronic/progressive multiple sclerosis. Neurology 1988;38:1826–1829.

Franklin GM, Nelson LM, Filley CM, Heaton RK. Cognitive loss in multiple sclerosis. Arch Neurol 1989;46:162–167.

Fraser CL, Arieff AI. Hepatic encephalopathy. N Engl J Med 1985;313:865–873.

Fraser TN. Cerebral manifestations of Addisonian pernicious anaemia. Lancet 1960;2:458–459.

Frazier CH. Tumor involving the frontal lobe alone. Arch Neurol Psychiatry 1936; 35:525–571.

Frederick MW. Cerebrovascular disease. In: Conn HL, Horwitz O, eds. Cardiac and vascular diseases. Lea & Febiger, Philadelphia, 1971:1473–1499.

Freeman JM. The clinical spectrum and early diagnosis of Dawson's encephalitis. J Pediatr 1969;75:590–603.

Freeman JW, Couch JR. Prolonged encephalopathy with arsenic poisoning. Neurology 1978;28:853–855.

Freemon FR. Evaluation of patients with progressive intellectual deterioration. Arch Neurol 1976;33:658–659.

Friede RL, Magee KR. Alzheimer's disease. Presentation of a case with pathologic and enzymatic-histochemical observations. Neurology 1962;12:213–222.

Friede RL, Magee KR, Mack EW. Idiopathic nonarteriosclerotic calcification of the cerebral vessels. Arch Neurol 1961;5:279–286.

Friedland RP, Budinger TF, Ganz E, Yano Y, Mathis CA, Koss B, Ober BA,

Huesman RH, Derenzo SE. Regional cerebral metabolic alterations in dementia of the Alzheimer type: Positron emission tomography with (^{18}F) fluorodeoxyglucose. J Computer Assisted Tomography 1983;7:590–598.

Friedland RP, Jagust WJ, Ober BA, Dronkers NF, Koss E, Simpson GV, Ellis WG, Budinger TF. The pathophysiology of Pick's disease: A comprehensive case study. Neurology 1986;36(Suppl. 1):268 (Abstr.).

Friedland RP, Koss E, Kumar A, Gaine S, Metzler D, Haxby JV, Moore A. Motor vehicle crashes in dementia of the Alzheimer type. Ann Neurol 1988;24:782–786.

Friedland RP, Prusiner S, Jagust W, Budinger TF. Bitemporal hypometabolism in Creutzfeldt-Jakob disease: Positron emission tomography with 1-2-fluorodeoxyglucose. J Computer Assisted Tomography 1984;8:978–981.

Friedman AS. Minimal effects of severe depression on cognitive functioning. J Abnorm Soc Psychol 1964;69:237–243.

Friedman H, Odom GL. Expanding intracranial lesions in geriatric patients. Geriatrics 1972;27:105–115.

Friedman LL, Signorelli JJ. Blastomycosis: a brief review of the literature and a report of a case involving the meninges. Ann Intern Med 1946;24:385–396.

Front D, Beks JWF, Penning L. Porencephaly diagnosed by isotope cisternography. J Neurol Neurosurg Psychiatry 1972;35:669–675.

Fujita M, Hosoki M, Miyazaki M. Brainstem auditory evoked responses in spinocerebellar degeneration and Wilson disease. Ann Neurol 1981;9:42–47.

Fuld PA. Psychological testing in the differential diagnosis of the dementias. In: Katzman R, Terry RD, Bick KL, eds. Alzheimer's disease, senile dementia and related disorders. Raven Press, New York, 1978:185–193.

Fuld PA, Katzman R, Davies P, Terry RD. Intrusions as a sign of Alzheimer dementia: chemical and pathological verification. Ann Neurol 1982;11:155–159.

Fulford KWM, Catterall RD, Delhanty JJ, Doniach D, Kremer M. A collagen disorder of the nervous system presenting as multiple sclerosis. Brain 1972; 95:373–386.

Fuller SC. Alzheimer's disease (senium praecox): the report of a case and review of published cases. J Nerv Ment Dis 1912;39:440–455, 536–557.

Fulton JS, Burton AN. After-effects of western equine encephalomyelitis infections in man. Can Med Assoc J 1953;69:268–272.

Funkenstein HH, Hicks R, Dysken MW, Davis JM. Drug treatment of cognitive impairment in Alzheimer's disease and the late life dementias. In: Miller NE, Cohen GD, eds. Clinical aspects of Alzheimer's disease and senile dementia. Raven Press, New York, 1981:139–158.

Furlan AJ, Henry CE, Sweeney PJ, Mitsumoto H. Focal EEG abnormalities in Heidenhain's variant of Jakob-Creutzfeldt disease. Arch Neurol 1981;38:312–314.

Gaan D, Brewis RAL, Mallick NP, Seedat YK, Mahoney MP. Cerebral damage from declotting Scribner shunts. Lancet 1969;2:77–79.

Gabuzda DH, Levy SR, Chiappa KH. Electroencephalography in AIDS and AIDS-related complex. Clin Electroenceph 1988;19:1–6.

Gado M. CT scanning in dementia. Paper presented at the 110th Annual Session, California Medical Association, Anaheim, Calif., March 13, 1981.

Gado MH, Coleman RE, Lec KS, Mikhael MA, Alderson PO, Archer CR. Correlation between computerized transaxial tomography and radionuclide cister-nography in dementia. Neurology 1976;26:555–560.

Gainotti G, Caltagirone C, Masullo C, Miceli G. Patterns of neuropsychologic impairment in various diagnostic groups of dementia. In: Amaducci L, Davison AN, Antuono P, eds. Aging of the brain and dementia. Raven Press, New York; 1980:245–250.

Gaitz CM, Varner RV, Overall JE. Pharmacotherapy for organic brain syndrome in late life. Arch Gen Psychiatry 1977;34:839–845.

Gajdusek DC. Unconventional viruses and the origin and disappearance of kuru. Science 1977;197:943–960.

Gajdusek DC, Gibbs CJ Jr, Asher DM, et al. Precautions in medical care of, and in handling materials from, patients with transmissible virus dementia (Creutz-feldt-Jakob disease). N Engl J Med 1977;297:1253–1258.

Gajdusek DC, Salazar AM. Amyotrophic lateral sclerosis and parkinsonian syn-dromes in high incidence among the Auyu and Jakai people of West New Guinea. Neurology 1982;32:107–126.

Galera GR, Greitz T. Hydrocephalus in the adult secondary to rupture of intracranial arterial aneurysms. J Neurosurg 1970;32:634–641.

von Gall M, Beckes H, Artmann H, Lerch G, Nemeth N. Results of computer tomography on chronic alcoholics, Neuroradiology 1978;16:329–331.

Gallassi R, Montagna P, Morreale A. Lorusso S, Tinuper P, Daidone R, Lugaresi E. Neuropsychological, electroencephalogram and brain computed tomography findings in motor neuron disease. Eur Neurol 1989;29:115–120.

Gamboa ET, Isaacs G, Harter DH. Chorea associated with oral contraceptive therapy. Arch Neurol 1971;25:112–114.

Gandy SE, Snow RB, Zimmerman RD, Deck MDF. Cranial nuclear magnetic resonance imaging in head trauma. Ann Neurol 1984;16;254-257.

Gannon WE, Cook AW, Browder EJ. Resolving subdural collections. J Neurosurg 1962;19:865–869.

Garcia-Bunuel L. Elliot DC, Blank NK. Apneic spells in progressive dialysis en-cephalopathy. Arch neurol 1980;37:594–596.

Gardner WJ, Smith JL, Padget DH. The relationship of Arnold-Chiari and Dandy-Walker malformations. J Neurosurg 1972;36:481–486.

Garland H, Pearce J. Neurological complications of carbon monoxide poisoning. Q J Med 1967;36:445–455.

Garron DC. Huntington's chorea with schizophrenia. Adv Neurol 1973;1:729–734.

Garruto RM, Yanagihara R, Gajdusek DC. Disappearance of high-incidence amy-otrophic lateral sclerosis and parkinsonism-dementia on Guam. Neurology 1985;35:193–198.

Gatewood JW, Organ CH Jr, Mead BT. Mental changes associated with hyper-parathyroidism. Am J Psychiatry 1975;132:129–132.

Gath I, Jorgensen A, Sjaastad O, Berstad J. Pneumoencephalographic findings in parkinsonism. Arch Neurol 1975;32:769–773.

Gath I, Vinje B. Pneumoencephalographic findings in Huntington's chorea. Neurol 1968;18:991–996.

Gauthier S, Masson H, Gauthier L, Bouchard R, Collier B, Bacher Y, Bailey R, Becker R, Bergman H, Charbonneau R, Dastoor D, Gayton D, Kennedy J,

Kissel C, Krieger M, Kushnir S, Lamontagne A, St-martin M, Morin J, Nair NPV, Neirinck L, Ratner J, Suissa S, Tesfaye Y. Vida S. Tetrahydroaminoacridine and lecithin in Alzheimer's disease. In: Giacobini E, Becker R, eds., Current research in Alzheimer therapy. Cholinesterase inhibitors. Taylor and Francis, New York, 1988:237–245.

Gawel MJ, Das P, Vincent S, Rose FC. Visual and auditory evoked responses in patients with Parkinson's disease. J Neurol Neurosurg Psychiatry 1981;44:227–232.

Gawler J, DuBoulay GH, Bull JWD, Omae T. Computerized tomography (the EMI scanner): a comparison with pneumoencephalography and ventriculography. J Neurol Neurosurg Psychiatry 1976;39:203–211.

Gaylord SA, Marsh GR. Age differences in the speed of a spatial cognitive process. J Gerontol 1975;30:674–678.

Geisser BS, Kurtzberg D, Vaughan HG Jr, Arezzo JC, Aisen ML, Smith CR, LaRocca NG, Scheinberg LC. Trimodal evoked potentials compared with magnetic resonance imaging in the diagnosis of multiple sclerosis. Arch Neurol 1987;44:281–284.

Gelenberg A. The catatonic syndrome. Lancet 1976;1:1339–341.

Gemmell HG, Sharp PF, Evans NTS, Beeson JAO, Lyall D, Smith FW. Single photon emission tomography with I-123 isopropylamphetamine in Alzheimer's disease and multi-infarct dementia. Lancet 1984;ii:1348.

Gershell WJ. Psychiatric manifestations and nutritional deficiencies in the elderly. In: Levenson AJ, Hall RCW, eds. Neuropsychiatric manifestations of physical disease in the elderly. Raven Press, New York, 1981:119–131.

Gershon S, Shaw FH. Psychiatric sequelae of chronic exposure to organophosphorus insecticides. Lancet 1961;1:1371–1374.

Gerson SN, Benson DF, Frazier SH. Diagnosis: schizophrenia versus posterior aphasia. Am J Psychiatry 1977;134:966–969.

Gertz H-J, Henkes H, Cervos-Navaro J. Creutzfeldt-Jakob disease: Correlation of MRI and neuropathologic findings. Neurology 1988;38:1481–1482.

Geschwind N. The mechanism of normal pressure hydrocephalus. J Neurol Sci 1968;7:481–493.

Geschwind N. The apraxias: neural mechanisms of disorders of learned movement. Am Sci 1975;63:188–195.

Geschwind N, Kaplan E. A human cerebral deconnection syndrome. Neurology 1962;12:675–685.

Geschwind N, Quadfasel FA, Segarra JM. Isolation of the speech area. Neuropsychology 1968;6:327–340.

Geschwind N, Segarra JM. Sensory radicular neuropathy ("Denny-Brown's disease"), dementia, and seizures. In: Locke S, ed. Modern neurology. J & A Churchill, London, 1969:509–514.

Gevins AS, Doyle JC, Cutillo BA, et al. Electrical potentials in human brain cognition: new method reveals dynamic patterns of correlation. Science 1981;213:918–922.

Ghatak NR, Hadfield G, Rosenblum WI. Association of central pontine myelinolysis and Marchiafava-Bignami disease. Neurology 1978;28:1295–1298.

Ghetti B, Tagliavini F, Masters CL, Beyreuther K, Giaccone G, Verga L. Farlow MR, Conneally PM, Dlouhy SR, Azzarelli B, Bugiani O. Gerstmann-Straussler-Scheinker disease. II. Neurofibrillary tangles and plaques with PrP-amyloid coexist in an affected family. Neurology 1989;39:1453–1461.

Gibb WRG, Luthert PT, Marsden CD. Corticobasal degeneration. Brain 1989; 112:1171–1192.

Gibbs CJ, Gajdusek DC. Amyotrophic lateral sclerosis, Parkinson's disease, and amyotrophic lateral sclerosis-parkinsonism-dementia complex on Guam: a review and summary of attempts to demonstrate infection as the aetiology. J Clin Pathol 1971;25(suppl 6);132–140.

Gibbs CJ Jr, Gajdusek DC. Subacute spongiform virus encephalopathies: the transmissible virus dementias. In: Katzman R, Terry RD, Bick KL, eds. Alzheimer's disease; senile dementia and related disorders. Raven Press, New York, 1978:559–575.

Gibson TP. Dialyzability of common therapeutic agents. Dialysis Transplant 1979;8:24–40.

Gierl B, Groves L, Lazarus LW. Use of the dexamethasone suppression test with depressed and demented elderly. J Am Geriatr Soc 1987;35:115–120.

Gierz M, Zweifach M, Jeste DV. Antidepressant agents. In: Cummings JL, Miller BL, eds. Alzheimer's disease. Treatment and long-term management. Marcel Dekker, New York, 1989:125–141.

Gilbert GJ. Correspondence: pneumoencephalograthy in normal pressure hydrocephalus. N Engl J Med 1971;285:177–178.

Gilbert GJ, Glaser GH. Neurologic manifestations of chronic carbon monoxide poisoning. N Engl J Med 1969;261:1217–1220.

Gilbert JJ, Feldman RG. L-dopa for progressive supranuclear palsy. Lancet 1969;2:494.

Gilbert JJ, Kish SJ, Chang L-J, Morito C, Shannak K, Hornykiewicz O. Dementia, parkinsonism, and motor neuron disease: neurochemical and neuropathological correlates. Ann Neurol 1988;24:688–691.

Gilden DH, Rorke LB, Tanaka R. Acute SSPE. Arch Neurol 1975;32:644–646.

Gillilan LA. The arterial and venous blood supplies of the forebrain (including the internal capsule) of primates. Neurology 1968;18:653–670.

Gimenez-Roldan S, Peraita P, Lopez Agreda JM, Abad JM, Esteban A. Myoclonus and photic-induced seizures in Alzheimer's disease. Eur Neurol 1971;5:215–224.

Ginn HE. Neurobehavioral dysfunction in uremia. Kidney Internat 1975;217(suppl 2):S217–S221.

Giombetti RJ, Miller BL, Daly JA, Garrett K, Boone K, Kniesley L. Villanueva-Meyer J, Mena I. Sleep apnea, neuropsychological deficits and cerebral blood flow changes. Bull Clin Neurosci 1989;54:133–136.

Giombetti RJ, Miller BL. Recognition and management of superimposed medical conditions. In: Cummings JL, Miller BL, eds. Alzheimer's disease. Treatment and long-term management. Marcel Dekker, New York, 1990:253–265.

Giordani B, Sackellares JC, Miller S, Berent S, Sutula T, Seidenberg M, Boll TJ, O'Leary D, Dreifuss FE. Improvement in neuropsychological performance in patients with refractory seizures after intensive diagnostic and therapeutic intervention. Neurology 1983;33:489–493

Glaser GH. Psychotic reactions induced by corticotropin (ACTH) and cortisone. Psychosomat Med 1953;15:280–291.

Glaser GH. Collagen diseases and the nervous system. Med Clin North Am 1963;47:1475–1495.

Glaser GH. Diphenylhydantoin toxicity. In: Woodbury DM, Penry JK, Schmidt RP, eds. Antiepileptic drugs. Raven Press, New York, 1973:219–226.

Glaser GH. Brain dysfunction in uremia. Res Publ Assoc Res Nerv Ment Dis 1974;53:173–197.

Glaser GH, Pincus JH. Limbic encephalitis. J Nerv Ment Dis 1969;149:59–67.

Glaser J. Neuro-ophthalmology. Harper & Row, New York, 1978.

Glaser MA, Imerman CP, Imerman SW. So-called hemorrhagic encephalitis and myelitis secondary to intravenous arsphenamins. Am J Med Sci 1935;189:64–79.

Glass RM, Uhlenhuth EH, Hartel FW, Matzas W, Fischman MW. Cognitive dysfunction and imipramine in outpatient depressives. Arch Gen Psychiatry 1981;38:1048–1051.

Glass JD, Reich SG, DeLong MR. Wilsons disease. Development of neurological disease after beginning penicillomine therapy. Arch Neurol 1990;47:595–596.

Glen AIM, Christie JE. Early diagnosis of Alzheimer's disease: working definitions for clinical and laboratory criteria. In: Glen AIM, Whalley LJ, eds. Alzheimer's disease: early recognition of potentially reversible deficits. Churchill Livingstone, Edinburgh, 1979:122–128.

Glenner GG. Current knowledge of amyloid deposits as applied to senile plaques and congophilic angiopathy. In: Katzman R, Terry RD, Bick KL, eds. Alzheimer's disease, senile dementia and related disorders. Raven Press, New York, 1978:493–501.

Gloor P, Kalabay O, Giard N. The electroencephalogram in diffuse encephalopathies: electroencephalographic correlates of grey and white matter lesions. Brain 1968;91:779–802.

Glowinski H. Cognitive deficits in temporal lobe epilepsy. J Nerv Ment Dis 1973;157:129–137.

Goebel HH, Zur PH-B. Central pontine myelinolysis. Brain 1972;95:495-504.

Goetz CG, Klawans HL. Neurologic aspects of other metals. In: Vinken PJ, Bruyn GW, eds. Intoxications of the nervous system. Part I, vol. 36. Handbook of clinical neurology. North-Holland, New York, 1979:319–345.

Goetz CG, Klawans HL, Cohen MM. Neurotoxic agents: In: Baker AB, Baker LH, eds. Clinical neurology. Harper & Row, New York, 1981:1–84.

Goetz I, Roberts E, Comings DE. Fibroblasts in Huntington's disease. N Engl J Med 1975;293:1225–1227.

Goffinet AM, De Volder AG, Gillain C, Rectem D, Bol A, Michel C, Cogneau M, Labar D, Laterre C. Positron tomography demonstrates frontal lobe hypometabolism in progressive supranuclear palsy. Ann Neurol 1989;25:131–139.

Golbe LI, Davis PH, Schoenberg BS, Duvoisin RC. Prevalence and natural history of progressive supranuclear palsy. Neurology 1988;38:1031–1034.

Gold MS, Pottash ALC, Extein I, et al. The TRH test in the diagnosis of major and minor depression. Psychoneuroendocrinology 1981;6:159–169.

Goldberg A. Acute intermittent porphyria. Q J Med 1959;33:183–209.

Goldberg E. Varieties of perseveration: a comparison of two taxonomies. J. Clin Exper Neuropsychol 1986;8:701–705.

Goldberg ID, Bloomer WD, Dawson DM. Nervous system toxic effects of cancer therapy. JAMA 1982;247:1437–1441.

Golden CJ. A standardized version of Luria's neuropsychological tests: a quantitative and qualitative approach to neuropsychological evaluation. In: Filskov SB, Boll TJ, eds. Handbook of clinical neuropsychology. John Wiley & Sons, New York, 1981.

Golden CJ, Graber B, Coffman J, Berg RA, Newlin DB, Bloch S. Structural brain deficits in schizophrenia. Arch Gen Psychiatry 1981;38:1014–1017.

Golden CJ, Graber B. Moses JA, Zatz LM. Differentiation of chronic schizophrenics with and without ventricular enlargement by the Luria-Nebraska neuropsychological battery. Int J Neurosci 1980a;11:131–138.

Golden CJ, Moses JA Jr, Zelazowski R, et al. Cerebral ventricular size and neuropsychological impairment in young chronic schizophrenics. Arch Gen Psychiatry 1980b;37:619–623.

Goldfarb AI. Prevalence of psychiatric disorders in metropolitan old age and nursing homes. J Am Geriatr Soc 1962;10:77–84.

Goldhammer Y, Bubis JJ, Sarova-Pinhas I, Braham J. Subacute spongiform encephalopathy and its relation to Jakob-Creutzfeldt disease: report on six cases. J Neurol Neurosurg Psychiatry 1972;35:1–10.

Goldin S, MacDonald JE. The Ganser state. J Ment Sci 1955;101:267–280.

Goldstein G. Dementia associated with alcoholism. In: Tarter RE, Van Thiel DH, eds. Alcohol and the brain. Chronic effects. Plenum Medical Book Company, New York, 1985:283–294.

Goldstein M. Traumatic brain injury: a silent epidemic. Ann Neurol 1990:27:327.

Goldstein NP. Pigmented corneal rings in a patient with primary biliary cirrhosis. Arch Neurol 1976;33:372.

Goldstein NP, Ewert JC, Randall RV, Gross JB. Psychiatric aspects of Wilson's disease (hepatolenticular degeneration): results of psychometric tests during long-term therapy. Am J Psychiatry 1968;124:1555–1561.

Goldstein NP, Randall RV, Gross JB, Rosevear JW, McGuckin WF. Treatment of Wilson's disease (hepatolenticular degeneration) with DL-penicillamine. Neurology 1962;12:231–244.

Goldstein SG, Kleinknecht RA, Gallo AE Jr. Neuropsychological changes associated with carotid endarterectomy. Cortex 1970;6:308–322.

Gomori AJ, Partnow MJ, Horoupian DS, Hirano A. The ataxic form of Creutzfeldt-Jakob disease. Arch Neurol 1973;29:318–323.

Gonatas NK, Anderson W. Evangelista I. The contribution of altered synapses in the senile plaque, an electron microscopic study in Alzheimer's dementia. J Neuropathol Exp Neurol 1967;26:25–39.

Gonatas NK, Terry RD. Weiss M. Electron microscopic study of two cases of Jakob Creutzfeldt disease. J Neuropathol Exp Neurol 1965;24:575–598.

Gonzalez - Vitale JC, Garcia Bunuel R. Meningeal carcinomatosis. CA 1976;37:2906–2911.

Good MI. Pseudodementia and physical findings masking significant psychopathology. Am J Psychiatry 1981;138:811–814.

Goodglass H, Benson DF, Helm N. Aphasia and Related Disorders: Assessment and Therapy. Cerebrovascular survey report, National Institute of Neurological and Communicative Disorders and Stroke. Whiting Press, Rochester, Minn., 1980.

Goodin DS, Aminoff MJ. Electrophysiological differences between subtypes of dementia. Brain 1986;109:1103–1113.

Goodin DS, Aminoff MJ. Electrophysiological differences between demented and nondemented patients with Parkinson's disease. Ann Neurol 1987;21:90–94.

Goodin DS, Squires KC, Starr A. Long latency event-related components of the auditory evoked potential in dementia. Brain 1978;101:635–648.

Goodman L. Alzheimer's disease. A clinico-pathologic analysis of twenty-three cases with a theory on causation. J Nerv Ment Dis 1953;117:97–130.

Goodnight SH, Kenoyer G, Rapaport SI, Patch MJ, Lee JA, Kurze T. Defibrination after brain-tissue destruction. N Engl J Med 1974;290:1043–1047.

Goodstein RK, Ferrell RB. Multiple sclerosis—presenting as depressive illness. Dis Nerv Syst 1977;38:127–131.

Goodwin FK. Psychiatric side effects of levodopa in man. JAMA 1971;218:1915–1920.

Gopinathan G, Teravainen H, Dambrosia JM, et al. Lisuride in parkinsonism. Neurology 1981;31:371–376.

Gordon BM. Parkinsonism occurring with methyldopa treatment. Br Med J 1963; 1:1001.

Gordon EB. Serial EEG studies in presenile dementia. Br J Psychiatry 1968;114:779–780.

Gordon EB, Sim M. The EEG in presenile dementia. J Neurol Neurosurg Psychiatry 1967;30:285–291.

Gordon M. Gryfe CI. Hyperthyroidism with painless subacute thyroiditis in the elderly. JAMA 1981;246:2354–2355.

Goto I, Tobimatsu S, Ohta M, Hosokawa S, Shibasaki H, Kuroiwa Y. Dentatorubropallidoluysian degeneration: clinical, neuro-ophthalmologic, biochemical, and pathologic studies on autosomal dominant form. Neurology 1982;32:1395–1399.

Goto K, Umegaki H, Suetsugu M. Electroencephalographic and clinicopathological studies in Creutzfeldt-Jakob syndrome. J Neurol Neurosurg Psychiatry 1976; 39:931–940.

Gottlieb GL, Piotrowski LS. Neuroleptic treatment. In: Cummings JL, Miller BL, eds. Alzheimer's disease. Treatment and long-term management. Marcel Dekker, New York, 1990:89–107.

Goudsmit J, Morrow CH, Asher DM, et al. Evidence for and against the transmissibility of Alzheimer disease. Neurology 1980;30:945–950.

Govan CD Jr, Walsh FB. Symptomatology of subdural hematoma in infants and in adults. Arch Ophthalmol 1947;37:701–715.

Grady CL, Haxby JV, Horwitz B, Sundaram M, Berg G, Schapiro M, Friedland RP, Rapoport SI. Longitudinal study of the early neuropsychological and cerebral metabolic changes in dementia of the Alzheimer type. J Clin Exp Neuropsychol 1988;10:576–596.

Graebner RW, Celesia GG. EEG findings in hydrocephalus and their relation to shunting procedures. Electroencephalogr Clin Neurophysiol 1973;35:517–521.

Graef JW. Clinical aspects of lead poisoning. In: Vinken PJ. Bruyn GW, eds.

Intoxications of the nervous system. Part I, vol. 36. Handbook of clinical neurology. North-Holland, New York, 1979:1–34.

Grafe MR, Wiley CA. Spinal cord and peripheral nerve pathology in AIDS: the roles of cytomegalovirus and human immunodeficiency virus. Ann Neurol 1989;25:561–566.

Graff-Radford N, Rezai K, Godersky JC, Eslinger P, Damasio H, Kirchner PT. Regional cerebral blood flow in normal pressure hydrocephalus. J Neurol Neurosurg Psychiat 1987;50:1589–1596.

Graff-Radford NR, Godersky JC. Normal pressure hydrocephalus: onset of gaot abnormality before dementia predicts good surgical outcome. Arch Neurol 1986;43:940–942.

Granacher RP, Baldessarini RJ. Physostigmine. Its use in acute anticholinergic syndrome with antidepressant and antiparkinson drugs. Arch Gen Psychiatry 1975;32:375–380.

Granholm E, Butters N. Associative encoding and retrieval in Alzheimer's and Huntington's disease. Brain Cognit 1988;7:335–347.

Grant HC, McMenemey WH. Giant cell encephalitis in a dement. Neuropathol Pol 1966;4(suppl):735–740.

Grant I, Adams KM, Reed R. Aging, abstinence, and medical risk factors in the prediction of neuropsychologic deficit among long-term alcoholics. Arch Gen Psychiatry 1984a;41:710–718.

Grant I, Atkinson JH, Hesselink JR, et al. Evidence for early central nervous system involvement in the acquired immunodeficiency syndrome (AIDS) and other human immunodeficiency virus (HIV) infections. Ann Intern Med 1987;107:828–836.

Grant I, Judd LL. Neuropsychological and EEG disturbances in polydrug users. Am J Psychiatry 1976;133:1039–1042.

Grant I, McDonald WI, Trimble MR, Smith E, Reed R. Deficient learning and memory in early and middle phases of multiple sclerosis. J Neurol Neurosurg Psychiatry 1984b;47:250–255.

Grant I, Mohns L, Miller M, Reitan RM. A neuropsychological study of polydrug users. Arch Gen Psychiatry 1976;33:973–978.

Gray AM. Addison's disease and diffuse cerebral sclerosis. J Neurol Neurosurg Psychiatry 1969;32:344–347.

Gray F, Gherardi R, Marshall A, Janota I, Poirier J. Adult polyglucosan body disease (APBD). J Neuropath Exp Neurol 1988;47:459–474.

Grcevic N. Concentric lacunar leukoencephalopathy. Arch Neurol 1960;2:266–273.

Greden Jf, Albala AA, Smokler IA, Gardner R, Carroll BJ. Speed pause time: a marker of psychomotor retardation among endogenous depressives. Biol Psychiatry 1981;16:851–859.

Greden JF, Carroll BJ. Decrease in speech pause times with treatment of endogenous depression. Biol Psychiatry 1980;15:575–587.

Greden JF, Carroll BJ. Psychomotor function in affective disorders: an overview of new monitoring techniques. Am J Psychiatry 1981;138:1441–1448.

Green GJ, Lessell S. Acquired cerebral dyschromatopsia. Arch Ophthalmol 1977; 95:121–128.

Green J, Morris JC, Sandson J, McKeel DW Jr, Miller TW. Progressive aphasia: A precursor of global dementia? Neurology 1990;40:423–429.

Green GR, Linsk NL, Pinkston EM. Modification of verbal behavior of the mentally impaired elderly by their spouses. J Appl Behav Anal 1986;19:329–336.

Green RL. Electroencephalographic changes in Parkinson's disease. J Neurosurg 1966;24:377–381.

Greenberg GD, Ryan JJ, Bourlier PF. Psychological and neuropsychological aspects of COPD. Psychosomatics 1985;26:29–33.

Greenberg HS, Halverson D. Lane B. CT scanning and diagnosis of adrenoleukodystrophy. Neurology 1977;27:884–886.

Greenblatt DJ, Sellars EM, Shader RI. Drug disposition in old age. N Engl J Med 1982;306:1081–1088.

Greenfield JG. Subacute spinocerebellar degeneration occurring in elderly patients. Brain 1934;57:161–176.

Greenfield JG. The spinocerebellar degenerations. Blackwell Scientific Publications, Oxford, Eng., 1954.

Greenfield JG, Bosanquet FD. The brain-stem lesions in parkinsonism. J Neurol Neurosurg Psychiatry 1953;16:213–226.

Greenhouse AH, Barr JW. The bilateral isodense subdural hematoma on computerized tomographic scan. Arch Neurol 1979;36:305–307.

Greenmayre JT, Penney JB, Young AB, D'Amato CJ, Shoulson I. Alterations in L-glutamate binding in Alzheimer's and Huntington's diseases. Science 1985; 227:1496–1499.

Greenwald BS, Mathe AA, Mohs RC, Levy MI, Johns CA, Davis KL. Cortisol and Alzheimer's disease, II: dexamethasone suppression, dementia severity, and affective symptoms. Am J Psychiatry 1986;143:442–446.

Greenwood RS, Nelson JS. Atypical neuronal ceroid-lipofuscinosis. Neurology 1978;29:710–717.

Greitz T. Effect of brain distension on cerebral circulation. Lancet 1969;1:863–865.

Greitz TVB, Grepe AOL, Kalmer MSF, Lopez J. Pre- and postoperative evaluation of cerebral blood flow in low-pressure hydrocephalus. J Neurosurg 1969;31:644–651.

Griffin DE, Moser HW, Mendoza Q. Moench TR, O'Toole S. Moser AE. Identification of the inflammatory cells in the central nervous system of patients with adrenoleukodystrophy. Ann Neurol 1985;18:660–664.

Griffin JW, Goren E, Schaumburg H, Engel WK, Loriaux L. Adrenomyeloneuropathy: a probable variant of adrenoleukodystrophy. Neurology 1977;27:1107–1113.

Griffin JW, Thompson RW, Mitchinson MJ, de Kiewiet JC, Welland FH. Lymphomatous leptomeningitis. Am J Med 1971;51:200–208.

Griffiths RA, Mortimer TF, Oppenheimer DR, Spalding JMK. Congophilic angiopathy of the brain: a clinical and pathological report on two siblings. J Neurol Neurosurg Psychiatry 1982;45:396–408.

Grinker RR. Parkinsonism following carbon monoxide poisoning. J Nerv Ment Dis 1926;64:18–28.

Grinker RR, Serota H, Stein SI. Myoclonic epilepsy. Arch Neurol Psychiatry 1938;40:968–980.

Grober E, Buschke H, Crustal H, Bang S, Dresener R. Screening for dementia by memory testing. Neurology 1988;39:900–903.

Groch SN, Sayre GP, Heck FJ. Cerebral hemorrhage in leukemia. Arch Neurol 1960;2:439–451.

Groen JJ, Endtz LJ. Hereditary Pick's disease. Second re-examination of a large family and discussion of other hereditary cases, with particular reference to electroencephalography and computed tomography. Brain 1982;105:443–459.

Gross M. L-dopa for progressive supranuclear palsy. Lancet 1969;2:1359–1360.

Growdon JH, Cohen El, Wurtman RJ. Huntington's disease: clinical and chemical effects of choline administration. Ann Neurol 1977;1:418–422.

Grubb RL, Raichle ME, Gado MH, Eichling JO, Hughes CP. Cerebral blood flow, oxygen utilization, and blood volume in dementia. Neurology 1977;27:905–910.

Gruenberg E. Epidemiology. In: Katzman R, Terry RD, Bick KL, eds. Alzheimer's disease, senile dementia and related disorders. Raven Press, New York, 1978:323–326.

Grundke-Iqbal I, Iqbal K, Tung Y-C, Quinlan M, Wisniewski HM, Binder LI. Abnormal phosphorylation of the microtubule-associated protein tau in Alzheimer cytoskeletal pathology. Proc Natl Acad Sci 1986;83:4913–4917.

Grunfeld O, Hinostroza G. Thallium poisoning. Arch Intern Med 1964;114:132–138.

Grunnet ML. Nuclear bodies in Creuzfeldt-Jakob and Alzheimer's diseases. Neurology 1975;25:1091–1093.

Guberman A, Stuss D. The syndrome of bilateral paramedian thalamic infarction. Neurology 1983;33:540–546.

Gumasekera L, Richardson AE. Computerized axial tomography in idiopathic hydrocephalus. Brain 1977;100:749–754.

Gunale SR. Dialysis dementia: asparagine deficiency? Lancet 1973;2:847.

Gunner-Svensson F, Jensen K. Frequency of mental disorders in old age. Acta Psychiatr Scand 1976;53:283–297.

Guseo A, Deak G, Szirmai I. An adult case of metachromatic leukodystrophy. Acta Neuropathol 1975;32:333–339.

Gusella JF, Wexlewr NS, Conneally PH, et al. A polymorphic DNA marker genetically linked to Huntington's disease. Nature 1983;306:234–238.

Gustafson L. Frontal lobe degeneration of the non-Alzhiemer type. II. clinical picture and differential diagnosis. Arch Gerontol Geriatr 1987;6:209–233.

Gustafson L, Hagberg B, Ingvar DH. Speech disturbances in presenile dementia related to local cerebral blood flow abnormalities in the dominant hemisphere. Brain Lang 1978;5:103–118.

Gustafson L, Risberg J. Regional cerebral blood flow related to psychiatric symptoms in dementia with onset in the presenile period. Acta Psychiatr Scand 1974;50:516–538.

Guthe T. Treponemal diseases. In: Beeson PB, McDermott W. eds. Cecil-Loeb: text book of medicine. 13th ed. WB Saunders, Philadelphia, 1971:655–675.

Guthrie A, Elliott WA. The nature and reversibility of cerebral impairment in alcoholism. J Stud Alcohol 1980;41:147–155.

Gutmann L, Lemli L. Ataxia-telangiectasia associated with hypogammaglobulinemia. Arch Neurol 1963;8:318–327.

Guze SB, Woodruff RA, Clayton PJ. A study of conversion symptoms in psychiatric outpatients. Am J Psychiatry 1971;128:643–646.

Gyldensted C. Computer tomography of the cerebrum in multiple sclerosis. Neuroradiology 1976;12:33–42.

Haan J, Thomeer RTWM. Predictive value of temporary external lumbar drainage in normal pressure hydrocephalus. Neurosurgery 1988;22:388–391.

Haase GR. Diseases presenting as dementia. In: Wells, CE, ed. Dementia. 2nd ed. FA Davis, Philadelphia, 1977:27–67.

Hachinski VC, Iliff LD, Zilhka E, et al. Cerebral blood flow in dementia. Arch Neurol 1975;32:632–637.

Hachinski VC, Lassen NA, Marshall J. Multi-infarct dementia. A cause of mental deterioration in the elderly. Lancet 1974;2:207–210.

Haddad FS, Risk WS. Isoprinosine treatment in 18 patients with subacute sclerosing panencephalitis: a controlled study. Ann Neurol 1980;7:185–188.

Haddad FS, Risk WS, Jabbour JT. Subacute sclerosing panencephalitis in the Middle East: report of 99 cases. Ann Neurol 1977;1:211–217.

Hadden WB. The nervous symptoms of myxedema. Brain 1882–1883;5:188–196.

Haerer AF, Currier RD, Jackson JF. Hereditary nonprogressive chorea of early onset. N Engl J Med 1967;276:1220–1224.

Hagberg B, Ingvar DH. Cognitive reduction in presenile dementia related to regional abnormalities of the cerebral blood flow. Br J Psychiatry 1976;128:209–222.

Hahn BH. Systemic lupus erythematosus. In: Braunwald E, Isselbacher KJ, Petersdorf RG, Wilson JD, Martin JB, Fauci AS, eds. Harrison's principles of internal medicine, 11th ed. McGraw-Hill, New York, 1987:1418–1423.

Hahn RD, Webster B. Weickhardt G, et al. Penicillin treatment of general paresis (dementia paralytica). Arch Neurol Psychiatry 1959;81:557–590.

Haid RW, Gutmann L. Grosby TW. Wernicke-Korsakoff encephalopathy after gastric plication. JAMA 1982;247:2566–2567.

Hakim AM, Mathieson G. Basis of dementia in Parkinson's disease. Lancet 1978;2:729.

Hakim AM, Mathieson G. Dementia in Parkinson disease: a neuropathologic study. Neurology 1979;29:1209–1214.

Hakim S. Some observations on CSF pressure: hydrocephalic syndrome in adults with "normal" CSF pressure. Unpublished, Ph.D. diss., Javeriana University School of Medicine, Bogota, Columbia, 1964.

Hakim S. Biomechanics of hydrocephalus. In: Harbert JC, ed. Cisternography and hydrocephalus. Springfield, Ill.: Charles C Thomas, 1972:25–55.

Hakola HPA. Neuropsychiatric and genetic aspects of a new hereditary disease characterized by progressive dementia and lipomembranous polycystic osteodysplasia. Acta Psychiatr Scand 1972; (suppl 232):1–173.

Haldeman S, Goldman JW, Hyde J, Pribrain HFW. Progressive supranuclear palsy, computed tomography, and response to antiparkinsonian drugs. Neurology 1981;31:442–445.

Halgin R, Riklan M, Misiak H. Levodopa, parkinsonism, and recent memory. J Nerv Ment Dis 1977;164:268–272.

Hall P. Cyclandelate in the treatment of cerebral arteriosclerosis. J Am Geriatr Soc 1976;24:41–45.

Hall RA, Jackson RB, Swain JM. Neurotoxic reactions resulting from chlorpromazine administration. JAMA 1956;161;214–218.

Hall SB. The mental aspect of epidemic encephalitis. Br Med J 1929;1:444–446.

Hall WJ. Psychiatric problems in the elderly related to organic pulmonary disease.

In: Levenson AJ, Hall RCW, eds. Neuropsychiatric manifestations of physical disease in the elderly. Raven Press, New York, 1981:41–48.

Halliday AM, McDonald WI, Mushin J. Delayed visual evoked response in optic neuritis. Lancet 1972;1:982–985.

Halperin JJ, Landis DMD, Kleinman GM. Whipple disease of the nervous system. Neurology 1982;32:612–617.

Halsey JH Jr, Scott TR, Farmer TW. Adult hereditary cerebello-retinal degeneration. Neurology 1967;17:87–90.

Halstead WC. Preliminary analysis of grouping behavior in patients with cerebral insults by the method of equivalent and non-equivalent stimuli. Am J Psychiatry 1940;96:1263–1294.

Haltia M, Kristensson K. Sourander P. Neuropathological studies in three Scandinavian cases of progressive myoclonus epilepsy. Acta Neurol Scand 1969;45:63–77.

Hamilton CR, Shelley WM, Tumulty PA. Giant cell arteritis and polymyalgia rheumatica. Medicine 1971;50:1–27.

Hamilton JD, Gross NJ. Unusual neurological and cardiovascular complications of respiratory failure. Br Med J 1963;2:1092–1096.

Hamilton M. Development of a rating scale for primary depressive illness. Brit J Soc. Clin Psychol 1967;6:278–296.

Hamilton M. Fish's schizophrenia. John Wright & Sons, Bristol, Eng., 1976.

Handin RI. Coagulation disorders. In: Braunwald E, Isselbacher KJ, Petersdorf RG, Wilson JD, Martin JB, Fauci AS, eds. Harrison's principles of internal medicine, 11th ed. McGraw-Hill, New York, 1987:1475–1480.

Hanfmann E. Analysis of the thinking disorder in a case of schizophrenia. Arch Neurol Psychiatry 1939;41:568–579.

Hankey GJ, Stewart-Wynne EG. Bilateral intracerebral haemorrhage presenting with supranuclear ophthalmoplegia, bradykinesia and rigidity. Clin Exp Neurol 1987;23:195–199.

Hanna SM. Hypopituitarism (Sheehan's syndrome) presenting with organic psychosis. J Neurol Neurosurg Psychiatry 1970;33:192–193.

Hannah JA. A case of Alzheimer's disease with neuropathological findings. Can Med Assoc J 1936;35:351–366.

Hansch EC, Syndulko K, Cohen SN, Goldberg ZI, Potvin AK, Tourtellotte WW. Cognition in Parkinson disease: an event-related potential perspective. Ann Neurol 1982;11:579–607.

Hansen LA, Deteresa R, Tobias H, Alford M, Terry RD. Neocortical morphometry and cholinergic neurochemistry in Pick's disease. Am J Pathol 1988;131:507–518.

Harbaugh RE. Intracerebroventricular bethanechol chloride administration in Alzheimer's disease. Ann N Y Acad Sci 1988;531:174–179.

Harding AE. Friedreich's ataxia: a clinical and genetic study of 90 families with an analysis of early diagnostic criteria and intrafamilial clustering of clinical features. Brain 1981;104:589–620.

Harding AE. The clinical features and classification of the late onset autosomal dominant cerebellar ataxias. Brain 1982;105:1–28.

Harding AE. The hereditary ataxias and related disorders. Churchill Livingstone, New York, 1984.

Hardman JM, Allen LW, Baughman FA Jr, Waterman DF. Subacute necrotizing encephalopathy in late adolescence. Arch Neurol 1968;18:478–486.

Hardyck C, Petrinovich LF. The pattern of intellectual functioning in Parkinson patients. J Consult Clin Psychol 1963;27:548.

Harenko A, Toivakka El. Myoclonus epilepsy (Unverricht-Lundborg) in Finland. Acta Neurol Scand 1961;37:282–296.

Harik SI, Pool MJD. Computed tomography in Wilson disease. Neurology 1981; 31:107–110.

Harner RN, EEG evaluation of the patient with dementia. In: Benson DF, Blumer D, eds. Psychiatric aspects of neurologic disease: Grune & Stratton, New York, 1975:63–82.

Harper CG, Giles M, Finlay-Jones R. Clinical signs in the Wernicke-Korsakoff complex: a retrospective analysis of 131 cases diagnosed at necropsy. J Neurol Neurosurg Psychiatry 1986;49:341–345.

Harries-Jones R, Knight R, Will RC, Cousens S, Smith PG, Matthews WB. Creutz-feldt-Jakob disease in England and Wales, 1980–1984: A case-control study of potential risk factors. J Neurol Neurosurg Psychiatry 1988;51:1113–1119.

Harriman DGF. Bacterial infections of the central nervous system. In: Blackwood W, Corsellis JAN, eds. Greenfield's neuropathology. Year Book Medical Publishers, Chicago, 1976:238–268.

Harriman DGF, Miller JHD. Progressive familial myoclonic epilepsy in three families: its clinical features and pathological basis. Brain 1955;78:325–349.

Hart MN, Malamud N, Ellis WG. The Dandy-Walker syndrome. Neurology 1972;22:771–780.

Hart RG, Sherman DG. The diagnosis of multiple sclerosis. JAMA 1982;247:498–503.

Hart RP, Kwentus JA, Leshner RT, Frazier R. Information procesing speed in Friedreich's ataxia. Ann Neurol 1985;17:612–614.

Hart RP, Kwentus JA. Psychomotor slowing and subcortical-type dysfunction in depression. J Neurol Neurosurg Psychiatry 1987;50:1263–1266.

Hart RP, Rose CS, Hamer RM. Neuropsychological effects of occupational exposure to cadmium. J Clin Exp Neuropsychol 1989;11:933–943.

Harter DH, Petersdorf RG. Viral diseases of the central nervous system: aseptic meningitis and encephalitis. In: Braunwald E, Isslbacher KJ, Petersdorf RG, Wilson JD, Martin JB, Fauci AS, eds. Harrison's principles of internal medicine, 11th ed. McGraw-Hill, New York, 1987:1987–1995.

Hartman DE. Neuropsychological toxicology. Pergamon Press, New York, 1988.

Hartmann A, Alberti E. Differentiation of communicating hydrocephalus and pre-senile dementia by continuous recording of cerebrospinal fluid pressure. J Neurol Neurosurg Psychiatry 1977;40:630–640.

Haruda F, Friedman JH, Ganti SR, Hoffman N, Chutorian AM. Rapid resolution of organic mental syndrome in sickle cell anemia in response to exchange transfusion. Neurology 1981;31:1015–1016.

Haskell CM, Canellos GP, Leventhal BG. et al. L-asparaginase: therapeutic and toxic effects in patients with neoplastic disease. N Engl J Med 1969;281:1028–1034.

Hassin GB, Levitin D. Pick's disease. Clinicopathologic study and report of a case. Arch Neurol Psychiatry 1941;45:814–833.

Hathaway BM, Ch'ien L. Marchiafava-Bignami disease. South Med J 1971;64:602–606.

Haug JO. Pneumoencephalographic evidence of brain damage in chronic alcoholics. Acta Psychiatr Scand 1968;(suppl 203):135–143.

Hauser WA, Morris ML, Heston LL, Anderson VE. Seizures and myoclonus in patients with Alzheimer's disease. Neurology 1986;36:1226–1230.

Hausser-Hauw C, Roullet E, Robert R, Marteau R. Oculo-facio-skeletal myorhythmia as a cerebral complication of systemic Whipple's disease. Movement Disorders 1988;3:179–184.

Hawkins RA, Mazziotta JC, Phelps ME. Wilson's disease studied with FDG and positron emission tomography. Neurology 1987;37:1707–1711.

Hawkins RA, Phelps ME, Mazziotta JC, Kuhl DE. A study of Wilson's disease with F-18 FDG and positron tomography. J Cerebral Blood Flow and Metab 1983;3(suppl.1):5498–5499.

Haxby JV, Duara R, Grady CL, Cutler NR, Rapoport Sl. Relations between neuropsyhological and cerebral metabolic asymmetries in early Alzheimer's disease. J Cereb Blood Flow Metab 1985;5:193–200.

Haxby JV, Grady CL, Duara R, Schlageter N, Berg G, Rapoport Sl. Neocortical metabolic abnormalities precede nonmemory cognitive defects in early Alzheimer's-type dementia. Arch Neurol 1986;43:882–885.

Haxby JV, Grady CL, Koss E, Horwitz B, Schapiro M, Frieldand RP, Rapoport Sl. Heterogeneous anterior-posterior metabolic patterns in dementia of the Alzheimer type. Neurology 1988;38:1853–1863.

Hay JW, Ernst RL. The economic costs of Alzheimer's disease. Am J Public Health 1987;77:1169–1175.

Hayden MR, Hewitt J, Stoessl AJ, Clark C, Ammann W, Martin WRW. The combined use of positron emission tomography and DNA polymorphisms for preclinical detection of Huntington's disease. Neurology 1987;37:1441–1447.

Hayden MR, Martin AJ, Stoessl AJ, Clark C, Hollenberg S, Adam MJ, Ammann W, Harrop R, Rogers J, Ruth T, Sayre C, Pate BD. Positron emission tomography in the early diagnosis of Huntington's disease. Neurology 1986; 36:888–894.

Hayden MR. Huntington's disease. Springer-Verlag, New York, 1981.

Hayflick L. The limited in vitro lifetime of human diploid cell strains. Exp Cell Res 1965;37:614–636.

Hayflick L. The biology of human aging. Adv Pathobiol 1976;7:80–99.

Haymaker W, Mehler WF, Schiller F. Extrapyramidal motor disorders. In: Haymaker W, ed. Bing's local diagnosis in neurological diseases. 15th ed. St. Louis: CV Mosby, 1969:404–440.

Hecaen H. Mental symptoms associated with tumors of the frontal lobe. In: Warren JM, Akert K, eds. The frontal granular cortex and behavior. McGraw-Hill, New York, 1964:335–352.

Hecaen H, de Ajuriaguerra J. Balint's syndrome (psychic paralysis of visual fixation) and its minor forms. Brain 1954;77:373–400.

Hecht F, McCaw BK, Koler RD. Ataxia-telangiectasia—clonal growth of translocation lymphocytes. N Engl J Med 1973;289:286–291.

Heck AF. Heart disease in Friedreick's ataxia. I. Clinical studies and review of the literature. Neurology 1963;13:587–600.

Heck AF, Hameroff SB, Hornick RB. Chronic *Listeria monocytogenes* meningitis and normotensive hydrocephalus. Neurology 1971;21:263–270.

Heffner RR Jr, Porro RS, Olson ME, Earle KM. A demyelinating disorder associated with cerebrovascular amyloid angiopathy. Arch Neurol 1976;33:501–506.

Heilman K. Apraxia. In: Heilman K, Valenstein E, eds. Clinical Neuropsychology. Oxford University Press, New York, 1979;159–185.

Heilman KM, Fisher WR. Hyperlipidemic dementia. Arch Neurol 1974;31:67–68.

Heilman KM, Gonzalez Rothi LJ. Apraxia. In: Heilman KM, Valenstein E, eds. Clinical neuropsychology, 2nd ed. Oxford University Press, New York, 1985:131–150.

Heilman KM, Safran A, Geschwind N. Closed head trauma and aphasia. J Neurol Neurosurg Psychiatry 1971;34:265–269.

Heindel WC, Butters N, Salmon DP. Impaired learning of a motor skill in patients with Huntington's disease. Behav Neurosci 1988;102:141–147.

Held D, Fencl V, Poppenheimer JR. Electrical potential of cerebrospinal fluid. J Neurophysiol 1964;27:942–959.

Helig CW, Knopman DS, Mastri AR, Frey W II. Dementia without Alzheimer pathology. Neurology 1985;35:762–765.

Heller GL, Kooi KA. The electroencephalogram in hepato-lenticular degeneration (Wilson's disease). Electroencephalogr Clin Neurophysiol 1962;14:520–526.

Helms PM. Efficacy of antipsychotics in the treatment of the behavioral complications of dementia: A review of the literature. J Am Geriatr Soc 1985;33:206–209.

Hemphill RE, Klein R, Contribution to the dressing disability as a focal sign and to the imperception phenomenon. J Ment Sci 1948;94:611–622.

Henderson AS. The epidemiology of Alzheimer's disease. Brit Med Bull 1986;42:3–10.

Henderson DK, MacLachlan SH. Alzheimer's disease. J Ment Sci 1930;76:646–661.

Henderson VW, Mack W, Williams BW. Spatial disorientation in Alzheimer's disease. Arch Neurol 1989;46:391–394.

Henderson VW, Wooten GF. Neuroleptic malignant syndrome: a pathogenetic role for dopamine receptor blockade? Neurology 1981;31:132–137.

Henschke PJ, Bell DA, Cape RDT. Alzheimer's disease and HLA. Tissue Antigens 1978;12:132–135.

Henson RA. The neurological aspects of hypercalcemia: with special reference to primary hyperparathyroidism. J R Coll Physicians Lond 1968;1:41–50.

Henson RA, Hoffman HL, Urich H. Encephalomyelitis with carcinoma. Brain 1965;88:449–464.

Hershey LA, Gado MH, Trotter JL. Computerized tomography in the diagnostic evaluation of multiple sclerosis. Ann Neurol 1979;5:32–39.

Hershey LA, Modic MT, Jaffe DF, Greenough PG. Natural history of the vascular dementias: a prospective study of seven cases. Can J Neurol Sci 1986;13:559–565.

Herzon H, Shelton JT, Bruyn HB. Sequelae of Western equine and other arthropodborne encephalitides. Neurology 1957;7:535–548.

Herzog AG, Kemper TL. Amygdaloid changes in aging and dementia. Arch Neurol 1980;37:625–629.

Heston LL. Alzheimer's disease, trisomy 21, and myeloproliferative disorders: associations suggesting a genetic diathesis. Science 1976;196:322–323.

Heston LL. Genetic studies of dementia: with emphasis on Parkinson's disease and Alzheimer's neuropathology. In: Mortimer JA, Schuman LM, eds. The epidemiology of dementia. Oxford University Press, New York, 1981:101–114.

Heston LL, Lowther DLW, Leventhal CM. Alzheimer's disease. Arch Neurol 1966;15:225–233.

Heston LL, Mastri AR. The genetics of Alzheimer's disease. Association with hematologic malignancy and Down's syndrome. Arch Gen Psychiatry 1977;34:976–981.

Heston LL, Mastri AR. Age of onset of Pick's and Alzheimer's dementia: implications for diagnosis and research. J Gerontol 1982;37:422–424.

Heston LL, Mastri AR, Anderson E, White J. Dementia of the Alzheimer type. Arch Gen Psychiatry 1981;38:1085–1090.

Heston LL, White JA, Mastri AR. Pick's disease. Clinical genetics and natural history. Arch Gen Psychiatry 1987;44:409–411.

Hicks LH, Birren JE. Aging, brain damage, and psychomotor slowing. Psychol Bull 1970;74:377–396.

Hier DB, Caplan LR. Drugs for senile dementia. Drugs 1980;20:74–80.

Hier DB, Hagenlocker K, Shindler AG. Language disintegration in dementia: effects of etiology and severity. Brain Lang 1985;25:117–133.

Hier DB, Warach JD, Gorelick PB, Thomas J. Predictors of survival in clinically diagnosed Alzheimer's disease and multi-infarct dementia. Arch Neurol 1989;46:1213–1216.

Hierons R. Changes in the nervous system in acute porphyria. Brain 1957;80:176–192.

Higginbottom MC, Sweetman L, Nyhan WL. A syndrome of methyl-malonic aciduria, homocystinuria, megaloblastic anemia and neurologic abnormalities in a vitamin B_{12}-deficient breast-fed infant of a strict vegetarian. N Engl J Med 1978;299:317–323.

Hilt DC, Uhl GR, Hedreen JC, Whitehouse PJ, Price DL. Pick disease: loss of neurons in the nucleus basalis. Neurology 1982;32(2):A229.

Hirano A, Arumugasamy N, Zimmerman HM. Amyotrophic lateral sclerosis. Arch Neurol 1967;16:357–363.

Hirano A, Kurland LT, Krooth RS, Lessell S. Parkinsonism-dementia complex, an endemic disease on the island of Guam. I. Clinical features. Brain 1961a;84:642–661.

Hirano A, Malamud N, Elizan TS, Kurland LT. Amyotrophic lateral sclerosis and parkinsonism-dementia complex on Guam. Arch Neurol 1966;15:35–51.

Hirano A, Malamud N, Kurland LT. Parkinsonism-dementia complex, an endemic disease on the island of Guam. II. Pathological features. Brain 1961b;84:662–679.

Hirano A, Tuazon R, Zimmerman HM. Neurofibrillary changes, granulovacuolar bodies and argentophilic globules observed in tuberous sclerosis. Acta Neuropathol 1968;11:257–261.

Hirano A, Zimmerman HM. Alzheimer's neurofibrillary changes. Arch Neurol 1962;7:227–242.

Hirose G, Bass NH. Metachromatic leukodystrophy in the adult. Neurology 1972;22:312–320.

Ho S, Berenberg RA, Kim KS, Dal Canto MC. Sarcoid encephalopathy with diffuse inflammation and focal hydrocephalus shown by sequential CT. Neurology 1979;29:1161–1165.

Hoaglund HC, Goldstein NP. Hematologic (cytopenic) manifestations of Wilson's disease (hepatolenticular degeneration). Mayo Clin Proc 1978;53:498–500.

Hoehn MM, Yahr MD. Parkinsonism: onset, progression, and mortality. Neurology 1967;17:427–442.

Hoffman NE. Gastrointestinal diseases presenting as psychiatric symptoms. In: Levenson AJ, Hall RCW, eds. Neuropsychiatric manifestations of physical disease in the elderly. Raven Press, New York, 1981:49–57.

Hoffman PM, Robbins DS, Nolte MT, Gibbs CJ Jr. Gajdusek DC. Cellular immunity in Guamanians with amyotrophic lateral scelosis and parkinsonism-dementia, N Engl J Med 1978;299:680–685.

Hoffman PM, Robbins DS, Oldstone MBA, Gibbs CJ Jr, Gajdusek DC. Humoral immunity in Guamanians with amyotrophic lateral sclerosis and parkinsonism-dementia. Ann Neurol 1981;10:193–196.

Hoffman SB, Platt CA, Barry KE, Hamill LA. When language fails: nonverbal communication abilities of the demented. In: Hutton JT, Kenny AD, eds. Senile dementia of the Alzheimer type. Alan R. Liss, New York, 1985:49–64.

Hogg JE, Massey EW, Schoenberg BS. Mortality from Huntington's disease in the United States. Adv Neurol 1979;23:27–35.

Holland AL, McBurney DH, Moossy J, Reinmuth OM. The dissolution of language in Pick's disease with neurofibrillary tangles: a case study. Brain Lang 1985;24:36–58.

Hollister LE. Psychotherapeutic drugs. In: Levenson AJ, ed. Neuropsychiatric side effects of drugs in the elderly. Raven Press, New York, 1979:79–88.

Hollister LE, Cull VL, Gonda VA, Kolb FO. Hepatolenticular degeneration. Clinical, biochemical and pathologic study of a patient with fulminant course aggravated by treatment with BAL and versenate. Am J Med 1960;28:623–630.

Holmes JM. Cerebral manifestations of vitamin B_{12} deficiency. Br Med J 1956;2:1394–1398.

Holmes MD, Brant-Zawadzki MM, Simon RP. Clinical features of meningovascular syphilis. Neurology 1984;34:553–556.

Hooper MW, Vogel FS. The limbic system in Alzheimer's disease. Am J Pathol 1976;85:1–13.

Hormes JT, Filley CM, Rosenberg NL. Neurologic sequelae of chronic solvent vapor abuse. Neurology 1986:36:698–702.

Horn S. Some psychological factors in Parkinsonism. J Neurol Neurosurg Psychiatry 1974;37:27–31.

Hombein TF, Townes BD, Schoene RB, Sutton JR, Houston CS. The cost to the central nervous system of climbing to extremely high altitude. N Engl J Med 1989;321:1714–1719.

Horner J, Heyman A, Dawson D, Rogers H. The relationship of agraphia to the severity of dementia in Alzheimer's disease. Arch Neurol 1988;45:760–763.

Horoupian DS, Powers JM, Schaumburg HH. Kuru-like neuropathological changes in a North American. Arch Neurol 1972;27:555–561.

Horoupian DS, Thal L, Katzman R, Terry RD, Davies P, Hirano A, DeTeresa R, Fuld P, Petito C, Blass J, Ellis JM. Dementia and motor neuron disease: morphometric, biochemical, and Golgi studies. Ann Neurol 1984;16:305–313.

Horowitz S, Benson DF, Kuhl DE, Cummings JL. FDG scan to confirm Creutzfeldt-Jakob diagnosis. Neurology 1982;32(2):A167.(Abstr.)

Hossain M. Neurological and psychiatric manifestations in idiopathic hypoparathyroidism: response to treatment. J Neurol Neurosurg Psychiatry 1970;33:153–156.

Hotson JR. Modern neurosyphilis: a paritally treated chronic meningitis. West J Med 1981;135:191–200.

Hotson JR, Langston JW. Disulfiram-induced encephalopathy. Arch Neurol 1976;33:141–142.

Hourani BT, Hamlin EM, Reynolds TB. Cerebrospinal fluid glutamine as a measure of hepatic encephalopathy. Arch Intern Med 1971;127:1033–1036.

Hovestadt A, de Jong GJ, Meerwaldt JD. Spatial disorientation as an early symptom of Parkinson's disease. Neurology 1987;37:485–487.

Huber M, Herholtz K, Pawlik G, Szelies B, Jurgens R, Heiss W-D. Cerebral glucose metabolism in the course of subacute sclerosing panencephalitis. Arc Neurol 1989a;46:97–100.

Huber SJ, Freidenberg DL, Shuttleworth EC, Paulson GW, Christy JA. Neuropsychological impairments associated with severity of Parkinson's disease. J Neuropsychiatry Clin Neurosci 1989b;1:154–158.

Huber SJ, Kissel JT, Shuttleworth EC, Chakeres DW, Clapp LE, Brogan MA. Magnetic resonance imaging and clinical correlates of intellectual impairment in myotonic dystrophy. Arch Neurol 1989c;46:536–540.

Huber SJ, Shuttleworth EC, Paulson GW, Bellchambers MJG, Clapp LE, Cortical vs subcortical dementia. Neuropsychological differences. Arch Neurol 1986a;43:392–294.

Huber SJ, Shuttleworth EC, Paulson GW. Dementia in Parkinson's disease. Arch Neurol 1986b;43:987–990.

Huckman MS. Normal pressure hydrocephalus: evaluation of diagnostic and prognostic tests. AJNR 1981;2:385–395.

Huckman MS, Fox JH, Topel JL. The validity of criteria for the evaluation of cerebral atrophy by computed tomography. Radiology 1975;116:85–92.

Hudson AJ. Amyotrophic lateral sclerosis and its association with dementia, parkinsonism and other neurological disorders: a review. Brain 1981;104:217–247.

Hudson AJ, Farrell MA, Kalnins R, Kaufmann JCE. Gerstmann-Straussler-Scheinker disease with coincidental familial onset. Ann Neurol 1983;14:670–678.

Huff FJ, Auerbach J. Chakravarti A, Boller F. Risk of dementia in relatives of patients with Alzheimer's disease. Neurology 1988;38:786–790.

Hughes CP, Siegel BA, Coxe WS, et al. Adult communicating hydrocephalus with and without shunting. J Neurol Neurosurg Psychiatry 1978;41:961–971.

Hughes JR. The electroencephalogram in Parkinsonism. J Neurosurg 1966;24:369–376.

Hughes JR, Schreeder MT. EEG in dialysis encephalopathy. Neurology 1980;30:1148–1154.

Hughes JT, Brownell B. Granulomatous giant-celled angiitis of the central nervous system. Neurology 1966;16:293–298.

Hughes JT, Brownell B. Traumatic thrombosis of the internal carotid artery in the neck. J Neurol Neurosurg Psychiatry 1968;31:307–314.

Hughes W. Alzheimer's disease. Gerontol Clin 1970;12:129–148.

Hughes W, Dodgson MCH, MacLennan DC. Chronic cerebral hypertensive disease. Lancet 1954;2:770–774.

Hunder GG, Disney TF, Ward LE. Polymyalgia rheumatica. Mayo Clin Proc 1969;44:849–875.

Hunt AL, Orrison WW, Yeo RA, Haaland KY, Rhyne RL, Garry PJ, Rosenberg GA. Clinical significance of MRI white matter lesions in the elderly. Neurology 1989;39:1470–1474.

Hunter R, Blackwood W, Bull J. Three cases of frontal meningiomas presenting psychiatrically. Br Med J 1968;3:9–16.

Hunter R, Dayan AD, Wilson J. Alzheimer's disease in one monozygotic twin. J Neurol Neurosurg Psychiatry 1972;35:707–710.

Hunter R, Jones M. Acute lethargica-type encephalitis. Lancet 1966;2:1023–1024.

Huntington G. On chorea. Med Surg Reporter 1872;26:317–321.

Huttenlocher PR, Mattson RH. Isoprinosine in subacute sclerosing panencephalitis. Neurology 1979;29:763–771.

Hutton JT. Atrial myxoma as a cause of progressive dementia. Arch Neurol 1981a;38:533.

Hutton JT. Results of clinical assessment for the dementia syndrome: implications for epidemiologic studies. In: Mortimer JA, Schuman LM, eds. The epidemiology of dementia. Oxford University Press, New York, 1981b:62–69.

Hutton JT, Nagel JA, Loewenson RB. Eye tracking dysfunction in Alzheimer-type dementia. Neurology 1984:34:99–102.

Hwang T-L, Yung A, Estey EH, Fields WS. Central nervous system toxicity with high-dose Ara-C. Neurology 1985;35:1475–1479.

Hyman BT, Van Hoesen GW, Damasio AR, Barnes CL. Alzheimer's disease: cell-specific pathology isolates the hippocampal formation. Science 1984;225:1168–1170.

Iivanainen M. Himberg T-J. Valproate and clonazepam in the treatment of severe progressive myoclonus epilepsy. Arch Neurol 1982;39:236–238.

Iizuka R, Hirayama K, Maehara K. Dentato-rubro-pallido-luysian atrophy: a clinicopathological study. J Neurol Neurosurg Psychiatry 1984;47:1288–1298.

Illingsworth RD, Logue V, Syman L, Uemura K. The ventriculocaval shunt in the treatment of adult onset hydrocephalus: results and complications in 101 patients. J Neurosurg 1971;35:681–685.

Illis S, Taylor FM. The electroencephalogram in herpes-simplex encephalitis. Lancet 1972;1:718–721.

Indravasu S, Dexter RA. Infantile neuroaxonal dystrophy and its relationship to Hallervorden-Spatz disease. Neurology 1968;18:693–699.

Ineichen B. Measuring the rising tide. How many dementia cases will there be by 2001? Brit J Psychiatry 1987;150:193–200.

Ines DF, Markand ON. Epileptic seizures and abnormal electroencephalographic findings in hydrocephalus and their relation to the shunting procedures. Electroencephalogr Clin Neurophysiol 1977;42:761–768.

Ingvar DH, Franzen G. Distribution of cerebral activity in chronic schizophrenia. Lancet 1974;2(No. 7895):1484–1486.

Ingvar DH, Gustafson L. Regional cerebral blood flow in organic dementia with early onset. Acta Neurol Scand 1970;46(suppl 43):42–73.

Ingvar DH, Risberg J, Schwartz MS. Evidence of subnormal function of association cortex in presenile dementia. Neurology 1975;25:964–974.

Inzelberg R, Treves T, Reider I, Gerlenter I, Korczyn AD. Computed tomography brain changes in parkinsonian dementia. Neuroradiology 1987;29:535–539.

Iqbal A, Alter M, Lee SH. Pseudoxanthoma elasticum: a review of neurological complications. Ann Neurol 1978;4:18–20.

Iqbal K, Wisniewski HM, Grunde-Iqbal I, Korthals JK, Terry RD. Chemical pathology of neurofibrils. Neurofibrillary tangles of Alzheimer's presenile-senile dementia. J Histochem Cytochem 1975;23:563–569.

Irey NS, McAllister HA, Henry JM. Oral contraceptives and stroke in young women: a clinicopathologic correlation. Neurology 1978;28:1216–1219.

Ironside R, Bosanquet FD, McMenemy WH. Central demyelination of the corpus callosum (Marchiafava-Bignami disease). Brain 1961;84:212–230.

Isaacs B, Kennie AT. The set test as an aid to the detection of dementia in old people. Br J Psychiatry 1973;123:467–470.

Isbell H, Altschul S, Kornetsky CH, Eisenman AJ, Flanary HG, Fraser HF. Chronic barbiturate intoxication. Arch Neurol Psychiatry 1950;64:1–28.

Ishii N, Hishahara Y, Imamura T. Why do frontal lobe symptoms predominate in vascular dementia with lacunes? Neurology 1986;36:340–345.

Ishii T. Distribution of Alzheimer's neurofibrillary changes in brainstem and hypothalamus of senile dementia. Acta Neuropathol 1966;6:181–187.

Ishino H, Higashi H, Kuroda S, Yabuki S, Hayahara T, Otsuki S. Motor nuclear involvement in progressive supranuclear palsy. J Neurol Sci 1974;22:235–244.

Ishino H, Ikeda H, Otsuki S. Contribution to clinical pathology of progressive supranuclear palsy (subcortical argyrophilic dystrophy). J Neurol Sci 1975;24: 471–481.

Itoyama Y, Webster HdeF, Sternberger NH, et al. Distribution of papovavirus, myelin-associated glycoprotein and myelin basic protein in progressive multifocal luekoencephalopathy lesions. Ann Neurol 1982;11:396–407.

Iversen SD. Behavior after neostriatal lesions in animals. In: Divac I, Oberg RGE, eds. The neostriatum. Pergamon Press, New York, 1979:195–210.

Ivnik RJ. Pseudodementia in tardive dyskinesia. Psychiatr Ann 1979;9:211–216.

Jackson JA, Free GBM, Pike HV. The psychic manifestations in paralysis agitans. Arch Neurol Psychiatry 1923;10:680–684.

Jackson JA, Jankovic J, Ford J. Progressive supranuclear palsy: clinical features and response to treatment in 16 patients. Ann Neurol 1983;13:273–278.

Jacob H. Muscular twitchings in Alzheimer's disease. In: Wolstenholme GEW, O'Connor M, eds. Alzheimer's disease and related conditions. J & A Churchill, London 1970:75–89.

Jacob JC, Gloor P, Elwan OH, Dossetor JB, Pateras VR. Electroencephalographic changes in chronic renal failure. Neurology 1965;15:419–429.

Jacobs JW, Bernard MR, Delgado A, Strain JJ. Screening for organic mental syndromes in the medically ill. Ann Intern Med 1977;86:40–46.

Jacobs L, Conti D, Kinkel WR, Manning EJ. "Normal pressure" hydrocephalus. JAMA 1976;235:510–512.

Jacobs L, Kinkel W. Computerized axial transverse tomography in normal pressure hydrocephalus. Neurology 1976;26:501–507.

Jacobs L, Kinkel WR, Polachini I, Kinkel RP. Correlations of nuclear magnetic resonance imaging, computerized tomography, and clinical profiles in multiple sclerosis. Neurology 1986;36:27–34.

Jacobson PL, Farmer TW. The "hypernormal" CT scan in dementia: bilateral isodense subdural hematomas. Neurology 1979;29:1522–1523.

Jaffe HW. The laboratory diagnosis of syphilis. Ann Intern Med 1975;83:846–850.

Jaffe R, Librot IE, Bender MB. Serial EEG studies in unoperated subdural hematoma. Arch Neurol 1968;19:325–330.

Jagust WJ, Budinger TF, Reed BR. The diagnosis of dementia with single photon emission computed tomography. Arch Neurol 1987;44:258–262.

Jagust WJ, Friedland RP, Budinger TF. Positron emission tomography with [18F] fluorodeoxyglucose differentiates normal pressure hydrocephalus from Alzheimer-type dementia. J Neurol Neurosurg Psychiatry 1985;48:1091–1096.

Jakob A. Concerning a disorder of the central nervous system clinically resembling multiple sclerosis with remarkable anatomic findings (spastic pseudosclerosis). EP Richardson Jr, trans, In: Rottenberg DA, Hochberg FH, eds. Neurological classics in modern translation. Hafner Press, New York, 1977:113–125.

Jambor KL. Cognitive functioning in multiple sclerosis. Br J Psychiatry 1969;115:765–775.

Jampel RS, Okazaki H, Bernstein H. Opthalmoplegia and retinal degeneration associated with spinocerebellar ataxia. Arch Opthalmol 1966;66:247–259.

Jana DK, Romano-Jana L. Hypernatremic psychosis in the elderly: case reports. J Am Geriatr Soc 1973;21:473–477.

Jandl JH. Pernicious anemia. In: Beeson PB, McDermott W, eds Cecil-Loeb: textbook of medicine, 13th ed. WB Saunders, Philadelphia, 1971:1466–1470.

Janeway R, Ravens JR, Pearce LA, Odor DL, Suzuki K. Progressive myoclonus epilepsy with Lafora inclusion bodies. Arch Neurol 1967;16:565–582.

Jankovic J, Kirkpatrick JB, Blomquist KA, Langlais PJ, Bird ED. Late-onset Hallervorden-Spatz disease presenting as familial parkinsonism. Neurology 1985; 35:227–234.

Janssen RS, Saykin AJ, Cannon L. Campbell J, Pinsky PF, Hessol NA, O'Malley PM, Lifson AR, Doll LS, Rutherford GW, Kaplan JE. Neurological and neuropsychological manifestations of HIV-1 infection: association with AIDS-related complex but not asymptomatic HIV-1 infection. Ann Neurol 1989;26:592–600.

Jarvik JG, Hesselink JR, Kennedy C, Teschke R, Wiley C, Spector S, Richman D, McCutchan JA. Acquired immunodeficiency syndrome. Magnetic resonance patterns of brain involvement with pathologic correlation. Arch Neurol 1988; 45:731–736.

Jarvik LF. Genetic factors and chromosomal aberrations in Alzheimer's disease, senile dementia, and related disorders. In: Katzman R, Terry RD, Bick KL, eds. Alzheimer's disease, senile dementia and related disorders. Raven Press, New York, 1978:273–277.

Jarvik LF, Matsuyama SS, Kessler JO. Philothermal response of polymorphonuclear leukocytes in dementia of the Alzheimer type. Neurobiol Aging 1982;3;93–99.

Jarvik LF, Perl M. Overview of physiologic dysfunctions related to psychiatric problems in the elderly. In: Levenson AJ, Hall RCW, eds. Neuropsychiatric manifestations of physical disease in the elderly. Raven Press, New York, 1981;1–15.

Javoy-Agid F, Agid Y. Is the mesocortical dopaminergic system involved in Parkinson disease? Neurology 1980;30:1326–1330.

Jebsen RH, Tenckhoff H, Honet JC. Natural history of uremic polyneuropathy and effects of dialysis. N Engl J Med 1967;277:327–333.

Jeffries GH. Disease of the hepatic system. In: Beeson PB, McDermott W, eds. Cecil-Loeb: textbook of medicine. 13th ed. WB Saunders, Philadelphia, 1971:1377–1404.

Jelgersma HC. A case of encephalopathia subcorticalis chronica (Binswanger's disease). Psychiatr Neurol (Basel) 1964;147:81–89.

Jelliffe SE. Oculogyric crises as compulsion phenomena in post-encephalitis: their occurrence, phenomenology and meaning. J Nerv Ment Dis 1929;69:59–68, 165–184, 278–297, 415–426, 531–551, 666–679.

Jellinger K. Neuropathological aspects of dementias resulting from abnormal blood and cerebrospinal fluid dynamics. Acta Neurol Belg 1976;76:83–102.

Jellinger K, Seitelberger F. Protracted post-traumatic encephalopathy. J Neurol Sci 1970;10:51–94.

Jenike MA. Handbook of geriatric psychopharmacology. PSG Publishing Company, Littleton, Mass., 1985.

Jenike MA, Albert MS. The dexamethasone suprression test in patients with pre-senile and senile dementia of the Alzheimer type. J Am Geriatr Soc 1984;32:441–444.

Jenkins RB. L-dopa for progressive supranuclear palsy. Lancet 1969;2:742.

Jenkins RB. Inorganic arsenic and the nervous system. Brain 1966;89:479–498.

Jenkins RB, Groh RH. Mental symptoms in parkinsonian patients treated with L-dopa. Lancet 1970;2:177–180.

Jenkins VE, Postlewaite JC. Coccidioidal meningitis: report of four cases with necropsy findings in three cases. Ann Intern Med 1951;35:1068–1083.

Jenkyn LR, Reeves AG. Neurologic signs in uncomplicated aging (senescence). Semin Neurol 1981;1(1):21–30.

Jennett B, Plum F. Persistent vegetative state after brain damage. Lancet 1972;1:734–737.

Jennett B, Teasdale G. Management of head injuries. FA Davis, Philadelphia, 1981.

Jensen ON, Olesen OV. Folic acid and anticonvulsive drugs. Arch Neurol 1969;21:208–214.

Jervis GA. Alzheimer's disease. Psychiatr Q 1937;11:5–18.

Jervis GA. Early senile dementia in mongoloid idiocy. Am J Psychiatry 1948;105:102–106.

Jervis GA. Huntington's chorea in childhood. Arch Neurol 1963;9:244–256.

Jervis GA. Alzheimer's disease. In: Minkler J, ed. Pathology of the nervous system. Vol. 2. McGraw-Hill, New York, 1971a:1385–1395.

Jervis GA. Pick's disease. In: Minkler J, ed. Pathology of the nervous system. Vol. 2. McGraw-Hill, New York, 1971b:1395–1401.

Jervis GA, Soltz SE. Alzheimer's disease—the so-called juvenile type. Am J Psychiatry 1936;93:39–56.

Jeste DV, Kleinman JE, Potkin SG, et al. Ex Uno Multi: subtyping the schizophrenic syndrome. Biol Psychiatry 1982;17:199–222.

Joffe RT, Lippert GP, Gray TA, Sawa G, Horvath Z. Mood disorder and multiple sclerosis. Arch Neurol 1987;44:376–378.

Johannesson G, Brun A, Gustafson I, Ingvar DH. EEG in presenile dementia related to cerebral blood flow and autopsy findings. Acta Neurol Scand 1977;56:89–103.

Johnson AH. Antibiotics. In: Levenson AJ, ed. Neuropsychiatric side effects of drugs in the elderly. Raven Press, New York, 1979:27–38.

Johnson DR, Chalgren WS. Polychthemia vera and the nervous system. Neurology 1950;1:53–67.

Johnson KA, Davis KR, Buonanno FS, Brady TJ, Rosen J, Growdon JH. Comparison of magnetic resonance and roentgen ray computed tomography in dementia. Arch Neurol 1987a;44:1075–1080.

Johnson KA, Holman L, Mueller SP, Rosen J, English R, Nagel S, Growdon JH. Single photon emission computed tomography in Alzheimer's disease. Arch Neurol 1988;45:392–396.

Johnson KA, Mueller ST, Wlashe TM, English RJ, Holman L. Cerebral perfusion imaging in Alzheimer's disease. Arch Neurol 1987b;44:165–168.

Johnson RT, Richardson EP. The neurological manifestations of systemic lupus erythematosus. Medicine 1968;47:337–369.

Johnson TN, Rosvold HE, Mishkin M. Projections from behaviorally defined sectors of the prefrontal cortex to the basal ganglia, septum, and diencephalon of the monkey. Exp Neurol 1968;21:20–34.

Johnstone EC, Crow TJ, Frith CD, Husband J, Kreel L. Cerebral ventricular size and cognitive impairment in chronic schizophrenia. Lancet 1976;2:924–926.

Johnstone EC, Crow TJ, Frith CD, Stevens M, Kreel L, Husband J. The dementia of dementia praecox. Acta Psychiatr Scand 1978;57:305–324.

Jolkkonen JT, Soininen HS, Riekkinen PJ. Beta-endorphin-like immunoreactivity in cerebrospinal fluid of patients with Alzheimer's disease and Parkinson's disease. J Neurol Sci 1987;77:153–159.

Jolliffe N, Bowman KM, Rosenblum LA, Fein HD. Nicotinic acid deficiency encephalopathy. JAMA 1940;114:307–312.

Jones B, Parsons OA. Impaired abstracting ability in chronic alcoholics. Arch Gen Psychiatry 1971;24:71–75.

Jones B, Parsons OA. Specific vs generalized deficits of abstracting ability in chronic alcoholics. Arch Gen Psychiatry 1972;26:380–384.

Jones DP. Nevin S. Rapidly progressive cerebral degeneration (subacute vascular encephalopathy) with mental disorder, focal disturbances, and myoclonic epilepsy. J Neurol Neurosurg Psychiatry 1954;17:148–159.

Jones HR, Hedley-Whyte ET, Freidberg SR, Baker RA. Ataxic Creutzfeldt-Jakob disease: Diagnostic techniques and neuropathologic observations in early disease. Neurology 1985;35:254–257.

Jones IH. Observations on schizophrenic stereotypes. Compr Psychiatry 1965;6:323–335.

Jones JA, Niessen LC, Hobbins MJ, Zocchi M. Oral health care for patients with Alzheimer's disease. In: Volicer L, Fabiszewski KJ, Rheaume YL, Lasch KE, eds. Clinical management of Alzheimer's disease. Aspen Publishers, Rockville, Md., 1988;111–126.

Jonker C, Eikelenboom P, Tavenier P. Immunological indices in the cerebrospinal fluid of patients with presenile dementia of the Alzheimer type. Br J Psychiatry 1982;140:44–49.

Joosten E, Hoes M, Gabreels-Festen A, Hommes O, Stekhoven HS, Sloof JL. Electron microscopic investigation of inclusion material in a case of adult metachromatic leukodystrophy; observations on kidney biopsy, peripheral nerve and cerebral white matter. Acta Neuropathol 1975;33:165–171.

Jordan BD. Neurologic aspects of boxing. Arch Neurol 1987;44:453–459.

Jorm AF, Korten AE, Henderson AS. The prevalence of dementia: a quantitative integration of the literature. Acta Psychiatr Scand 1987;76:465–479.

Josiassen RC, Curry L, Roemer RA, Bease C, Mancall EL. Patterns of intellectual deficit in Huntington's disease. J Clin Neuropsychol 1982;4:173–183.

Joynt RJ, Zimmerman G, Khalifeh R. Cerebral emboli from cardiac tumors. Arch Neurol 1965;12:84–91.

Judd BW, Meyer JS, Rogers RL, Gandhi S, Tanahashi N, Mortel KF, Tawakina T. Cognitive performance correlates with cerebrovascular impairments in multi-infarct dementia. J Am Geriatr Soc 1986;34:355–360.

Judd LL, Grant I. Intermediate duration organic mental disorder among polydrug abusing patients. Psychiatr Clin North Am 1978;1:153–167.

Judge RD, Currier RD, Gracie WA, Figley MM. Takayasu's arteritis and the aortic arch syndrome. Am J Med 1962;32:379–392.

Kaell AT, Shetty M, Lee BCP, Lockshin MD. The diversity of neurologic events in systemic lupus erythematosus. Arch Neurol 1986;43:273–276.

Kahan J, Kemp B, Staples FR, Brummel-Smith K. Decreasing the burden in families caring for a relative with a dementing illness. J Am Geriatr Soc 1985;33:664–670.

Kahana E, Leibowitz U, Alter M. Cerebral multiple sclerosis. Neurology 1971;21:1179–1185.

Kahn E, Thompson LJ. Concerning Pick's disease. Am J Psychiatry 1933—1934; 90:937–946.

Kahn RL, Zarit SH, Hilbert NM, Niederehe G. Memory complaint and impairment in the aged. Arch Gen Psychiatry 1975;32:1569–1573.

Kaiya H, Takeuchi TK, Adachi MS, Shirakawa, Ueki H, Namba M. Decreased level of beta-endorphin-like immunoreactivity in cerebrospinal fluid of patients with senile dementia of Alzheimer type. Life Sci 1983;33:1039–1043.

Kak VK, Taylor AR. Hydrocephalus due to elongated basilar artery. Lancet 1967; 1:874–877.

Kakulas BA, Finlay-Jones LR. A lymphoma with central nervous system involvement. Neurology 1962;12:495–500.

Kalambonkis Z, Molling P. Symmetrical calcification of the brain in the predominance in the basal ganglia and cerebellum. J Neuropathol Exp Neurol 1962;21:364–371.

Kalimo H, Lundberg PO, Olsson Y. Familial subacute necrotizing encephalomyelopathy of the adult form (adult Leigh syndrome). Ann Neurol 1979;6:200–206.

Kamo H, McGeer PL, Harrop R, McGeer EG, Calne DB, Martin WRW, Pate BD. Positron emission tomography and histopathology in Pick's disease. Neurology 1987;37:439–445.

Kamp PE, Den Hartog Jager WA, Maathuis J, De Groot PA, De Jong JMBV, Bolhuis PA. Brain gangliosides in the presenile dementia of Pick. J Neurol Neurosurg Psychiatry 1986;49:881–885.

Kanazawa I, Bird ED, Gale JS, et al. Substance P: decrease in substantia nigra and globus pallidus in Huntington's disease. Adv Neurol 1979;23:495–504.

Kanazawa I, Kwak S, Sasaki H, Muramoto O, Mizutani T, Hori A, Nukina N. Studies on neurotransmitter markers of the basal ganglia in Pick's disease, with special reference to dopamine reduction. J Neurol Sci 1988;83:63–74.

Kantarjian AD. A syndrome clinically resembling amyotrophic lateral sclerosis following chronic mercurialism. Neurology 1961;11:639–644.

Kaplan E. The process approach to neuropsychological assessment of psychiatric patients. J Neuropsychiat Clin Neurosci 1990;2:72–87.

Kaplan JG, Katzman R, Horoupian DS, Fuld PA, Mayeux R, Hays AP. Progressive dementia, visual deficits, amyotrophy, and microinfarcts. Neurology 1985;35:789–796.

Kaplan JG, Sterman AB, Horoupian D, Leeds NE, Zimmerman RD, Gade R. Luetic meningitis with gumma: clinical, radiographic and neuropathologic features. Neurology 1981;31:464–467.

Kark RAP. Clinical and neurochemical aspects of inorganic mercury intoxication. In: Vinken PJ, Bruyn GW, eds. Intoxications of the nervous system. Part I, vol. 36. Handbook of clinical neurology. North-Holland, New York, 1979:147–197.

Kark RAP, Poskanzer DC, Bullock JD, Boylen G. Mercury poisoning and its treatment with N-acetyl-D, L-penicillamine. N Engl J Med 1971;285:10–16.

Kark RAP, Rodriquez-Budelli MM. Clinical correlations of partial deficiency of lipoamide dehydrogenase. Neurology 1979;29:1006–1013.

Karpati G, Frame B. Neuropsychiatric disorders in primary hyperparathyroidism. Arch Neurol 1964;10:387–397.

Kartzinel R, Hunt RD, Calne DB. Bromocriptine in Huntington chorea. Arch Neurol 1976;33:517–518.

Kasanin J, Crank RP. Alzheimer's disease. Arch Neurol Psychiatry 1933;30:1180–1183.

Kasanin J, Crank RP. A case of extensive calcification in the brain. Arch Neurol Psychiatry 1935;34:164–178.

Kase M, Warabi T, Tashiro K. A case of progressive supranuclear palsy: electrophysiological analysis of the abnormal oculomotor function. Jpn J Ophthalmol 1976;20:466–473.

Kaszniak AW, Fox J, Gandell DL, Garron DC, Huckman MS, Ramsey RG. Predictors of mortality in presenile and senile dementia. Ann Neurol 1978;3:246–252.

Katona CLE, Aldridge CR. The dexamethasone suppression test and depressive signs in dementia. J Affect Dis 1985;8:83–89.

Katz DI, Alexander MP, Mandell AM. Dementia following strokes in the mesencephalon and diencephalon. Arch Neurol 1987;444:1127–1133.

Katz IR, Greenberg WH, Barr GA, Garbarino C, Buckley P, Smith D. Screening for cognitive toxicity of anticholinergic drugs. J Clin Psychiatry 1985;46:323–326.

Katz M. Carbon monoxide asphyxia, a common clinical entity. Can Med Assoc J 1958;78:182–186.

Katzman R. A reversible form of dementia? Med World News Rev 1974;1:65

Katzman R. Normal pressure hydrocephalus. In: Wells CE, ed. Dementia. 2nd ed. FA Davis, Philadelphia, 1977:69–92.

Katzman R. Annual course, Neurology of Aging. American Academy of Neurology, Washington D.C., April 26, 1982.

Katzman R, Brown T, Thal LJ, Fuld PA, Aronson M, Butters N, Klauber MR, Wiederholt W, Pay M, Renbing X, Ooi W, Hofstetter R, Terry RD. Comparison of rate of annual change of mental status score in four independent studies of patients with Alzheimer's disease. Ann Neurol 1988;24:384–389.

Katzman R, Hussey F. A simple constant-infusion manometric test for measurement of CSF absorption. Neurology 1970;20:534–544.

Katzman R, Karasu TB. The differential diagnosis of dementia. In: Fields WS, ed. Neurological and sensory disorders of the elderly. Stratton, New York, 1975.

Katzman R, Pappius HM. Brain electrolytes and fluid metabolism. Williams & Wilkins, Baltimore, 1973.

Katzman R, Thal LJ. Neurochemistry of Alzheimer's disease. In: Siegel GJ, Agranoff BW, Albers RW, Molinoff PB, eds. Basic neurochemistry: Molecular, cellular, and medical aspects, 4th ed. Raven Press, New York, 1989:827–838.

Kaufman B, Pearson OH, Chamberlin WB. Radiographic features of intrasellar masses and progressive, asymmetrical non-tumorous enlargement of the sella turcica. The "empty" sella syndrome. In: Diagnosis and treatment of pituitary tumors. International Congress Series no. 303. Excerpta Medica, Amsterdam, 1973:100–129.

Kaufman DM, Zimmerman RD, Leeds NE. Computed tomography in herpes simplex encephalitis. Neurology 1979;29:1392–1396.

Kawamura M, Shiota J, Yagishita T, Hirayama K. Marchiafava-Bignami disease: Computed tomographic scan and magnetic resonance imaging. Ann Neurol 1985;18:103–104.

Kay AD, Milstien S, Kaufman S, Creasey H, Haxby JV, Cutler NR, Rapoport SI. Cerebrospinal fluid biopterin is decreased in Alzheimer's disease. Arch Neurol 1986;43:996–999.

Kay DWK, Bergmann K, Foster EM, McKechnie AA, Roth M. Mental illness and hospital usage in the elderly: a random sample followed up. Compr Psychiatry 1970;11:26–35.

Kay DWK, Roth M. Hopkins B. Affective disorders arising in the senium. J Ment Sci 1955;101:302–318.

Kaye EM, Kolodny EH, Ligigian EL, Ullman MD. Nervous system involvement in Fabry's disease: clinicopathological and biochemical correlation. Ann Neurol 1988;23:505–509.

Kaye WH. Sitaram N, Weingartner H, Ebert MH, Smallberg S, Gillin JC. Modest facilitation of memory in dementia with combined lecithin and anticholinesterase treatment. Biol Psychiatry 1982;17:275–280.

Kazniak AW, Garron DC, Fox JH, Bergen D, Huckman M. Cerebral atrophy, EEG slowing, age, education, and cognitive functioning in suspected dementia. Neurology 1978;29:1273–1279.

Keen PE, Weitzner S. Inflammatory pseudotumor of mesentery: a complication of ventriculoperitoneal shunt. J Neurosurg 1973;38:371–373.

Keimowitz RM, Annis BL. Disseminated intravascular coagulation associated with massive brain injury. J Neurosurg 1973;39:178–180.

Kelly MP, Garron DC, Javid H. Carotid artery disease, carotid endarterectomy, and behavior. Arch Neurol 1980;37:743–748.

Kempler D, Curtiss S, Jackson C. Syntactic preservation in Alzheimer's disease. J Speech Hear Res 1987;30:343–350.

Kempler D, Metter EJ, Riege WH, Jackson CA, Benson DF, Hanson WR. Slowly progressive aphasia: Three cases with language, memory, CT and PET data. J Neurol Neurosurg Psychiatry 1990;53:987–993.

Kendell RE. The stability of psychiatric diagnoses. Br J Psychiatry 1974;124:352–356.

Kennedy J, Fisher J, Shoulson I, Caine E. Language impairment in Huntington disease. Neurology 1981;31(2):81–82.

Kepes JJ, Chou SM, Price LW Jr. Progressive multifocal leukoencephalopathy with a 10-year survival in a patient with nontropical sprue. Neurology 1975;25:1006–1012.

Kerr DNS. Chronic renal failure. In: Beeson PB, McDermott W, eds. Cecil-Loeb: textbook of medicine. 13th ed. WB Saunders, Philadelphia, 1971:1144–1168.

Kertesz A, Black SE, Tokar G, Benke T, Carr T, Nicholson L. Periventricular and subcortical hyperintensities on magnetic resonance imaging. Arch Neurol 1988;45:404–408.

Kertesz A, Polk M, Carr T. Cognitive and white matter changes on magnetic resonance imaging in dementia. Arch Neurol 1990;47:387–391.

Keschner M, Bender MB, Strauss I. Mental symptoms in cases of tumor of the temporal lobe. Arch Neurol Psychiatry 1936;35:572–596.

Keschner M, Bender MB, Strauss I. Mental symptoms associated with brain tumor. JAMA 1938;110:714–718.

Kessler JT, Jortner BS, Adapon BD. Cerebral vasculitis in a drug abuser. J Clin Psychiatry 1978;39:559–564.

Key A, Retzius G. Studien in der anatomie des nervensystems und des bindegewebes. Samson & Wallin, Stockholm, 1875.

Khachaturian ZS. Diagnosis of Alzheimer's disease. Arch Neurol 1985;42:1097–1105.

Khurana RK, Garcia JH. Autonomic dysfunction in subacute spongiform encephalopathy. Arch Neurol 1981;38:114–117.

Khurana RK, Nelson E, Azzarelli B, Garcia JH. Shy-Drager syndrome: diagnosis and treatment of cholinergic dysfunction. Neurology 1980;30:805–809.

Kibler RF, Couch RSC, Crompton MR. Hydrocephalus in the adult following spontaneous subarachnoid haemorrhage. Brain 1961;84:45–60.

Kidd M. Alzheimer's disease—an electron microscopical study. Brain 1964;87:307–320.

Kiloh LG. Pseudo-dementia. Acta Psychiatr Scand 1961;37:336–351.

Kiloh LG, McComas AJ, Osselton JW. Clinical electroencephalography. 3rd ed. Butterworths, London, 1972.

Kinsella G, Moran C, Ford B, Ponsford J. Emotional disorder and its assessment within the severe head injured population. Psychol Med 1988;18:57–63.

Kipowski ZJ. Delirium in the elderly patient. New Engl J Med 1989;320:578–582.

Kirkegaard C, Bjorum N, Cohn D, Lauridsen UB. Thyrotropin-releasing hormone (TRH) stimulation test in manic-depressive illness. Arch Gen Psychiatry 1978;35:1017–1021.

Kirschbaum WR. Jakob-Creutzfeldt disease. American Elsevier, New York, 1968.

Kirshner HS, Tanridag O, Thurman L, Whetsell WO Jr. Progressive aphasia without dementia: two cases with focal spongiform degeneration. Ann Neurol 1987;22:527–532.

Kirshner HS, Tsai SI, Runge VM, Price AC. Magnetic resonance imaging and other techniques in the diagnosis of multiple sclerosis. Arch Neurol 1985;42:859–863.

Kish SJ, Chang LJ, Mirchandani L, Shannak K, Hornykiewicz O. Progressive supranuclear palsy: relationship between extrapyramidal disturbances, dementia, and brain neurotransmitter markers. Ann Neurol 1985;18:530–536.

Kish SJ, El-Awar M, Schut L, Leach L, Oscar-Berman M, Freedman M. Cognitive deficits in olivopontocerebellar atrophy: Implications for the cholinergic hypothesis of Alzheimer's dementia. Ann Neurol 1988a;24:200–206.

Kish SJ, Robitaille Y, El-Awar M, Deck JHN, Simmons J, Schut L, Chang L-J, DiStafano L, Freedman M. Non-Alzheimer-type pattern of brain cholineacetyltransferase reduction in dominantly inherited olivopontocerebellar atrophy. Ann Neurol 1989;26:352–367.

Kish SJ, Shannak K, Hornykiewicz O. Elevated serotonin and reduced dopamine in subregionally divided Huntington's disease striatum. Ann Neurol 1987;22:386–389.

Kish SJ, Shannak K, Hornykiewicz O. Uneven pattern of dopamine loss in the striatum of patients with idiopathic Parkinson's disease. N Engl J Med 1988; 318:876–880.

Kitagawa Y, Meyer JS, Tachibana H, Mortel KF, Rogers RL. CT-CBF correlations of cognitive deficits in multi-infarct dementia. Stroke 1984;15:1000–1009.

Kitamura J, Kubuki Y, Tsuruta K, Kurihara T, Matsukura S. A new family with Joseph disease in Japan. Arch Neurol 1989;46:425–428.

Kito S, Itoga E, Hiroshige Y, Matsumoto N, Miwa S. A pedigree of amyotrophic chorea with acanthocytosis. Arch Neurol 1980;37:514–517.

Kiyosawa M, Bosley TM, Alavi A, Gupta N, Rhodes CH, Chawluk J, Kushner M, Savino PJ, Sergott RC, Schatz NJ, Reivich M. Positron emission tomography in a patient with progressive multifocal leukoencephalopathy. Neurology 1988;38:1864–1867.

Klatzo I, Wisniewski H, Stretcher E. Experimental production of neurofibrillary degeneration. I. Light microscopic observations. J Neuropathol Exp Neurol 1965;24;187–199.

Klawans HL Jr. A pharmacologic analysis of Huntington's chorea. Eur Neurol 1970;4:148–163.

Klawans HL, Goetz CG, Perlik S. Presymptomatic and early detection in Huntington's disease. Ann Neurol 1980;8:343–347.

Klawans HL, Lupton M, Simon L. Calcification of the basal ganglia as a cause of levodopa-resistant parkinsonism. Neurology 1976;26:221–225.

Klawans HL, Paulson GW, Barbeau A. Predictive test for Huntington's chorea. Lancet 1970;2:1185–1186.

Klawans HL Jr, Ringel SDP. Observations on the efficacy of L-dopa in progressive supranuclear palsy. Eur Neurol 1971;5:115–129.

Klawans HL, Stein RW, Tanner CM, Goetz CG. A pure parkinsonian syndrome following acute carbon monoxide intoxication. Arch Neurol 1982;39:302–304.

Klonoff DC, Andrews BT, Obana WG. Stroke associated with cocaine use. Arch Neurol 1989;46:989–993.

Kluin KJ, Gilman S, Markel DS, Koeppe RA, Rosenthal G, Junck L. Speech disorders in olivopontocerebellar atrophy correlate with positron emission tomography findings. Ann Neurol 1988;23:547–554.

Klüver H, Bucy PC. Preliminary analysis of functions of the temporal lobes in monkeys. Arch Neurol Psychiatry 1939;42:979–1000.

Knehr CA, Bearn AG. Psychological impairment in Wilson's disease. J Nerv Ment Dis 1956;124:251–255.

Knee ST, Razani J. Acute organic brain syndrome: a complication of disulfiram therapy. Am J Psychiatry 1974;131:1281–1282.

Knights EB, Folstein MF. Unsuspected emotional and cognitive disturbance in medical patients. Ann Intern Med 1977;87:723–724.

Knopman DS, Christensen KJ, Schut LJ, Harbaugh RE, Reeder T, Ngo T, Frey W II. The spectrum of imaging and neuropsychological findings in Pick's disease. Neurology 1989;39:362–368.

Knopman DS, Mastri AR, Frey WH II, Sung JH, Rustan T. Dementia lacking distinctive histologic features: A common non-Alzheimer degenerative dementia. Neurology 1990;40:251–256.

von Knorring J, Erma M, Lindstrom D. The clinical manifestations of temporal arteritis. Acta Med Scand 1966;179:691–702.

Knopp W, Paulson G, Allen JN, Smeltzer D, Brown FD, Kose W. Parkinson's disease: L-dopa treatment and handwriting area. Cur Ther Res 1970;12:115–125.

Knuth WP, Kisner P. Symmetrical cerebral calcification associated with parathyroid adenoma. JAMA 1956;162:462–464.

Koch TK, Yee MCH, Hutchinson HT, Berg BO. Magnetic resonance imaging in subacute necrotizing encephalomyelopathy (Leigh's disease). Ann Neurol 1986;19:605–607.

Koenig H. Dementia associated with the benign form of multiple sclerosis. Trans Am Neurol Assoc 1968;93:227–228.

Koeppen AH, Barron KD. Marchiafava-Bignami disease. Neurology 1978;28:290–294.

Kohler J, Heilmeyer H, Volk B. Multiple sclerosis presenting as chronic atypical psychosis. J Neurol Neurosurg Psychiatry 1988;51:281–284.

Kokman E, Beard M, Offord KP, Kurland LT. Prevalence of medically diagnosed dementia in a defined United States population: Rochester, Minnesota, January 1, 1975. Neurology 1989;39:773–776.

Koller WC. Classification of parkinsonism. In: Koller WC, ed., Handbook of Parkinson's disease. Marcel Dekker, New York, 1987:51–80.

Kolodny A. Symptomatology of tumor of the frontal lobe. Arch Neurol Psychiatry 1929;21:1107–1127.

Kolodny EH, Cable WJL. Inborn errors of metabolism. Ann Neurol 1982;11:221–232.

Kolodny EH, Rebeiz JJ, Caviness VS Jr, Richardson EP Jr. Granulomatous angiitis of the central nervous system. Arch Neurol 1968;19:510–524.

Konigsmark BW, Weiner LP. The olivopontocerebellar atrophies: a review. Medicine 1970;49:227–241.

Kondo K, Kuroiwa Y. A case control study of Creutzfeldt-Jakob disease: association with physical injuries. Ann Neurol 1982;11:377–381.

Koponen H, Hurri L, Stenback U, Riekkinen PJ. Acute confusional states in the elderly: a radiological evaluation. Acta Psychiatr Scand 1987;76:726–731.

Kornhuber HH. Cerebral cortex, cerebellum, and basal ganglia: an introduction to their motor functions. In: Schmitt FO, Worden FG, eds. The neurosciences. Third study program. MIT Press, Cambridge, Mass., 1974:267–280.

Kosaka K, Oyanagi S, Matsushita M, Hori A, Iwase S. Presenile dementia with Alzheimer, Pick, and Lewy-body changes. Acta Neuropathol 1976;36:221–233.

Koskiniemi M, Donner M, Majuri H, Haltia M, Norio R. Progressive myoclonus epilepsy. Acta Neurol Scand 1974a;50:307–332.

Koskiniemi M, Toivakka E, Donner M. Progressive myoclonus epilepsy. Acta Neurol Scand 1974b;50:333–359.

Koss E, Friedland RP, Ober BA, Jagust WJ. Differences in lateral hemispheric asymmetries of glucose utilization between early- and late-onset Alzheimer-type dementia. Am J Psychiatry 1985;142:638–640.

Koudouris SD, Stern TN, Utterback RA. Involvement of central nervous system in Whipple's disease. Neurology 1963;13:397–404.

Kowlessar OD. Diseases of the pancreas. In: Beeson PB, McDermott W, eds. Cecil-Loeb: textbook of medicine. 13th ed. WB Saunders, Philadelphia, 1971:1312–1327.

Kozin F, Haughton V, Bernhard GC. Neuro-Behçet disease: two cases and neuro-radiologic findings. Neurology 1977;27:1148–1152.

Kraepelin E. General paresis. Moore JW, trans. Journal of Nervous and Mental Disease Publishing Company, New York, 1913. Reprinted. Johnson Reprint, New York, 1970.

Kral VA. The relationship between senile dementia (Alzheimer type) and depression. Canad J Psychiatry 1983;28:304–306.

Kramer JH, Delis DC, Blusewicz MJ, Brandt J, Ober BA, Strauss M. Verbal memory errors in Alzheimer's and Huntington's dementias. Develop Neuropsychol 1988;4:1–15.

Kramer S, Lee KF. Complications of radiation therapy: the central nervous system. Semin Roentgenol 1974;9:75–83.

Krauthammer C, Klerman GL. Secondary mania. Arch Gen Psychiatry 1978;35:1333–1339.

Krawiecki NS, Dyken PR, Gammal TE, DuRant RH, Swift A. Computed tomography of the brain in subacute sclerosing panencephalitis. Ann Neurol 1984;15:489–493.

Kremzner LT, Berl S, Stellar S, Cote LJ. Amino acids, peptides, and polyamines in cortical biopsies and ventricular fluid in patients with Huntington's disease. Adv Neurol 1979;23:537–546.

Krigman MR, Feldman RG, Bensch K. Alzheimer's presenile dementia. A histochemical and electron microscopic study. Lab Invest 1965;14:381–396.

Kristensen V, Olsen M, Theilgaard A. Levodopa treatment of presenile dementia. Acta Psychiatr Scand 1977;55:41–51.

Krop HD, Block AJ, Cohen E. Neuropsychologic effects of continuous oxygen therapy in chronic obstructive pulmonary disease. Chest 1973;64:317–322.

Krupp LB, Lipton RB, Swerdlow ML, Leeds NE, Llena J. Progressive multifocal leukoencephalopathy: Clinical and radiographic features. Ann Neurol 1985; 17:344–349.

Kuhl DE, Edwards RQ, Ricci AR, Reich M. Quantitative section scanning using orthogonal tangent correction. J Nucl Med 1973;14:196–200.

Kuhl DE, Engel J, Phelps ME, Selin C. Epileptic patterns of local cerebral metabolism and perfusion in man determined by emission computed tomography of [18]FDG and [13]NH$_3$. Ann Neurol 1980a;8:348–360.

Kuhl DE, Metter EJ, Riege WH. Patterns of local cerebral glucose utilization determined in Parkinson's disease by [^{18}F]fluorodeoxyglucose method. Ann Neurol 1984;15:419–424.

Kuhl DE, Metter EJ, Riege WH, Hawkins RA, Mazziotta JC, Phelps ME, Kling AS. Local cerebral glucose utilization in elderly patients with depression, multiple infarct dementia and Alzheimer's disease. J Cerebral Blood Flow and Metabolism 1983;3(Suppl. 1):S494–S495.

Kuhl DE, Phelps ME, Kowell AP, Metter EJ, Selin C, Winter J. Effects of stroke on local cerebral metabolism and perfusion: mapping by emission computed tomography of [18]FDG and [13]NH$_3$. Ann Neurol 1980b;8:47–60.

Kuhl DE, Phelps ME, Markham CH, Metter EJ, Riege WH, Winter J. Cerebral metabolism and atrophy in Huntington's disease determined by [18]FDG and computed tomographic scan. Ann Neurol 1982;12:425–434.

Kumar A, Koss E, Metzler D, Moore A, Friedland RP. Behavioral Symptomatology in dementia of the Alzheimer type. Alzheimer Dis Assoc Dis 1988;2:363–365.

Kurland LT. The epidemiologic characteristics of multiple sclerosis. In: Vinken PJ, Bruyn GW, eds. Multiple sclerosis and other demyelinating diseases. Vol. 9. Handbook of clinical neurology. New York: American Elsevier, 1970:63–84.

Kurland LT, Faro SN, Siedler H. Minamata disease. World Neurol 1960;1:370–392.

Kurland ML. Organic brain syndrome with propranolol. N Engl J Med 1979;300:366.

Kuroiwa Y, Celesia GG. Clinical significance of periodic EEG patterns. Arch Neurol 1980;37:15–20.

Kurtze JF. Clinical manifestations of multiple sclerosis. In: Vinken PJ, Bruyn GW, eds. Multiple sclerosis and other demyelinating diseases. Vol. 9. Handbook of clinical neurology. American Elsevier, New York, 1970:161–216.

Kutt H, Winters W, Kokenge R, McDowell F. Diphenylhydantoin metabolism, blood levels, and toxicity. Arch Neurol 1964;11:642–648.

Kuzuhara S, Kanazawa I, Sasaki H, Nakanishi T, Shimamura K. Gerstmann-Straussler-Scheinker's disease. Ann Neurol 1983;14:216–225.

Kvale JN. Amitriptyline in the management of progressive supranuclear palsy. Arch Neurol 1982;39:387–388.

Ladurner G, Iliff LD. Lechner H. Clinical factors associated with dementia in ischaemic stroke. J Neurol Neurosurg Psychiatry 1982;45:97–101.

Lai F, Williams RS. A prospective study of Alzheimer disease in Down syndrome. Arch Neurol 1989;46:849–853.

Lambie CG, Latham O, McDonald GL. Olivo-ponto-cerebellar atrophy (Marie's ataxia). Med J Aust 1947;2:626–632.

Lamoureux G, Giard JN, St-Hilaire M, Duplantis F. Cerebrospinal fluid protein in multiple sclerosis. Neurology 1975;25:537–546.

Lampe TH, Plymate SR, Risse SC, Kopeikin H, Cubberley L, Raskind MA. TSH responses to two TRH doses in men with Alzheimer's disease. Psychoneuroendocrin 1988;13:245–254.

Lampert P, Tom MI, Cummings JN. Encephalopathy in Whipple's disease. Neurology 1962;12:65–71.

Lance JW, Adams RD. The syndrome of intention or action myoclonus as a sequel to hypoxic encephalopathy. Brain 1963;86:111–134.

Lance JW, McLeod JG. A physiological approach to clinical neurology. Butterworths, Stoneham, Mass.; 1975.

Lance JW, Schwab RS, Peterson EA. Action tremor and the cogwheel phenomenon in Parkinson's disease. Brain 1963;86:95–109.

Landau WM, Gitt JJ. Hereditary spastic paraplegia and hereditary ataxia. Arch Neurol Psychiatry 1951;66:346–354.

Landau WM, Luse SA. Relapsing inclusion encephalitis (Dawson type) of eight years' duration. Neurology 1958;8:669–676.

Landis DMD, Williams RS, Masters CL. Golgi and electronmicroscopic studies of spongiform encephalopathy. Neurology 1981;31:538–549.

Landis T, Cummings JL, Benson DF, Palmer EP. Loss of topographic familiarity. An environmental agnosia. Arch Neurol 1986;43:132–136.

Landis T, Graves R, Benson DF, Hebben N. Visual recognition through kinaesthetic mediation. Psychol Med 1982;12:515–531.

Landrigan PJ, Baloh RW, Barthel WF, Whitworth RH, Staehling NW, Rosenblum BF. Neuropsychological dysfunction in children with chronic low-level lead absorption. Lancet 1975;1:708–712.

Landy PJ, Bain BJ. Alzheimer's disease in siblings. Med J Aust 1970;2:832–834.

Lane B, Carroll BA, Pedley TA. Computerized cranial tomography in cerebral diseases of white matter. Neurology 1978;28:534–544.

Lang AW, Moore RA. Acute toxic psychosis concurrent with phenothiazine therapy. Am J Psychiatry 1961;117:939–940.

Langston JW, Dorfman LJ, Forno LS. "Encephalomyeloneuritis" in the absence of cancer. Neurology 1975;25:633–637.

Langston JW, Forno LS. The hypothalamus in Parkinson disease. Ann Neurol 1978;3:129–133.

Larrsen T, Sjøgren T. Essential tremor. Acta Psychiatr Scand (Suppl) 1960;144:1–176.

Larrsen T, Sjøgren T, Jacobson G. Senile dementia. Acta Psychiatr Scand 1963;(suppl 167):1–259.

Larsen TA, Dunn HG, Jan JE, Caine DB. Dystonia and calcification of the basal ganglia. Neurology 1985;35:533–537.

Larson EB, Reifler BV, Featherstone HJ, English DR. Dementia in elderly outpatients: a prospective study. Ann Intern Med 1984;100:417–423.

La Rue A, Spar J, Hill CD. Cognitive impairment in late-life depression: clinical correlates and treatment implications. J Affect Dis 1986;11:179–184.

Latovitzki N, Abrams G, Clark C, Mayeux R, Ascherl G Jr, Sciarra D. Cerebral cysticercosis. Neurology 1978;28:838–842.

Laurence KM, Coates S. The natural history of hydrocephalus: detailed analysis of 182 unoperated cases. Arch Dis Child 1962a;37:345–362.

Laurence KM, Coates S. Further thoughts on the natural history of hydrocephalus. Dev Med Child Neurol 1962b;4:263–267.

Laurence KM, Coates S. Spontaneously arrested hydrocephalus. Dev Med Child Neurol (Suppl) 1967;13:4–13.

Laurence KM, Tew BJ. Follow-up of 65 survivors from the 435 cases of spina bifida born in South Wales between 1956 and 1962. Dev Med Child Neurol 1967;(suppl 13):1–3.

Lavin P, Alexander CP. Dementia associated with clonidine therapy. Br Med J 1975;1:628.

Lavis VR. Psychiatric manifestations of endocrine disease in the elderly. In: Levenson AJ, Hall RCW, eds. Neuropsychiatric manifestations of physical disease in the elderly. Raven Press, New York, 1981:59–81.

Lavy S, Melamed E, Cooper G, Bentin S, Rinot Y. Regional cerebral blood flow in patients with Parkinson's disease. Arch Neurol 1979;36:344–348.

Lawson JS, Barker MG. The assessment of nominal dysphasia in dementia: the use of reaction-time measures. Br J Med Psychol 1968;41:411–414.

Leaf A. Posterior pituitary. In: Beeson PB, McDermott W, eds. Cecil-Loeb: textbook of medicine. 13th ed. WB Saunders, Philadelphia, 1971:1748–1752.

Leanderson R, Meyerson BA, Persson A. Effect of L-dopa on speech in parkinsonism. J Neurol Neurosurg Psychiatry 1971;34:679–681.

Learoyd BM. Psychotropic drugs and the elderly patient. Med J Aust 1972;1:1131–1133.

Leavitt S, Tyler HR. Studies in asterixis. Arch Neurol 1964;10:360–368.

Lebensohn ZM, Jenkins RB. Improvement in parkinsonism in depressed patients treated with ECT. Am J Psychiatry 1975;132:283–285.

Lechevalier B, Andersson JC, Morin P. Hemispheric disconnection syndrome with a "crossed avoiding" reaction in a case of Marchiafava-Bignami disease. J Neurol Neurosurg Psychiatry 1977;40:483–497.

Lederman RJ, Henry CE. Progressive dialysis encephalopathy. Ann Neurol 1978;4:199–204.

Lee K, Hardt F, Moller L, Haubek A, Jensen E. Alcohol-induced brain damage and liver damage in young males. Lancet 1979;2:759–761.

Lee RG, Blair RDG. Evolution of EEG and visual evoked response changes in Jakob-Creutzfeldt disease. Electroencephalogr Clin Neurophysiol 1973;35:133–142.

Leenders KL, Frackowiak RSJ, Lees AJ. Steele-Richardson-Olszewski syndrome. Brain energy metabolism, blood flow and fluorodopa uptake measured by positron emission tomography. Brain 1988;111:615–630.

Leenders KL, Palmar AJ, Quinn N, Clark JC, Firnau G, Garnett ES, Nahmias C, Jones T, Marsden CD. Brain dopamine metabolism in patients with Parkinson's disease measured with positron emission tomography. J Neurol Neurosurg Psychiatry 1986;49:853–860.

Lees AJ. Progressive supranuclear palsy (Steele-Richardson-Olszewski syndrome). In: Cummings JL, ed. Subcortical dementia. Oxford University Press, New York, 1990:123–131.

Lehrer GM, Levitt MF. Neuropsychiatric presentation of hypercalcemia. J Mount Sinai Hosp 1960;27:10–18.

LeMay M, Hochberg FH. Ventricular differences between hydrostatic hydrocephalus and hydrocephalus ex vacuo by computed tomography. Neuroradiology 1979;17:191–195.

LeMay M, New PFJ. Radiological diagnosis of occult normal-pressure hydrocephalus. Radiology 1970;96:347–358.

Lennox WG. Brain injury, drugs, and environment as causes of mental decay in epilepsy. Am J Psychiatry 1942;99:174–180.

Leonard A, Shapiro FL. Subdural hematoma in regularly hemodialyzed patients. Ann Intern Med 1975;82:650–658.

Leonard DP, Kidson MA, Shaunon PJ, Brown J. Double-blind trial of lithium carbonate and haloperidol in Huntington's chorea. Lancet 1974;2:1208–1209.

Lepore FE, Steele JC, Cox TA, Tillson G, Calne DB, Duvoisin RC, Lavine L, McDarby JV. Supranuclear disturbances of ocular motility in Lytico-Bodig. Neurology 1988;38:1849–1853.

Lesse S, Hoefer PFA, Austin JH. The electroencephalogram in diffuse encephalopathies. Arch Neurol Psychiatry 1958;79:359–375.

Lessell S. Higher disorders of visual function: positive phenomena. In: Glaser JS, Smith JL, eds. Neuro-ophthalmology. Vol. 8. CV Mosby, St. Louis, 1975:27–44.

Lessell S, Hirano A, Torres J, Kurland LT. Parkinsonism-dementia complex. Arch Neurol 1962;7:377–385.

Letemendia F, Pampiglione G. Clinical and electroencephalographic observations in Alzheimer's disease. J Neurol Neurosurg Psychiatry 1958;21:167–172.

Leuchter AF, Spar JE, Walter DO, Weiner H. Electroencephalographic spectra and coherence in the diagnosis of Alzheimer's-type and multi-infarct dementia. Arch Gen Psychiatry 1987;44:993–998.

Levenson AJ, Hall RCW. Preface: a statement of the problem. In: Levenson AJ, Hall RCW, eds. Neuropsychiatric manifestations of physical disease in the elderly. Raven Press, New York, 1981:v–vi.

Levin BE, Llabre MM, Weiner WJ. Cognitive impairments associated with early Parkinson's disease. Neurology 1989;39:557–561.

Levin BE, Nordgren RE, Sachs E Jr, McBeath J. Correctable atherosclerotic dementia with improvement. Neurology 1976a;26:355.

Levin HS. Memory deficit after closed-head injury. J Clin Exp Neuropsychol 1989;12:129–153.

Levin HS, Amparo E, Eisenberg HM, Williams DH, High WM Jr, McArdle CB, Weiner RL. Magnetic resonance imaging and computerized tomography in relation to the neurobehavioral sequelae of mild and moderate head injuries. J Neurosurg 1987;66:706–713.

Levin HS, Grossman RG. Behavioral sequelae of closed head injury. Arch Neurol 1978;35:720–727.

Levin HS, Handel SF, Goldman AM, Eisenberg HM, Guinto FC Jr. Magnetic resonance imaging after 'diffuse' nonmissile head injury. Arch Neurol 1985; 42:963–968.

Levin HS, Rodnitzky RL, Mick DL. Anxiety associated with exposure to organophosphate compounds. Arch Gen Psychiatry 1976b;32:225–228.

Levin P, Kunin AS, Donaghy RMP, Hamilton WH, Maurer JJ. Intracranial calcification and hypoparathyroidism. Neurology 1961;11:1076–1080.

Levine AM. Buspirone and agitation in head injury. Brain Injury 1988;2:165–167.

Levine J, Swanson PD. Nonatherosclerotic causes of stroke. Ann Intern Med 1969;70:807–816.

Levita E, Riklan M. Integrative functions in parkinsonism. Percept Mot Skills 1970;31:379–385.

Levita E, Riklan M, Cooper IS. Cognitive and perceptual performance in parkinsonism as a function of age and neurological impairment. J Nerv Ment Dis 1964;139:516–520.

Levy NL, Auerbach PS, Hayes EC. A blood test for multiple sclerosis based on the adherence of lymphocytes to measles-infected cells. N Engl J Med 1976;294:1423–1427.

Levy RM, Bredesen DE, Rosenblum ML. Neurological manifestations of the acquired immunodeficiency syndrome (AIDS): experience at UCSF and review of the literature. J Neurosurg 1985;62:475–495.

Levy RM, Janssen RS, Bush TJ, Rosenblum ML. Neuroepidemiology of acquired immunodeficiency syndrome. In: Rosenblum ML, Levy RL, Bredesen DE, eds. AIDS and the nervous system, Raven Press, New York, 1988:13–27.

Lewey FH, Govons SR. Hemochromatotic pigmentation of the central nervous system. J Neuropathol Exp Neurol 1942;1:129–138.

LeWitt PA, Forno LS, Brant-Zawadzki M. Neoplastic angioendotheliosis: a case with spontaneous regression and radiographic appearance of cerebral arteritis. Neurology 1983;33:39–44.

Lezak MD. Neuropsychological assessment. Oxford University Press, New York, 1976.

Lezak MD. Neuropsychological assessment, 2nd ed. Oxford University Press, New York, 1983.

Lhermitte F, Marteau R, Serdaru M, Chedru F. Signs of interhemispheric disconnection in Marchiafava-Bignami disease. Arch Neurol 1977;34:254.

Liddell DW. Investigations of EEG findings in presenile dementia. J Neurol Neurosurg Psychiatry 1958;21:173–176.

Liddell DW, Northfield DWC. The effect of temporal lobectomy upon two cases of an unusual form of mental deficiency. J Neurol Neurosurg Psychiatry 1954;17:267–275.

Liddle GW. Adrenal cortex. In: Beeson PB, McDermott W, eds. Cecil-Loeb: textbook of medicine. 13th ed. WB Saunders, Philadelphia, 1971:1780–1799.

Lieberman A, Dziatolowski M, Kupersmith M, et al. Dementia in Parkinson disease. Ann Neurol 1979a;6:355–359.

Lieberman A, Dziatolowski M, Neophytides A, et al. Dementias of Huntington's and Parkinson's disease. Adv Neurol 1979b;23:273–280.

Lieberman A, Kupersmith M, Estey E, Goldstein M. Treatment of Parkinson's disease with bromocriptine. N Engl J Med 1976;295:1400–1404.

Lieberman A, Kupersmith M, Neophytides A, et al. Long-term efficacy of bromo-criptine in Parkinson disease. Neurology 1980;30:518–532.

Lilly R, Cummings JL, Benson DF, Frankel M. Clinical occurrence of the Klüver-Bucy syndrome. Neurology 1982;32(2):A96.

Lima L, Coutinho P. Clinical criteria for diagnosis of Machado-Joseph disease: report of a non-Azorean Portuguese family. Neurology 1980;30:319–322.

Lin JT-Y, Ziegler DK. Psychiatric symptoms with initiation of carbidopa-levodopa treatment. Neurology 1976;26:699–700.

Lindenbaum J, Healton EB, Savage DG, Brust JCM, Garrett TJ, Podell ER, Marcell PD, Stabler SP, Allen RH. Neuropsychiatric disorders caused by cobalamin deficiency in the absence of anemia or macrocytosis. N Engl J Med 1988;318:1720–1728.

Lindenberg R, Freytag E. The mechanism of cerebral contusions. Arch Pathol 1960;69:440–469.

Lindvall O, Bjorklund A, Moore RY, Stenevi U. Mesencephalic dopamine neurons projecting to neocortex. Brain Res 1974;81:325–331.

Lipowski ZJ. Delirium. Acute brain failure in man. Charles C Thomas, Springfield, Ill, 1980a.

Lipowski ZJ. Delirium updated. Compr Psychiatry 1980b;21:190–196.

Lipowski ZJ. Transient cognitive disorders (delirium, acute confusional states) in the elderly. Am J Psychiatry 1983;140:1426–1436.

Lipowski ZJ. Delirium (acute confusional states). JAMA 1987;258:1789–1792.

Lisak RP, Keshgegian AA. Oligoclonal immunoglobulins in cerebrospinal fluid in multiple sclerosis. Clin Chem 1980;26:1340–1345.

Lishman WA. Brain damage in relation to psychiatric disability after head injury. Brit J Psychiatry 1968;114:373–410.

Lishman WA. Organic psychiatry. Blackwell Scientific Publications, London, 1978.

Lishman WA. Cerebral disorder in alcoholism. Syndromes of impairment. Brain 1981;104:1–20.

Lishman WA. Organic Psychiatry, 2nd ed. Blackwell Scientific Publications, Oxford, 1987.

Liss L. Histopathology of the mamillary bodies in alcoholic psychosis. Neurology 1958;8:832–838.

Liston EH Jr. Occult presenile dementia. J Nerv Ment Dis 1977;164:263–267.

Liston EH, La Rue A. Clinical differentiation of primary degenerative and multi-infarct dementia: a critical review of the evidence. Part I: Clinical studies. Biol Psychiatry 1983a:18:1451–1465.

Liston EH, La Rue A. Clinical differentiation of primary degenerative and multi-infarct dementia: a critical review of the evidence. Part II: Pathological studies. Biol Psychiatry 1983b;18:1467–1484.

Little BW, Brown PW, Rodgers-Johnson P, Perl DP, Gajdusek DC. Familial my-oclonic dementia masquerading as Creutzfeldt-Jakob disease. Ann Neurol 1986;20:231–239.

Little JR, Dale AJD, Okazaki H. Meningeal carcinomatosis. Arch Neurol 1974;30:138–143.

Little JR, MacCarty CS. Colloid cysts of the third ventricle. J Neurosurg 1974;39:230–235.

Littrup PJ, Gebarski SS. MR imaging of Hallervorden-Spatz disease. J Comput Assist Tomog 1985;9:491–493.

Litvan I, Grafman J, Golmez C, Chase TN. Memory impairment in patients with progressive supranuclear palsy. Arch Neurol 1989;46:756–767.

Lloyd GG, Lishman WA. Effect of depression on the speed of recall of pleasant and unpleasant experiences. Psychol Med 1975;5:173–180.

Lo B, Dornbrand L. Guiding the hand that feeds. N Engl J Med 1984;311:402–404.

Locke S. Progressive personality changes and hemiparesis in a middle-aged man (clinical pathological conference). JAMA 1973;225:143–153.

Locke S, Foley JM. A case of cerebellar ataxia with a discussion of classification. Arch Neurol 1960;3:279–289.

Loeb C, Gandolfo C. Diagnostic evaluation of degenerative and vascular dementia. Stroke 1983;14:399–401.

Logothetis J. Neurologic and muscular manifestations of hyperthyroidism. Arch Neurol 1961;5:533–544.

Logothetis J. Psychotic behavior as the initial indicator of adult myxedema. J Nerv Ment Dis 1963;136:561–568.

Logothetis J. Silverstein P, Coe J. Neurologic aspects of Waldenstroms's macroglobulinemia. Arch Neurol 1960;5:564–573.

Lombes A, Mendell JR, Nakase H, Barohn RJ, Bonilla E, Zevani M, Yates AJ, Omerza J, Gales TL, Nakahara K, Rizzuto R, Engel WK, DiMauro S. Myoclonic epilepsy and ragged-red fibers with cytochrome oxidase deficiency: neuropathology, biochemistry, and molecular genetics. Ann Neurol 1989;26:20–33.

Longo VG. Behavioral and electroencephalographic effects of atropine and related compounds. Pharmacol Rev 1966;18:965–996.

Longstreth WT Jr, Farrell DF, Bolen JW, Bird JD, Daven JR. Adult dystonic lipidosis: clinical, histologic, and biochemical findings of a neurovisceral storage disease. Neurology 1982;32(2):A141.

Lopez RI, Collins GK. Wernicke's encephalopathy: a complication of chronic hemodialysis. Arch Neurol 1968;18:248–259.

Lorand B, Nagy T, Tariska S. Subacute progressive panencephalitis. World Neurol 1962;3:376–394.

Loranger AW, Goodell H, Lee JE, McDowell F. Levodopa treatment of Parkinson's syndrome. Arch Gen Psychiatry 1972a;26:163–168.

Loranger AW, Goodell H, McDowell FH, Lee JE, Sweet RD. Intellectual impairment in Parkinson's syndrome. Brain 1972b;95:405–412.

Lorenz M, Cobb S. Language behavior in manic patients. Arch Neurol Psychiatry 1952;67:763–770.

Lou HOC, Reske-Nielsen E. The central nervous system in Fabry's disease. Arch Neurol 1971;25:351–359.

Loudon RG, Lawson RA Jr. Recurrent neurological relapse in a case treated with amphotericin B. Ann Intern Med 1961;55:139–146.

Low PA, Allsop JL, Halmagyi GM. Huntington's chorea: the rigid form (Westphal variant) treated with levodopa. Med J Aust 1974;1:393–394.

Lowenberg K. Pick's disease. A clinicopathologic contribution. Arch Neurol Psychiatry 1936;36:768–789.

Lowenberg K, Boyd DA Jr, Salon DD. Occurrence of Pick's disease in early adult years. Arch Neurol Psychiatry 1939;41:1004–1020.

Lowenberg K, Waggoner RW. Familial organic psychosis (Alzheimer's type). Arch Neurol Psychiatry 1934;31:737–754.

Lowenstein RJ, Weingartner H, Gillin JC, et al. Disturbances of sleep and cognitive functioning in patients with dementia. Neurobiol Aging 1982;3:371–377.

Lowenthal A, Bruyn GW. Calcification of the striopallidodentate system. In: Vinken PJ, Bruyn GW, eds. Diseases of the basal ganglia. Vol 6. Handbook of clinical neurology. American Elsevier, New York, 1968:703–725.

Lucas-Blaustein MJ, Filipp L, Dungan C, Tune L. Driving in patients with dementia. J Am Geriatr Soc 1988;36:1987–1991.

Luke RA, Stern BJ, Krumholz A, Johns CJ. Neurosarcoidosis: the long-term clinical course. Neurology 1987;37:461–463.

Lunzer M, James IM, Weinman J, Sherlock S. Treatment of chronic hepatic encephalopathy with levodopa. Gut 1974;15:555–561.

Luque FA, Selhorst JB, Petruska P. Parkinsonism induced by high-dose cytosine arabinoside. Movement Disorders 1987;2:219–222.

Luria AR. Disorders of "simultaneous perception" in a case of bilateral occipito-parietal brain injury. Brain 1959;82:437–449.

Luria AR. Neuropsychology in the local diagnosis of brain damage. Cortex 1964;1:3–18.

Luria AR. Higher cortical functions in man. Basic Books, New York, 1966.

Luse SA, Smith KR Jr. The ultrastructure of senile plaques. Am J Pathol 1964;44:553–563.

Lusins JO, Szilagyi PA. Clinical features of chorea associated with systemic lupus erythematosus. Am J Med 1975;58:857–861.

Luxon L, Lees AJ, Greenwood RJ. Neurosyphilis today. Lancet 1979;1:90–93.

Lyle OE, Gottesman II. Subtle cognitive deficits as 15- to 20-year precursors of Huntington's disease. Adv Neurol 1979;23:227–238.

Lyle WH. Dialysis dementia. Lancet 1973;2:271.

Lyon-Caen O, Jouvent R, Hauser S, Chaunu M-P, Benoit N, Widlocher D, Lhermitte F. Cognitive function in recent-onset demyelinating diseases. Arch Neurol 1986;43:1138–1141.

McAllister TW, Ferrell RB, Price TRP, Neville MB. The dexamethasone suppression test in two patients with severe depressive pseudodementia. Am J Psychiatry 1982;139:479–481.

McAllister TW, Hays LR. TRH tests, DST, and response to desipramine in primary degenerative dementia. Biol Psychiatry 1987;22:189–193.

McAllister TW, Price TPR. Severe depressive pseudodementia with and without dementia. Am J Psychiatry 1982;139:626–629.

McAlpine D. The pathology of the parkinsonian syndrome following encephalitis lethargica, with a note on the occurrence of calcification in this disease. Brain 1923;46:255–280.

McAlpine D, Araki S. Minimata disease. An unusual neurological disorder caused by contaminated fish. Lancet 1958;2:629–631.

MacAlpine I, Hunter R. The "insanity" of King George III: a classic case of porphyria. Br Med J 1966;1:65–71.

MacAlpine I, Hunter R, Rimington C. Porphyria in the royal houses of Stuart, Hanover, and Prussia. Br Med J 1968;1:7–18.

McArthur JC. Neurologic manifestations of AIDS. Medicine 1987;66:407–437.

McArthur JC, Cohen BA, Selnes OA, Kumar AJ, Cooper K, McArthur JH, Soucy G, Cornblath DR, Chmiel JS, Wang M-C, Starkey DL, Ginzburg H, Ostrow DG, Johnson RT, Phair JP, Polk BF. Low prevalence of neurological and neuropsychological abnormalities in otherwise healthy HIV-1-infected individuals: results from the Multicenter AIDS Cohort Study. Ann Neurol 1989;26:601–611.

McAuley DLF, Lecky BRF, Earl CJ. Gold encephalopathy. J Neurol Neurosurg Psychiatry 1977;40:1021–1022.

McCaughey WTE. The pathologic spectrum of Huntington's chorea. J Nerv Ment Dis 1961;133:91–103.

Macchi G, Abbamondi AL, Di Trapani G, Sbriccoli A. On the white matter lesions of the Creutzfeldt-Jakob disease. J Neurol Sci 1984;63:197–206.

McCormick WF, Danneel CM. Central pontine myelinolysis. Arch Intern Med 1967;119:444–478.

McCullough DC, Fox JL. Negative intracranial pressure hydrocephalus in adults with shunts and its relationship to the production of subdural hematoma. J Neurosurg 1974;40:372–375.

McDaniel K. Thalamic dementia. In: Cummings JL, ed. Subcortical dementia. Oxford University Press, New York, 1990:132–144.

McDermott JR, Smith AI, Iqbal K, Wisniewski HM. Aluminum and Alzheimer's disease. Lancet 1977;2:710–711.

McDermott JR, Smith AI, Iqbal K, Wisniewski HM. Brain aluminum in aging and Alzheimer disease. Neurology 1979;29:809–814.

McDowell FH, Lee JE, Sweet RD. Extrapyramidal disease. In: Baker AB, Baker LH, eds. Clinical neurology. Harper & Row, New York, 1978:1–67.

Mace NL, Rabins PV. The 36-hour day. Johns Hopkins University Press, Baltimore, 1981.

McEntee WJ, Mair RG. Memory enhancement in Korsakoff's psychosis by clonidine: further evidence for a noradrenergic deficit. Ann Neurol 1980;7:466–470.

McEvoy CL. Behavioral treatment. In: Cummings JL, Miller BL, eds. Alzheimer's disease. Treatment and long-term management. Marcel Dekker, New York, 1990:207–224.

McEvoy JP, Wells CE. Case studies in neuropsychiatry. II. Conversion pseudodementia. J Clin Psychiatry 1979;40:447–449.

McFarland HR, Good WG, Drowns BV, Meneses ACO. Papulosis atrophicans maligna (Kohlmeier-Degos disease): a disseminated occlusive vasculopathy. Ann Neurol 1978;3:388–392.

McFarlin DE, Strober W, Waldmann TA. Ataxia-telangiectasia. Medicine 1972;51:281–314.

McGeachie RE, Fleming JO, Sharer LR, Hyman RA. Diagnosis of Pick's disease by computed tomography. J Comput Assist Tomogr 1979;3:113–115.

McGee DA, van Patter HJ, Moretta J, Olszewski J. Subpial cerebral siderosis. Neurology 1962;12:108–113.

McGeer EG, McGeer PL. Neurotransmitter metabolism in the aging brain. In: Terry

RD, Gershon S, eds. Neurobiology of aging. Raven Press, New York, 1976:389–403.

McGeer PL, McGeer EG, Fibiger HC. Choline acetylase and glutamic acid decarboxylase in Huntington's chorea. Neurology 1973;23:912–917.

McHugh PR. Occult hydrocephalus. Q J Med 1964;33:297–308.

McHugh PR. Depression and dementia. Alzheimer's disease and related disorders. Mini-White House Conference on Aging, Washington, D.C., January 15, 1981.

McHugh PR, Folstein MF. Psychiatric syndromes of Huntington's chorea: a clinical and phenomenologic study. In: Benson DF, Blumer D, eds. Psychiatric aspects of neurologic disease. Grune & Stratton, New York, 1975:267–285.

McHugh PR, Folstein MF. Psychopathology of dementia: implications for neuropathology. In: Katzman R, ed. Congenital and acquired cognitive disorders. Raven Press, New York, 1979:17–30.

McIntosh GC, Jameson D, Markesbery WR. Huntington disease associated with Alzheimer disease. Ann Neurol 1978;3:545–548.

McIntyre HD, McIntyre AP. The problem of brain tumor in psychiatric diagnosis. Am J Psychiatry 1942;98:720–726.

Mackay RP. Course and prognosis in amyotrophic lateral sclerosis. Arch Neurol 1963;8:117–127.

McKhann G, Drachman D, Folstein M, Katzman R, Price D, Stadlan EM. Clinical diagnosis of Alzheimer's disease: report of the NINCDS-ADRDA Work Group, Department of Health and Human Services Task Force on Alzheimer's Disease. Neurol 1984;34:939–944.

McKissock W, Paine KWE. Primary tumours of the thalamus. Brain 1958;81:41–63.

MacLean AR, Berkson J. Mortality and disability in multiple sclerosis. JAMA 1951;146:1367–1369.

McLennan JE, Nakano K, Tyler HR, Schwab RS. Micrographia in Parkinson's disease. J Neurol Sci 1972;15:141–152.

McMenemy WH. Alzheimer's disease. J Neurol Psychiatry 1940;3:211–240.

McMenemy WH, Worster-Drought C, Flind J, Williams HG. Familial presenile dementia. Report of case with clinical and pathological features of Alzheimer's disease. J Neurol Psychiatry 1939;2:293–303.

Macrae D, Trolle E. The defect of function in visual agnosia. Brain 1956;79:94–110.

McQuinn BA, Kemper TL. Sporadic case resembling autosomal-dominant motor system degeneration (Azorean disease complex). Arch Neurol 1987;44:341–344.

Madison DP, Baehr ET, Bazell M, Hartman RW, Mahurkar SD, Dunea G. Communicative deterioration in dialysis dementia: two case studies. J Speech Hear Disord 1977;42:238–246.

Madow L, Alpers BJ. Encephalitic form of metastatic carcinoma. Arch Neurol Psychiatry 1951;65:161–173.

Magnaes B. Communicating hydrocephalus in adults. Neurology 1978;28:478–484.

Maher ER, Lees AJ. The clinical features and natural history of the Steele-Richardson-Olszewski syndrome (progressive supranuclear palsy). Neurology 1986;36:1005–1008.

Maher ER, Smith EM, Lees AJ. Cognitive deficits in Steele-Richardson-Olszewski syndrome (progressive supranuclear palsy). J Neurol Neurosurg Psychiatry 1985;48:1234–1239.

Mahurkar SD, Meyers L Jr, Cohen J, Kamath RV, Dunea G. Electroencephalographic and radionuclide studies in dialysis dementia. Kidney Int 1978;13:306–315.

Mahurkar SD, Salta R, Smith EC, Dhar SK, Meyers L Jr, Dunea G. Dialysis dementia. Lancet 1973;1:1412–1415.

Malamud N. Neuromuscular system disease. In: Minckler J, ed. Diseases of the nervous system. McGraw-Hill, New York, 1968:712–725.

Malamud N, Boyd DA Jr. Pick's disease with atrophy of the temporal lobes. Arch Neurol Psychiatry 1940;43:210–222.

Malamud N, Hirano A, Kurkland LT. Pathoanatomic changes in amyotrophic lateral sclerosis on Guam. Arch Neurol 1961;5:401–415.

Malamud N, Lowenberg K. Alzheimer's disease. Arch Neurol Psychiatry 1929;21:805–827.

Malamud N, Skillicorn SA. Relationship between the Wernicke and Korsakoff syndromes. Arch Neurol Psychiatry 1956;76:585–596.

Malamud N, Waggoner RW. Genealogic and clinicopathologic study of Pick's disease. Arch Neurol Psychiatry 1943;50:288–303.

Maletta GJ. Management of behavior problems in elderly patients with Alzheimer's disease and other dementias. Clin Geriatr Med 1988;4:719–747.

Maletta GJ, Pirozzolo FT, Thompson G, Mortimer JA. Organic mental disorders in a geriatric outpatient population. Am J Psychiatry 1982;139:521–523.

Mallette LE, Bilezikian JP, Health DA, Aurbach GD. Primary hyperparathyroidism: clinical and biochemical features. Medicine 1974;53:127–146.

Malloy FW, Small IF, Miller MJ, Milstein V, Stout JR. Changes in neuropsychological test performance after electroconvulsive therapy. Biol Psychiatry 1982;17:61–67.

Mancall EL. Progressive multifocal leukoencephalopathy. Neurology 1965;15:693–699.

Mandell AJ, Markham C, Fowler W. Parkinson's syndrome, depression, and imipramine. Calif Med 1961;95(1):12–14.

Mandell AJ, Markham CH, Tallman FF, Mandell MP. Motivation and ability to move. Am J Psychiatry 1962;119:544–549.

Mandell AM, Alexander MP, Carpenter S. Creutzfeldt-Jakob disease presenting as isolated aphasia. Neurology 1989;39:55–58.

Mandybur TI. The incidence of cerebral amyloid angiopathy in Alzheimer's disease. Neurology 1975;25:120–126.

Mandybur TI. Cerebral amyloid angiopathy: possible relationship to rheumatoid vasculitis. Neurology 1979;29:1336–1340.

Mandybur TI, Nagpaul AS, Pappas Z, Niklowitz WJ. Alzheimer neurofibrillary change in subacute sclerosing panencephalitis. Ann Neurol 1977;1:103–107.

Mann DMA, Neary D, Yates PO, Lincoln J, Snowden JS, Stanworth P. Alterations in protein synthetic capability of nerve cells in Alzheimer's disease. J Neurol Neurosurg Psychiatry 1981;44:97–102.

Mann DMA, Yates PO, Hawkes J. The noradrenergic system in Alzheimer and multi-infarct dementias. J Neurol Neurosurg Psychiatry 1982;45:113–119.

Manowitz P, Kling A, Kohn H. Clinical course of adult metachromatic leukodystrophy presenting as schizophrenia. J Nerv Ment Dis 1978;166:500-506.

Manuelidis EE, Rorke LB. Transmission of Alper's disease (chronic progressive encephalopathy) produces experimental Creutzfeldt-Jakob disease in hamsters. Neurology 1989;39:615–621.

Manyam BV, Katz L, Hare TA, Kanefski K, Tremblay RD. Isoniazid-induced elevation of CSF GABA levels and effects on chorea in Huntington's disease. Ann Neurol 1981;10:35–37.

Marc-Vergenes JP, Celsis P, Puel M, Angiel A, Clerret M, Roscol A. SPECT study of blood flow changes in normal and demented patients during memorizing. J Cereb Blood Flow Metab 1985;5(suppl.1):133–134.

Margolin D, Hammerstad J, Orwoll E, McClung M, Calhoun D. Intracranial calcification in hyperparathyroidism associated with gait apraxia and parkinsonism. Neurology 1980;30:1005–1007.

Margolis MT, Newton TH. Methamphetamine ("speed") arteritis. Neuroradiology 1971;2:179–182.

Markand ON, Panszi JG. The electroencephalogram in subacute sclerosing panencephalitis. Arch Neurol 1975;32:719–726.

Markesbery WR, Ehmann WD, Hossain TIM, Alauddin M, Goodin DT. Instrumental neutron activation analysis of brain aluminum in Alzheimer disease and aging. Ann Neurol 1981;10:511–516.

Markowitz AM, Slanetz CA Jr, Frantz VK. Functioning islet cell tumors of the pancreas. Ann Surg 1961;154:877–884.

Marlowe WB, Mancall EL, Thomas JJ. Complete Klüver-Bucy syndrome in man. Cortex 1975;11:53–59.

Maroon JC, Campbell RL. Subdural hematoma. Arch Neurol 1970;22:234–239.

Marries-Jones R, Knight R, Will RG, Cousens S, Smith PG, Matthews WB. Creutzfeldt-Jakob disease in England and Wales, 1980–1984: a case-control study of potential risk factors. J Neurol Neurosurg Psychiatry 1988;51:1113–1119.

Marsden CD, Harrison MJG. Outcome of investigation of patients with presenile dementia. Br Med J 1972;2:249–252.

Marsden CD, Tarsy D, Baldessarini RJ. Spontaneous and drug-induced movement disorders in psychotic patients. In: Benson DF, Blumer D, eds. Psychiatric aspects of neurologic disease. In Grune & Stratton, New York, 1975:219–265.

Marsh, DO. Organic mercury: methylmercury compounds. In: Vinken PJ, Bruyn GW, eds. Intoxications of the nervous system. Part I, vol. 36. Handbook of clinical neurology. North-Holland, New York, 1979:73–81.

Marsh GG, Markham CH. Does levodopa alter depression and psychopathology in parkinsonism patients? J Neurol Neurosurg Psychiatry 1973;36:925–935.

Marsh GG, Markham CM, Ansel R. Levodopa's awakening effect on patients with parkinsonism. J Neurol Neurosurg Psychiatry 1971;34:209–218.

Marshall DW, Brey RL, Cahill WT, Houk RW, Zajac RA, Boswell RN. Spectrum of cerebrospinal fluid findings in various stages of human immunodeficiency virus infection. Arch Neurol 1988;45:954–958.

Marshall G, Roessmann U, van den Noort S. Invasive Hodgkin's disease of brain. Cancer 1968;22:621–630.

Martilla RJ, Rinne UK. Dementia in Parkinson's disease. Acta Neurol Scand 1976;54:431–441.

Martin JB, Gusella JF. Huntington's disease. Pathogenesis and management. N Engl J Med 1986;315:1267–1276.

Martin JB, Reichlin S, Brown GM. Clinical neuroendocrinology. FA Davis, Philadelphia, 1977a.

Martin JJ, Ceuterick C, Martin L, Libert J. Skin and conjunctival biopsies in adrenoleukodystrophy. Acta Neuropathol (Berlin) 1977b;38:247–250.

Martin JJ, Ceuterick C, Martin L, Libert J. Skin and conjunctival nerve biopsies in adrenoleukodystrophy and its variants. Ann Neurol 1980;8:291–295.

Martin, JP. Wilson's disease. In: Vinken PJ, Bruyn GW, eds. Diseases of the basal ganglia. Vol 6. Handbook of clinical neurology. American Elsevier, New York, 1968:267–278.

Martin RL, Gerteis G, Gabrielli Jr. A family-genetic study of dementia of Alzheimer type. Arch Gen Psychiatry 1988;45:894–900.

Martin WE, Resch JA, Baker AB. Juvenile parkinsonism. Arch Neurol 1971;25:494–500.

Martland HS. Punch drunk. JAMA 1928;91:1103–1107.

Martone M, Butters N, Payne M, Becker JT, Sax DS. Dissociations between skill learning and verbal recognition in amnesia and dementia. Arch Neurol 1984;41:965–970.

Marzewski DJ, Towfighi J, Harrington MG, Merril CR, Brown P. Creutzfeldt-Jakob disease following pituitary-derived human growth hormone therapy: a new American case. Neurology 1988;38:1131–1133.

Mas J-L, Bousser M-G, Lacombe C, Agar N. Hyperlipidemic dementia. Neurology 1985;35:1385–1387.

Mastaglia FL, Grainger KMR. Internuclear ophthalmoplegia in progressive supranuclear palsy. J Neurol Sci 1975;25:303–308.

Mastaglia FL, Grainger KMR, Kee F, Sadka M, Lefroy R. Progressive supranuclear palsy (the Steele-Richardson-Olszewski syndrome) clinical and electrophysiological observations in eleven cases. Proc Aust Assoc Neurol 1973;10:35–44.

Mastaglia FL, Savas S, Kakulas BA. Intracranial thrombosis of the internal carotid artery after closed head trauma. J Neurol Neurosurg Psychiatry 1969;32:383–388.

Masters CL, Gajdusek C, Gibbs CJ Jr. Creutzfeldt-Jakob disease virus isolations from the Gerstmann-Straussler syndrome with an analysis of the various forms of amyloid plaque deposition in the virus-induced spongiform encephalopathies. Brain 1981a;104:559–588.

Masters CL, Gajdusek C, Gibbs CJ Jr. The familial occurrence of Creutzfeldt-Jakob disease and Alzheimer's disease. Brain 1981b;104:535–538.

Masters CL, Harris JO, Gajdusek C, Gibbs CJ Jr, Bernoulli C, Asher DM. Creutzfeldt-Jakob disease: patterns of worldwide occurrence and the significance of familial and sporadic clustering. Ann Neurol 1979;5:177–188.

Masters CL, Richardson EP Jr. Subacute spongiform encephalopathy (Creutzfeldt-Jakob disease). Brain 1978;101:333–344.

Mathew NT, Meyer JS, Achari AN, Dodson RF. Hyperlipidemic neuropathy and dementia. Eur Neurol 1976;14:370–382.

Mathew NT, Meyer JS, Hartmann A, Ott EO. Abnormal cerebrospinal fluid-blood flow dynamics. Arch Neurol 1975;32:657–664.

Mathew RJ, Meyer JS, Francis DJ, Semchuk KM, Mortel K, Claghorn JL. Cerebral blood flow in depression. Am J Psychiatry 1980;137:1449–1450.

Mathews T, Wisotzkey H, Moossy J. Multiple central nervous system infections in progressive multifocal leukoencephalopathy. Neurology 1976;26:9–14.

Matison R, Mayeux R, Rosen J, Fahn S. "Tip-of-the-tongue" phenomenon in Parkinson disease. Neurology 1982;32:567–570.

Mattern WD, Krigman MR, Blythe WB. Failure of successful renal transplantation to reverse the dialysis-associated encephalopathy syndrome. Clin Nephrol 1977;7:275–278.

Mattis S. Mental status examination for organic mental syndrome in the elderly patient. In: Bellak L, Karasu TB, eds. Geriatric Psychiatry. Grune & Stratton, New York, 1976.

Matthews CG, Haaland KY. The effect of symptom duration on cognitive and motor performance in parkinsonism. Neurology 1979;29:951–956.

Matthews WB. Sarcoidosis of the nervous system. J Neurol Neurosurg Psychiatry 1965;28:23–29.

Matthews WB, Howell DA, Stevens DL. Progressive myoclonus epilepsy without Lafora bodies. J Neurol Neurosurg Psychiatry 1969;32:116–122.

Matuk F, Kalyanaraman K. Syndrome of inappropriate secretion of antidiuretic hormone in patients treated with psychotherapeutic drugs. Arch Neurol 1977;34:374–375.

Matushita M, Oyanagi S, Hanawa S, Shiraki H, Kosaka K. Nasu-Hakola's disease (membranous lipodystrophy). Acta Neuropathol 1981;54:89–93.

Mawdsley C, Ferguson FR. Neurological disease in boxers. Lancet 1963;2:795–801.

May C, Rapoport SI, Tomai TP, Chrousos GP, Gold PW. Cerebrospinal fluid concentrations of corticotropin-releasing hormone (CRH) and corticotropin (ACTH) are reduced in patient's with Alzheimer's disease. Neurology 1987;37:535–538.

May RH, Voegele GE, Paolino AF. The Ganser syndrome: a report of three cases. J Nerv Ment Dis 1960;130:331–339.

May WW. Creutzfeldt-Jakob disease. Acta Neurol Scand 1968;44:1–32.

May WW, Itabashi HH, DeJong RN. Creutzfeldt-Jakob disease. II. Clinical, pathologic, and genetic study of a family. Arch Neurol 1968;19:137–149.

Mayer-Gross W, Critchley M, Greenfield JG, Meyer A. Discussion on the presenile dementias: symptomatology, pathology, and differential diagnosis. Proc R Soc Med 1937–1938;31:1443–1454.

Mayeux R, Hunter S, Fahn S. More on myoclonus in Alzheimer disease. Ann Neurol 1981a;9:200.

Mayeux R, Stern Y, Rosen J, Benson DF. Is "subcortical dementia" a recognizable clinical entity? Ann Neurol 1983;14:278–283.

Mayeux R, Stern Y, Rosen J, Leventhal J. Depression, intellectual impairment, and Parkinson disease. Neurol 1981b;31:645–650.

Mayeux R, Stern Y, Spanton S. Heterogeneity in dementia of the Alzheimer type: evidence of subgroups. Neurology 1985;35:453–461.

Mazurek MF, Beal MF, Bird ED, Martin JB. Vasopressin in Alzheimer's disease: a study of postmortem brain concentrations. Ann Neurol 1986a;20:665–670.

Mazurek MF, Beal MF, Martin JB. Neuropeptides in Alzheimer's disease. Neurol Clin 1986b;4:753–768.

Mazurek MF, Growdon JH, Beal MF, Martin JB. CFS vasopressin concentration is reduced in Alzheimer's disease. Neurology 1986c;36:1133–1137.

Mazziotta JC, Phelps ME, Pahl JJ, Huang S-C, Baxter LR, Riege WH, Hoffman JM, Kuhl DE, Lanto AB, Wapenski JA, Markham CH. Reduced cerebral glucose metabolism in asymptomatic subjects at risk for Huntington's disease. N Engl J Med 1987;316:357–362.

Meadows JC. The anatomical basis of prosopagnosia. J Neurol Neurosurg Psychiatry 1974;37:489–501.

Medalia A, Isaacs-Glaberman K, Scheimberg H. Neuropsychological impairment in Wilson's disease. Arch Neurol 1988;45:502–504.

Medalia A, Merriam A, Sandberg M. Neuropsychological deficits in choreoacantho-cytosis. Arch Neurol 1989;46:573–575.

Mehta PD, Kane A, Thormar H. Further characterization of bound measles-specific IgG eluted from SSPE brains. Ann Neurol 1978;3:552–555.

Meier MJ, Martin WE. Intellectual changes associated with levodopa therapy. JAMA 1970;213:465–466.

Melchior JC, Benda CE, Yakovlev PI. Familial idiopathic cerebral calcification in childhood. Am J Dis Child 1960;99:787–803.

Mena I. Manganese poisoning. In: Vinken PJ, Bruyn GW, eds. Intoxications of the nervous system. Part I, vol. 36. Handbook of clinical neurology. North-Holland, New York, 1979:217–237.

Mena I, Marin O, Fuenzalida S, Cotzias GC. Chronic manganese poisoning. Neurology 1967;17:128–136.

Mendell JR, Chase TN, Engel WK. Modification by L-dopa of a case of progressive supranuclear palsy. Lancet 1970;1:593–594.

Menkes, JH. Textbook of child neurology. Lea & Febiger, Philadelphia, 1974.

Menkes JH, Hanoch A. Huntington's disease—growth of fibroblast cultures in lipid-deficient medium: a preliminary report. Ann Neurol 1977;1:423–425.

Mensing JWA, Hoogland PH, Sloof JL. Computed tomography in the diagnosis of Wernicke's encephalopathy: a radiological-neuropathological correlation. Ann Neurol 1984;16:363–365.

Mercer B, Wagner W, Gardner H, Benson DF. A study of confabulation. Arch Neurol 1977;34:429–433.

Merriam AE, Aronson MK, Gaston P, Wey-S-L, Katz I. The psychiatric symptoms of Alzheimer's disease. J Am Geriatr Soc 1988;36:7–12.

Merritt HH, Springlova M. Lissauer's dementia paralytica. Arch Neurol Psychiatry 1932;27:987–1030.

Merritt HH, Weisman AD. Primary degeneration of the corpus callosum (Marchiafava-Bignami's disease). J Neuropathol Exp Neurol 1945;4:155–163.

Merskey, H. The analysis of hysteria. Bailliere Tindall, London, 1979.

Merskey H, Buhrich NA. Hysteria and organic brain disease. Br J Med Psychol 1975;48:359–366.

Messert B, Baker NH. Syndrome of progressive spastic ataxia and apraxia associated with occult hydrocephalus. Neurology 1966;16:440–452.

Messert B, Van Nuis C. A syndrome of paralysis of downward gaze, dysarthria, pseudobulbar palsy, axial rigidity of neck and trunk and dementia. J Nerv Ment Dis 1966;143:47–54.

Messert B, Wannamaker BB. Reappraisal of the adult hydrocephalus syndrome. Neurology 1974;24:224–231.

Messert B, Wannamaker BB, Dudley AW Jr. Reevaluation of the size of the lateral ventricles of the brain. Neurology 1972;22:941–951.

Metcalf DR, Holmes JH. EEG, psychological, and neurological alterations in humans with organophosphorus exposure. Ann NY Acad Sci 1969;160:357–365.

Mesulam M-M. Slowly progressive aphasia without generalized dementia. Ann Neurol 1982;11:592–598.

Metter EJ. Speech Disorders. Spectrum, New York, 1985.

Metter EJ, Mazziotta JC, Itabashi HH, Mankovich NJ, Phelps ME, Kuhl DE. Comparison of glucose metabolism, x-ray CT, and postmortem data in a patient with multiple cerebral infarcts. Neurology 1985;35:1695–1701.

Metzer WS, Angtuaco E. Long-term followup computed tomography and magnetic resonance imaging findings in hepatolenticular degeneration: case report and summary of the literature. Movement Disorders 1986;1:145–149.

Meyer A, Leigh D, Bagg CE. A rare presenile dementia associated with cortical blindness (Heidenhain's syndrome). J Neurol Neurosurg Psychiatry 1954;17:129–133.

Meyer JS, Barron DW. Apraxia of gait: a clinico-physiological study. Brain 1960; 83:261–284.

Meyer JS, Judd BW, Tawaklna T, Rogers RL, Mortel KF. Improved cognition after control of risk factors for multi-infarct dementia. JAMA 1986;256:2203–2209.

Meyer JS, McClintic KL, Rogers RL, Sims P, Mortel KF. Aetiological considerations and risk factors for multi-infarct dementia. J Neurol Neurosurg Psychiatry 1988a;51:1489–1497.

Meyer JS, Rogers RL, Judd BW, Mortel KF, Sims P. Cognition and cerebral blood flow fluctuate together in multi-infarct dementia. Stroke 1988b;19:163–169.

Meyer JS, Rogers RL, McClintic K, Mortel KF, Lofti J. Randomized clinical trial of daily aspirin therapy in multi-infarct dementia. J Am Geriatr Soc 1989;37:549–555.

Meyer JS, Welch KMA, Deshmukh VD, et al. Neurotransmitter precursor amino acids in the treatment of multi-infarct dementia and Alzheimer's disease. J Am Geriatr Soc 1977;25:289–298.

Micheli F, Pardal MF, Gatto M, Torres M, Paradiso G, Parera IC, Giannaula R. Flunarizine- and cinnarizine-induced extrapyramidal reactions. Neurology 1987;37:881–884.

Miller AE, Neighbor A, Katzman R, Aronson M, Lipkowitz R. Immunological studies in senile dementia of the Alzheimer type: evidence for enhanced suppressor cell activity. Ann Neurol 1981;10:506–510.

Miller BL, Benson DF, Goldberg MA, Gould R. The misdiagnosis of hysteria. Amer Fam Physician 1986a;34:157–160.

Miller BL, Benson DF, Cummings JL, Neshkes R. Late-life paraphrenia: an organic delusional syndrome. J Clin Psychiat 1986b;47:204–207.

Miller E. On the nature of the memory disorder in presenile dementia. Neuropsychology 1971;9:75–81.

Miller E. Efficiency of coding and the short-term memory defect in presenile dementia. Neuropsychology 1972;10:133–136.

Miller E, Hague F. Some characteristics of verbal behaviour in presenile dementia. Psychol Med 1975;5:255–259.

Miller E, Lewis P. Recognition memory in elderly patients with depression and dementia. J Abnorm Psychol 1977;86:84–86.

Miller EN, Selnes OA, McArthur JC, Satz P, Becker JT, Cohen BA, Sheridan K, Machado AM, Van Gorp WG, Visscher B. Neuropsychological performance in HIV-1-infected homosexual men: the multicenter AIDS cohort study (MACS). Neurology 1990;40:197–203.

Miller GA. The magical number seven, plus or minus two: some limits on our capacity for processing information. Psychological Review, 1956;63:81–97.

Miller H. Mental sequelae of head injury. Proc R Soc Med 1966;59:257–261.

Miller H, Stern G. The long-term prognosis of severe head injury. Lancet 1965;1:225–229.

Miller MD. Opportunities for psychotherapy in the management of dementia. J Geriatr Psychiatry Neurol 1989;2:11–17.

Miller WR. Psychological defeat in depression. Psychol Bull 1975;82:238–260.

Mindham RHS. Psychiatric symptoms in parkinsonism. J Neurol Neurosurg Psychiatry 1970;33:188–191.

Mindham RIIS, Marsden CD, Parkes JD. Psychiatric symptoms during L-dopa therapy for Parkinson's disease and their relationship to physical disability. Psychol Med 1976;6:23–33.

Minski L. The mental symptoms associated with 58 cases of cerebral tumour. J Neurol Psychopathol 1933;13:330–343.

Mintz G, Fraga A. Arteritis in systemic lupus erythematosus. Arch Intern Med 1965;116:55–66.

Miranda AF, Ishii S, DiMauro S, Shay JW. Cytochrome c oxidase deficiency in Leigh's syndrome: genetic evidence for a nuclear DNA-encoded mutation. Neurology 1989;39:697–702.

Miyajima H, Nishimura Y, Mizoguchi K, Sakamoto M, Shimizu T, Honda N. Familial apoceruloplasmin deficiency associated with blepharospasm and retinal degeneration. Neurology 1987;37:761–767.

Miyatake T, Atsumi T, Obayashi T, et al. Adult type neuronal storage disease with neuraminidase deficiency. Ann Neurol 1979;6:232–244.

Mizutani T, Okumura A, Oda M, Shiraki H. Panencephalopathic type of Creutzfeldt-Jakob disease: primary involvement of the cerebral white manner. J Neurol Neurosurg Psychiatry 1981;44:103–115.

Mohs RC, Breitner JCS, Silverman JM, Davis KL. Alzheimer's disease. Morbid risk among first-degree relatives approximates 50 percent by 90 years. Arch Gen Psychiatry 1987;44:405–408.

Mohs RC, Davis BM, Johns CA, Mathe AA, Greenwald BS, Horvath TB, Davis KL. Oral physostigmine treatment of patients with Alzheimer's disease. Am J Psychiatry 1985;142:28–33.

Molsa PA, Paljarvi L, Rinne JO, Rinne UK, Sako E. Validity of clinical diagnosis in dementia: a prospective clinicopathological study. J Neurol Neurosurg Psychiatry 1985;48:1085–1090.

Montamat SC, Susack BJ, Vestal RE. Management of drug therapy in the elderly. N Engl J Med 1989;321:303–309.

de la Monte SM. Disproportionate atrophy of cerebral white matter in chronic alcoholics. Arch Neurol 1988;45:990–992.

Monteiro MLR, Swanson RA, Coppeto JR, Cuneo RA, DeArmond SJ, Prusiner SB. A microangiopathic syndrome of encephalopathy, hearing loss, and retinal arteriolar occlusions. Neurology 1985;35:1113–1121.

Moore EW, Thomas LB, Shaw RK, Freireich EJ. The central nervous system in acute leukemia. Arch Intern Med 1960;105:451–488.

Moore GRW, Neumann PE, Suzuki K, Litjmaer HN, Traugott U, Raine CS. Balo's concentric sclerosis: new observations on lesion development. Ann Neurol 1985;17:604–611.

Moore MT. Progressive akinetic mutism in cerebellar hemangioblastoma with "normal pressure hydrocephalus." Neurology 1969;19:32–36.

Moore V, Wyke MA. Drawing disability in patients with senile dementia. Psychol Med 1984;14:97–105.

Morariu MA. Progressive supranuclear palsy and normal pressure hydrocephalus. Neurology 1979;29:1544–1546.

Morariu MA, Wilkins DE, Patel S. Multiple sclerosis and serial computerized tomography. Arch Neurol 1980;37:189–190.

Morgagni GB. The seats and causes of diseases investigated by anatomy. Alexander B, trans. A Millar & T Caddell, London, 1769.

Morgan JP, Rivera-Calimlim L, Messiha F, Sundaresau PR, Trabert N. Imipramine-mediated interference with levodopa absorption from the gastrointestinal tract in man. Neurology 1975;25:1029–1034.

Morgan MY, Jakobivits A, Elithorn A, James IM, Sherlock S. Successful use of bromocriptine in the treatment of a patient with chronic portoasystemic encephalopathy. N Engl J Med 1977;296:793–794.

Mori S, Hamada C, Kumanishi T, Fukuhara N, Ichihashi Y, Ikuta F, Miyatake T, Tsubaki T. A Creutzfeldt-Jakob disease agent (Echigo-1 strain) recovered from brain tissue showing the 'panencephalopathic type' disease. Neurology 1989;39:1337–1342.

Morimatsu M, Hirai S, Muramatsu A, Yoshikawa M. Senile degenerative brain lesions and dementia. J Am Geriatr Soc 1975;23:390–406.

Morishita L. Wandering behavior. In: Cummings JL, Miller BL, eds. Alzheimer's disease. Treatment and long-term management. Marcel Dekker, New York, 1990:157–176.

Morris JC, Cole M, Banker BQ, Wright D. Hereditary dysphasic dementia and the Pick-Alzheimer spectrum. Ann Neurol 1984;16:455–466.

Morris HH III, McCormick WF, Reinarz JA. Neuroleptic malignant syndrome. Arch Neurol 1980;37:462–463.

Mortell EJ. Idiopathic hypoparathyroidism with mental deterioration: effect of treatment on intellectual function. J Clin Endocrinol 1946;6:266–274.

Mortimer JA, Pirozzolo FJ, Hansch EC, Webster DD. Relationship of motor symptoms to intellectual deficits in Parkinson disease. Neurology 1982;32:133–137.

Mortimer JA, Schuman LM, French LR. Epidemiology of dementing illness. In: Mortimer JA, Schuman LM, eds. The epidemiology of dementia. Oxford University Press, New York, 1981:3–23.

Mosberg WH Jr, Arnold JG Jr. Torulosis of the central nervous sytem: review of the literature and report of five cases. Ann Intern Med 1950;32:1153–1183.

Moscovitch M, Moscovitch J, Crapper-Maclachlan D. Memory disorders in patients with Alzheimer's disease. Neurology 1981;31(4;2):62.

Moser HW, Moser AB, Kawamura N, et al. Adrenoleukodystrophy: elevated C26 fatty acid in cultured skin fibroblasts. Ann Neurol 1980;7:542–549.

Moser HW, Moser AE, Singh I, O'Neill BP. Adrenoleukodystrophy: survey of 303 cases: biochemistry, diagnosis, and therapy. Ann Neurol 1984a;16:628–641.

Moses AM, Miller M. Drug-induced dilutional hyponatremia. N Engl J Med 1974;291:1234–1238.

Mosher HW, Tutschka PJ, Brown FR III, Moser AE, Yeager Am, Singh I, Mark SA, Kumar AAJ, McDonnell JM, White CL III, Maumenee IH, Green WR, Powers JM, Santos GW. Bone marrow transplant in adrenoleukodystrophy. Neurology 1984b;34:1410–1417.

Moskowitz MA, Winickoff RN, Heinz ER. Familial calcification of the basal ganglions. N Engl J Med 1971;285:72–77.

Mozai T, Watanabe H, Yoshizawa K, et al. Abnormal copper metabolism and Kayser-Fleischer ring associated with schistosoma infection. Neurology 1962; 12:540–546.

Mueller J, Hotson Jr, Langston JW. Hyperviscosity-induced dementia. Neurology 1983;33:101–103.

Muenter MD, Whisnant JP. Basal ganglia calcification, hypoparathyroidism, and extrapyramidal motor manifestations. Neurology 1968;18:1075–1083.

Mukoyama M, Gimple K, Poser CM. Aspergillosis of the central nervous system. Neurology 1969;19:967–973.

Mulder DW, Pavrott M, Thaler M. Sequelae of western equine encephalitis. Neurology 1951;1:318–327.

Muller D, Pilz H, TerMeulen V. Studies on adult metachromatic leukodystrophy. l. Clinical, morphological and histochemical observations in two cases. J Neurol Sci 1969;9:567–584.

Mueller SP, Johnson KA, Hamil D, English RJ, Nagel SJ, Ichise M, Holman BL. Assessment of I-123 IMP SPECT in mild/moderate and severe Alzheimer's disease. J Nuc Med 1986;27:889 (Abstr.).

Munoz-Garcia D, Ludwin SK. Adult-onset neuronal intranuclear hyaline inclusion disease. Neurology 1986;36:785–790.

Munoz-Garcia D, Ludwin SK. Classic and generalized variants of Pick's disease: a clinicopathological, ultrastructural, and immunocytochemical comparative study. Ann Neurol 1984;16:467–480.

Mur J, Kumpel G, Dostal S. An anergic phase of disseminated sclerosis with psychotic course. Confin Neurol 1966;28:37–49.

Murayama S, Mori H, Ihara Y, Tomonaga M. Immunocytochemical and ultrastructural studies of Pick's disease. Ann Neurol 1990;27:394–405.

Murphy MJ, Goldstein MN. Diphenylhydantoin-induced asterixis. JAMA 1974; 229:538–540.

Murray RM, Greene JG, Adams JH. Analgesic abuse and dementia. Lancet 1971; 2:242–245.

Mutoh T, Sobue I, Naoi M, Matsuoka Y, Kiuchi K, Sugimura K. A family with beta-galactosidase deficiency: three adults with atypical clinical patterns. Neurology 1986;36:54–59.

Myers RH, Vonsattel JP, Stevens TJ, Cupples LA, Richardson EP, Martin JB, Bird

ED., Clinical and neuropathologic assessment of severity in Huntington's disease. Neurology 1988;38:341–347.

Myrianthopoulos NC. Huntington's chorea. J Med Genet 1966;3:298–314.

Myrianthopoulos NC, Smith JK. Amyotrophic lateral sclerosis with progressive dementia and with pathologic findings of Creutzfeldt-Jakob syndrome. Neurology 1962;12:603–610.

Nadel AM, Wilson WP. Dialysis encephalopathy: a possible seizure disorder. Neurology 1976;26:1130–1134.

Naef RW, Berry RG, Schlezinger NS. Neurologic aspects of porphyria. Neurology 1959;9:313–20.

Naeser MA, Albert MS, Kleefield J. New methods in the CT scan diagnosis of Alzheimer's disease: examination of white and gray matter mean CT density numbers. In: Corkin S, Davis KL, Growdon JH, Usdin E, Wurtman RJ, eds. Alzheimer's disease: a report of progress in research. Raven Press, New York, 1982:63–78.

Naeser MA, Gebhardt C, Levine HL. Decreased computerized tomography numbers in patients with presenile dementia. Arch Neurol 1980;37:401–409.

Nag TK, Falconer MA. Non-tumoral stenosis of the aqueduct in adults. Br Med J 1966;2:1168–1170.

Nagel JS, Johnson KA, Ichise M, English RJ, Walshe TM, Morris JH, Holman Bl. Decreased iodine-123 IMP caudate nucleus uptake in patients with Huntington's disease. Clin Nuclear Med 1988;13:486–490.

Nahor A, Benson DF. A screening test for organic brain disease in emergency psychiatric evaluation. Behav Psychiatry 1970;2:23–26.

Naito H, Oyanagi S. Familial myoclonus epilepsy and choreoathetosis: hereditary dentatorubral-pallidoluysian atrophy. Neurology 1982;32:798–807.

Nakano I, Hirano A. Neuron loss in the nucleus basalis of Meynert in parkinsonism-dementia complex of Guam. Ann Neurol 1983;13:87–91.

Nakano KK, Dawson DM, Spence A. Machado disease. Neurology 1972;22:49–55.

Nakano KK, Zubick H, Tyler HR. Speech defects in parkinsonian patients. Neurology 1973;23:865–870.

Namba T, Nolte CT, Jackrel J, Grob D. Poisoning due to organophosphate insecticides. Am J Med 1971;50:475–492.

Nandy, K. Brain-reactive antibodies in aging and senile dementia. In: Katzman R, Terry RD, Bick KL, eds. Alzheimer's disease: senile dementia and related disorders. Raven Press, New York, 1978:503–512.

Narayan O, Penney JB Jr, Johnson RT, Herndon RM, Weiner LP. Etiology of progressive multifocal leukoencephalopathy. N Engl J Med 1973;289:1278–1282.

Nardizzi LR. Computerized tomographic correlate of carbon monoxide poisoning. Arch Neurol 1979;36:38–39.

Nasrallah HA, McChesney CM. Psychopathology of corpus callosum tumors. Biol Psychiatry 1981;16:663–669.

Nasu T, Tsukahara Y, Terayama K. A lipid metabolic disease—"membranous lipodystrophy"—an autopsy case demonstrating numerous peculiar membrane structures composed of compound lipid in bone and bone marrow and various adipoid tissues. Acta Pathol Jpn 1973;23:539–558.

Nath A, Jankovic J, Petigrew LC. Movement disorders and AIDS. Neurology 1987;37:37–41.

Nausieda PA, Koller WC. Weiner WJ, Klawans HL. Chorea induced by oral contraceptives. Neurology 1979;29:1605–1609.

Nausieda PA, Weiner WJ, Klawans HL. Dystonic foot response in parkinsonism. Arch Neurol 1980;37:132–136.

Nauta WJH. The problem of the frontal lobe: a reinterpretation. J Psychiatr Res 1971;8:167–187.

Nauta WJH. A proposed conceptual reorganization of the basal ganglia and telencephalon. Neuroscience 1979;4:1875–1881.

Navia BA, Cho E-S, Petito CK, Price RW. The AIDS demetia complex: II. Neuropathology. Ann Neurol 1986a, 19:525–535.

Navia BA, Jordan BD, Price RW. The AIDS dementia complex: I. Clinical features. Ann Neurol 1986b;19:517–524.

Navia BA. AIDS dementia complex. In: Cummings JL, ed. Subcortical dementia Oxford University Press, New York, 1990.

Navon R, Argov Z, Brand N, Sandbank U. Adult GM_2 gangliosidosis in association with Tay-Sachs disease: a new phenotype. Neurology 1981;31:1397–1401.

Neary D, Snowden JS, Northen B, Goulding P. Dementia of frontal lobe type. J Neurol Neurosurg Psychiat 1988;51:353–361.

Neary D, Snowden JS, Shields RA, Burjan AW, Northen B, MacDermott N, Prescott MC, Tests HJ. Single photon emission tomography using 99m-Tc-HM-PAO in the investigation of dementia. J Neurol Neurosurg Psychiatry 1987;50:1101–1109.

Nee LE, Eldridge R, Sunderland T, Thomas CB, Katz D, Thompson KE, Weingartner H, Weiss H, Julian C, Cohen R. Dementia of the Alzheimer type: clinical and family study of 22 twin pairs. Neurology 1987;37:359–363.

Needleman HL, Gunnoe C, Leviton A, et al. Deficits in psychologic and classroom performance of children with elevated dentine lead levels. N Engl J Med 1979;300:689–695.

Neff IH. A report of 13 cases of ataxia in adults with hereditary history. Am J Insanity 1894–1895;51:365–373.

Nelson JS, Woolsey RM, Broun GO Jr. Cortical degeneration associated with myeloma and dementia. J Neuropathol Exp Neurol 1966;25:489–497.

Nelson RF, Guzman DA, Grahovac Z, Howse DCN. Computerized cranial tomography in Wilson disease. Neurology 1979;29:866–868.

Nelson RF, Pullicino P, Kendall BE, Marshall J. Computed tomography in patients presenting with lacunar syndromes. Stroke 1980;11:256–261.

Neophytides AN, DiChiro G, Barron SA, Chase TN. Computed axial tomography in Huntington's disease and persons at risk for Huntington's disease. Adv Neurol 1979;23:185–191.

Neophytides A, Lieberman AN, Goldstein M, et al. The use of lisuride, a potent dopamine and serotonin agonist, in the treatment of progressive supranuclear palsy. J Neurol Neurosurg Psychiatry 1982;45:261–263.

Neshige R, Barrett G, Shibaski H. Auditory long latency event-related potentials in Alzheimer's disease and multi-infarct dementia. J Neurol Neurosurg Psychiatry 1988;51:1120–1125.

Netsky MG. Degenerations of the cerebellum and its pathways. In: Mickler J, ed. Pathology of the nervous system. McGraw-Hill, New York, 1968:1163–1185.

Neubuerger KT. Lesions of the human brain following circulatory arrest. J Neuropathol Exp Neurol 1954;13:144–160.

Neufeld R, Inzelberg R, Korczyn AD. EEG in demented and non-demented parkinsonian patients. Acta Neurol Scand 1988;78:1–5.

Neumann MA. Chronic progressive subcortical encephalopathy—report of a case. J Gerontol 1947;2:57–64.

Neumann MA. Hemochromatosis of the central nervous system. J Neuropathol Exp Neurol 1948;7:19–34.

Neumann MA. Pick's disease. J Neuropathol Exp Neurol 1949;8:255–282.

Neumann MA. Combined amyloid vascular changes and argyrophilic plaques in the central nervous system. J Neuropathol Exp Neurol 1960;19:370–382.

Neumann MA. Iron and calcium dysmetabolism in the brain. J Neuropathol Exp Neurol 1963;22:148–163.

Neumann MA. Cholesterinosis of the basal ganglia associated with olivocerebellar atrophy in an adult. J Neuropathol Exp Neurol 1971;30:390–411.

Neumann MA, Cohn R. Incidence of Alzheimer's disease in a large mental hospital. Arch Neurol Psychiatry 1953;69:615–636.

Neumann MA, Cohn R. Progressive subcortical gliosis; a rare form of presenile dementia. Brain 1967;90:405–418.

Nevin S, McMenemey WH, Behrman S, Jones DP. Subacute spongiform encephalopathy—a subacute form of encephalopathy attributable to vascular dysfunction (spongiform cerebral atrophy). Brain 1960;83:519–563.

Newhouse PA, Sunderland T, Tariot PN, Mueller EA, Murphy DL, Coehn RM. Prolactin response to TRH in Alzheimer's disease and elderly controls. Biol Psychiatry 1986;21:963–967.

Newman GC. Treatment of progressive supranuclear palsy with tricyclic antidepressants. Neurology 1985;35:1189–1193.

Newman N, Gay AJ, Stroud MH, Brooks J. Defective rapid eye movements in progressive supranuclear palsy. Brain 1970;93:775–784.

Newman SE. The EEG manifestations of chronic ethanol abuse: relation to cerebral cortical atrophy. Ann Neurol 1978;3:299–304.

Nichols IC, Weigner WC. Pick's disease—a specific type of dementia. Brain 1938; 61:237–249.

Nickel SN, Frame B. Neurologic manifestations of myxedema. Neurology 1958;8:511–517.

Nickerson, M. Drugs inhibiting adrenergic nerves and structures innervated by them. In: Goodman LS, Gilman A, eds. The pharmacological basis of therapeutics. 4th ed. Macmillan, New York, 1970:549–584.

Nicklowitz WJ. Neurofibrillary changes after acute experimental lead poisoning. Neurology 1975;25:927–934.

Nielsen J. Geronto-psychiatric period-prevalence investigation in a geographically delimited population. Acta Psychiatr Scand 1962;38:307–330.

Nielsen SL. Davis RL. Neuropathology of acquired immunodeficiency syndrome. In: Rosenblum ML, Levy RM, Bredesen DE, eds. AIDS and the nervous system. Raven Press, New York, 1988:155–181.

Nightingale S, Mitchell KW, Howe JW. Visual evoked cortical potentials and pattern electroretinograms in Parkinson's disease and control subjects. J Neurol Neurosurg Psychiatry 1986;49:1280–1287.

Nikaido T, Austin J, Trueb L, Rinehart R. Studies in aging of the brain. II. Microchemical analyses of the nervous system in Alzheimer patients. Arch Neurol 1972;27:549–554.

Nino HE, Noreen HJ, Dubey DP, et al. A family with hereditary ataxia: HLA typing. Neurology 1980;30:12–30.

Nishimura RN, Barranger JA. Neurologic complications of Gaucher's disease, type 3. Arch Neurol 1980;37:92–93.

Noad KB, Lance JW. Familial myoclonic epilepsy and its association with cerebellar disturbance. Brain 1960;83:618–629.

Nobuyoshi I, Nishihara Y. Pellagra among chronic alcoholics: clinical and pathological study of 20 necropsy cases. J. Neurol Neurosurg Psychiatry 1981;44:209–215.

Norberg A, Melin E, Asplund K. Reactions to music, touch and object presentation in the final stage of dementia. An exploratory study. Int J Nurs Stud 1986;23:315–323.

Norbiato G, Bevilacqua M, Carella F, Chebat E, Raggi U, Bertora P, Grassi MP, Mangoni A. Alterations in vasopressin regulation in Alzheimer's disease. J Neurol Neurosurg Psychiatry 1988;51:903–908.

Noriega-Sanchez A, Martinez-Maldonado M. Haiffe RM. Clinical and electroencephalographic changes in progressive uremic encephalopathy. Neurology 1978;28:667–669.

Norman DD, Miller ZR. Coccidioidomycosis of the central nervous system. Neurology 1954;4:713–717.

Noronha ABC, Roos RP, Antel JP, Arnason BGW. Huntington's disease: abnormality of lymphocyte capping. Ann Neurol 1979;6:447–450.

Norrell H, Wilson CB, Slagel DE, Clark DB. Leukoencephalopathy following the administration of methotrexate into the cerebrospinal fluid in the treatment of primary brain tumors. Cancer 1974;33:923–932.

Norris JR, Chandrasekar S. Anoxic brain damage after cardiac resuscitation. J Chron Dis 1971;24:585–590.

Nott PN, Fleminger JJ, Presenile dementia: the difficulties of early diagnosis. Acta Psychiatr Scand 1975;51:210–217.

Novak DJ, Victor M. The vagus and sympathetic nerves in alcoholic polyneuropathy. Arch Neurol 1974;30:273–284.

Nugent GR, AL-Meffy D, Chou S. Communicating hydrocephalus as a cause of aqueductal stenosis. J Neurosurg. 1979;51:812–818.

Nurick S, Blackwood W, Mair WGP. Giant cell granulomatous angiitis of the central nervous system. Brain 1972;95:133–142.

Nutt JG, Gillespie MM, Chase TN. Treatment of Huntington's disease with alpha- and beta-adrenergic antagonists. Adv Neurol 1979;23:777–784.

Nutt JG, Rosin A, Chase TN. Treatment of Huntington disease with a cholinergic agonist. Neurol 1978a;28:1061–1064.

Nutt JG, Rosin AJ, Eisler T, Calne DB, Chase TN. Effect of an opiate antagonist on movement disorders. Arch Neurol 1978b;35:810–811.

Nutting PA, Cole BR, Schimke RN. Benign, recessively inherited choreoathetosis of early onset. J Med Genet 1969;6:408–410.

Nyback H, Nyman H, Ohman G, Nordgren I, Lindstrom B. Preliminary experiences and results with THA for the amelioration of symptoms of Alzheimer's disease. In: Giacobini E. Becker R, eds. Current research in Alzheimer therapy. Cholinesterase inhibitors. Taylor and Francis, New York, 1988;231–236.

Oberg RGE, Divac I. "Cognitive" functions of the neostriatum. In: Divac I, Oberg RGE, eds. The neostriatum. Pergamon Press, New York, 1979:291–313.

Obler LK. Narrative discourse in the elderly. In: Obler LK, Albert ML, eds. Language and communication in the elderly. D.C. Heath, Lexington, Mass, 1980.

Obler LK, Cummings JL, Albert ML. Subcortical dementia: speech and language functions. Am Geriatr Soc, Washington, D.C., 1979.

Oblu N. Gumma of the brain. In: Vinken PJ, Bruyn GW, eds. Tumors of the brain and skull. Part III, vol. 18, Handbook of clinical neurology. North-Holland, New York, 1975;427–434.

O'Brien MD. Vascular disease and dementia in the elderly. In: Smith WL. Kinsbourne M, eds. Aging and dementia. Spectrum, New York, 1977:77–90.

Obrist WD, Chivian E, Cronquist S, Ingvar DH. Regional cerebral blood flow in senile and presenile dementia. Neurology 1970;20:315–322.

O'Connor JF, Musher DM. Central nervous system involvement in systemic lupus erythematosus. Arch Neurol 1966;14:157–164.

Odell, WD. Humoral manifestations of nonendocrine neoplasms. In: Williams RH, ed. Textbook of endocrinology. 4th ed. WB Saunders, Philadelphia, 1968:1211–1222.

Odell WD, Wolfsen AR. Humoral syndromes associated with cancer. Ann Rev Med 1978;29:379–406.

O'Donnell VM, Pitts WM, Fann WE. Noradrenergic and cholinergic agents in Korsakoff's syndrome. Clin Neuropharm 1986;9:65–70.

Office of Technology Assessment Task Force. Confronting Alzheimer's disease and other dementias. JB Lippincott Company, Philadelphia, 1988.

Offner H, Konat G, Clausen J. A blood test for multiple sclerosis. N Engl J Med 1977;296:451–452.

Ohta K, Tsuji S, Mizuno Y, Atsumi T, Yahagi T, Miyatake T. Type 3 (adult) GM1 gangliosidosis: case report. Neurology 1985;35:1490–1494.

Ojemann RG, Fisher CM, Adams RD, Sweet WH, New PFJ. Further experience with the syndrome of "normal" pressure hydrocephalus. J Neurosurg 1969; 31:279–294.

Okazaki H, Reagan TJ, Campbell RJ. Clinicopathalogic studies of primary cerebral amyloid angiopathy. Mayo Clin Proc 1979;54:22–31.

Okinaka S, Yoshikawa M, Mozai T, et al. Encephalomyelopathy due to an organic mercury compound. Neurology 1964;14:69–76.

Okuma T, Kishimoto A, Inoue K, et al. Anti-manic and prophylactic effects of carbamazepine (Tegretol) on manic depressive psychosis. Folia Psychiatr Neurol Jpn 1973;27:283–297.

Oldendorf WH. The quest for an image of the brain. Raven Press, New York, 1980.

O'Leary MR, Radford LM, Chaney EF, Schau EJ. Assessment of cognitive recovery in alcoholics by use of the trail-making test. J Clin Psychol 1977;33:579–582.

Olivarius BdeF, Roder E. Reversible psychosis and dementia in myxedema. Acta Psychiatr Scand 1970;46:1–13.

Oliver J, Dewhurst K. Childhood and adolescent forms of Huntington's disease. J Neurol Neurosurg Psychiatry 1969;32:455–459.

Oliveros JC, Jandali MK, Timsit-Berthier M, et al. Vasopressin in amnesia. Lancet 1978;1:42.

Olmos-Lau N, Ginsberg MD, Geller JB. Aphasia in multiple sclerosis. Neurology 1977;27:623–626.

Olsen PZ, Stoier M, Sierksbaek-Nielson K, Hansen JM, Shioler M, Kristensen M. Electroencephalographic findings in hyperthyroidism. Electroencephalogr Clin Neurophysiol 1972;32:171–177.

Olson MI, Shaw C-M. Presenile dementia and Alzheimer's disease in mongolism. Brain 1969;92:147–156.

Olsson Y, Sourander P. The reliability of the diagnosis of metachromatic leukodystrophy by peripheral nerve biopsy. Acta Pediatr Scand 1969;58:15–24.

Olszewski J. Subcortical arteriosclerotic encephalopathy. World Neurol 1962;3:359–375.

O'Neill B, Butler AB, Young E, Falk PM, Bass NH. Adult-onset GM$_2$ gangliosidosis. Neurology 1978;28:1117–1123.

O'Neill BP, Moser HW, Marmion LC. Adrenoleukodystrophy: elevated C26 fatty acid in cultured skin fibroblasts and correlation with disease expression in three generations of a kindred. Neurology 1982;32:540–542.

Oppenheimer DR. Demyelinating disease. In: Blackwood W, Corsellis JAN, eds. Greenfield's neuropathology. Year Book Medical Publishers, Chicago, 1976a:470–499.

Oppenheimer DR. Diseases of the basal ganglia, cerebellum, and motor neurons. In: Blackwood W, Corsellis JAN, eds. Greenfield's neuropathology. Year Book Medical Publishers, Chicago, 1976b:608–651.

Oppler W. Manic psychosis in a case of parasagittal meningioma. Arch Neurol Psychiatry 1950;64:417–430.

O'Reilly S. Problems in Wilson's disease. Neurology 1967;17:137–146.

Osetowska E, Torck P. Subacute sclerosing leukoencephalitis. World Neurol 1962;3:566–578.

Ostuni E, Pietro MJS. Getting through: communicating when someone you care for has Alzheimer's disease. The Speech Bin, Plainsboro, N.J., 1986.

Ouslander JG. Drug therapy in the elderly. Ann Int Med 1981;95:711–722.

Ouslander JG. Incontinence. In: Cummings JL, Miller BL, eds. Alzheimer's disease. Treatment and long-term management. Marcel Dekker, New York, 1990;177–206.

Overman W Jr. Stoudemire A. Guidelines for legal and financial counseling of Alzheimer's disease patients and their families. Am J Psychiatry 1988;145:1495–1500.

Owens D, Dawson JC, Losin S. Alzheimer's disease in Down's syndrome. Am J Ment Defic 1971;75:600–612.

Packer RJ, Cornblath DR, Gonatas NK, Bruno LA, Ashbury AK. Creutzfeldt-Jakob disease in a 20-year-old woman. Neurology 1980;30:492–496.

Page RD, Linden JD, "Reversible" organic brain syndrome in alcoholics. J Stud Alcohol 1974;35:98–107.

Pallis CA, Fudge BJ. The neurological complications of Behçet's syndrome. Arch Neurol Psychiatry 1956;75:1–14.

Pallis CA, Lewis PD. The neurology of gastrointestinal disease. WB Saunders, Philadelphia, 1974.

Palmer A, Sims NR, Dowen DM, Neary D, Palo J, Wikstron J, Davison AN. Monoamine metabolite concentrations in lumbar cerebrospinal fluid of patients with histologically verified Alzheimer's disease. J Neurol Neurosurg Psychiatry 1984;467:481–484.

Palmer AM, Francis PT, Bowen DM, Benton JS, Neary D, Mann DMA, Snowden JS. Catecholaminergic neurones assessed ante-mortem in Alzheimer's disease. Brain Res 1987;414:365–375.

Pan GD, Stern Y, Sano M, Mayeux R. Clock-drawing in neurological disorders. Behav Neurol 1989;2:39–48.

Panella JJ Jr, Lilliston BA, Bruch D, McDowell FH. Day care for dementia patients: an analysis of a four-year program. J Am Geriatr Soc 1984;32:883–886.

Panitch HS, Gomez-Plascencia J, Norris FH, Cantell K, Smith RA. Subacute sclerosing panencephalitis: remission after treatment with intraventricular interferon. Neurology 1986;36:562–566.

Pant SS, Asbury AK, Richardson EP Jr. The myelopathy of pernicious anemia. Acta Neurol Scand 1968;44 (suppl 35):8–36.

Paone JF, Jeyasingham K. Remission of cerebellar dysfunction after pneumonectomy for bronchogenic carcinoma. N Engl J Med 1980;302:156.

Park BE, Netsky MG, Betsill WL Jr. Pathogenesis of pigment and spheroid formation in Hallervorden-Spatz syndrome and related disorders. Neurology 1975;25:1172–1178.

Parker HL, Kernohan JW. Parenchymatous cortical cerebellar atrophy (chronic atrophy of Purkinje's cells). Brain 1933;56:191–212.

Parkes JD, Marsden CD, Rees JE, et al. Parkinson's disease, cerebral arteriosclerosis, and senile dementia. Q J Med 1974;43:49–61.

Parkinson Study Group. Effect of deprenyl on the progression of disability in early Parkinson's disease. N Engl J Med 1989;321:1364–1371.

Parr D. Diagnostic problems in pre-senile dementia illustrated by a case of Alzheimer's disease proven histologically during life. J Ment Sci 1955;101:387–390.

Parrillo OJ, Meiberger M, Elston H. Candida meningitis complicating Hodgkin's disease. JAMA 1962;182:189–191.

Parry SW, Schuhmacher JF, Llewellyn RC. Abdominal pseudocysts and ascites formation after ventriculoperitoneal shunt procedures. J Neurosurg 1975;43:476–480.

Pascuzzi RM, Roos KL, Davis TE Jr. Mental status abnormalities in temporal arteritis: a treatable cause of dementia in the elderly. Arth Rhem 1989;32:1308–1311.

Passer JA. Cerebral atrophy in end-stage uremia. Proc Dialysis Transplant Forum 1977;7:91–94.

Patel CD, Matloub H. Vaginal perforation as a complication of ventriculoperitoneal shunt. J Neurosurg 1973;38:761–762.

Patrick H. Hereditary cerebellar ataxia, with report of a case. J Nerv Ment Dis 1902;29:129–152.

Pattison EM. Uveomeningoencephalitic syndrome (Vogt-Koyanagi-Harada). Arch Neurol 1965;12:197–205.

Paulley JW, Hughes JP. Giant-cell arteritis, or arteritis of the aged. Br Med J 1960;2:1562–1567.

Paulson, GW. The neurological examination in dementia. In: Wells CE, ed. Dementia. 2nd ed. FA Davis, Philadelphia, 1977:169–188.

Paulson GW, Boesel CP, Evans WE. Fibromuscular dysplasia. Arch Neurol 1978;35:287–290.

Paulson GW, Kapp J, Cook W. Dementia associated with bilateral carotid artery disease. Geriatrics 1966;21:159–166.

Pavlakis SG, Rowland LP, De Vivo DC, Bonilla E, DiMauro S. Mitochondrial myopathies and encephalomyopathies. In: Plum F, ed. Advances in contemporary neurology. FA Davis Company, Philadelphia, 1988;95–133.

Payne CE, Brains of boxers. Neurochirurgia 1968;11:173–188.

Pearce I, Heathfield KWG, Pearce JMS. Valproate sodium in Huntington chorea. Arch Neurol 1977;34:308–309.

Pearlman RL, Towfighi J, Pezeshkpour GH, Tenser RB, Turel AP. Clinical significance of types of cerebellar amyloid plaques in human spongiform encephalopathies. Neurology 1988;38:1249–1254.

Pearlson GD, Rabins PV, Kim WS, Speedie LJ, Moberg PJ, Burns A, Bascom MJ. Structural brain CT changes and cognitive deficits in elderly depressive with and without reversible dementia ('pseudodementia'). Psychol Med 1989;19:573–584.

Penalver R. Manganese poisoning. Ind Med Surg 1955;24:1–7.

Penn RD, Martin EM, Wilson RS, Foc JH, Savoy SM. Intraventricular bethanechol infusion for Alzheimer's disease: results of double-blind and escalating-dose trials. Neurology 1988;38:219–222.

Penttila M, Partanen JV, Soininen H, Riekkinen PJ. Quantitative analysis of occipital EEG in different stages of Alzheimer's disease. EEG Clin Neurophysiol 1985;60:1–6.

Percy AK, Kaback MM. Infantile and adult-onset metachromatic leukodystrophy. N Engl J Med 1971;285:785–787.

Percy AK, Kaback MM, Herndon RM. Metachromatic leukodystrophy: comparison of early- and late-onset forms. Neurology 1977;27:933–941.

Percy AK, Nobrega FT. Kurland LT. Optic neuritis and multiple sclerosis. Arch Ophthalmol 1972;87:135–139.

Perdices M, Cooper DA. Simple and choice reaction time in patients with human immunodeficiency virus infection. Ann Neurol 1989;25:460–467.

Peress NS, DiMauro S, Roxburgh VA. Adult polysaccharidosis. Arch Neurol 1979;36:840–845.

Perez FI, Rivera VM, Meyer JS, Gay JRA, Taylor RL, Mather NT. Analysis of intellectual and cognitive performance in patients with multi-infarct dementia, vertebro-basilar insufficiency with dementia and Alzheimer's disease. J Neurol Neurosurg Psychiatry 1975;38:533–540.

Perl DP, Brody AR. Alzheimer's disease: X-ray spectrometric evidence of aluminum accumulation in neurofibrillary tangle-bearing neurons. Science 1980;208:297–299.

Perlmutter I, Gobles C. Subdural hematoma in older patients. JAMA 1961;176:212–214.

Perlstein MA, Attala R. Neurologic sequelae of plumbism in children. Clin Pediatr 1966;5:292–298.

Perry EK, Perry RH, Blessed G, Tomlinson BE. Necropsy evidence of central cholinergic deficits in senile dementia. Lancet 1977;1:189.

Perry EK, Tomlinson BE, Blessed G, Gergmann K, Gibson PH, Perry RH. Correlation of cholinergic abnormalities with senile plaques and mental test scores in senile dementia. Br Med J 1978;2:1457–1459.

Perry S, Belsky-Barr D, Barr WB, Jacobsberg L. Neuropsychological function in physically asymptomatic, HIV-seropositive men. J Neuropsychiatr Clin Neurosci 1989;1:296–302.

Perry TL, Bratty PJA, Hansen S, Kennedy J, Urguhart N, Dolman CL. Hereditary mental depression and parkinsonism with taurine deficiency. Arch Neurol 1975;32:108–113.

Perry TL, Hansen S, Jones K. Brain amino acids and glutathione in progressive supranuclear palsy. Neurology 1988;38:943–946.

Perry TL, Hansen S, Kloster M. Huntington's chorea. Deficiency of gamma-aminobutyric acid in brain. N Engl J Med 1973;288:337–342.

Perry TL, Wright JM, Hansen S, MacLeod PM. Isoniazid therapy of Huntington disease. Neurology 1979;29:370–375.

Perry TL, Norman MG, Yong VW, Whiting S, Crichton JU, Hansen S, Kish SJ. Hallervorden-Spatz disease: cysteine accumulation and cysteine dioxygenase deficiency in the globus pallidus. Ann Neurol 1985;18:482–489.

Perry TL. Wright JM, Hansen S, et al. A double-blind clinical trial of isoniazid in Huntington disease. Neurology 1982;32:354–358.

Peters A, Palay SL, Webster HdeF. The fine structure of the nervous system: the neurons and supporting cells. WB Saunders, Philadelphia, 1976;96–102.

Peters BH, Levin HS. Effects of physostigmine and lecithin on memory in Alzheimer disease. Ann Neurol 1979;6:219–221.

Peterson HdeC, Swanson AG. Acute encephalopathy occurring during hemodialysis. Arch Intern Med 1964;113:877–880.

Peterson I, Hambert O. Clinical and electroencephalographic studies of responses to lidocaine and chlormethiazole in progressive myoclonus epilepsy. Act Psychiatr Scand 1966;42(suppl 192):45–64.

Peterson P. Psychiatric disorders in primary hyperparathyroidism. J Clin Endocrinol Metabol 1968;28:1491–1495.

Peterson PL, Saad J, Nigro MA. The treatment of Friedreich's ataxia with amantadine hydrochloride. Neurology 1988;38:1478–1480.

Petito CK, Gottlieb GJ, Dougherty JH, Petito FA. Neoplastic angioendotheliosis: ultrastructural study and review of the literature. Ann Neurol 1978;3:393–399.

Petrie WM, Maffucci RJ, Woosley RL. Propranolol and depression. Am J Psychiatry 1982;139:92–94.

Petry S, Cummings JL, Hill MA, Shapira J. Personality alterations in dementia of the Alzheimer type. Arch Neurol 1988,45:1187–1190.

Petry S, Cummings JL, Hill MA, Shapira J. Personality alterations in dementia of the Alzheimer type: a three-year follow-up study. J Geriatr Psychiatry Neurol 1989;2:203–207.

Pettegrew JW, Nichols JS, Stewart RM. Membrane studies in Huntington's disease:

steady-state fluorescence studies of intact erythrocytes. Ann Neurol 1980;8:381–386.

Peyser JM, Edwards KR, Poser CM, Filskov SB. Cognitive function in patients with multiple sclerosis. Arch Neurol 1980;37:577–579.

Plaffenbach DD, Layton DD Jr, Kearns TP. Ocular manifestations in progressive supranuclear palsy. Am J Ophthalmol 1972;74:1179–1184.

Pfeiffer JAF. A case of hereditary ataxia (Friedreich) with anatomic findings. Arch Neurol Psychiatry 1922;7:341–348.

Pfeffer RI, Afifi AA, Chance JM. Prevalence of Alzheimer's disease in a retirement community. Am J Epidemiology 1987;125:420–436.

Phelps ME. Emission computed tomography. Semin Nucl Med 1977;7:337–365.

Phelps ME, Hoffman EJ, Huang SC, Kuhl DE. ECAT: a new computerized imaging system for positron-emitting radiopharmaceuticals. J Nucl Med 1978;19:635–647.

Phelps ME, Huang SC, Hoffman EJ, Selin C, Sokoloff L, Kuhl DE. Tomographic measurement of local cerebral glucose metabolism in humans with (F-18)2-fluoro-2-deoxy-D-glucose: validation of method. Ann Neurol 1979;6:371–388.

Pick A. On the relation between aphasia and senile atrophy of the brain (1892). In: Rottenberg DA, Hochberg FH, eds. (Schoene WC, trans.) Neurological classics in modern translation. Hafner Press, New York, 1977:35–40.

Piercy M, Smyth VOG. Right hemisphere dominance for certain non-verbal intellectual skills. Brain 1962;85:775–790.

Pierides AM, Ward MK, Kerr DNS. Haemodialysis encephalopathy: possible role of phosphate depletion. Lancet 1976;1:1234–1235.

Pierot L, Desnos C, Blin J, Raisman R, Scherman D, Javoy-Agid F, Ruberg M, Agid Y. D_1 and D_2-type dopamine receptors in patients with Parkinson's disease and progressive supranuclear palsy. J Neurol Sci 1988;86:291–306.

Pilleri G. A case of morbus Fahr (nonarteriosclerotic, idiopathic intracerebral calcification of the blood vessels) in three generations. Psychiatr Neurol Basel 1966;152:43–58.

Pilleri G. The Klüver-Bucy syndrome in man. Psychiatr Neurol Basel 1966;152:65–103.

Pincus JH, Chutorian A. Familial benign chorea with intention tremor: a clinical entity. J Pediatr 1967;70:724–729.

Pincus JH, Reynolds EH, Glaser GH. Subacute combined system degeneration with folate deficiency. JAMA 1972;221:496–497.

Pillon B, Dubois B, Lhermitte F, Agid Y. Heterogeneity of cognitive impairment in progressive supranuclear palsy, Parkinson's disease, and Alzheimer's disease. Neurology 1986;36:1179–1185.

Pinkston EM, Linsk NL, Young RN. Home-based behavioral family treatment of the impaired elderly. Behav Therapy 1988;19:331–344.

Pirozzolo FJ, Hansch EC, Mortimer JA, Webster DA, Kuskowski MA. Dementia in Parkinson's disease: a neuropsychological analysis. Brain Cognit 1982;1:71–83.

Pizzolato G, Borsato N, Saitta B, Da Col C, Perlotto N, Zanco P, Ferlin G, Battistin L. [99mTc]-HM-PAO SPECT in Parkinson's disease. J Cereb Blood Flow Metab 1988;8:S101–S108.

Plaitakis A, Nicklas WJ, Desnick RJ. Glutamate dehydrogenase deficiency in three patients with spinocerebellar syndrome. Ann Neurol 1980;7:297–303.

Plato CC, Garruto RM, Fox KM, Gajdusek DC. Amyotrophic lateral sclerosis and parkinsonism-dementia on Guam: a 25-year prospective case-control study. Am J Epidemiol 1986;124:643–656.

Platts MM, Moorhead PJ, Grech P. Dialysis dementia. Lancet 1973;2:159.

Plum F. Dementia: an approaching epidemic. Nature 1979;279:372–373.

Plum F, Posner JB, Hain RF. Delayed neurological deterioration after anoxia. Arch Intern Med 1962;110:18–25.

Podoll K, Caspary P, Lange HW, Noth J. Language functions in Huntington's disease. Brain 1988;111:1475–1503.

Poeck, K. Pathophysiology of emotional disorders associated with brain damage. In: Vinken PJ, Bruyn GW, eds. Disorders of higher nervous activity. Vol 3. Handbook of clinical neurology. American Elsevier, New York, 1969:343–367.

Poeck K, Luzzatti C. Slowly progressive aphasia in three patients. Brain 1988;111:151–168.

Polatin P, Hoch PH, Horwitz WA, Roizin L. Presenile psychosis. Am J Psychiatry 1948;105:96–101.

Pollay M. CSF formation and mechanism of change. In: Harbert JC ed. Cisternography and hydrocephalus. Charles C Thomas, Springfield, Ill., 1972:13–24.

Pollock M, Hornabrook RW. The prevalence, natural history and dementia of Parkinson's disease. Brain 1966;89:429–488.

Pomara N, Oxenkrug GF, McIntyre IM, Block R, Stanley M, Gershon S. Does severity of dementia modulate response to dexamethasone in individuals with primary degenerative dementia? Biol Psychiatry 1984;19:1481–1487.

Pons VG, Jacobs RA, Hollander H. Nonviral infections of the central nervous system in patients with acquired immunodeficiency syndrome. In: Rosenblum ML, Levy RM, Bredesen DE, eds. AIDS and the nervous system. Raven Press, New York, 1988:263–283.

Popoff N, Weinberg S, Feigin I. Pathologic observations in lead encephalopathy. Neurology 1963;13:101–112.

Portnoy HD, Croissant PD. Two unusual complications of a ventriculoperitoneal shunt. J Neurosurg 1973;39:775–776.

Poser CM. Diffuse-disseminated sclerosis in the adult. J Neuropathol Exp Neurol 1957;16:61–78.

Poser CM. Diseases of the myelin sheath. In: Baker AB, Baker LH, eds. Clinical neurology. Harper & Row, New York, 1978:1–188.

Posmer TB. Paraneoplastic syndromes involving the nervous system. In: Aminoff MT, ed, Neurology and general medicine. Churchill Livingstone, New York, 1989;341–364.

Powell AL, Cummings JL, Hill MA, Benson DF. Speech and language alterations in multi-infarct dementia. Neurology 1988;38:717–719.

Powell HC, London GW, Lampert PW. Neurofibrillary tangles in progressive supranuclear palsy. J Neuropathol Exp Neurol 1974;33:98–106.

Powell HC, Tindall R, Schultz P, Paa D, O'Brien J, Lampert P. Adrenoleukodystrophy. Arch Neurol 1975;32:250–260.

Powers JM, Schaumburg HH. Adreno-leukodystrophy. Arch Neurol 1974;30:406–408.

Powers JM, Schaumburg HH, Gaffney CL. Klüver-Bucy syndrome caused by adrenoleukodystrophy. Neurology 1980;30:1231–1232.

Pratt RTC. The genetics of Alzheimer's disease. In: Wolstenholme GEW, O'Connor M, eds. Alzheimer's disease and related conditions. J & A Churchill, London, 1970:137–139.

Preston FE, Malia RG, Sworn MJ, Timperley WR, Blackburn EK, Disseminated intravascular coagulation as a consequence of cerebral damage. J Neurol Neurosurg Psychiatry 1974;37:241–248.

Prevey ML, Mattson RH, Cramer JA. Improvement in cognitive functioning and mood state after conversion to valproate monotherapy. Neurology 1989;39:1640–1641.

Price RW, Brew B, Sidtis J, Rosenblum M, Scheck AC, Cleary P. The brain in AIDS: central nervous system HIV-1 infection and AIDS dementia complex. Science 1988a;239:586–592.

Price RW, Sidtis JJ, Navia BA, Pumarola-Sune T, Ornitz DB. The AIDS dementia complex. In: Rosenblum ML, Levy RM, Bredesen DE, eds. AIDS and the nervous system. Raven Press, New York, 1988b:203–219.

Price TRP, Tucker GJ. Psychiatric and behavioral manifestations of normal pressure hydrocephalus. J Nerv Ment Dis 1977;164:51–55.

Prick JJG. Thallium poisoning. In: Vinken PJ, Bruyn GW, eds. Intoxications of the nervous system. Part I, vol. 36. Handbook of clinical neurology. North-Holland, New York, 1979:239–278.

Prinz PN, Reskind ER, Vitaliano PP, et al. Changes in the sleep and waking EEG's of nondemented and demented elderly subjects. J Am Geriatr Soc 1982;20:86–93.

Pro JD, Smith CH, Sumi SM. Presenile Alzheimer disease: amyloid plaques in the cerebellum. Neurology 1980;30:832–835.

Pro JD, Wells CE. The use of the electroencephalogram in the diagnosis of delirium. Dis Nerv Sys 1977;38:804–808.

Prockop L. Neurotoxic volatile substances. Neurology 1979;29:862–865.

Prohovnik I, Mayeux R, Sackeim HA, Smith G, Stern Y, Alderson PO. Cerebral perfusion as a diagnostic marker of early Alzheimer's disease. Neurology 1988;38:931–937.

Pruchno RA, Potashnik SL. Caregiving spouses. J Am Geriatr Soc 1989;37:697–705.

Prull G, Rompel K. EEG changes in acute poisoning with organic tin compounds. Electroencephalogr Clin Neurophysiol 1970;29:215.

Prusiner SB. Prions and neurodegenerative diseases. N Engl J Med 1987;317:1571–1581.

Pullicino P, Nelson RF, Kendall BE, Marshall J. Small deep infarcts diagnosed on computed tomography. Neurology 1980;30:1090–1096.

Pulsinelli WA, Hamill RW. Chorea complicating oral contraceptive therapy. Am J Med 1978;65:557–559.

Purdie FR, Honigman B, Rosen P. Acute organic brain syndrome: a review of 100 cases. Ann Emerg Med 1981;10:455–461.

Quadfasel AF, Pruyser PW. Cognitive deficit in patients with psychomotor epilepsy. Epilepsia 1955;4:80–90.

Rabins PV. The prevalence of reversible dementia in a psychiatric hospital. Hosp Community Psychiatry 1981;32:490–492.

Rabins PV. Establishing Alzheimer's disease units in nursing homes: pros and cons. Hosp Commun Psychiatry 1986;37:120–121.

Rabins PV. Family-directed therapy. In: Cummings JL, Miller BL, eds. Alzheimer's disease. Treatment and long-term management. Marcel Dekker, New York, 1990:225–233.

Rabins PV, Folstein MF. Delirium and dementia: diagnostic criteria and fatality rates. Br J Psychiatry 1982;140:149–153.

Rabins PV, Mace NL, Lucas MJ. The impact of dementia on the family. JAMA 1982;248:333–335.

Rabins PV, Merchant A, Nestedt G. Criteria for diagnosing reversible dementia caused by depression: validation by 2-year follow-up. Br J Psychiatry 1984; 144:488–492.

Rafal RD, Grimm RJ. Progressive supranuclear palsy: functional analysis of the response to methysergide and antiparkinsonian agents. Neurology 1981;31:1507–1518.

Rahman AN, Lindenberg R. The neuropathology of hereditary dystopic lipidosis. Arch Neurol 1963;9:373–385.

Rainero I, Kay JA, Freidland RP, Rapoport SI. CSG alpha-MSH in dementia of the Alzheimer type. Neurology 1988;38:1281–1284.

Rajjoub RK, Wood JH, Ommaya AK. Granulomatous angiitis of the brain: a successfully treated case. Neurology 1977;27:588–591.

Rall DP, Tower DB. Environmental hazards and neurological disease. Ann Neurol 1977;1:209–210.

Ramani PS. Extrusion of abdominal catheter of ventriculoperitoneal shunt into the scrotum. J Neurosurg 1974;40:772–773.

Ramos M, Mandybur TI. Cerebral vasculitis in rheumatoid arthritis. Arch Neurol 1975;32:271–275.

Ramsdell JW, Swart JA, Jackson JE, Renvall M. The yield of a home visit in the assessment of geriatric patients. J Am Geriatr Soc 1989;37:17–24.

Rand KH, Johnson KP, Rubinstein LJ, et al. Adenine arabinoside in the treatment of progressive multifocal leukoencephalopathy: use of virus-containing cells in the urine to assess response to therapy. Ann Neurol 1977;1:458–462.

Rao SM. Neuropsychology of multiple sclerosis: a critical review. J Clin Exp Neuropsychol 1986;8:503–542.

Rao SM, Hammeke TA, McQuillen MP, Khatri BO, Lloyd D. Memory disturbance in chronic progressive multiple sclerosis. Arch Neurol 1984;41:625–631.

Rao SM, Leo GJ, Haughton VM, St. Aubin-Faubert P, Bernardin L. Correlation of magnetic resonance imaging with neuropsychological testing in multiple sclerosis. Neurology 1989a;39:161–166.

Rao SM, St. Aubin-Faubert P, Leo GJ. Information processing speed in patients with multiple sclerosis. J Clin Exp Neuropsychol 1989b;11:471–477.

Rapcsak SZ, Arthur SA, Bliklen DA, Rubens AB. Lexical agraphia in Alzheimer's disease. Arch Neurol 1989a;46:65–68.

Rapcsak SZ, Croswell SC, Rubens AB. Apraxia in Alzheimer's disease. Neurology 1989b;39:664–668.

Rapin I, Suzuki K, Suzuki K, Valsamis MP. Adult (chronic) GM_2 gangliosidosis. Arch Neurol 1976;33:120–130.

Rappaport EB. Iatrogenic Creutzfeldt-Jakob disease. Neurology 1987;37:1520–1522.

Raskin N, Ehrenberg R. Senescence, senility, and Alzheimer's disease. Am J Psychiatry 1958;113:133–137.

Raskin NH, Fishman RA. Neurologic disorders in renal failure. N Engl J Med 1976;294:143–148, 204–210.

Raskind M, Peskind E, Rivard M-F, Veith R, Barnes R. Dexamethasone suppression test and cortisol circadian rhythm in primary degenerative dementia. Am J Psychiatry 1982;139:1468–1471.

Raskind MA, Peskind ER, Lampe TH, Risse SC, Taborsky GJ Jr, Dorsa D. Cerebrospinal fluid vasopressin, oxytocin, somatostatin, and beta-endorphin in Alzheimer's disease. Arch Gen Psychiatry 1986;43:382–388.

Ratner J, Rosenberg G, Kral VA, Engelsmann F. Anticoagulant therapy for senile dementia. J Am Geriatr Soc 1972;20:556–559.

Rawls WE, Dyck PJ, Klass DW, Greer HD III, Herrmann ED Jr. Encephalitis associated with herpes simplex virus. Ann Intern Med 1966;64:104–115.

Ray WA, Federspiel CF, Schaffner W. A study of antipsychotic drug use in nursing homes: epidemiologic evidence suggesting misuse. Am J Public Health 1980; 70:485–491.

Ray WA, Griffin MR, Schaffner W, Baugh DK, Melton LJ III. Psychotoropic drug use and the risk of hip fracture. N Engl J Med 1987;316:363–369.

Read AE, Sherlock S, Laidlaw J, Walker JG. The neuro-psychiatric syndromes associated with chronic liver disease and an extensive portal-systemic collateral circulation. Q J Med 1967;36:135–150.

Read S. Community resources. In Cummings JL, Miller BL, eds. Alzheimer's disease. Treatment and long-term management. Marcel Dekker, New York, 1990:235–244.

Reagan TJ, Okazaki H. The thrombotic syndrome associated with carcinoma. Arch Neurol 1974;31:390–395.

Rebeiz JJ, Kolodny EH, Richardson E P Jr. Corticodentatonigral degeneration with neuronal achromasia. Arch Neurol 1968;18:20–33.

Reches A, Tietler J, Lavy S. Parkinsonism due to lithium carbonate poisoning. Arch Neurol 1981;38:471.

Reed D, Crawley J, Faro SN, Pieper SJ, Kurland LT. Thallotoxicosis. JAMA 1963;183:516–522.

Reed H, Lindsay A, Silversides JL, Speakman J, Monckton G, Rees DL. The uveoencephalitic syndrome or Vogt-Koyanagi-Harada disease. Can Med Assoc J 1958a;79:451–459.

Reed TE, Chandler JH, Hughes EM, Davidson RT. Huntington's chorea in Michigan. I. Demography and genetics. Am J Hum Genet 1958b;10:201–225.

Reese HW, Rodeheaver D. Problem solving and complex decision making. In Birren J, Schaie KW, eds. Handbook of the Psychology of Aging. Van Nostrand Reinhold, New York, 1985;474–499.

Reeves AG, Plum F. Hyperphagia, rage, and dementia accompanying a ventromedial hypothalamic neoplasm. Arch Neurol 1969;20:616–624.

Refsum S, Skre H. Neurological approaches to the inherited ataxias. Adv Neurol 1978;21:1–13.

Regard M, Oelz O, Brugger P, Biol D, Landis T. Persistent cognitive impairment in climbers after repeated exposure to extreme altitude. Neurology 1989;39:210–213.

Reich P, Regestein QR, Murawski BJ, DeSilva RA, Lown B. Unrecognized organic mental disorders in survivors of cardiac arrest. Am J Psychiatry 1983;140:1194–1197.

Reid IC, Besson JAO, Best PV, Sharp PF, Gemmell HG, Smith FW. Imaging of cerebral blood flow markers in Huntington's disease using single photon emission computed tomography. J Neurol Neurosurg Psychiatry 1988;51:1264–1268.

Reifler BV, Larson E, Hanley R. Coexistence of cognitive impairment and depression in geriatric outpatients. Am J Psychiatry 1982;139:623–626.

Reik L Jr, Korn JH. Cryoglobulinemia with encephalopathy: successful treatment by plasma exchange. Ann Neurol 1981;10:488–490.

Reik L Jr, Smith L, Khan A, Nelson W. Demyelinating encephalopathy in Lyme disease. Neurology 1985;35:267–269.

Reinherz EL, Weiner HL, Hauser SL, Cohen JA, Distaso JA, Schlossman SF. Loss of suppressor T cells in active multiple sclerosis. N Engl J Med 1980;303:125–129.

Reinikainen KJ, Kiekkinen PJ, Jolkkonen J, Kosma V-M, Soininen H. Decreased somatostatin-like immunoreactivity in cerebral cortex and cerebrospinal fluid in Alzheimer's disease. Brain Res 1987;402:103–108.

Reisberg B, Borenstein J, Salob SP, Ferris SH, Franssen E, Georgotas A. Behavioral symptoms in Alzheimer's disease: phenomenology and treatment. J Clin Psychiatry 1987;48(Suppl):9–15.

Reitan RM. Investigation of the validity of Halstead's measures of biological intelligence. Arch Neurol Psychiatry 1955;73:28–35.

Reitan RM. Psychological deficits resulting from cerebral lesions in man. In: Warren JM. Akert K, eds. The frontal granular cortex and behavior. McGraw-Hill, New York, 1964:295–312.

Reitan RM, Boll TJ. Intellectual and cognitive functions in Parkinson's disease. J Consult Clin Psychol 1971;37:364–369.

Reitan RM, Davison LA, eds. Clinical neuropsychology: current status and applications. John Wiley & Sons, New York, 1974.

Remick RA, O'Kane J, Sparling TC. A case report of toxic psychosis with low-dose propranolol therapy. Am J Psychiatry 1981;138:850–851.

Rennick PM, Nolan DC, Bauer RB, Lerner AM. Neuropsychologic and neurologic follow-up after herpes virus hominis encephalitis. Neurology 1973;23:42–47.

Renvoize EB, Jerram T. Choline in Alzheimer's disease. N Engl J Med 1979;301:330

Resnick L, Berger JR, Shapshak P, Tourtellotte WW. Early penetration of the blood-brain barrier by HIV. Neurology 1988;38:9–14.

Rewcastle MB, Ball MJ. Electron microscopic structure of the "inclusions bodies" in Pick's disease. Neurology 1968;18:1205–1213.

Reynolds CF III, Hoch CC, Stack J, Campbell D. The nature and management of sleep/wake disturbance in Alzheimer's dementia. Psychopharm Bull 1988;24:43–48.

Reynolds EH, Rothfeld P, Pincus JH. Neurological disease associated with folate deficiency. Br Med J 1973;2:398–400.

Reynolds EH, Travers RD. Serum anticonvulsant concentrations in epileptic patients with mental symptoms. Br J Psychiatry 1974;124:440–445.

Rezek DL. Olfactory deficits as a neurologic sign in dementia of the Alzheimer type. Arch Neurol 1987;44:1030–1032.

Rice E, Gendelman S. Psychiatric aspects of normal pressure hydrocephalus. JAMA 1973;233:409–412.

Richards F II, Cooper MR, Pearce LA, Cowan RJ, Spurr CL. Familial spinocerebellar degeneration, hemolytic anemia, and glutathione deficiency. Arch Intern Med 1974;134:534–537.

Richardson, EP Jr. Progressive multifocal leukoencephalopathy. In: Vinken PJ, Bruyn GW, eds. Multiple sclerosis and other demyelinating diseases. Vol 9. Handbook of clinical neurology. American Elsevier, New York, 1970:485–499.

Richardson EP Jr. Our evolving understanding of progressive multifocal leukoencephalopathy. Ann NY Acad Sci 1974;230:358–364.

Richardson JC, Chambers RA, Heywood PM. Encephalopathies of anoxia and hypoglycemia. Arch Neurol 1959;1:178–190.

Richardson JC, Steele J, Olszewski J. Supranuclear ophthalmoplegia, pseudobulbar palsy, nuchal dystonia and dementia. Trans Am Neurol Assoc 1963;88:25–27.

Richter JA, Perry EK, Tomlinson BE. Acetylcholine and choline levels in postmortem human brain tissue: preliminary observations in Alzheimer's disease. Life Sci 1980;26:1683–1689.

Richter R. A clinico-pathologic study of parenchymatous cortical cerebellar atrophy: report of a familial case. J Nerv Ment Dis 1940;91:37–46.

Ridley A. Porphyric neuropathy. In: Dyck PJ, Thomas PK, Lambert EH, eds. Peripheral neuropathy. Philadelphia: WB Saunders, 1975:942–955.

Riegel K. Changes in psycholinguistic performances with age. In: Talland GA, ed. Human aging and behavior. Academic Press, New York, 1968:239–279.

Riehl J-L. The idiopathic arteritis of Takayasu. Neurology 1963;13:873–884.

Riggs JE. Neurological manifestations of electrolyte disturbances. In: Aminoff MJ, ed. Neurology and general medicine. Churchill Livingstone, New York, 1989:247–256.

Rigrodsky S, Morrison EB. Speech changes in parkinsonism during L-dopa therapy: preliminary findings. J Am Geriatr Soc 1970;18:142–151.

Riley HA. Epidemic encephalitis. Arch Neurol Psychiatry 1930;24:574–604.

Riley T. Neurological aspects of sleep. In: Aminoff MJ, ed. Neurology and general medicine. Churchill Livingstone, New York, 1989;431–447.

Riley V. Dialysis dementia: probably not asparagine deficiency. Lancet 1973;2:1275.

Rinne JO, Rummukainen J, Paljarvi L, Rinne UK. Dementia in Parkinson's disease is related to neuronal loss in the medial substantia nigra. Ann Neurol 1989;26:47–50.

Risberg J. Regional cerebral blood flow measurements by ^{133}Xe-inhalation: methodology and applications in neuropsychology and psychiatry. Brain Lang 1980;9:9–34.

Risberg J. Frontal lobe degeneration of the non-Alzheimer type. III. Regional cerebral blood flow. Arch Gerontol Geriatr 1987;6:225–233.

Risk WS, Haddad FS. The variable natural history of subacute sclerosing panencephalitis. Arch Neurol 1979;36:610–614.

Risse SC, Barnes R. Pharmacologic treatment of agitation associated with dementia. J Am Geriatr Soc 1986;34:368–376.

Rivera VM, Meyer JS, Baer PE, Faibish GM, Mathew NT, Hartmann A. Vertebrobasilar arterial insufficiency with dementia. Controlled trials of treatment with betahistine hydrochloride. J Am Geriatr Soc 1974;22:397–406.

Rizzo WB, Leshner RT, Odone A, Dammann AL, Craft DA, Jensen ME, Jennings SS, Davis S, Jaitly R, Sgro JA. Dietary erucic acid therapy for x-linked adrenoleukodystrophy. Neurology 1989;39:1415–1422.

Robbins, SL. Pathology. 3rd ed. WB Saunders, Philadelphia, 1967.

Roberts GW. Immunocytochemistry of neurofibrillary tangles in dementia pugilistica and Alzheimer's disease: evidence of common genesis. Lancet 1988;2:1456–1458.

Roberts GW, Losthouse R, Allsop D, Landon M, Kidd M, Prusiner SB, Crow TJ. CNS amyloid proteins in neurodegenerative diseases. Neurology 1988;38:1534–1540.

Roberts MA, Caird FI, Grossart KW, Steven JL. Computerized tomography in the diagnosis of cerebral atrophy. J Neurol Neurosurg Psychiatry 1976;39:909–915.

Robertson EE, le Roux A, Brown JH. The clinical differentiation of Pick's disease. J Ment Sci 1958;104:1000–1024.

Robertson WC Jr, Clark DB, Markesbery WR. Review of 38 cases of subacute sclerosing panencephalitis: effect of amantadine on the natural course of the disease. Ann Neurol 1980;8:422–425.

Robinson KC, Kallberg MH, Crowley MF. Idiopathic hypoparathyroidism presenting as dementia. Br Med J 1954;2:1203–1206.

Robinson RG, Benson DF. Depression in aphasic patients: frequency, severity, and clinical-pathological correlations. Brain Lang 1981;14:282–291.

Robinson RG, Szetela B. Mood change following left hemisphere brain injury. Ann Neurol 1981;9:447–453.

Robitaille Y, Carpenter S, Karpati G, DiMauro S. A distinct form of adult-polyglucosan body disease with massive involvement of central and peripheral neuronal processes and astrocytes. Brain 1980;103:315–336.

Roca RP, Klein LE, Kirby SM, McArthur JC, Vogelsang GB, Folstein MF, Smith CR. Recognition of dementia among medical patients. Arch Intern Med 1984;144:73–75.

Rocca WA, Amaducci LA, Schoenberg BS. Epidemiology of clinically diagnosed Alzheimer's disease. Ann Neurol 1986;19:415–424.

Rochford G. A study of naming errors in dysphasic and in demented patients. Neuropsychology 1971;9:437–443.

Rodgers-Johnson P, Garruto RM, Yanagihara R, Chen K-M, Gajdusek DC, Gibbs CJ Jr. Amyotrophic lateral sclerosis and parkinsonism-dementia on Guam: a 30-year evaluation of clinical and neuropathological trends. Neurology 1986;36:7–13.

Rodriguez M. Multiple sclerosis: basic concepts and hypothesis. Mayo Clin Proc 1989;64:570–576.

Rodriguez-Budelli MM, Kark RAP, Blass JP, Spence MA. Action of physostigmine on inherited ataxias. Adv Neurol 1978;21;195–202.

Rogers D, Lees AJ, Smith E, Trimble M, Stern GM. Bradyphrenia in Parkinson's disease and psychomotor retardation in depressive illness. Brain 1987;110:761–776.

Roizin L, Stellar S, Liu JC. Neuronal nuclear-cytoplasmic changes in Huntington's chorea: electron microscopic investigations. Adv Neurol 1979;23:95–122.

Roman GC. Senile dementia of the Binswanger type. JAMA 1987;258:1782–1788.

Romano J, Engel GL. Delirium. I. Electroencephalographic data. Arch Neurol Psychiatry 1944;51;356–377.

Romanul, FCA. Examination of the brain and spinal cord. In: Tedeschi CG, ed. Neuropathology. Little, Brown, Boston, 1970:131–214.

Romanul FCA, Abramowicz A. Changes in brain and pial vessels in arterial border zones. Arch Neurol 1964;11:40–65.

Romanul FCA, Fowler HL, Radvany J, Feldman RG, Feingold M. Azorean disease of the nervous system. N Engl J Med 1977a;296:1505–1508.

Romanul FCA, Radvany J, Rosales RK. Whipple's disease confined to the brain: a case studied clinically and pathologically. J Neurol Neurosurg Psychiatry 1977b;40:901–909.

Ron MA. Brain damage in chronic alcoholism: a neuropathological, neuroradiological and psychological review. Psychol Med 1977;7:103–112.

Ron MA, Toone BK, Garralda ME, Lishman WA. Diagnostic accuracy in presenile dementia. Br J Psychiatry 1979; 134:161–168.

Ronnov-Jessen V, Kirkegaard C. Hyperthyroidism—a disease of old age? Br Med J 1973;1:41–43.

Roos R, Gajdusek DC, Gibbs CJ Jr. The clinical characteristics of transmissible Creutzfeldt-Jakob disease. Brain 1973;96:1–20.

Roos RP, Johnson RT. Viruses and dementia. In: Wells CE, ed. Dementia. 2nd ed. FA Davis, Philadelphia, 1977:93–112.

Ropper AH, Williams RS. Relationship between plaques, tangles, and dementia in Down syndrome. Neurology 1980;30:639–655.

Rose FC, Symonds CP. Persistent memory defect following encephalitis. Brain 1960;83:195–212.

Roseman E. Dilantin toxicity. Neurology 1961;11:912–921.

Rosen WG. Verbal fluency in aging and dementia. J Clin Neuropsychol 1980;2:135–146.

Rosen WG, Terry RD, Fuld PA, Katzman R, Peck A. Pathological verification of ischemic score in differentiation of dementias. Ann Neurol 1980;7:486–488

Rosenbaum D. Psychosis with Huntington's chorea. Psychiatr Q 1941;15:93–99.

Rosenbek JC, McNeil MR, Lemme ML, Prescott TE, Alfrey AC. Speech and language findings in a chronic hemodialysis patient: a case report. J Speech Hear Disord 1975;40:245–252.

Rosenberg GA, Johnson SF, Brenner RP. Recovery of cognition after prolonged vegetative state. Ann Neurol 1977;2:167–168.

Rosenberg GA, Kornfeld M, Stovring J, Bicknell JM. Subcortical arteriosclerotic encephalopathy (Binswanger): computerized tomography. Neurology 1979; 29:1102–1106.

Rosenberg NL, Kleinschmidt-DeMasters BK, Davis KA, Dreisbach JN, Hormes JT, Filley CM. Toluene abuse causes diffuse central nervous system white matter changes. Ann Neurol 1988; 23:611–614.

Rosenberg RN, Fowler HL. Autosomal dominant motor system disease of the Portuguese: a review. Neurology 1981;31:1124–1126.

Rosenberg RN, Nyhan WL, Bay C, Shore P. Autosomal dominant striatonigral degeneration. Neurology 1976;26:703–714.

Rosenblum ML, Levy RM, Bredesen DE. Overview of AIDS and the nervous system. In: Rosenblum ML, Levy RM, Bredesen DE, eds. AIDS and the nervous system. Raven Press, New York, 1988:1–12.

Rosenblum WI, Ghatak NR. Lewy bodies in the presence of Alzheimer's disease. Arch Neurol 1979;36:170–171.

Rosenthal G, Gilman S, Koeppe RA, Kluin KJ, Markel DS, Junck L, Gebarski SS. Motor dysfunction in olivopontocerebellar atrophy is related to cerebral metabolic rate studied with positron emission tomography. Ann Neurol 1988;24:414–419.

Ross ED. The aprosodias. Arch Neurol 1981;38:561–569.

Ross ED, Mesulam M-M. Dominant language features of the right hemisphere? Prosody and emotional gestures. Arch Neurol 1979;36:144–148.

Ross ED, Rush AJ. Diagnosis and neuroanatomical correlates of depression in brain-damaged patients. Arch Gen Psychiatry 1981;38:1344–1354.

Ross RJ, Cole M, Thompson JS, Kim KH. Boxers—computer tomography, EEG, and neurological evaluation. JAMA 1983;249:211–213.

Ross WD, Gechman AS, Sholiton MC, Paul HS. Need for alertness to neuropsychiatric manifestations of inorganic mercury poisoning. Compr Psychiatry 1977;18:595–598.

Rossi GF, Galli G, DiRocco C, Maira G, Meglio M, Troncone L. Normotensive hydrocephalus. The relations of pneumoencephalography and isotope cisternography to the results of surgical treatment. Acta Neurochir (Wien) 1974;30:69–83.

Rosselli A, Rosselli M, Ardila A, Penagos B. Severe dementia associated with neurocysticercosis. Intern J Neurosci 1988;41:87–95.

Rosselli M. Wilson's disease, a reversible dementia: Case report. J Clin Exp Neuropsychol 1987;9:399–406.

Rossor MN, Emson PC, Iversen LL, et al. Neuropeptides and neurotransmitters in cerebral cortex in Alzheimer's disease. In: Corkin S, Davis KL, Growdon JH, Usdin E, Wurtman RJ, eds. Alzheimer's disease: a report of progress in research. Raven Press, New York, 1982:15–24.

Rosvold HE. The frontal lobe system: cortical-subcortical interrelationships. Acta Neurobiol Exp 1972;32:439–460.

Roth, M. Epidemiological studies. In: Katzman R, Terry RD, Bick KL, eds. Alzheimer's disease, senile dementia and related disorders. Raven Press, New York, 1978:337–339.

Roth M, Tomlinson BE, Blessed G. Correlation between scores for dementia and counts of senile plaques in cerebral grey matter of elderly subjects. Nature 1966;209:109–110.

Roth N. The neuropsychiatric aspects of porphyria. Psychosomat Med 1945;7:291–301.

Roth RL, Bebin J. Cerebral hemispheric tumors and extrapyramidal signs and symptoms. Neurology 1958;8:277–284.

Rothermich ND, von Haam E. Pancreatic encephalopathy. J Clin Endocrinol 1941;1:872–881.

Rothschild D. Alzheimer's disease. Am J Psychiatry 1934;91:485–518.

Rothschild D. The clinical differentiation of senile and arteriosclerotic psychoses. Am J Psychiatry 1941;98:324–333.

Rothschild D, Kasanin J. Clinicopathologic study of Alzheimer's disease. Arch Neurol Psychiatry 1936;36:293–321.

Rottenberg DA, Horten B, Kim J-H, Posner JB. Progressive white matter destruction following irradiation of an extracranial neoplasm. Ann Neurol 1980;8:76–78.

Rottenberg DA, Moeller JR, Strother SC, Sidtis JJ, Navia BA, Dhawan V, Ginos JZ, Price RW. The metabolic pathology of the AIDS dementia complex. Ann Neurol 1987;22:700–706.

Rovner BW, Kafonek S, Filipp L, Lucas MJ, Folstein MF. Prevalence of mental illness in a community nursing home. Am J Psychiatry 1986;143:1446–1449.

Rowe JW, Kahn RL. Human aging: Usual and successful. Science 1987;237:143–149.

Roy S, Datta CK, Hirano A, Ghatak NR, Zimmerman HM. Electron microscopic study of neurofibrillary tangles in Steele-Richardson-Olszewski syndrome. Acta Neuropathol 1974;29:175–179.

Rozas VV, Port FK, Rutt WM. Progressive dialysis encephalopathy from dialysate aluminum. Arch Intern Med 1978;138:1375–1377.

Rozdilsky B, Cummings JN, Huston AF. Hallervorden-Spatz disease—late infantile and adult types, report of two cases. Acta Neuropathol 1968;10:1–16.

Rubens AB. Aphasia with infarction in the territory of the anterior cerebral artery. Cortex 1975;11:239–250.

Rubens AB, Geschwind N, Mahowald MW, Mastri A. Post-traumatic cerebral hemispheric disconnection syndrome. Arch Neurol 1977;34:750–755.

Ruberg RM, Javoy-Agid F, Hirsh E, Scatton B, LHeureux R, Hauw J-J, Duychaerts C, Gray F, Morel-Maroger A, Rascol A, Serdaru M, Agid Y. Dopaminergic and cholinergic lesions in progressive supranuclear palsy. Ann Neurol 1985;18:523–529.

Rubin EH, Drevets WC, Burke WJ. The nature of psychotic symptoms in senile dementia of the Alzheimer type. J Geriatr Psychiatry Neurol 1988;1:16–20.

Rubin EH, Morris JC, Berg L. The progression of personality changes in senile dementia of the Alzheimer type. J Am Geriatr Soc 1987a;37:721–725.

Rubin EH, Morris JC, Storandt M, Berg L. Behavioral changes in patients with mild senile dementia of the Alzheimer's type. Psychiatr Res 1987b;21:55–62.

Ruff RM, Buchsbaum MS, Troster AZ, Marshall LF, Lottenberg S. Somers LM, Tobias MD. Computerized tomography, neuropsychology, and positron emission tomography in the evaluation of head injury. Neuropsychiatry, Neuropsychol, Behav Neurol 1989;2:103–123.

Rumble B, Retallack R, Hilbich C, Simms G, Multhaup G, Martins R, Hockey A, Montgomery P, Beyreuther K, Masters CL. Amyloid A4 protein and its precursors in Down's syndrome and Alzheimer's disease. N Engl J Med 1989;320:1446–1452.

Russell DN, Keller FS, Whitaker JN. Episodic confusion and tremor associated with extrahepatic portacaval shunting in cirrhotic liver disease. Neurology 1989;39:403–405.

Russell DS. Observations on the pathology of hydrocephalus. His Majesty's Stationery Office, London, 1949.

Russell DS, Rubinstein LJ. Pathology of tumours of the nervous system. Williams & Wilkins, Baltimore, 1977.

Russell RWR. The traumatic amnesias. Oxford University Press, London, 1971.

Russell RWR. Supranuclear palsy of eyelid closure. Brain 1980;103:71–82.

Rustam H, Hamdi T. Methylmercury poisoning in Iraq. Brain 1974;97:499–510.

Sachias BA, Logue JN, Carey MS. Baclofen, a new antispastic drug. Arch Neurol 1977;34:422–428.

Sachdev HS. Forno LS. Kane CA. Joseph disease: a multisystem degenerative disorder of the nervous system. Neurology 1982;32:192–195.

Sachs E Jr. Meningiomas with dementia as the first presenting feature. J Ment Sci 1950;96:998–1007.

Sachs H, Russell JAG, Christman DR, Cook B. Alteration of regional cerebral glucose metabolic rate in non-Korsakoff chronic alcoholism. Arch Neurol 1987;44:1242–1251.

Sacks, OW. Awakenings. Vintage Books, New York, 1976.

Sacks, OW, Aguilar MJ, Brown WJ. Hallervorden-Spatz disease. Its pathogenesis and place among the axonal dystrophies. Acta Neuropathol 1966;6:164–174.

Sacks OW, Kohl MS. Messeloff CR, Schwartz WF. Effects of levodopa in parkinsonian patients with dementia. Neurology 1972;22:516–519.

Sacks OW, Messeloff CR, Schwartz WF. Long-term effects of levodopa in the severely disabled patient. JAMA 1970a;213:2270.

Sacks OW, Messeloff C, Schwartz W, Goldfarb A, Kohl M. Effects of L-dopa in patients with dementia. Lancet 1970b;1:1231.

Sagar HJ, Cohen EV, Sullivan EV, Corkin S, Growdon JH. Remote memory function in Alzheimer's disease and Parkinson's disease. Brain 1988a;111:185–206.

Sagar HJ, Sullivan EV, Gabrieli JDE, Corkin S, Growdon JH. Temporal ordering and short-term memory defects in Parkinson's disease. Brain 1988b;111:525–539.

Sage JI, Weinstein MP, Miller DC. Chronic encephalitis possibly due to herpes simplex virus: Two cases. Neurology 1985;35:1470–1472.

Sagel J, Matisonn R. Neuropsychiatric disturbance as the initial manifestation of digitalis toxicity. S Afr Med J 1972;46:512–514.

Sahakian BJ, Morris RG, Evenden JL, Heald A, Levy R, Philpot M, Robbins TW. A comparative study of visuospatial memory and learning in Alzheimer-type dementia and Parkinson's disease. Brain 1988;111:695–718.

Sahs AL, Joynt RJ. Bacterial meningitis. In: Baker AB, Baker LH, eds. Clinical neurology. Harper & Row, New York, 1981:1–90.

St. Clair D, Whalley LJ. Hypertension, multi-infarct dementia and Alzheimer's disease. Br J Psychiatry 1983;143:274–276.

Saint-Cyr JA, Taylor AE, Lang AE. Procedural learning and neostriatal dysfunction in man. Brain 1988;111:941–959.

Sakai T, Mawatari S, Iwashita H, Goto I, Kuroiwa Y. Choreoacanthocytosis. Clues to clinical diagnosis. Arch Neurol 1981;38:335–338.

Sakoda TH, Maxwell JA, Brackett CE Jr. Intestinal volvulus secondary to a ventriculoperitoneal shunt. J Neurosurg 1971;35:95–96.

Salazar AM, Masters CL, Gajdusek DC, Gibbs CJ Jr. Syndromes of amyotrophic lateral sclerosis and dementia: relation to transmissible Creutzfeldt-Jakob disease. Ann Neurol 1983;14:17–26.

Salguero LF, Itabashi HH, Gutierrez NB. Childhood multiple sclerosis with psychotic manifestations. J Neurol Neurosurg Psychiatry 1969;32:572–579.

Salmon DP, Shimamura AP, Butters N, Smith S. Lexical and semantic priming in patients with Alzheimer's disease. J Clin Exp Neuropsychol 1988;10:477–494.

Salmon JH, Armitage JL. Surgical treatment of hydrocephalus ex-vacou: ventriculoatrial shunt for degenerative brain disease. Neurology 1968;18:1223–1226.

Salthouse T. Speed of behavior and its implications for cognition. In: Birren J, Schaie KW, eds. Handbook for the Psychology of Aging, 2nd ed. Van Nostrand Reinhold Company, New York, 1985:400–426.

Salthouse TA. Speed and age: multiple rates of decline. Exp Aging Res 1976;2:349–359.

Salvini M, Binaschi S, Riva M. Evaluation of the psychophysiological functions in humans exposed to trichloroethylene. Br J Ind Med 1971;28:293–295.

Sanchez JE, Lopez VF. Sex-linked sudanophilic leukodystrophy with adrenocortical atrophy (so-called Schilder's disease). Neurology 1976;26:261–269.

Sanders J, Schenk VWD, Van Veen P. A family with Pick's disease. Uitgave van de NV, ed. Noord-Hollandsche, Amsterdam, 1939.

Sanders V. Neurologic manifestations of myxedema. N Engl J Med 1962;266:547–552, 599–603.

Santamaria J, Tolosa E, Valles A. Parkinson's disease with depression: possible subgroup of idiopathic parkinsonism. Neurology 1986;36:1130–1133.

Saric M, Markicevic A, Hrustic O. Occupational exposure to manganese. Br J Ind Med 1977;34:114–118.

Sawa M, Ueki Y, Arita M, Harada T. Preliminary report on the amygdalectomy on the psychotic patients, with interpretation of oral-emotional manifestations of schizophrenia. Folia Psychiatr Neurol Jpn 1954;7:309–329.

Sax DS, Bird Ed, Gusella JF, Myers RH. Phenotypic variation in 2 Huntington's disease families with linkage to chromosome 4. Neurology 1989;39:1332–1336.

Saxon A, Stevens RH, Golde DW. Helper and suppressor T-lymphocyte leukemia in ataxia telangiectasia. N Engl J Med 1979;300:700–704.

Scarf JE. Treatment of hydrocephalus: an historical and critical review of methods and results. J Neurol Neurosurg Psychiatry 1963;26:1–26.

Schaffert DA, Johnsen SD, Johnson PC, Drayer BP. Magnetic resonance imaging in pathologically proven Hallervorden-Spatz disease. Neurology 1989;39:440–442.

Schaltenbrand G, Putnam T. Untersuchungen zum Kreislauf de liquor cerebrospinalis mit hilfe intravenoser fluoreseineinspritzunger. Dtsch Z Nervenheilk 1927;96:123–132.

Scharenberg K. The histologic structure of the "inclusion bodies" of the neurons in Pick's disease. J Neuropathol Exp Neurol 1958;17:346–351.

Schaumburg HH, Powers JM, Raine CS, Suzuki K, Richardson EP Jr. Adrenoleukodystrophy. Arch Neurol 1975;32:577–591.

Schaumburg HH, Powers JM, Suzuki K, Raine CS. Adreno-leukodystrophy (sex-linked Schilder disease). Arch Neurol 1974;31:210–213.

Scheibel AB. Structural aspects of the aging brain: spine systems and the dendritic arbor. In: Katzman R, Terry RD, Bick KL, eds. Alzheimer's disease, senile dementia and related disorders. Raven Press, New York, 1978:353–373.

Scheibel ME, Tomiyasu U, Scheibel AB. The aging human Betz cell. Exp Neurol 1977;56:598–609.

Scheinberg IH, Sternlieb I. The long-term management of hepatolenticular degeneration (Wilson's disease). Am J Med 1960;29:316–333.

Schenk VWD. Re-examination of a family with Pick's disease. Ann Hum Genet 1958–1959;23:325–333.

Schenk VWD, Stolk PJ. Psychosis following arsenic (possibly thallium) poisoning. Psychiatr Neurol Neurochir 1967;70:31–37.

Schenk VWD, van Mansvelt T. The cortical degeneration in Pick's syndrome. Folia Psychiatr Neurol Neurochir Neerland 1955;58:42–62.

Scherokman BJ. Triphasic delta waves in a patient with acute hyperthyroidism. Arch Neurol 1980;37:731.

Schiffer RB, Babigian HM. Behavioral disorders in multiple sclerosis, temporal lobe epilepsy, and amyotrophic lateral sclerosis. Arch Neurol 1984;41:1067–1069.

Schiffer RB, Herndon RM, Rudick RA. Treatment of pathologic laughing and weeping with amitriptyline. N Engl J Med 1985;312:1480–1482.

Schilder P. Psychic disturbances after head injuries. Am J Psychiatry 1934;90:155–188.

Schildkraut JJ. Neuropsychopharmacology and the affective disorders. N Engl J Med 1969;281:197–201, 248–255, 302–308.

Schildkraut JJ, Schanberg SM, Breese GR, Kopin IJ. Norepinephrine metabolism and drugs used in the affective disorders: a possible mechanism of action. Am J Psychiatry 1967;124:600–608.

Schlegel U, Clarenbach P. Cordt A, Steudel A. Cerebral sarcoidosis presenting as supranuclear gaze palsy with hypokinetic rigid syndrome. Movement Disorders 1989;4:274–277.

Schlesser MA, Winokur G, Sherman BM. Hypothalamic-pituitary-adrenal axis activity in depressive illness. Arch Gen Psychiatry 1980;37:737–743.

Schmid R. Porphyria. In: Beeson PB, McDermott W, eds. Cecil-Loeb: textbook of medicine. 13th ed. WB Saunders, Philadelphia, 1971:1704–1709.

Schmidt RP, Gonyea EF. Neurosyphilis. In: Baker AB, Baker LH, eds. Clinical neurology. Harper & Row, Philadelphia, 1980:1–26.

Schmitt FA, Bigley JW, McKinnis R, Logue PE, Evans RW, Drucker JL, and the AZT Collaborative Working Group. Neuropsychological outcome of zidovudine (AZT) treatment of patients with AIDS and AIDS-related complex. N Engl J Med 1988;319:1573–1578.

Schmitt HP, Emser W, Heimes C. Familial occurrence of amyotrophic lateral sclerosis, parkinsonism, and dementia. Ann Neurol 1984;16:642–648.

Schneck SA, Penn I. Cerebral neoplasms associated with renal transplantation. Arch Neurol 1970;22:226–233.

Schneck SA, Penn I. De-novo brain tumors in renal-transplant recipients. Lancet 1971;1:983–986.

Schnur JA, Chase TN, Brody JA. Parkinsonism-dementia of Guam: treatment with L-dopa. Neurology 1971;21:1236–1242.

Schochet SS Jr. Earle KM. Pick's disease with compound intraneuronal inclusion bodies. Acta Neuropathol 1970;15:293–297.

Schochet SS Jr, Lampert PW, Lindenberg R. Fine structure of the Pick and Hirano bodies in a case of Pick's disease. Acta Neuropathol 1968;11:330–337.

Schoenberg BS. Epidemiology of Alzheimer's disease and other dementing illnesses. J Chronic Dis 1986;39:1095–1104.

Schoenberg BS, Anderson DW, Haerer AF. Severe dementia: prevalence and clinical features in a biracial US population. Arch Neurol 1985;42:740–743.

Schoenberg BS, Kokmen E, Okazaki H. Alzheimer's disease and other dementing illnesses in a defined United States population: incidence rates and clinical features. Ann Neurol 1987;22:724–729.

Schreiner GE. Mental and personality changes in the uremic syndrome. Med Ann Dist Columbia 1959;28:316–362.

Schuler P, Oyanguren H, Maturana V, et al. Manganese poisoning. Ind Med Surg 1957;26:167–173.

Schulman S. Wilson's disease. In: Minkler J, ed. Pathology of the nervous system. McGraw-Hill, New York, 1968:1139–1152.

Schut JW. Hereditary ataxia. Arch Neurol Psychiatry 1950;63:535–568.

Schulz PE, Weiner SP, Belmont JW, Fishman MA. Basal ganglia calcifications in a case of biotinidase deficiency. Neurology 1988;38:1326–1328.

Schwab RS, England AC Jr. Parkinson syndromes due to various specific causes. In: Vinken PJ, Bruyn GW, eds. Diseases of the basal ganglia. Vol 6. Handbook of clinical neurology. American Elsevier, New York, 1968:227–247.

Schwab RS, Poskanzer DC, England AC Jr, Young RR. Amantadine in Parkinson's disease. JAMA 1972;222:792–795.

Schwankaus JD, Patronas N, Dorwart R, Eldridge R, Schlesinger S, McFarland H. Computed tomography and magnetic resonance imaging in adult-onset leukodystrophy. Arch Neurol 1988;45:1004–1008.

Schwartz GE, Fair PL, Salt P, Mandel MR, Klerman GL. Facial muscle patterning to affective imagery in depressed and nondepressed subjects. Science 1976;199:489–491.

Schwartz MA, Selhorst JB, Ochs AL, Beck RW, Campbell WW, Harris JK, Waters B, Velasco ME. Oculomasticatory myorhythmia: a unique movement disorder occurring in Whipple's disease. Ann Neurol 1986;20:677–683.

Schwartz MF, Marin OSM, Saffran EM. Dissociations of language function in dementia: a case study. Brain Lang 1979;7:277–306.

Schwartz, WB. Disorders of fluid, electrolyte, and acid-base balance. In: Beeson PB, McDermott W, eds. Cecil-Loeb: textbook of medicine. 13th ed. WB Saunders, Philadelphia, 1971:1618–1639.

Schwartz GA, Yanoff M. Lafora's disease. Arch Neurol 1965;12:172–188.

Scicutella A, Davies P. Marked loss of cerebral galactolipids in Pick's disease. Ann Neurol 1987;22:606–609.

Scott DF, Heathfield KWG, Toone B. Margerison JH. The EEG in Huntington's chorea: a clinical and neuropathological study. J Neurol Neurosurg Psychiatry 1972;35:97–102.

Scott JP, Roberto KA, Hutton JT. Families of Alzheimer's victims. J Am Geriatr Soc 1986;34:348–354.

Scrimshaw NS. Deficiencies of individual nutrients: vitamin diseases. In: Beeson PB, McDermott W, eds. Cecil-Loeb: textbook of medicine. 13th ed. WB Saunders, Philadelphia, 1971:1438–1448.

Sears ES, Hammerberg EK, Norenberg MD, Wilson B, Nellhaus G. Supranuclear ophthalmoplegia and dementia in olivopontocerebellar atrophy: a clinicopathologic study. Neurology 1975;25:395.

Selnes OA, Miller E, McArthur J, Gordon B, Munoz A, Sheridan K, Fox R, Saah AJ, and the Multicenter AIDS Cohort Study. HIV-1 infection: no evidence of cognitive decline during the asymptomatic stages. Neurology 1990;40:204–208.

Selby G. Parkinson's disease. In: Vinken PJ, Bruyn GW, eds. Diseases of the basal ganglia. Vol. 6. Handbook of clinical neurology. American Elsevier, New York, 1968:173–211.

Selby G, Walker GL. Cerebral arteritis in cat-scratch fever. Neurology 1979;29:1413–1418.

Selecki BR. Cerebral mid-line tumours involving the corpus callosum among mental hospital patients. Med J Aust 1964;2:954–960.

Selecki BR. Intracranial space-occupying lesions among patients admitted to mental hospitals. Med J Aust 1965;1:383–390.

Selekler K, Kansy T, Zileli T. Computed tomography in Wilson's disease. Arch Neurol 1981;38:727–728.

Selkoe DJ. Altered protein composition in isolated human cortical neurons in Alzheimer disease. Ann Neurol 1980;8:468–478.

Selkoe DJ, Brown BA, Salazar FJ, Marotta CA. Myelin basic protein in Alzheimer disease neuronal fractions and mammalian neurofilament preparations. Ann Neurol 1981;10:429–436.

Sellars EM, Kalant H. Alcohol intoxication and withdrawal. N Engl J Med 1976; 294:757–762.

Sells CJ, Loeser JD. Peritonitis following perforation of the bowel: a rare complication of a ventriculoperitoneal shunt. J Pediatr 1973;83:823–824.

Seltzer B, Benson DF. The temporal pattern of retrograde amnesia in Korsakoff's disease. Neurology 1974;24:527–530.

Seltzer B, Sherwin I. "Organic brain syndromes": an empirical study and critical review. Am J Psychiatry 1978;135:13–21.

Seltzer B, Sherwin I. A comparison of clinical features in early- and late-onset primary degenerative dementia. Arch Neurol 1983;40:143–146.

Sensenbach W, Madison L, Eisenberg S, Ochs L. The cerebral circulation and metabolism in hyperthyroidism and myxedema. J Clin Invest 1954;33:1434–1440.

Sercl M, Jaros O. The mechanisms of cerebral concussion in boxing and their consequences. World Neurol 1962;3:351–358.

Sergaroglu P, Yazici H, Ozdemir C, Yurdakul S, Bahar S, Aktin E. Neurologic involvement in Behcet's syndrome. Arch Neurol 1989;46:265–269.

Sergent JS, Lockshin MD, Klempner MS, Lipsky BA. Central nervous system disease in systemic lupus erythematosus. Am J Med 1975;58:644–654.

Sethi KD, Adams RJ, Loring DW, Gammal TE. Hallervorden-Spatz syndrome: clinical and magnetic resonance imaging correlations. Ann Neurol 1988;24:692–694.

Shabas D, Gerard G, Cunha B, Rossi D. MRI appearance of AIDS subacute encephalopathy. Comput Radiol 1987;11:69–73.

Shafey S, Scheinberg P. Neurological syndromes occurring in patients receiving synthetic steroids (oral contraceptives). Neurology 1966;16:205–211.

Shagass C. The EEG in affective psychoses. In: Wilson WP, ed. Applications of electroencephalography in psychiatry. Duke University Press, Durham, N.C., 1965:146–167.

Shallat RF, Pawl RP, Jerva MJ. Significance of upward gaze palsy (Parinaud's syndrome) in hydrocephalus due to shunt malfunction. J Neurosurg 1973;38:717–721.

Shapiro MD, Field J, Post F. An inquiry into the determinants of a differentiation between elderly "organic" and "non-organic" psychiatric patients on the Bender-Gestalt test. J Ment Sci 1957;103:364–374.

Shapiro SK. Psychosis due to bilateral carotid artery occlusion. Minn Med 1959;42:25–27.

Shapiro WR. Remote effects of neoplasm on the central nervous system: encephalopathy. Adv Neurol 1976;15:101–117.

Sharp PF, Gemmell HG, Cherryman G, Besson JAO, Crawford J, Smith FW. The application of 123-I labelled isopropyl-amphetamine to the study of dementia. J Nuc Med 1986;27:761–768.

Shaw RK, Moore EW, Fredreich EJ, Thomas LB. Meningeal leukemia. Neurology 1960;10:823–833.

Shelanski ML, Wisniewski H. Neurofibrillary degeneration induced by vincristine therapy. Arch Neurol 1969;20:199–206.

Shenkin HA, Greenberg J, Borizarth WF, Gutterman P, Morales JO. Ventricular shunting for relief of senile symptoms. JAMA 1973;225:1486–1489.

Shepherd M. Report of a family suffering from Friedreich's disease, peroneal muscular atrophy, and schizophrenia. J Neurol Neurosurg Psychiatry 1955;18:297–304.

Sheremata W, Cosgrove JBR, Eylar EH. Cellular hypersensitivity to basic myelin (A₁) protein and clinical multiple sclerosis. N Engl J Med 1974;291:14–17.

Sherlock S, Summerskill WHJ, White LP, Phear EA. Portal-systemic encephalopathy. Lancet 1954;2:453–457.

Shibasaki H, Motomura S, Yamashita Y, Shii H, Kuroiwa Y. Periodic synchronous discharge and myoclonus in Creutzfeldt-Jakob disease: diagnostic application of jerk-locked averaging method. Ann Neurol 1981;9:150–156.

Shih WJ, Markesbery WR, Clark DB, Goldstein CS, Domstad PA, Coupal JJ, Kung H, DeKosky ST, DeLand FH. Iodine-123 HIPDM brain imaging findings in subacute spongiform encephalopathy (Creutzfeldt-Jakob disease). J Nucl Med 1987;28:1484–1487.

Shimamoto T, Murase H, Numano F. Treatment of senile dementia and cerebellar disorders with phthalazinol. Cyclic AMP-increasing agent, phthalazinol, in therapeutic trials in hitherto incurable morbid conditions. Mech Aging Dev 1976;5:241–250.

Shiraki H. Neuropathological aspects of organic mercury intoxication, including Minamata disease. In: Vinkin PJ, Bruyn GW, eds. Intoxications of the nervous system. Part I, vol. 36. Handbook of clinical neurology. North-Holland, New York, 1979:83–145.

Shoji H, Teramoto H, Satowa S, Satowa H, Narita Y. Partial Klüver-Bucy syndrome following probable herpes simplex encephalitis. J Neurol 1979;221:163–167.

Shopsin B, Johnson G, Gershon S. Neurotoxicity with lithium: differential drug responsiveness. Int Pharmacopsychiatry 1970;5:170–182.

Shore D, Millson M, Holtz JL, Wing SW, Bridge TP, Wyatt RJ. Serum aluminum in primary degenerative dementia. Biol Psychiatry 1980;15:971–977.

Shoulson I, Goldblatt D, Charlton M, Joynt RJ. Huntington's disease: treatment with muscimol, a GABA-mimetic drug. Ann Neurol 1978;4:279–284.

Shoulson I, Kartzinel R, Chase TN. Huntington's disease: treatment with dipropylacetic acid and gamma-aminobutyric acid. Neurology 1976;26:61–63.

Shraberg D. The myth of pseudodementia: depression and the aging brain. Am J Psychiatry 1978;135:601–603.

Shrubsall FC. The sequelae of encephalitis lethargica. Br J Med Psychol 1927;7:210–220.

Shy GM, Drager GA. A neurological syndrome associated with orthostatic hypotension. Arch Neurol 1960;2:511–527.

Sibley WA. Diagnosis and course of multiple sclerosis. In: Rao SM, ed. Neurobehavioral aspects of multiple sclerosis. Oxford University Press, New York, 1990;5–14.

Siedler H, Malamud N. Creutzfeldt-Jakob's disease. J Neuropathol Exp Neurol 1963;22:381–402.

Silva CA, Paula-Barbosa MM, Pereira S, Cruz C. Two cases of rapidly progressive subacute sclerosing panencephalitis. Arch Neurol 1981;38:109–113.

Silverberg GD, Castellino RA, Goodwin DA. Porencephalic cysts demonstrated by encephalography with radioiodinated serum albumin. N Engl J Med 1969; 280:315–316.

Silverman D. Some observations on the EEG in hepatic coma. Electroencephalogr Clin Neurophysiol 1962;14:53–59.

Silverstein A, Feuer MM, Siltzbach LE. Neurologic sarcoidosis. Arch Neurol 1965; 12:1–11.

Sim M. Alzheimer's disease: a forgotten entity. Geriatrics 1965;20:668–674.

Sim M. Early diagnosis of Alzheimer's disease. In: Glen AIM, Whalley LJ, eds. Alzheimer's disease: early recognition of potentially reversible deficits. Edinburgh: Churchill Livingstone, 1979:78–85.

Sim M, Sussman I. Alzheimer's disease: its natural history and differential diagnosis. J Nerv Ment Dis 1962;135:489–499.

Sim M, Turner E, Smith WT. Cerebral biopsy in the investigation of presenile dementia. I. Clinical aspects. Br J Psychiatry 1966;112:119–125.

Simon RP. Neurosyphilis. Arch Neurol 1985;42:606–613.

Simpson DM, Foster D. Improvement in organically disturbed behavior with trazodone treatment. J Clin Psychiatry 1986;47:191–193.

Simpson GM, Amuso D, Blair JH, Farkas T. Phenothiazine-produced extrapyramidal system disturbance. Arch Gen Psychiatry 1964;10:199–208.

Sipe JC. Leigh's syndrome: the adult form of subacute necrotizing encephalomyelopathy with predilection for the brainstem. Neurology 1973;23:1030–1038.

Sjaastad O, Skalpe IO, Engeset A. The width of the temporal horn in the differential diagnosis between pressure hydrocephalus and hydrocephalus ex-vacuo. Neurology 1969;19:1087–1093.

Sjøgren H. Twenty-four cases of Alzheimer's disease. Acta Med Scand 1950;(suppl 246):225–233.

Sjøgren T, Sjogren H, Lindgren AGH. Morbus Alzheimer and morbus Pick. Acta Psychiatr Neurol Scand 1952;(suppl 82):1–152.

Skre H. Spino-cerebellar ataxia in western Norway. Clin Genet 1974;6:265–288.

Slaby AE, Wyatt RJ. Dementia in the presenium. Charles C Thomas, Springfield, Ill., 1974.

Slater E. Diagnosis of "hysteria." Br Med J 1965;1:1395–1399.

Slater E, Beard AW. The schizophrenia-like psychoses of epilepsy. I. Psychiatric aspects. Br J Psychiatry 1963;109:95–112.

Slater E, Beard AW, Clithero E. The schizophrenia-like psychoses of epilepsy. Br J Psychiatry 1963;109:95–150.

Slyter H. Idiopathic hypoparathyroidism presenting as dementia. Neurology 1979; 29:393–394.

Smith AD. Adult age differences in cued recall. Devel Psychol 1977;13:326–331.

Smith ADM. Megaloblastic madness. Br Med J 1960;2:1840–1845.

Smith ADM, Miller JW. Treatment of inorganic mercury poisoning with N-acetyl-D, L-penicillamine. Lancet 1961;1:640–642.

Smith CCT, Bowen DM, Francis PT, Snowden JS, Neary D. Putative amino acid transmitters in lumbar cerebrospinal fluid of patients with histologically verified Alzheimer's dementia. J Neurol Neurosurg Psychiatry 1985;48:469–471.

Smith CK, Barish J, Correa J, Williams RH. Psychiatric disturbance in endocrinologic disease. Psychosomat Med 1972;34:69–86.

Smith CM, Swash M. Possible biochemical basis of memory disorder in Alzheimer disease. Ann Neurol 1978;3:471–473.

Smith CM, Swash M, Exton-Smith AN, et al. Choline therapy in Alzheimer's disease. Lancet 1978;2:318.

Smith CR, Simon AAF, Salif IE, Gentili F. Progressive multifocal leukoencephalopathy: failure of cytarabine therapy. Neurology 1982;32:200–203.

Smith FW, Besson JAO, Gemmell HG, Sharp PF. The use of Technetium-99m-HM-PAO in the assessment of patients with dementia and other neuropsychiatric conditions. J Cereb Blood Flow Metab 1988a;8:S116–S122.

Smith JB, Westmoreland BF, Reagan TJ, Sandok BA. A distinctive clinical EEG profile in herpes simplex encephalitis. Mayo Clin Proc 1975;50:469–474.

Smith JK, Gonada VE, Malamud N. Unusual form of cerebellar ataxia. Neurology 1958;8:205–209.

Smith JS, Kiloh LG. The investigation of dementia: results in 200 consecutive admissions. Lancet 1981;1:824–827.

Smith JS, Kiloh LG, Ratnavale GS, Grant DA. The investigation of dementia. Med J Aust 1976;2:403–405.

Smith S, Butters N, White R, Lyon L, Granholm E. Priming semantic relations in patients with Huntington's disease. Brain Cognit 1988b;33:27–40.

Smith T, Jakobsen J, Gaub J, Helweg-Larsaen S, Trojaborg W. Clinical and epectrophysiological studies of human immunodeficiency virus—seropositive men without AIDS. Ann Neurol 1988c;23:295–297.

Smith WL, Lowrey JB, Davis JA. The effects of cyclandelate on psychological test performance in patients with cerebral vascular insufficiency. Curr Ther Res 1968;10:613–618.

Smith WT. Intoxications, poisons and related metabolic disorders. In: Blackwood

W, Corsellis JAN, eds. Greenfield's neuropathology. Year Book Medical Publishers, Chicago, 1976a:148–193.

Smith WT. Nutritional deficiencies and disorders. In: Blackwood W, Corsellis JAN, eds. Greenfield's neuropathology. Year Book Medical Publishers, Chicago, 1976b:194–237.

Smith WT, Turner E, Sim M. Cerebral biopsy in the investigation of presenile dementia. II. Pathological aspects. Br J Psychiatry 1966;112:127–133.

Smyers-Verbeke J, Michotte Y, Pelsmaeckers J, et al. The chemical composition of idiopathic nonarteriosclerotic cerebral calcifications. Neurology 1975;25:48–57.

Smyth GE, Stern K. Tumours of the thalamus—a clinico-pathological study. Brain 1938;61:339–374.

Snider WD, DeMaria AA Jr, Mann JD. Diazepam and dialysis encephalopathy. Neurology 1979;29:414–415.

Snider WD, Simpson DM, Nielsen S, Gold JWM, Metroka CE, Posner JB. Neurological complications of acquired immune deficiency syndrome: analysis of 50 patients. Ann Neurol 1983;14:403–418.

Snow RM, Dismukes WE. Cryptococcal meningitis. Arch Intern Med 1975;135:1155–1157.

Snowden JS, Goulding PJ, Neary D. Semantic dementia: a form of circumscribed cerebral atrophy. Behav Neurol 1989;2:167–182.

Snyder BD, Harris S. Treatable aspects of the dementia syndrome. J Am Geriatr Soc 1976;24:179–184.

Snyder RD. The involuntary movements of chronic mercury poisoning. Arch Neurol 1972;26:379–381.

Snyder SH, Banerjee SP, Yamamura HI, Greenberg D. Drugs, neurotransmitters and schizophrenia. Science 1974;184:1243–1253.

So NK, O'Neill BP, Frytak S, Eagan RT, Earnest F IV, Lee RE. Delayed leukoencephalopathy in survivors with small cell lung cancer. Neurology 1987;37:1198–1201.

Sobin P, Schneider L, McDermott H. Fluoxetine in the treatment of agitated dementia. Am J Psychiatry 1989;146:1636.

Soeters PB, Fischer JE. Insulin, glucagon, aminoacid imbalance, and hepatic encephalopathy. Lancet 1976;2:880–882.

Sokoloff L. Circulation and energy metabolism of the brain. In: Siegel GJ, Albers RW, Katzman R, Agranoff BW, eds. Basic neurochemistry. 2nd ed. Little, Brown, Boston, 1976:388–413.

Solitare GB, Lamarche JB. Alzheimer's disease and senile dementia as seen in mongoloids: neuropathological observations. Am J Ment Defic 1966;70:840–848.

Solitare GB, Lopez VF. Louis-Bar's syndrome (ataxia telangiectasia). Neurology 1967;17:23–31.

Solomon S, Hotchkiss E, Saravay SM, Bayer C, Ramsey P, Blum RS. Impairment of memory function by antihypertensive medication. Arch Gen Psychiatry 1983;40:1109–1112.

Sorenson PS, Jansen EC, Gjerris F. Motor disturbances in normal-pressure hydrocephalus: special reference to stance and gait. Arch Neurol 1986;43:34–38.

Souetre E, Salvati E, Krebs B, Belugou J-L, Darcourt G. Abnormal melatonin response to 5-methoxypsoralen in dementia. Am J Psychiatry 1989;146:1037–1040.

Sourander P. Sjøgren H. The concept of Alzheimer's disease and its clinical implications. In: Wolstenholme GEW, O'Connor M, eds. Alzheimer's disease and related conditions. J & A Churchill, London, 1970:11–32.

Sourander P, Svennerholm L. Sulphatide lipidosis in the adult with the clinical picture of progressive organic dementia with epileptic seizures. Acta Neuropathol 1962;1:384–396.

Sourkes TL. Parkinson's disease and other disorders of the basal ganglia. In: Siegel GJ, Albers RW, Katzman R, Agranoff BW, eds. Basic neurochemistry. 2nd ed. Little, Brown, Boston, 1976:668–684.

Spar JE, Gerner R. Does the dexamethasone suppression test distinguish dementia from depression? Am J Psychiatry 1982;139:238–240.

Specola N, Vanier MT, Goutieres F, Mikol J, Aicardi J. The juvenile and chronic forms of GM2 gangliosidosis: clinical and enzymatic heterogeneity. Neurology 1990;40:145–150.

Spellman GG. Report of familial cases of parkinsonism. JAMA 1962;179:160–162.

Spencer CA. Clinical utility and cost-effectiveness of sensitive thyrotropin assays in ambulatory and hospitalized patients. Mayo Clin Proc 1988;63:1214–1222.

Spillane JD. Nutritional disorders of the nervous system. Williams & Wilkins, Philadelphia, 1947.

Spillane JD. Nervous and mental disorders in Cushing's syndrome. Brain 1951;74:72–94.

Spillane JD. Developmental abnormalities in the region of the foramen magnum. In: Bowman PW, Mautner HV, eds. Mental retardation. Grune & Stratton, New York, 1960:194–210.

Spillane JD. Five boxers. Br Med J 1962;2:1205–1210.

Spiller WG. Two cases of partial internal hydrocephalus from closure of the interventricular passages. Am J Med Sci 1902;124:44–55.

Spokes EGS. Dopamine in Huntington's disease: a study of postmortem brain tissue. Adv Neurol 1979;23:481–493.

Sponzilli EE, Smith JK, Malamud N, McCulloch JR. Progressive multifocal leukoencephalopathy: a complication of immunosuppressive treatment. Neurology 1975;25:664–668.

Sroka H, Elizan TS, Yahr MD, Burger A, Mendoza MR. Organic mental syndrome and confusional states in Parkinson's disease. Arch Neurol 1981;38:339–342.

Staal A, Went LN. Juvenile amyotrophic lateral sclerosis-dementia complex in a Dutch family. Neurology 1968;18:800–806.

Stahl WL, Swanson PD. Biochemical abnormalities in Huntington's chorea brains. Neurology 1974;24:813–819.

Stam FC, Op den Velde W. Haptoglobin types in Alzheimer's disease and senile dementia. In: Katzman R, Terry RD, Bick KL, eds. Alzheimer's disease, senile dementia and related conditions. Raven Press, New York, 1978:279–285.

Starkman MN, Schteingart DE. Neuropsychiatric manifestations of patients with Cushing's syndrome. Arch Intern Med 1981;141:215—219.

Starkstein SE, Brandt J, Folstein S, Strauss M, Berthier ML, Pearlson G, Wong D,

McDonnell A, Folstein M. Neuropsychological and neuroradiological correlates in Huntington's disease. J Neurol Neurosurg Psychiatry 1988;51:1259–1263.

Starkstein SE, Pearlson GD, Boston J, Robinson RG. Mania after brain injury. Arch Neurol 1987;44:1069–1073.

Starkstein SE, Rabins PV, Berthier ML, Cohen BJ, Folstein MF, Robinson RG. Dementia of depression among patients with neurological disorders and functional depression. J Neuropsychiatry Clin Neurosci 1989;1:263–268.

Starkstein SE, Robinson RG, Price TR. Comparison of cortical and subcortical lesions in the prediction of poststroke mood disorders. Brain 1987;110:1045–1059.

Starosta-Rubinstein S, Young AB, Kluin K, Hill G, Aisen AM, Gabrielsen T, Brewer GJ. Clinical assessment of 31 patients with Wilson's disease. Correlations with structural changes on magnetic resonance imaging. Arch Neurol 1987;44:365–370.

Starr A. A disorder of rapid eye movements in Huntington's chorea. Brain 1967;90:545–564.

Starr A, Achor J. Auditory brain stem responses in neurologic disease. Arch Neurol 1975;32:761–768.

Steckelberg JM, Cockerill FR III. Serologic testing for human immunodeficiency virus antibodies. Mayo Clin Proc 1988;63:373–380.

Steel R. GPI in an observation ward. Lancet 1960;1:121–123.

Steele C, Lucas J, Tune L. Haloperidol versus thioridazine in the treatment of behavioral symptoms in senile dementia of the Alzheimer's type: preliminary findings. J Clin Psychiatry 1986;47:310–312.

Steele JC. Progressive supranuclear palsy. Brain 1972;95:693–704.

Steele JC, Guzman T. Observations about amyotrophic lateral sclerosis and the parkinsonism-dementia complex of Guam with regard to epidemiology and etiology. Can J Neurol Sci 1987;14:358–362.

Steele JC, Richardson JC, Olszewski J. Progressive supranuclear palsy. Arch Neurol 1964;10:333–359.

Stefansson JG, Messina JA, Meyerowitz S. Hysterical neurosis, conversion type: clinical and epidemiological considerations. Acta Psychiatr Scand 1976;53:119–138.

Steere AC. Lyme disease. N Engl J Med 1989;321:586–596.

Stein SC, Langfitt TW. Normal pressure hydrocephalus. J Neurosurg 1974;41:463–470.

Steinberg D, Hirsch SR, Marston SP, Reynolds K, Sutton RNP. Influenza infection causing manic psychosis. Br J Psychiatry 1972;120:531–535.

Stell R, Bronstein AM, Plant GT, Harding AE. Ataxia telangiectasia: a reappraisal of the ocular motor features and their value in the diagnosis of atypical cases. Movement Disorders 1989;4:320–329.

Stengel E. A study of the symptomatology and differential diagnosis of Alzheimer's disease and Pick's disease. J Ment Sci 1943;89:1–20.

Stern BJ, Krumholz A, Johns C, Scott P, Nissim J. Sarcoidosis and its neurological manifestations. Arch Neurol 1985;42:909–917.

Stern K, Dancey TE. Glioma of the diencephalon in a manic patient. Am J Psychiatry 1942;98:716–719.

Stern K, Reed GE. Presenile dementia (Alzheimer's disease). Am J Psychiatry 1945;102:191–197.

Stern Y, Langston JW. Intellectual changes in patients with MPTP-induced parkinsonism. Neurology 1985;35:1506–1509.

Stern Y, Mayeux R, Rosen J. Contribution of perceptual motor dysfunction to construction and tracing disturbances in Parkinson's disease. J Neurol Neurosurg Psychiatry 1984;47:983–989.

Stern Y, Mayeux R. Effects of oral physostigmine in Alzheimer's disease. Ann Neurol 1987;22:306–310.

Stern Y, Mayeux R. Long-term administration of oral physostigmine in Alzheimer's disease. Neurology 1988;38:1837–1841.

Sternberg DE, Jarvik ME. Memory functions in depression. Arch Gen Psychiatry 1976;33:219–224.

Sternlieb I, Scheinberg IH. Prevention of Wilson's disease in asymptomatic patients. N Engl J Med 1968;278:352–359.

Stevens H, Forster FM. Effect of Carbon tetrachloride on the nervous system. Arch Neurol Psychiatry 1953;70:635–649.

Stevens JR. Motor disorders in schizophrenia. N Engl J Med 1974;290:110.

Stevens JR. Disturbances of ocular movements and blinking in schizophrenia. J Neurol Neurosurg Psychiatry 1978;41:1024–1030.

Stewart JM, Houser OW, Baker HL Jr, O'Brien PC, Rodriguez M. Magnetic resonance imaging and clinical relationships in multiple sclerosis. Mayo Clin Proc 1987;62:174–184.

Stiel JN, Hales IB, Reeve TS. Thyrotoxicosis in an elderly population. Med J Aust 1972;2:986–988.

Stotsky BA, Stotsky ES. Nursing homes: improving a flawed community facility. Hosp Commun Psychiatry 1983;34:238–242.

Strachan RW, Henderson JG. Psychiatric syndromes due to avitaminosis B_{12} with normal blood and marrow. Q J Med 1965;34:303–317.

Strachan RW, Henderson JG. Dementia and folate deficiency. Q J Med 1967;36:189–204.

Strang RR. Imipramine in treatment of parkinsonism: a double-blind placebo study. Br Med J 1965;2:33–34.

Strang RR. Parkinsonism occurring during methyldopa therapy. Can Med Assoc J 1966;95:928–929.

Strassman G. Iron and calcium deposits in the brain; their pathologic significance. J Neuropathol Exp Neurol 1949;8:428–439.

Straumanis JJ, Shagass C, Schwartz M. Visually evoked cerebral response changes associated with chronic brain syndromes and aging. J Gerontol 1965;20:498–506.

Strauss I, Keschner M. Mental symptoms in cases of tumor of the frontal lobe. Arch Neurol Psychiatry 1935;33:986–1005.

Streletz LJ, Cracco J. The effect of isoprinosine in subacute sclerosing panencephalitis (SSPE). Ann Neurol 1977;1:183–184.

Strich SJ. Diffuse degeneration of the cerebral white matter in severe dementia following head injury. J Neurol Neurosurg Psychiatry 1956;19:163–185.

Strich SJ. Shearing of nerve fibers as a cause of brain damage due to head injury. Lancet 1961;2:443–448.

Strobos RRJ, De La Toore E, Martin JF. Symmetrical calcification of the basal ganglia with familial ataxia and pigmentary macular degeneration. Brain 1957;80:313–318.

Stroop JR. Studies of interference in serial verbal reactions. J Exper Paychol 1935;18:643–662.

Strouth JC, Donahue S, Ross A, Aldred A. Neoplastic angioendotheliosis. Neurology 1965;15:644–648.

Strub RL. Acute confusional state. In: Benson DF, Blumer D, eds. Psychiatric aspects of neurologic disease. Vol. 2. Grune & Stratton, New York, 1982:1–21.

Strub RL, Black FW. The mental status examination in neurology. FA Davis, Philadelphia, 1977.

Strub RL, Black FW. Organic brain syndromes: an introduction to neurobehavioral disorders. FA Davis, Philadelphia, 1981.

Studler JM, Javoy-Agid F, Cesselin F, Legrand JC, Agid Y. CCK-8-immunoreactivity distribution in human brain: selective decrease in the substantia nigra from parkinsonian patients. Brain Res 1982;243:176–179.

Stumpf DA, Hayward A, Haas R, Frost M, Schaumburg HH. Adrenoleukodystrophy. Failure of immunosuppression to prevent neurological progression. Arch Neurol 1981;38:48–49.

Stusss DT, Benson DF. The Frontal Lobes. Raven Press, New York, 1986.

Stuteville P, Welch K. Subdural hematoma in the elderly person. JAMA 1958; 168:1445–1449.

Su PC, Goldensohn ES. Progressive supranuclear palsy. Electroencephalographic studies. Arch Neurol 1973;29:183–186.

Sudarsky L, Simon S. Gait disorder in late-life hydrocephalus. Arch Neurol 1987;44:263–267.

Sulkava R, Erkinjuntti T. Vascular dementia due to cardiac arrhythmias and systemic hypotension. Acta Neurol Scand 1987;76:123–128.

Sulkava R, Haltia M, Paetau A, Wikstrom J, Palo J. Accuracy of clinical diagnosis in primary degenerative dementia: correlation with neuropathological findings. J Neurol Neurosurg Psychiatry 1983;46:9–13.

Sulkava R, Koskimies S, Wikstrom J, Palo J. HLA antigens in Alzheimer's disease. Tissue Antigens 1980;16:191–194.

Sulkava R, Wikstrom J, Aromaa A, Raitasalo R, Lehtenen V, Lehtela K, Palo J. Prevalence of severe dementia in Finland. Neurology 1985;35:1025–1029.

Sullivan PA, Murnighan DJ, Callaghan N. Dialysis dementia: recovery after transplantation. Br Med J 1977;2:740.

Sultzer DL, Cumings JL. Drug-induced mania—causative agents, clinical characteristics and management. Med Toxicol Adv Drug Exp 1989;4:127–143.

Summers WK, Majovski LV, March GM, Tachiki K, Kling A. Oral tetrahydroaminoacridine in long-term treatment of senile dementia, Alzheimer type. N Engl J Med 1986;315:1241–1245.

Summers WK, Viesselman JO, Marsh GM, Candelorg K. Use of THA in treatment of Alzheimer-like dementia: pilot study in twelve patients. Biol Psychiatry 1981;16:145–153.

Summerskill WHJ. Aguecheek's disease. Lancet 1955;2:288.

Sunderland T, Rubinow DR, Tariot PN, Cohen RM, Newhouse PA, Mellow AM, Mueller EA, Murphy DL. CSF somatostatin in patients with Alzheimer's disease, older depressed patients, and age-matched control subjects. Am J Psychiatry 1987;144:1313–1316.

Suranyi-Cadotte BE, Nestoros JN, Nair NPV, Lai S, Gauthier S. Parkinsonism induced by high doses of diazepam. Biol Psychiatry 1985;20:451–460.

Surridge D. An investigation into some psychiatric aspects of multiple sclerosis. Br J Psychiatry 1969;115:749–764.

Susac JO, Hardman JM, Selhorst JB. Microangiopathy of the brain and retina. Neurology 1979;29:313–316.

Suter CC, Westmoreland BF, Sharbrough FW, Hermann RC Jr. Electroencephalographic abnormalities in interferon encephalopathy: a preliminary report. Mayo Clin Proc 1984;59:847–850.

Suzuki J, Takaku A. Cerebrovascular "Moyamoya" disease. Arch Neurol 1969;20:288–299.

Suzuki K, Chen G. Chemical studies on Jakob-Creutzfeldt disease. J Neuropathol Exp Neurol 1966;25:396–408.

Suzuki K, David E, Kutschman B. Presenile dementia with "lafora-like" intraneuronal inclusions. Arch Neurol 1971;25:69–80.

Suzuki K, Katzman R, Korey SR. Chemical studies on Alzheimer's disease. J Neuropathol Exp Neurol 1965;24:211–224.

Suzuki K, Terry RD. Fine structure localization of acid phosphatase in senile plaques in Alzheimer's presenile dementia. Acta Neuropathol 1967;8:276–281.

Suzuki S, Kobayashi T, Goto I, Kuroiwa Y. Dietary treatment of adrenoleukodystrophy. Neurology 1986;36:104–106.

Swain JM. Electroencephalographic abnormalities in presenile atrophy. Neurology 1959;9:722–727.

Swanson JW. Multiple sclerosis: update in diagnosis and review of prognostic factors. Mayo Clin Proc 1989;64:577–586.

Swanson JW, Kelly JJ Jr, McConahey WM. Neurologic aspects of thyroid dysfunction. Mayo Clin Proc 1981;56:504–512.

Swanson PD, Cromwell LD. Magnetic resonance imaging in cerebrotendinous xanthomatosis. Neurology 1986;36:124–126.

Swanson PD, Luttrell CN, Magladery JW. Myoclonus—a report of 67 cases and review of the literature. Medicine 1962;41:339–356.

Swash M, Roberts AH, Zakko H, Heathfield KWG. Treatment of involuntary movement disorders with tetrabenazine. J Neurol Neurosurg Psychiatry 1972;35:186–191.

Swearer JM, Drachman DA, O'Donnell BF, Mitchell AL. Troublesome and disruptive behaviors in dementia. J Am Geriatr Soc 1988;36:784–790.

Sweeney VP, Perry TL, Price JDE, Reeve CE, Godolphin WJ, Kish SJ. Brain gamma-aminobutyric acid deficiency in dialysis encephalopathy. Neurology 1985;35:180–184.

Sweet RD, McDowell FH, Feigenson JS, Loranger AW, Goodell H. Mental symptoms in Parkinson's disease during chronic treatment with levodopa. Neurology 1976;26:305–310.

Sydenstricker VP. The neurological complications of malnutrition. Psychic manifestations of nicotinic acid deficiency. Proc R Soc Med 1943;36:169–171.

Symon L, Dorsch NWC, Stephens RJ. Pressure waves in so-called low pressure hydrocephalus. Lancet 1972;2:1291–1292.

Symonds C. Disorders of memory. Brain 1966;89:625–644.

Syndulko K, Gilden ER, Hansch EC, Potvin AR, Tourtellotte WW, Potvin JH. Decreased verbal memory associated with anticholinergic treatment in Parkinson's disease patients. Intern J Neuroscience 1981;14:61–66.

Syndulko K, Hansch EC, Cohen SN, et al. Long-latency event-related potentials in normal aging and dementia. In: Courjan J, Mauguiere F, Revol M, eds. Clinical applications of evoked potentials in neurology. Raven Press, New York, 1982:279–285.

Sypert GW, Leffman H, Ojemann GA. Occult normal pressure hydrocephalus manifested by parkinsonism-dementia complex. Neurology 1973;23:234–238.

Tabaton M, Whitehouse PJ, Perry G, Davies P, Autilio-Gambetti L, Gambetti P. Alz 50 recognizes abnormal filaments in Alzheimer's disease and progressive supranuclear palsy. Ann Neurol 1988;24:407–413.

Taber LH, Greenberg SB, Perez FL, Couch RB. Herpes simplex encephalitis treated with Vidarabine (adenine arabinoside). Arch Neurol 1977;34:608–610.

Taclob L, Needle M. Drug-induced encephalopathy in patients on maintenance haemodialysis. Lancet 1976;2:704–705.

Takahashi H, Ohama E, Naito H, Takeda S, Nakashima S, Makifuchi T, Ikuta F. Hereditary dentatorubral-pallidoluysian atrophy: clinical and pathologic variants in a family. Neurology 1988;38:1065–1070.

Talalla A. Halbrook H, Barbour BH, Kurze T. Subdural hematoma associated with long-term hemodialysis for chronic renal disease. JAMA 1970;212:1847–1849.

Talland GA. Cognitive function in Parkinson's disease. J Nerv Ment Dis 1962;135:196–205.

Talland GA, Schwab RS, Performance with multiple sets in Parkinson's disease. Neuropsychology 1964;2:45–53.

Talley BJ, Faber R. Mitochondrial encephalomyopathic dementia in a young adult. Neuropsychiatry Neuropsychol Behav Neurol 1989;2:49–60.

Tanahashi N, Meyer JS, Ishikawa Y, Kandula P, Mortel KF, Rogers RL, Gandhi S, Walker M. Cerebral blood flow and cognitive testing correlate in Huntington's disease. Arch Neurol 1985;42:1169–1175.

Taquet H, Javoy-Agid F, Cesselin F, Hamon M, Legrand JC, Agid Y. Microtopography of methionine-enkephalin, dopamine and noradrenalin in the ventral mesencephalon of human control and parkinsonian brains. Brain Res 1982; 235:303–314.

Tariska I. Circumscribed cerebral atrophy in Alzheimer's disease: a pathological study. In: Wolstenholme GEW, O'Connor M, eds. Alzheimer's disease and related conditions. J & A Churchill, London, 1970:51–69.

Tarsy D, Bralower M. Deanol acetamidobenzoate treatment in choreiform movement disorders. Arch Neurol 1977;34:756–758.

Tarsy D, Holden EM, Segarra JM, Calabresi P, Feldman RG. 5-iodo-2'-deoxyuridine (IUDR;NSC-39661) given intraventricularly in the treatment of progressive multifocal leukoencephalopathy. Cancer Chemother Rep 1973;57:73–78.

Tarsy D, Lieberman B, Chirico-Post J, Benson DF. Unilateral asterixis associated with mesencephalic syndrome. Arch Neurol 1977;34:446–447.

Taylor AE, Saint-Cyr JA, Lang AE. Frontal lobe dysfunction in Parkinson's disease. The cortical focus of neostriatal outflow. Brain 1986;109:845–883.

Taylor AE, Saint-Cyr JA, Lange AE. Parkinson's disease. Cognitive changes in relation to treatment response. Brain 1987;110:35–51.

Taylor JR, Calabrese VP, Blanke RV. Organochlorine and other insecticides. In: Vinken PJ, Bruyn GW, eds. Intoxications of the nervous system. Part I, vol. 36. Handbook of clinical neurology, North-Holland, New York, 1979:391–455.

Tellez-Nagel I, Wisniewski HM. Ultrastructure of neurofibrillary tangles in Steele-Richardson-Olszewski syndrome. Arch Neurol 1973;29:324–327.

Tennison MB, Bouldin TW, Whaley RA. Mineralization of the basal ganglia detected by CT in Hallervorden-Spatz syndrome. Neurology 1988;38:154–155.

Teri L, Larson EB, Reifler BV. Behavioral disturbance in dementia of the Alzheimer's type. J Am Geriatr Soc 1988;36:1–6.

Terrence CF, Delaney JF, Alberts MC. Computed tomography for Huntington's disease. Neuroradiology 1977;13:173–175.

Terry RD. Ultrastructural alterations in senile dementia. In: Katzman R, Terry RD, Bick KL, eds. Alzheimer's disease, senile dementia and related disorders. Raven Press, New York, 1978:375–382.

Terry RD, Gonatas NK, Weiss M. Ultrastructure studies in Alzheimer's presenile dementia. Am J Pathol 1964;44:269–297.

Terry RD, Peck A, DeTeresa R, Schechter R, Horoupian DS. Some morphometric aspects of the brain in senile dementia of the Alzheimer type. Ann Neurol 1981;10:184–192.

Terzano MG, Montanari E, Calzetti S, Mancia D, Lechi A. The effect of amantadine on arousal and EEG patterns in Creutzfeldt-Jakob disease. Arch Neurol 1983;40:555–559.

Terzian H, Dalle Ore G. Syndrome of Klüver and Bucy. Neurology 1955;5:373–380

Testa HJ, Snowden JS, Neary D, Shields RA, Burjan AWI, Prescott MC, Northen B, Goulding P. The use of [^{99m} Tc]-HM-PAO in the diagnosis of primary degenerative dementia. J Cerebral Blood Flow and Metabolism 1988;8:S123–S126.

Tetrud JW, Langston JW. The effect of deprenyl (selegiline) on the natural history of Parkinson's disease. Science 1989;245:519–522.

Teuber H-L, Proctor F. Some effects of basal ganglia lesions in subhuman primates and man. Neuropsychology 1964;2:85–93.

Thal LJ. Changes in cerebrospinal fluid associated with dementia. Ann New York Acad Sci 1985;444:235–241.

Thal LJ, Grundman M, Klauber MR. Dementia. characteristics of a referral population and factors associated with progression. Neurology 1988;38:1083–1090.

Theander S, Grenholm L. Sequelae after spontaneous subarachnoid hemorrhage with special reference to hydrocephalus and Korsakoff's syndrome. Acta Neurol Scand 1967;43:479–488.

Theodore WH, Gendelman S. Meningeal carcinomatosis. Arch Neurol 1981;38:696–699.

Thiebaut, F. Sydenham's chorea. In: Vinken PJ, Bruyn GW, eds. Diseases of the basal ganglia. Vol 6. Handbook of clinical neurology. American Elsevier, New York; 1968:409–434.

Thienhaus OJ, Zemlan FP, Bienenfeld D, Hartford JT, Bosmann HB. Growth hormone response to edrophonium in Alzheimer's disease. Am J Psychiatry 1987;144:1049–1052.

Thomas FB, Mazzaferri EL, Skillman TG. Apathetic thyrotoxicosis: a distinctive clinical and laboratory entity. Ann Intern Med 1970;72:679–685.

Thomas JE, Schirger A. Idiopathic orthostatic hypotension. Arch Neurol 1970;22:289–293.

Thompson PD, Marsden CD. Gait disorder of subcortical arteriosclerotic encephalopathy: Binswanger's disease. Movement Disorders 1987;2:1–8.

Thompson TL II, Moran MG, Nies AS. Psychotropic drug use in the elderly. N Engl J Med 1983;308:134–138,194–199.

Thompson WG, Babitz L, Cassino C, Freedman M, Lipkin M Jr. Evaluation of current criteria used to measure vitamin B_{12} levels. Am J Med 1987;82:291–294.

Thomsen AM, Borgeson SE, Bruhn P, Gjerris F. Prognosis of dementia in normal pressure hydrocephalus after a shunt operation. Ann Neurol 1986;20:304–310.

Thornton WE. Dementia induced by methyldopa and haloperidol. N Engl J Med 1976;294:1222.

Thorpe FT. Pick's disease (circumscribed senile atrophy) and Alzheimer's disease. J Ment Sci 1932;78:302–314.

Thorpe FT. Familial degeneration of the cerebellum in association with epilepsy. Brain 1935;58:97–114.

Tierney MC, Fisher RH, Lewis AJ, Zorzitto ML, Snow WG, Reid DW, Nieustraten. The NINCDS-ADRDA Work Group criteria for the clinical diagnosis of probable Alzheimer's disease: a clinicopathologic study of 57 cases. Neurology 1988;38:359–364.

Tierney MC, Snow G, Reid DW, Zorzitto ML, Fisher RH. Psychometric differentiation of dementia. Arch Neurol 1987;44:720–722.

Timberlake WH, Vance MA. Four-year treatment of patients with parkinsonism using amantadine alone or with levodopa. Ann Neurol 1978;3:119–128.

Tintner R, Brown P, Hedley-Whyte ET, Rappaport EB, Piccardo CP, Gajdusek DC. Neuropathologic verification of Creutzfeldt-Jakob disease in the exhumed American recipient of human pituitary growth hormone: epidemiologic and pathogenetic implications. Neurology 1986;36:932–936.

Tishler PV, Woodward B, O'Connor J, Holbrook DA, Seidman LJ, Hallett M, Knighton DJ. High prevalence of intermittent acute porphyria in a psychiatric patient population. Am J Psychiatry 1985;142:1430–1436.

Tissenbaum MJ, Harter HM, Friedman AP. Organic neurological syndromes diagnosed as functional disorders. N Engl J Med 1951;147:1519–1521.

Tobo M, Mitsuyama Y, Ikari K, Itoi K. Familial occurrence of adult-type neuronal ceroid lipofuscinosis. Arch Neurol 1984;41:1091–1094.

Tom MI, Richardson JC. Hypoglycaemia from islet cell tumor of pancreas with amyotrophy and cerebrospinal nerve cell changes. J Neuropathol Exp Neurol 1951;10:57–66.

Tomlinson BE. The pathology of dementia. In: Wells CE, ed. Dementia. 2nd ed. FA Davis, Philadelphia, 1977:113–153.

Tomlinson BE, Blessed G, Roth M. Observations on the brains of demented old people. J Neurol Sci 1970;11:205–242.

Tomlinson BE, Kitchner D. Granulovacuolar degeneration of hippocampal pyramidal cells. J Pathol 1972;106:165–185.

Tomlinson BE, Pierides AM, Bradley WG. Central pontine myelinolysis. Q J Med 1976;45:373–386.

Tomlinson BE, Walton JN. Superficial haemosiderosis of the central nervous system. J Neurol Neurosurg Psychiat 1964;27:332–339.

Tomonaga M. Ultrastructure of neurofibrillary tangles in progressive supranuclear palsy. Acta Neuropathol 1977;37:177–181.

Toole JF, Patel AN. Cerebrovascular disorders. 2nd ed. McGraw-Hill, New York; 1974.

Toone B. Psychoses of epilepsy. In: Reynolds EH, Trimble MR, eds. Epilepsy and psychiatry. Churchill Livingstone, New York, 1981:113–137.

Toro G, Roman G. Cerebral malaria. Arch Neurol 1978;35:271–275.

Torvik A, Endresen GKM, Abrahamsen AF, Godal HC. Progressive dementia caused by an unusual type of generalized small vessel thrombosis. Acta Neurol Scand 1971;47:137–150.

Tourtellotte WW. Cerebrospinal fluid in multiple sclerosis. In: Vinken PJ, Bruyn GW, eds. Multiple sclerosis and other demyelinating diseases. Vol. 9. Handbook of clinical neurology. American Elsevier, New York, 1970:324–382.

Tourtellotte WW, Ma Bl, Brandes DB, Walsh MJ, Potvin AR. Quantification of de novo central nervous system IgG measles antibody synthesis in SSPE. Ann Neurol 1981;9:551–556.

Towfighi J. Early Pick's disease. A light and ultrastructural study. Acta Neuropathol 1972;21:224–231.

Townsend JJ, Baringer JR, Wolinsky JS, et al. Progressive rubella panencephalitis. N Engl J Med 1975;292:990–993.

Townsend JJ, Stroop WG, Baringer JR, Wolinsky JS, McKerrow JH, Berg BO. Neuropathology of progressive rubella panencephalitis after childhood rubella. Neurology 1982;32:185–190.

Townsend JJ, Wolinsky JS, Baringer JR. The neuropathology of progressive rubella panencephalitis of late onset. Brain 1976;99:81–90.

Traub R, Gajdusek DC, Gibbs CJ Jr. Transmissible virus dementia: the relation of transmissible spongiform encephalopathy to Creutzfeldt-Jakob disease. In: Smith WL, Kinsbourne M, eds. Aging and dementia. Spectrum, New York, 1977:91–146.

Trauner DA. Olivopontocerebellar atrophy with dementia, blindness, and chorea. Arch Neurol 1985;42:757–758.

Trautner RJ, Cummings JL, Read SL, Benson DF. Idiopathic basal ganglia calcification and organic mood disorder. Am J Psychiatry 1988;145:350–353.

Trelles JO. Cerebral cysticercosis. World Neurol 1961;2:488–494.

Treptow KR, Affleck DG, Roehl CA, Soelling WM, Nylidrin hydrochloride in senile arteriosclerosis. Arch Neurol 1963;9:142–146.

Tresch DD, Folstein MF, Rabins PV, Hazzard WR. Prevalence and significance of cardiovascular disease and hypertension in elderly patients with dementia and depression. J Am Geriatr Soc 1985;33:530–537.

Trethowan WH, Cobb S, Neuropsychiatric aspects of Cushing's syndrome. Arch Neurol Psychiatry 1952;67:283–309.

Treves T, Korczyn AD, Zilber N, Kahann E, Leibowitz Y, Alter M, Schoenberg BS. Presenile dementia in Israel. Arch Neurol 1986;43:26–29.

Trimble M. Neuropsychiatry. John Wiley & Sons, New York, 1981.

Trimble MR, Corbett JA, Donaldson D. Folic acid and mental symptoms in children with epilepsy. J Neurol Neurosurg Psychiatry 1980;43:1030–1034.

Trimble MR, Cummings JL. Neuropsychiatric disturbances following brainstem lesions. Br J Psychiatry 1981;138:56–59.

Trimble MR, Reynolds EH. Anticonvulsant drugs and mental symptoms: a review. Psychol Med 1976;6:169–178.

Troost BT, Daroff RB. The ocular motor defects in progressive supranuclear palsy. Ann Neurol 1977;2:397–403.

Troost BT, Daroff RB, Dell'Osso LF. Quantitative analysis of the ocular motor deficit in progressive supranuclear palsy (PSP). Trans Am Neurol Assoc 1976;101:60–64.

Truex RC, Carpenter MB. Human neuroanatomy. 6th ed. Williams & Wilkins, Baltimore, 1969.

Tschudy DP, Valsamis M, Magnussen CR. Acute intermittent porphyria: clinical and selected research aspects. Ann Intern Med 1975;83:851–864.

Tsukamoto T, Yamamoto H, Iwasaki Y, Yoshie O, Terunuma H, Suzuki H. Antineural autoantibodies in patients with paraneoplastic cerebellar degeneration. Arch Neurol 1989;46:1225–1229.

Tu J-b, Blackwell RQ, Hou T-y. Tissue copper levels in Chinese patients with Wilson's disease. Neurology 1963;13:155–159.

Tu J-b, Copper WC, Blackwell RQ, Hou T-y. Treatment of hepatolenticular degeneration (Wilson's disease) in the asymptomatic stage. Neurology 1965;15:402–408.

Tune L, Gucker S, Folstein M, Oshida L, Coyle JT. Cerebrospinal fluid acetylcholinesterase activity in senile dementia of the Alzheimer type. Ann Neurol 1985;17:46–48.

Turner B. Pathology of paralysis agitans. In: Vinken PJ, Bruyn GW, eds. Diseases of the basal ganglia. Vol. 6. Handbook of clinical neurology. American Elsevier, New York, 1968:212–217.

Tweedy J. Reding M. Garcia C, Schulman P, Deutsch G, Antin S. Significance of cortical disinhibition signs. Neurology 1982;32:169–173.

Tyler HR. Neurological complications of dialysis, transplantation, and other forms of treatment in chronic uremia. Neurology 1965;15:1081–1088.

Tyler HR. Abnormalities of perception with defective eye movements (Balint's syndrome). Cortex 1968a;4:154–171.

Tyler HR. Neurologic disorders in renal failure. Am J Med 1968b;44:734–748.

Tyndel M. Some aspects of the Ganser state. J Ment Sci 1956;102:324–329.

Tynes BS, Crutcher JC, Utz TP. Histoplasma meningitis. Ann Intern Med 1963;59:615–621.

Tyrer JH. Friedreich's ataxia. In: Vinken PJ, Bruyn GW, eds. System disorders and atrophies. Part I, vol. 21. Handbook of clinical neurology. American Elsevier, New York, 1975:319–364.

Udani PM, Dastur DK. Tuberculous encephalopathy with and without meningitis. Clinical features and pathological correlations. J Neurol Sci 1970;10:541–561.

Udvarhelyi GB, Wood JH, James AE Jr, Bartelt D. Results and complications in 55 shunted patients with normal pressure hydrocephalus. Surg Neurol 1975;3:271–275.

Uhl GR, Hilt DC, Hedreen JC, Whitehouse PJ, Price DL. Pick's disease (lobar sclerosis): depletion of neurons in the nucleus basalis of Meynert. Neurology 1983;33:1470–1473.

Ungerstedt U. Stereotaxic mapping of the monoamine pathways in the rat brain. Acta Physiol Scand 1971;(suppl 367):1–48.

Upton A, Gumpert J. Electroencephalography in diagnosis of herpes-simplex encephalitis. Lancet 1970;1:650–652.

Utz JP. Histoplasma and cryptococcus meningitis. Res Publ Assoc Res Nerv Ment Dis 1964;44:378–388.

Utz JP. The mycoses. In: Beeson PB, McDermott W, eds. Cecil-Loeb: textbook of medicine. 13th ed. WB Saunders, Philadelphia, 1971:683–698.

Uyematsu S. On the pathology of senile psychosis. J Nerv Ment Dis 1923;57:1–25, 131–156, 237–260.

Uzman LL, Jakus MA. The Kayser-Fleischer ring. Neurology 1957;7:341–355.

Vakili S, Drew AL, Von Schuching S, Becker D, Zeman W. Hallervorden-Spatz syndrome. Arch Neurol 1977;34:729–738.

Valenstein E, Rosman NP, Carter AP. Schilder's disease. JAMA 1971;217:1699–1700.

Vallarta JM, Bell DB, Reichert A. Progressive encephalopathy due to chronic hydantoin intoxication. Am J Dis Child 1974;128:27–34.

Valpey R, Sumi M, Copass MK, Goble GJ. Acute and chronic progressive encephalopathy due to gasoline sniffing. Neurology 1978;28:507–510.

Van Bogaert L. DeWulf A. Diffuse progressive leukodystrophy in the adult. Arch Neurol Psychiatry 1939;42:1083–1097.

Vanderzant C, Bromberg M, MacGuire A, McCune J. Isolated small-vessel angiitis of the central nervous system. Arch Neurol 1988;45:683–687.

Van Gorp W, Cummings JL, Mitrushina M, Satz P, Buckingham S. Normal aging and the subcortical encephalopathy of AIDS: A neuropsychological comparison. Paper presented at the IV International Conference on AIDS, Stockholm, 1988.

Van Gorp W, Mitrushina M, Cummings JL, Satz P, Modesitt J. Normal aging and the subcortical encephalopathy of AIDS. Neuropsychiatry Neuropsychol Behav Neurol 1989;2:5–20.

Van Gorp W, Satz P, Mitrushina M. Neuropsychological processes associated with normal aging. Develop Neuropsychol 1990;5:279–290.

Van Gorp WG, Mahler MM. Subcortical features of normal aging. In Subcortical Dementia. Cummings JL, ed. Oxford University Press, New York, 1990:231–250.

Van Horn G, Bastian FO, Moake JL. Progressive multifocal leukoencephalopathy: failure of response to transfer factor and cytarabine. Neurology 1978;28:794–797.

Vanneste J, Hyman R. Non-tumoral aqueduct stenosis and normal pressure hydrocephalus in the elderly. J Neurol Neurosurg Psychiatry 1986;49:529–535.

Van Putten T, Mutalipassi LR, Malkin MD. Phenothiazine-induced decompensation. Arch Gen Psychiatry 1974;30:102–105.

Vartdal F, Vandvik B, Michaelsen TE, Loe K, Norrby E. Neurosyphilis: intrathecal synthesis of oligoclonal antibodies to treponoma pallidum. Ann Neurol 1982;11:35–40.

Vejjajiva A, Foster JB, Miller H. Motor neuron disease. A clinical study. J Neurol Sci 1967;4:299–314.

Vereker R. The psychiatric aspects of temporal arteritis. J Ment Sci 1957;98:280–286.

Verity MA, Wechsler AF. Progressive subcortical gliosis of Neumann: a clinicopathologic study of two cases with review. Arch Gerontol Geriatr 1987;6:245–261.

Vernon RJ, Ferguson RK. Effects of trichloroethylene on visual-motor performance. Arch Environ Health 1969;18:894–900.

Veroff AE. The neuropsychology of aging. Psychological Research 1980;41:259–268.

Verwoerdt A. Individual psychotherapy in senile dementia. In: Miller NE, Cohen GD, eds. Clinical aspects of Alzheimer's disease and senile dementia. Raven Press, New York, 1981;187–208.

Vesalius A. Opera omnia anatomica et chirurgica. Cura Hermanni Boerhoave et Bernhardi Siegfried Albini. Vol. 1. Lugd Bat, J du Vivie et J. et H Verbeek, 1725:16.

Vick N, Schulman S, Dau P. Carcinomatous cerebellar degeneration, encephalomyelitis, and sensory neuropathy (radiculitis). Neurology 1969;19:425–441.

Victor M. Neurologic changes in liver disease. Res Publ Assoc Nerv Ment Dis 1974;53:1–12.

Victor M. Neurologic disorders due to alcoholism and malnutrition. In: Baker AB, Baker LH, eds. Clinical neurology. Harper & Row, New York, 1979:1–83.

Victor M, Adams RD, Cole M. The acquired (non-Wilsonian) type of chronic hepatocerebral degeneration. Medicine 1965;44:345–396.

Victor M, Adams RD, Collins GH. The Wernicke-Korsakoff syndrome. FA Davis, Philadelphia, 1971.

Victor M, Hope JM. The phenomenon of auditory hallucinations in chronic alcoholism. J Nerv Ment Dis 1958;126:451–481.

Victor M. Lear AA. Subacute combined degeneration of the spinal cord. Am J Med 1956;20:896–911.

Victor M, Yakovlev PI. SS Korsakoff's psychic disorder in conjunction with peripheral neuritis. Neurology 1955;5:394–406.

Victoratos GC, Lenman JAR, Herzberg L. Neurological investigation of dementia. Br J Psychiatry 1977;130:131–133.

Vigliani EC. Carbon disulfide poisoning in viscose rayon factories. Br J Ind Med 1954;11:235–244.

Vignaendra V, Lin CL, Chen ST. Subacute sclerosing panencephalitis with unusual ocular movements: polygraphic studies. Neurology 1978;28:1052–1056.

Vinters HV, Hudson AJ, Kaufmann JCE. Gerstmann-Straussler-Scheinker disease: autopsy study of a familial case. Ann Neurol 1986;20:540–543.

Visser SL, Stam FC, van Tilburg W, Den Velde OP. Blom JL, De Rijke W. Visual evoked response in senile and presenile dementia. Electroencephalogr Clin Neurophysiol 1976;40:385–392.

Visser SL, van Tilburg W, Jonker C, De Rijke. Visual evoked potentials (VEPs) in senile dementia (Alzheimer's type) and in non-organic behavioural disorders in the elderly: comparison with EEG parameters. Electroenceph Clin Neurophysiol 1985;60:115–121.

Vita G. Dattola R, Santoro M, Toscano A, Ventuo C, Carrozza G. Baradello A.

Peripheral neuropathy in amyotrophic chorea-acanthocytosis. Ann Neurol 1989;26:583–587.

Vollersten RS, McDonald TJ, Young BR, Banks PM, Stanson AW, Ilstrup DM. Cogan's syndrome: 18 cases and a review of the literature. Mayo Clin Proc 1986;61:344–361.

Voltoline EJ, Thompson SI, Tisue J. Acute organic brain syndrome with propranolol. Clin Toxicol 1971;4:357–359.

Voris HC. Postmeningitic hydrocephalus. Neurology 1955;5:72–75.

Voris HC. Craniocerebral trauma. In: Baker AB, Baker LH, eds. Clinical neurology. Harper & Row, New York, 1976:1–45.

Vroom FQ, Greer M. Mercury vapour intoxication. Brain 1972;95:305–318.

Wada T, Yoshida T, Sakurada S, Sato K. Myoclonus epilepsy: clinical and electroencephalographical study on hereditary and pathophysiological factors. Folia Psychiatr Neurol Jpn 1960;14:268–281.

Wade JPH, Mirsen TR, Hachinski VC, Fisman M, Lau C, Merskey H. The clinical diagnosis of Alzheimer's disease. Arch Neurol 1987;44:24–29.

Wadia NH, Swami RK. A new form of heredofamilial spinocerebellar degeneration with slow eye movements (nine families). Brain 1971;94:359–374.

Wadia NH, Williams E. Behcet's syndrome with neurological complications. Brain 1957;80:59–71.

Wagshul A, Daroff RB. L-dopa for progressive supranuclear palsy. Lancet 1969;2:105–106.

Waldenström J. Acute thyrotoxic encephalo- or myopathy, its cause and treatment. Acta Med Scand 1945;121:251–294.

Walker AE, Diamond EL, Moseley J. The neuropathological findings in irreversible coma. J Neuropathol Exp Neurol 1975;34:295–323.

Wallack EM, Revis WM Jr, Hall CD. Primary brain stem retriculum cell sarcoma causing dementia. Dis Nerv Sys 1977;38:744–747.

Walsh AC. Arterial insufficiency of the brain: progression prevented by long-term anticoagulant therapy in eleven patients. J Am Geriatr Soc 1969a;17:93–104.

Walsh AC. Prevention of senile and presenile dementia by bishydroxy-coumarin (Dicumarol) therapy. J Am Geriatr Soc 1969b;17:477–487.

Walsh AC, Walsh BH. Presenile dementia: further experience with an anticoagulant-psychotherapy regimen. J Am Geriatr Soc 1974;22:467–472.

Walsh FB, Hoyt WF. Clinical neuro-opthalmology. 3rd ed. Williams & Wilkins, Baltimore, 1969.

Walsh KW. Neuropsychology. A clinical approach. Churchill Livingstone, New York, 1978:312–316.

Walshe JM. The physiology of copper in man and its relation to Wilson's disease. Brain 1967;90:149–176.

Walton JN, Gardner-Medwin D. Progressive muscular dystrophy and the myotonic disorders. In: Walton JN, ed. Disorders of voluntary muscle. 3rd ed. Churchill Livingstone, New York, 1974:561–613.

Waltz G, Harik SI, Kaufman B. Adult metachromatic leukodystrophy. Value of computed tomographic scanning and magnetic resonance imaging of the brain. Arch Neurol 1987;44:225–227.

Wanzer SH, Adelstein SJ, Cranford RE, Federman DD, Hook ED, Moertel CG,

Safar P, Stone A, Taussig HB, van Eys J. The physician's responsibility toward hopelessly ill patients. N Engl J Med 1984;310:955–959.

Warburton JW. Depressive symptoms in parkinsonism patients referred for thalamotomy. J Neurol Neurosurg Psychiatry 1967a;30:368–370.

Warburton JW. Memory disturbance and the Parkinson syndrome. Br J Med Psychol 1967b;40:169–171.

Warren KG, Ball MJ, Paty DW, Banna M. Computer tomography in disseminated sclerosis. J Can Sci Neurol 1976;3:211–216.

Wasch HH, Estrin WJ, Yip P, Bowler R, Cone JE. Prolongation of the P-300 latency associated with hydrogen sulfide exposure. Arch Neurol 1989;46:902–904.

Waters BGH, Lapierre YD. Secondary mania associated with sympathomimetic drug use. Am J Psychiatry 1981;138:837–838.

Waters C. Cognitive enhancing agents: current status in the treatment of Alzheimer's disease. Can J Neurol Sci 1988;15:249–256.

Watson CP. Clinical similarity of Alzheimer and Creutzfeldt-Jakob disease. Ann Neurol 1979;6:368–369.

Watson CW, Denny-Brown D. Myoclonus epilepsy as a symptom of diffuse neuronal disease. Arch Neurol Psychiatry 1953;70:151–168.

Weaver JA, Jones A, Smith RA. Thyrotoxic coma (apathetic crisis). Br Med J 1956;1:20–23.

Weber FP, Greenfield JG. Cerebello-olivary degeneration: an example of heredo-familial incidence. Brain 1942;65:220–231.

Wechsler AF. Presenile dementia presenting as aphasia. J Neurol Neurosurg Psychiatry 1977;40:303–305.

Wechsler AF, Verity M, Rosenschein S, Fried I, Scheibel AB. Pick's disease. Arch Neurol 1982;39:287–290.

Wechsler D. A standardized memory scale for clinical use. J Psychol 1945;19:87–95.

Wechsler D. Manual for the Wechsler Adult Intelligence Scale. The Psychological Corporation, New York, 1955.

Weddington WW Jr. Dementia dialytica. Psychosomatics 1978;19:367–370.

Weed LH. Forces concerned in the absorption of CSF. An J Physiol 1935;114:40–45.

Weil ML. Infections of the nervous system. In: Menkes JH, ed. Textbook of child neurology. Lea & Febiger, Philadephia, 1974:213–282.

Weil ML, Itabashi HH, Cremer NE, Oshiro LS, Lennette EH, Carnay L. Chronic progressive panencephalitis due to rubella virus simulating subacute sclerosing panencephalitis. N Engl J Med 1975;292:994–998.

Weiler PG, Mungas D, Bernick C. Propranolol for the control of disruptive behavior in senile dementia. J Geriatr Psychiatry Neurol 1988;1:226–230.

Weinberger DR. The pathogenesis of schizophrenia: a neurodevelopmental theory. In: Nasrallah HA, Weinberger DR, eds. Handbook of Schizophrenia. Volume 1. The neurology of schizophrenia. Elsevier, New York, 1986;397–406.

Weinberger J, Gordon J, Hodson AK, Goldberg HI, Reivich M. Effect of intracerebral vasculitis on regional cerebral blood flow. Arch Neurol 1979;36:681–685.

Weiner H, Braiman A. The Ganser Syndrome. Am J Psychiatry 1955;111:767–773.

Weiner H, Schuster DB. The electroencephalogram in dementia—some preliminary observations and correlations. Electroencephalogr Clin Neurophysiol 1950;8:479–488.

Weiner LP, Konigsmark BW, Stall J Jr, Magladery JW. Hereditary olivocerebellar atrophy with retinal degeneration. Arch Neurol 1967;16:364–376.

Weingartner H. Burns S, Diebel R, LeWitt PA. Cognitive impairments in Parkinson's disease: distinguishing between effort-demanding and automatic cognitive processes. Psychiatry Res 1984;11:223–235.

Weingartner H, Caine ED, Ebert MH. Encoding processes, learning, and recall in Huntington's disease. Adv Neurol 1979;23:215–226.

Weingartner H, Cohen RM, Murphy DL, Martello J, Gerdt C. Cognitive processes in depression. Arch Gen Psychiatry 1981a;38:42–47.

Weingartner H, Kaye W, Smallberg SA, Ebert MH, Gilin JC, Sitaram N. Memory failures in progressive idiopathic dementia. J Abnor Psychol 1981b; 90:187–196.

Weinstein EA, Kahn RL. Non-aphasic misnaming (paraphasia) in organic brain disease. Arch Neurol Psychiatry 1952;67:72–79.

Weisberg LA. Cerebral computerized tomography in intracranial inflammatory disorders. Arch Neurol 1980;37:137–142.

Weisberg LA. Lacunar infarcts. Arch Neurol 1982;39:37–40.

Weiss AD. Sensory functions. In: Brinen TE, ed. Handbook of aging and the individual. University of Chicago Press, Chicago, 1959.

Weiss GM, Nelson RL, O'Neill BP, Carney A, Edis AJ. Use of adrenal biopsy in diagnosing adrenoleukomyeloneuropathy. Arch Neurol 1980;37:634–636.

Weiss HD, Walker MD, Wiernik PH. Neurotoxicity of commonly used antineoplastic agents. N. Engl J Med 1974;291:75–81, 127–133.

Weiss JH, Choi DW. Beta-N-methylamino-L-alanine neurotoxicity: requirement for bicarbonate as a cofactor. Science 1988;241:973–975.

Welford AT. Motor performance. In: Birren JE, Schaie KW, eds. Handbook of the psychology of aging. Charles C Thomas, Springfield, Ill., 1965.

Wells CE. Pseudodementia. Am J Psychiatry 1979;136:895–900.

Wells CE. A deluge of dementia. Psychosomatics 1981;22:837–838.

Wells CE, Duncan GW. Danger of overreliance on computerized cranial tomography. Am J Psychiatry 1977;134:811–13.

Wells CE, Silver RT. The neurologic manifestations of the acute leukemias: a clinical study. Ann Intern Med 1957;46:439–449.

Welsh JD, Cassidy D, Prigatano GP, Gunn CG. Chronic hepatic encephalopathy in a patient with lactose malabsorption. N Engl J Med 1974;291:240–241.

Welsh JE, Tyson GW, Winn HR, Jane JA. Chronic subdural hematoma presenting as transient neurologic deficits. Stroke 1979;10:564–567.

Welti W. Delirium with low serum sodium. Arch Neurol Psychiatry 1956;76:559–564.

Wernicke C. Acute hemorrhagic polioencephalitis superior. Bohne WHO, Rottenberg DA, trans. In: Rottenberg DA, Hochberg FH, eds. Neurological classics in modern translation. Hafner Press, New York, 1977:63–75.

Westmoreland BF, Gomez MR, Blume WT. Activation of periodic complexes of subacute sclerosing panencephalitis by sleep. Ann Neurol 1977;1:185–187.

Westmoreland BF, Sharbrough FW, Donat JR. Stimulus-induced EEG complexes and motor spasms in subacute sclerosing panencephalitis. Neurology 1979; 29:1154–1157.

Westreich G, Alter M. Lundgren S. Effect of cyclandelate on dementia. Stroke 1975;6:535–538.

Whalley LJ, Urbaniak SJ, Darg C, Peutherer JF, Christie JE. Histocompatibility antigens and antibodies to viral and other antigens in Alzheimer presenile dementia. Acta Psychiatr Scand 1980;61:1–7.

Wheelan L. Familial Alzheimer's disease. Ann Hum Genet 1959;23:300–310.

Whelihan WM, Lesher EL. Neuropsychological changes in frontal functions with aging. Develop Neuropsychol 1985;1:371–380.

White JC. Periodic EEG activity in subcortical arteriosclerotic encephalopathy (Binswanger's type). Arch Neurol 1979;36:485–489.

White JC, Cobb S. Psychological changes associated with giant pituitary neoplasms. Arch Neurol Psychiatry 1955;74:383–396.

White P. Goodhardt MJ, Keet JP, et al. Neocortical cholinergic neurons in elderly people. Lancet 1977;1:668–670.

Whitecar JP Jr. Bodey GP, Harris JE, Freireich EJ. L-asparaginase. N. Engl J Med 1970;282:732–734.

Whitehead A. Verbal learning and memory in elderly depressives. Br. J Psychiatry 1973;123:203–208.

Whitehouse PJ, Hedreen JC, White C, DeLong M, Price DL. Loss of neurons in the nucleus basalis in the dementia of Parkinson disease. Neurology 1982a; 32(2):A228.

Whitehouse PJ, Hedreen JC, White CL III, Price DL. Basal forebrain neurons in the dementia of Parkinson's disease. Ann Neurol 1983;1:243–248.

Whitehouse PJ, Martino AM, Marcus KA, Zweig RM, Singer HS, Price DL, Kellar KJ. Reductions in acetylcholine and nicotine binding in several degenerative diseases. Arch Neurol 1988;45:722–724.

Whitehouse PJ, Price DL, Clark AW, Coyle JT, DeLong MR. Alzheimer disease: evidence for selective loss of cholinergic neurons in the nucleus basalis. Ann Neurol 1981;10:122–126.

Whitehouse PJ, Price DL, Struble RG, Clark AW, Coyle JT, DeLong MR. Alzheimer's disease and senile dementia: loss of neurons in the basal forebrain. Science 1982b;215:1237–1239.

Whitehouse PJ, Trifiletti RR, Jones BE, Folstein S, Price DL, Snyder SH, Kuhar MJ. Neurotransmitter receptor alterations in Huntington's disease: autoradiographic and homogenate studies with special reference to benzodiazepine receptor complexes. Ann Neurol 1985;18:202–210.

Whitehouse PJ, Vale WW, Zweig RM, Singer HS, Mayeux R, Kuhar MJ, Price DL, De Souza EB. Reductions in corticotropin releasing factor-like immunoreactivity in cerebral cortex of Alzheimer's disease, Parkinson's disease, and progressive supranuclear palsy. Neurology 1987;37:905–909.

Whitfield CL, Ch'ien LT, Whitehead JD. Lead encephalopathy in adults. Am J Med 1972;52:289–298.

Whitley RJ, Soong S-j, Dolin R, et al. Adenine arabinoside therapy of biopsy-proved herpes simplex encephalitis. N Engl J Med 1977;297:289–294.

Whitley RJ, Soong S-j, Hirsch MS, et al. Herpes simplex encephalitis. N Engl J Med 1981;304:313–318.

Whitlock FA. The aetiology of hysteria. Acta Psychiatr Neurol Scand 1967a;43:144–162.

Whitlock FA. The Ganser syndrome. Br J Psychiatry 1967b;113:19–29.

Whitlock FA, Siskind MM. Depression as a major symptom of multiple sclerosis. J Neurol Neurosurg Psychiatry 1980;43:861–865.

Whittier J, Haydu G, Crawford J. Effect of imipramine (Tofranil) on depression and hyperkinesia in Huntington's disease. Am J Psychiatry 1961;118:79.

Whitty CWM. Mental changes as a presenting feature in subcortical cerebral lesions. J Ment Sci 1956;102:719–725.

Whitty CWM, Zangwill OL. Amnesia. Butterworths, Woburn, Mass., 1977:118–135.

Whitworth RH, Larson CM. Differential diagnosis and staging of Alzheimer's disease with an aphasia battery. Neuropsychiatry, Neuropsychol, Behav Neurol 1989;1:255–265.

Whybrow PC, Akiskal HS, McKinney WT Jr. Mood disorders. Toward a new psychobiology. Plenum Press, New York, 1984.

Whybrow PC, Prange AJ Jr, Treadway CR. Mental changes accompanying thyroid gland dysfunction. Arch Gen Psychiatry 1969;20:48–63.

Whytt R. Observations on the dropsy of the brain. Balfour, Auld & Smellie, Edinburgh, 1768.

Wiederholt WC, Siekert RG. Neurological manifestations of sarcoidosis. Neurology 1965;15:1147–1154.

Wiesert KN, Hendrie HC, Secondary mania? A case report. Am J Psychiatry 1977;134:929–930.

Wigboldus JM, Bruyn GW. Hallervorden-Spatz disease. In: Vinken PJ, Bruyn GW, eds. Diseases of the basal ganglia. Vol. 6. Handbook of clinical neurology. American Elsevier, New York, 1968:604–631.

Wikstrom J, Paetau A, Palo J, Sulkava R, Haltia M. Classic amyotrophic lateral sclerosis with dementia. Arch Neurol 1982;39:681–683.

Wilkins RH, Brody IA. Alzheimer's disease. Arch Neurol 1969;21:109–110.

Wilkinson HA, LeMay M, Drew JH. Adult aqueductal stenosis. Arch Neurol 1966;15:643–648.

Wilkinson IMS, Russell RWR. Arteritis of the head and neck in giant cell arteritis. Arch Neurol 1972;27:378–391.

Will RG, Lees AJ, Gibb W, Barnard RO. A case of progressive subcortical gliosis presenting clinically as Steele-Richardson-Olszewski syndrome. J Neurol Neurosurg Psychiatry 1988;51:1224–1227.

Will RG, Matthews WB. Evidence for case-to-case transmission of Creutzfeldt-Jakob disease. J Neurol Neurosurg Psychiatry 1982;45:235–238.

Williams D. The electroencephalogram in affective disorders. Proc R Soc Med 1954;47:779–782.

Williams FJB, Walshe JM. Wilson's disease. Brain 1981;104:735–752.

Williams GH, Dluhy RG. Diseases of the adrenal cortex. In: Braunwald E, Isselbacher KJ, Petersdorf RG, Wilson JD, Martin JB, Fauci AS, eds. Harrison's principles of internal medicine, 11th ed. McGraw-Hill, New York, 1987;1753–1754.

Williams HW. The peculiar cells of Pick's disease. Arch Neurol Psychiatry 1935;34:508–519.

Williams M, McGee TF. Psychological study of carotid occlusion and endarterectomy. Arch Neurol 1964;10:293–297.

Williams M, Smith HV. Mental disturbances in tuberculous meningitis. J Neurol Neurosurg Psychiatry 1954;17:173–182.

Williams RH. Metabolism and mentation. J Clin Endocrinol Metabol 1970;31:461–479.

Wilner EC, Brody JA. An evaluation of the remote effects of cancer on the nervous system. Neurology 1968;18:1120–1124.

Wilson CB, Bertan V. Perforation of the bowel complicating peritoneal shunt for hydrocephalus. Am Surg 1966;32:601–603.

Wilson RS, Fox JH, Huckman MS, Bacon LD, Lobick JJ. Computed tomography in dementia. Neurology 1982;32:1054–1057.

Wilson RS, Kasniak AW, Klawans HL, Garron DG. High-speed memory scanning in parkinsonism. Cortex 1980;16:67–72.

Wilson SAK. Progressive lenticular degeneration: a familial nervous disease associated with cirrhosis of the liver. Brain 1912;34:295–509.

Wilson WP, Musella L, Short MJ. The electroencephalogram in dementia. In: Wells CE, ed. Dementia. 2nd ed. FA Davis, Philadelphia, 1977:205–221.

Winblad B, Adolfson R, Carlsson A, Gottfries C-G. Biogenic amines in brains of patients with Alzheimer's disease. In: Corkin S, Davis KL, Growdon JH, Usdin E, Wurtman RJ. Alzheimer's disease: a report of progress in research. Raven Press, New York, 1982:25–33.

Winkleman NW, Book MH. Asymptomatic extrapyramidal involvement in Pick's disease. J Neuropathol Exp Neurol 1949;8:30–42.

Winkelman NW, Moore MT. Disseminated necrotizing panarteritis (periarteritis nodosa). J Neuropathol Exp Neurol 1950;9:60–77.

Winterstein CE. Head injuries attributable to boxing. Lancet 1937;2:719–720.

Wise D, Wallace HJ, Jellinek EH. Angiokeratoma corporis diffusum. Q J Med 1962;31:177–206.

Wisniewski HM, Coblentz JM, Terry RD. Pick's disease. A clinical and ultrastructural study. Arch Neurol 1972;26:97–108.

Wisniewski HM, Rabe A, Zignan W, Silverman W. Editorial: neuropathological diagnosis of Alzheimer disease. J Neuropath Exper Neurol 1989;48:606–609.

Wisniewski HM, Sturman JA, Shek JW. Aluminum chloride induced neurofibrillary changes in the developing rabbit: a chronic animal model. Ann Neurol 1980;8:479–490.

Wisniewski H, Terry RD, Hirano A. Neurofibrillary pathology. J Neuropathol Exp Neurol 1970;29:163–176.

Wisniewski K, Jervis GA, Moretz RC, Wisniewski HM. Alzheimer neurofibrillary tangles in diseases other than senile and presenile dementia. Ann Neurol 1979;5:288–294.

Wisniewski KE, Wisniewski HM, Wen GY. Occurrence of neuropathological changes and dementia of Alzheimer's disease in Down's syndrome. Ann Neurol 1985;17:278–282.

Wolff HG, Curran D. Nature of delirium and allied states. Arch Neurol Psychiatry 1935;33:1175–1215.

Wolfson LI, Leenders KL, Brown LL, Jones T. Alterations of regional cerebral blood flow and oxygen metabolism in Parkinson's disease. Neurology 1985;35:1399–1405.

Wolinsky JS, Barnes BD, Margolis MT. Diagnostic tests in normal pressure hydrocephalus. Neurology 1973;23:706–713.

Wolinsky JS, Berg BO, Maitland CJ. Progressive rubella panencephalitis. Arch Neurol 1976;33:722–723.

Wolinsky JS, Swoveland P, Johnson KP, Baringer JR. Subacute measles encephalitis complicating Hodgkin's disease in an adult. Ann Neurol 1977;1:452–457.

Wood JH, Bartlet D, James AE Jr, Udvarhelyi GB. Normal-pressure hydrocephalus: diagnosis and patient selection for shunt surgery. Neurology 1974;24:517–526.

Wood PL, Etienne P, Lal S, Nair NPV, Finlayson MH, Gauthier S, Palo J, Haltia M, Paetau A, Bird ED. A post-mortem comparison of the cortical cholinergic system in Alzheimer's disease and Pick's disease. J Neurol Sci 1983;62:211–217.

Woodward JS. Clinicopathologic significance of granulovacuolar degeneration in Alzheimer's disease. J Neuropathol Exp Neurol 1962;21:85–91.

Woodhouse MA, Dayan AD, Burston J, et al. Progressive multifocal leukoencephalopathy: electron microscope study of four cases. Brain 1967;90:863–870.

Woods BT, Schaumburg HH. Nigro-spino-dentatal degeneration with nuclear ophthalmoplegia. J Neurol Sci 1972;17:149–166.

Woodward JB III, Heaton RK, Simon DB, Ringel SP. Neuropsychological findings in myotonic dystrophy. J Clin Neuropsychol 1982;4:335–342.

Woodworth JA, Beckett RS, Netsky MG. A composite of hereditary ataxias. Arch Intern Med 1959;104:594–606.

Woolsey RM, Nelson JS. Progressive multifocal leukoencephalopathy. Neurology 1965;15:662–666.

Worster-Drought C, Greenfield JG, McMenemey WH. A form of familial presenile dementia with spastic paralysis. Brain 1940;63:237–254.

Worster-Drought C, Greenfield JG, McMenemey WH. A form of familial presenile dementia with spastic paralysis. Brain 1944;67:38–43.

Wragg RE, Jeste DV. Overview of depression and psychosis in Alzheimer's disease. Am J Psychiatry 1989;146:577–587.

Wu J-Y, Bird ED, Chen MS, Huang WM. Studies of neurotransmitter enzymes in Huntington's chorea. Adv Neurol 1979;23:527–536.

Wu S, Schenkenberg T, Wing SD, Osborn AG. Cognitive correlates of diffuse cerebral atrophy determined by computed tomography. Neurology 1981;31:1180–1184.

Wulff CH, Trojaborg W. Adult metachromatic leukodystrophy: neurophysiologic findings. Neurology 1985;35:1776–1778.

Yahr MD, Goldensohn SS, Kabat EA. Further studies on the gamma globulin content of cerebrospinal fluid in multiple sclerosis and other neurological diseases. Ann NY Acad Sci 1954;58:613–624.

Yakovlev PI. Paraplegias of hydrocephalics (a clinical note and interpretation). Am J Ment Defic 1947;51:561–576.

Yakovlev PI. Paraplegia in flexion of cerebral origin. J Neuropathol Exp Neurol 1954;13:267–296.

Yamaguchi F, Meyer JS, Yamamoto M, Sakai S, Shaw T. Noninvasive regional cerebral blood flow measurements in dementia. Arch Neurol 1980;37:410–418.

Yamamoto T, Hirose G, Shimazaki K, Takado S, Kosoegawa H, Saeki M. Movement disorders of familial neuroacanthocytosis syndrome. Arch Neurol 1982;39:298–301.

Yarchoan R, Berg G, Brouwers P, Fischl MA, Spitzer AR, Wichman A, Grafman J, Thomas RV, Safai B, Brunetti A, Perno CF, Schmidt PJ, Larson SM, Myers CE, Samuel Broder. Response of human immunodeficiency-virus-associated neurological disease to 3-azido-3-deoxythymidine. Lancet 1987;1:132–135.

Yarnell PR, Spann JF Jr, Dougherty J, Mason DT. Episodic central nervous system ischemia of undetermined cause: relation to occult left atrial myxoma. Stroke 1971;2:35–40.

Yaryura-Tobias JA, Diamond B, Merlis S. Psychiatric manifestations of levodopa. Can Psychiatr Assoc J 1972;17(suppl 2):SS123–128.

Yasargil MG, Yonekawa Y, Zumstein B, Stahl HJ. Hydrocephalus following spontaneous subarachnoid hemorrhage. J Neurosurg 39;1973;474–479.

Yates, CM. Aluminum and Alzheimer's disease. In: Glen AIM, Whalley LJ, eds. Alzheimer's disease. Early recognition of potentially reversible deficits. Churchill Livingstone, London, 1979:53–56.

Yates, PO. Vascular disease of the central nervous system. In: Blackwood W, Corsellis JAN, eds. Greenfield's neuropathology. Year Book Medical Publishers, Chicago, 1976:86–147.

Yokoi S, Kobori H, Yoshihara H. Clinical and neuropathological studies of myoclonic epilepsy. Acta Neuropathol 1965;4:370–379.

Young AB, Greenamyre JT, Hollingsworth Z, Albin R, D'Amato C, Shoulson I, Penney JB. NMDA receptor losses in putamen from patients with Huntington's disease. Science 1988;241:981–983.

Young AB, Penney JB, Starosta-Rubinstein S, Markel DS, Berent S, Giodani B, Ehkrenkaufer R, Jewett D, Hichwa R. PET scan investigations of Huntington's disease: cerebral metabolic correlates of neurological features and functional decline. Ann Neurol 1986;20:296–303.

Young AC, Saunders J, Ponsford JR. Mental change as an early feature of multiple sclerosis. J Neurol Neurosurg Psychiatry 1976;39:1008–1013.

Young SM, Fisher M, Sigsbee A, Errichetti A. Cardiogenic brain embolism and lupus anticoagulant. Ann Neurol 1989;26:390–392.

Younger DS, Hays AP, Brust JCM, Rowland LP. Granulomatous angiitis of the brain. An inflammatory reaction of diverse etiology. Arch Neurol 1988;45:514–518.

Yuasa T, Ohama E, Harayama H, Yamada M, Kawase Y, Wakabayashi M, Atsumi T, Miyatake T. Joseph's disease: clinical and pathological studies in a Japanese family. Ann Neurol 1986;19:152–157.

Yufe R, Karpati G, Carpenter S. Cardiac myxoma: a diagnostic challenge for the neurologist. Neurology 1976;26:1060–1065.

Yunis JY, Bloomfield CD, Ensrud K. All patients with acute nonlymphocytic leukemia may have a chromosomal defect. N Engl J Med 1981;305:135–139.

Zarit SH, Orr NK, Zarit JM. The hidden victims of Alzheimer's disease. New York University Press, New York, 1985.

Zarit SH, Reeever KE, Bach-Peterson J. Relatives of the impaired elderly: correlates of feelings of burden. Gerontologist 1980;20:649–655.

Zarit SH, Todd PA, Zarit JM. Subjective burden of husbands and wives as caregivers: a longitudinal study. Gerontologist 1986;26:260–266.

Zatuchni J, Hong K. Methyl bromide poisoning seen initially as psychosis. Arch Neurol 1981;38:529–530.

Zimmerman HM, Netsky MG. The pathology of multiple sclerosis. Res Publ Assoc Res Nerv Ment Dis 1950;28:271–312.

Zimmerman SL, Frutchey L, Gibbs JH. Meningitis due to *Candida* (monilia) albicans with recovery. JAMA 1947;135:145–147.

Zubenko GS, Huff J, Beyer J, Auerbach J, Teply I. Familial risk of dementia associated with a biologic subtype of Alzheimer's disease. Arch Gen Psychiatry 1988a;45:889–893.

Zubenko GS, Marquis JK, Volicer L, Direnfeld LK, Langlais PJ, Nixon RA. Cerebrospinal fluid level of angiotensin-converting enzyme, acetylcholinesterase, and dopamine metabolites in dementia associated with Alzheimer's disease and Parkinson's disease: a correlative study. Biol Psychiatry 1986;21:1365–1381.

Zubenko GS, Moossy J, Hamin I, Martinez J, Rao GR, Kopp U. Bilateral symmetry of cholinergic deficits in Alzheimer's disease. Arch Neurol 1988b:45:255–259.

Zucker DK, Livingston RL, Nakra R, Clayton PJ. B_{12} deficiency and psychiatric disorders: case report and literature review. Biol Psychiatry 1981;16:197–205.

Zu Rhein GM, Padgett BL, Walker DL, Chun RWM, Horowitz SD, Hong R. Progressive multifocal leukoencephalopathy in a child with severe combined immunodeficiency. N Engl J Med 1978;299:256–257.

Zung WWK. A self-rating depression scale. Arch Gen Psychiatry 1965;12:63–70.

Zweig RM, Whitehouse PJ, Casanova MF, Walker LC, Jankel WR, Price DL. Loss of pedunculopontine neurons in progressive supranuclear palsy. Ann Neurol 1987;22:18–25.

Index

Acalculia, 29, 384
Acetylcholine, 70, 252
Acquired dementias, 307–322
Acquired immunodeficiency syndrome
    (AIDS), 177
  clinical features of, 182
  cryptococcal meningitis with, 207
  dementia complex with, 178–179; *see also*
    human immunodeficiency virus (HIV)
    encephalopathy
  laboratory features and diagnosis of, 182–
    184
  progressive multifocal
    leukoencephalopathy (PML) with, 203
  risk factors for, 179
  treatment of, 188–189
Acute confusional state, 2
  chronic dementia syndromes and, 16
  differential diagnosis of dementia
    syndrome with, 14–17
  metabolic or toxic conditions and, 217
  state of awareness in, 21, 22
  toxic and metabolic conditions seen with,
    16
Addison's disease, 232–233, 248
Adenoma, pituitary, 247
Adrenoleukodystrophy (ALD), 325–327
Adrenomyeloneuropathy, 325
Adult polyglucosan body disease, 329–330
Affective changes

epilepsy and, 322
Huntington's disease and, 96
mental status examination of, 23–24
Pick's disease and, 77–78
pseudodementia and, 294
Age-associated memory impairment, 337
Age at onset
  alcoholic dementia and, 258
  cerebellar and olivopontocerebellar
    degeneration and, 146
  dementia of the Alzheimer's type (DAT)
    and, 46–47
  Friedreich's syndrome and, 144
  Hallervorden-Spatz syndrome and, 136
  Huntington's disease and, 96
  idiopathic calcification of the basal
    ganglia (ICBG) and, 150
  Jakob-Creutzfeldt disease and, 189–190
  metabolic disturbances and, 219
  multiple sclerosis and, 315
  Pick's disease and, 75
  progressive supranuclear palsy (PSP) and,
    108
  Wilson's disease and, 129
Aging
  incidence of dementia and, 383–384
  long-term care and, 366
  pharmacotherapy and, 369
  senility and, 335–344
Agnosias, 53–54, 384

Agraphia, 24, 27, 54
AIDS, *see* Acquired immunodeficiency
    syndrome (AIDS)
AIDS dementia complex (ADC), 178–179;
    see also human immunodeficiency
    virus (HIV) encephalopathy
AIDS-related complex (ARC), 182
Alcohol use and alcoholism
    cirrhosis with, 229–230
    dementias associated with, 257–260
    Wernicke-Korsakoff syndrome and, 240
Alexia, 24
Alper's disease, 178, 200
Alpha-galactosidase deficiency, 329
ALS, *see* Amyotrophic lateral sclerosis
    (ALS)-parkinsonism-dementia
    complex
Aluminum intoxication
    dementias associated with, 71, 72, 263,
        387
    dialysis dementia and, 227
Alzheimer's disease
    autopsy studies of prevalence of, 8
    classification of, 9
    diagnostic criteria for, 7–8
    differential diagnosis of, 89, 343
    prevalence of dementia with, 7–8
    specialized tests for, 42
    systematic approach to diagnosis of, 11–
        12
    see also Dementia of the Alzheimer's
        type (DAT)
Alzheimer's Association, 386
Alzheimer's Disease and Related Disorders
    Association (ADRDA), 8, 58, 386
Amnesia, 2, 384
    dementia of the Alzheimer's type (DAT)
        with, 57
    differential diagnosis of dementia
        syndrome with, 13–14
    herpes encephalitis with, 206
    intracranial neoplasms with, 312
    Pick's disease with, 88
    posttraumatic dementia and, 308, 309
    retrieval problems in, 33
    Wernicke-Korsakoff syndrome and, 239,
        240
Amphetamines, 255
Amyloid angiopathy, in dementia of the
    Alzheimer's type (DAT), 64, 68, 71
Amyotrophic lateral sclerosis (ALS)-
    parkinsonism-dementia complex, 139–
    142
    dementia with, 139–140
    differential diagnosis of, 141–142
    frontal lobe degeneration in, 90–91
    laboratory evaluation of, 140
    neurofibrillary tangles in, 66
    neuropathology of, 140–141

parkinsonism in, 128
Amyotrophic type, Jakob-Creutzfeldt
    disease, 191
Anemia
    anoxia with, 221–222
    vitamin B_{12} deficiency and, 241
Aneuploidy, in dementia of the Alzheimer's
    type (DAT), 59–60, 73
Angiography, diagnosis with, 357
Angular gyrus syndrome, 165
Anomia
    dementia of the Alzheimer's type (DAT)
        and, 52, 53
    Pick's disease and, 78
Anosognosia, 30
Anoxia, chronic, 220–222
Antibiotics, 255
Anticholinergic compounds, 252
Anticonvulsants, 253, 322
Antidepressants, 251, 370, 372
Antihypertensive agents, 252–253
Antineoplastic therapies, 253–255
Anxiety neurosis, 306, 372
Aphasia, 2, 24, 384
    cerebral trauma and, 309
    classification of dementias and, 9
    comprehension of spoken language in,
        25–26
    dementia of the Alzheimer's type (DAT)
        with, 48, 53, 57, 62
    differential diagnosis of dementia
        syndrome with, 13
    finger agnosia with, 30
    herpes encephalitis with, 206
    intracranial neoplasms with, 312
    Jakob-Creutzfeldt disease with, 190
    mental status examination and, 25–26, 27
    Pick's disease with, 75, 76–77
    posterior cortical atrophy with, 92
    primary progressive, 92
    progressive supranuclear palsy (PSP) and,
        109
    specialized tests for, 42
Appearance, in mental status examination,
    22–23
Appetite disturbances, in dementia of the
    Alzheimer's type (DAT), 56
Apraxia, 384
    dementia of the Alzheimer's type (DAT)
        with, 48, 53–54
    intracranial neoplasms with, 312
    mental status examination of, 28–29, 31
Arsenic, 262, 348
Arteriosclerosis
    parkinsonism with, 127
    vascular dementia with, 165
Arteriosclerotic encephalopathy, 341
L-asparaginase, 254
Aspergillus, 208

Assessment, *see* Mental status examination;
    Neuropsychological testing
Asterixis, 230, 384
Ataxia
    dementia pugilistica and, 310
    differential diagnosis of dementia with,
        147–148
    hereditary spastic, 144
    senility and, 341
Ataxia telangiectasia, 147–148
Ataxic type, Jakob-Creutzfeldt disease, 191
Atherosclerosis
    hydrocephalic dementia and, 277
    vascular dementia and, 169, 173
Attention disturbances
    acute confusional states with, 14
    differential diagnosis of dementia
        syndrome with, 14, 16
    mental status examination of, 20–22
    metabolic or toxic conditions and, 217
    specialized tests of, 42
Autotopagnosia, 30
Autopsy studies, 350
Awareness
    immediate recall and, 30–31
    mental status examination of, 20–22, 39
    types of, 20
Axial rigidity, in progressive supranuclear
    palsy (PSP), 109–110
Azorean disease, 148–149

Babcock sentence, 33
Bacterial meningitis, 207, 209–211
Balint's syndrome, 92, 165
Barbiturates, 253, 256
Basal ganglia, idiopathic calcification of the,
    128, 150–152
Basilar impression, 351
Bassen-Kornzweig syndrome, 107
Behavioral changes
    depression and, 295–296
    mental status examination of, 22–23
    subacute sclerosing panencephalitis
        (SSPE) with, 200
Behavioral management, and long-term care,
    368–373
Behavior modification techniques, 373
Benign senescent forgetfulness, 336
Benzodiazepines, 371, 372
Binswanger's disease, 156, 161–163, 341, 356
Bipolar disorder, 295
Bismuth, 263
Blastomycosis, 208
Blessed Dementia Scale, 43
Blood tests, and diagnosis, 346–348
Body awareness, in mental status
    examination, 30, 36–37, 54
Body changes, and aging, 339–340, 342
Border-zone infarctions, 168

Bradyphrenia, in senility, 336
Brain biopsy, 349
Brain death, 222
Brainstem tumors, 313
Brain trauma
    epilepsy and, 321
    posttraumatic dementia and, 307–308
Brain tumors
    dementia with, 312–314
    endocrine abnormalities with, 236–237
Butyrophenone drugs, 251–252

Calcium abnormalities, 233–234, 246–247
Calculation ability
    dementia of the Alzheimer's type (DAT)
        and, 54
    mental status examination of, 34
    specialized tests of, 42
Candida fungi, 208
Capgras syndrome, 55
Carbamazepine, 253, 256
Carbon dioxide poisoning, 220, 264
Carcinomas
    cerebellar degeneration with, 149–150
    Cushing's disease and, 247
    limbic encephalitis with, 205
Cardiac disease, and anoxia, 221
Caregivers
    day care and, 376–377
    home care and, 374–376
    respite care and, 377
Category naming, 26–27
Centers for Disease Control classification of
    human immunodeficiency virus (HIV)
    infection, 180
Central nervous system (CNS)
    definition of dementia and, 2–3, 9
    malignancies and infections associated
        with, 237
    superficial hemosiderosis of the, 319–321
    syphilis and, 212–214
Cerebellar degeneration, 145–150
    clinical characteristics of, 146–147
    dementia in, 145–146
    differential diagnosis of, 147–150
    paraneoplastic, 149–150
Cerebral blood vessels, and vascular
    dementia, 154, 156, 163–165, 174
Cerebral disturbances
    EEG studies in diagnosis of, 358
    endocrine abnormalities with, 237
    hydrocephalic dementia with, 278–279
    posttraumatic dementia and, 308–310
    systemic malignancies and, 235–238
Cerebrospinal fluid (CSF) tests
    bacterial meningitis and, 207
    dementia of the Alzheimer's type (DAT)
        and, 59, 60, 72
    diagnosis and, 348–349, 384, 388

Huntington's disease and, 99
hydrocephalic dementia and, 269–272,
    283–285
multiple sclerosis and, 316–317
progressive rubella encephalitis and, 203
subacute sclerosing panencephalitis
    (SSPE) and, 201, 202
Cerebrotendinous xanthomatosis, 328
Ceruloplasmin synthesis, in Wilson's disease,
    131, 134
Chemotherapy, 253–254
Chorea, in Huntington's disease, 98–99,
    105–106
Chromosomal abnormalities
    adrenoleukodystrophy (ALD) and, 327
    dementia of the Alzheimer's type (DAT)
        and, 48, 59–60, 73
Cirrhosis
    alcohol-induced, 229–230
    hepatocerebral degeneration with, 231
    Wilson's disease and, 133
Cisternography, and diagnosis, 361–362
Clonidine, 253
CNS, see Central nervous system (CNS)
Cobalamin deficiency, 238, 240–242
Coccidioidomycosis, 208
Cognition and cognitive functions
    calculating ability and, 34
    cerebellar and olivopontocerebellar
        degeneration and, 146
    cerebral trauma and, 309–310
    definition of dementia and, 2
    dementia of the Alzheimer's type (DAT)
        and, 48
    depression and, 295
    Friedreich's syndrome and, 143
    mental status examination of, 33–35
    metabolic or toxic conditions and, 217
    Parkinson's disease and, 114, 123–124
    postanoxic dementia and, 222
    proverb interpretation and, 34–35
    senility and, 338
    similarities and differences testing and,
        35
    subcortical dementias and, 10–11
    therapeutic agents and, 219
Community resources, 373–377
Comprehension
    dementia of the Alzheimer's type (DAT)
        and, 52, 53
    mental status examination of, 25–26
    primary progressive aphasia and, 92
    subcortical dementias with, 10
Computerized tomography (CT)
    aging and changes on, 341
    alcoholic dementia on, 258
    angular gyrus syndrome on, 165
    Binswanger's disease on, 163
    cerebral trauma on, 310

dementia of the Alzheimer's type (DAT)
    on, 60, 61–62, 63, 354
dementia pugilistica on, 311
depression on, 297
diagnosis with, 352–355, 384
dialysis dementia on, 226
Gerstmann-Straussler-Scheinker disease
    (GSSD) on, 199
Hallervorden-Spatz disease on, 137
Huntington's disease on, 99–100
hydrocephalic dementia on, 282
idiopathic calcification of the basal
    ganglia (ICBG) on, 150
Jakob-Creutzfeldt disease on, 193
multiple sclerosis on, 317
Parkinson's disease on, 119
Pick's disease on, 79, 354
progressive multifocal
    leukoencephalopathy (PML) on,
    204
subacute sclerosing panencephalitis
    (SSPE) on, 201
vascular dementia evaluation with, 175
Wernicke-Korsakoff syndrome on, 240
Wilson's disease on, 131
Confabulation, 33, 50
Confusional states
    differential diagnosis of dementia
        syndrome with, 14–17
    definition of dementia and, 2
    systematic approach to diagnosis of, 12–
        13
Conversion hysteria, 304–305
Copper levels in Wilson's disease, 133, 134–
    135
Copying tests, 27–28
Cortical dementias, 45–93
    classification of, 9
    clinical features of, 9–10
    differential diagnosis of, 14–15
    infarctions and, 163–168
    Jakob-Creutzfeldt disease with, 190
    specialized tests for, 42
    systematic approach to diagnosis of, 11–
        12
Corticobasal degeneration, 90
Corticodentatonigral degeneration, 90, 128
Cortisol
    Addison's disease with, 248
    Cushing's disease with, 247
Cryptococcal meningitis, 207–208
Cushing's disease, 247–248
Cysts, cerebral, 278–279, 357
Cytosine arabinoside (Ara-C), 254

DAT, see Dementia of the Alzheimer's type
    (DAT)
Dawson encephalitis, 200
Day care, 376–377

Deafness, and aging, 339
Deep white-matter lesions (DWMLs), 341
Deficiency states
    folate, 242–243
    niacin, 243
    testing for, 348
    thiamine, 238–240
    vitamin B$_{12}$, 240–242
Delirium
    differential diagnosis of, 15–16
    long-term care issues and, 367
Delusions
    dementia of the Alzheimer's type (DAT)
        with, 55
    mental status examination of, 36
Dementia
    amyotrophic lateral sclerosis (ALS)-
        parkinsonism-dementia complex with,
        139–140
    cerebellar and olivopontocerebellar
        degeneration with, 145–146
    classification of, 9
    clinical characteristics of, 9–10
    definition of, 1–3
    diagnostic approaches to, 11–13
    differential diagnosis of, 3, 13–17
    early use of term, 2
    epidemiology of, 3–8
    Friedreich's syndrome with, 143–144
    Hallervorden-Spatz disease with, 136–
        137, 138
    human immunodeficiency virus (HIV)
        encephalopathy with, 180–182
    Huntington's disease with, 96–98
    idiopathic calcification of the basal
        ganglia (ICBG) with, 150
    lacunar state with, 160
    Parkinson's disease with, 114–117
    paraneoplastic cerebellar degeneration
        with, 149
    prevalence of, 3–8
    progressive supranuclear palsy (PSP)
        with, 109
    specialized tests for, 42–44
    systemic lupus erythematosus (SLE) with,
        171
    Wilson's disease with, 129
Dementia of the Alzheimer's type (DAT),
    45, 46–75
    age at onset of, 46–47
    changing concepts of, 386–387
    clinical characteristics of, 48–58
    daily management of, 74–75
    DAT inventory for, 58
    depression compared with, 295, 296–297
    diagnosis of, 57–58, 349, 354
    differential diagnosis of, 88, 197, 311, 343
    distribution of pathologic changes in, 69–
        70

early work with, 46
epidemiology of, 46–47
etiology of, 71–73
family inheritance of, 47–48
incidence of, 47
laboratory investigation of, 58–64
length of survival after diagnosis of, 47
neuropathology of, 64–71, 90
Parkinson's disease with, 115
prevalence of, 46–47
progression of, 57
treatment of, 73–75
twin studies of, 48
vascular dementia and, 154, 165
Dementia pugilistica, 310–311
Demyelination
    adrenoleukodystrophy (ALD) with, 326
    anoxic cerebral insult and, 222
    metachromatic leukodystrophy (MLD)
        with, 324
    multiple sclerosis and, 318, 319, 320
Denny-Brown disease, 333
Dentatorubral-pallidoluysian atrophy, 149
Depersonalization, 37
Depression, 384
    acquired immunodeficiency syndrome
        (AIDS) and, 188–189
    aging and senility and, 339, 341, 342
    behavioral characteristics of, 295–296
    caregivers and, 379–380
    classification of dementia and, 7
    clinical characteristics of, 300–301
    comparison of Parkinson's disease and
        DAT and, 295, 296–297
    definition of dementia and, 3
    dementia of the Alzheimer's type (DAT)
        with, 55, 74
    Friedreich's syndrome with, 143
    Hallervorden-Spatz disease with, 136
    Huntington's disease with, 96, 97
    hydrocephalic dementia with, 281
    Jakob-Creutzfeldt disease with, 190
    laboratory investigation of, 297–298
    mental status examination of, 23–24
    multiple sclerosis with, 316
    natural history of, 296
    neuropsychological assessment of, 64, 297
    parkinsonism and, 128
    Parkinson's disease with, 115–116, 124,
        125
    pathophysiology of, 298–299
    postencephalitic parkinsonism with, 125
    prevalence of dementia with, 7
    pseudodementia and, 295–301
    specialized tests for, 44
    subcortical dementias with, 11
    systematic approach to diagnosis of, 12
    treatment of, 299, 372, 385
    vascular dementias with, 154

Dexamethasone suppression text (DST), in dementia of the Alzheimer's type (DAT), 56
Diagnostic and Statistical Manual of Mental Disorders
  DSM-IIIR, 3, 58
  DSM III, 386
Diagnostic criteria
  Alzheimer's disease and, 7–8
  dementia of the Alzheimer's type (DAT) and, 57–58, 68–70
  future trends in, 388–389
  Huntington's disease and, 104–105
  laboratory aids in, 345–364
  Pick's disease and, 79–80
  psychological testing with, 40
  systematic approach to, 11–13
Dialysis
  dementia with, 224–228
  disequilibrium syndrome with, 228–229
Digitalis toxicity, 255
Dilapidation, in subcortical dementias, 10
Disequilibrium syndrome, in dialysis, 228–229
Disulfiram, 255
Dopamine
  depression and, 298
  Parkinson's disease and, 121–122
Down's syndrome, and dementia of the Alzheimer's type (DAT), 48, 71, 73
Drawing tests
  dementia of the Alzheimer's type (DAT) and, 50
  mental status examination with, 27–28, 39
  senility and, 338
Dressing disturbances, 30, 50
Driving, 376
Drugs
  cognitive function and, 219
  dementia and, 250–257
  depression and, 299–300
  list of principal, 251
  long-term care issues with, 368–372
  see also specific agents and drugs
Dysarthria, 24
Dysgraphia, 29
Dystonia musculorum deformans, 138
Dystrophia myotonica, 333–334

Eastern equine encephalitis, 206
Echolalia
  dementia of the Alzheimer's type (DAT) and, 52, 62
  Pick's disease and, 78
Ectatic basilar artery, 277
Elderly
  alcoholic dementia and, 258

differential diagnosis of dementia syndrome in, 15–16
hypernatremia in, 233
hyperthyroidism and, 244
metabolic disturbances in, 219
pharmacotherapy and, 369
prevalence of dementia in, 4, 5
state of awareness in, 22
toxic dementias in, 249
see also Senility
Electroencephalography (EEG)
  aging and changes on, 340–341
  chronic renal failure on, 224
  dementia of the Alzheimer's type (DAT) on, 60–61, 387
  depression on, 297
  diagnosis with, 357–360, 384
  dialysis dementia on, 224, 225–226
  differential diagnosis of dementia syndrome with, 14–15
  Hallervorden-Spatz disease on, 137
  Huntington's disease on, 99
  hyperthyroidism on, 245
  Jakob-Creutzfeldt disease on, 190, 192, 193, 358
  lacunar state on, 160
  Parkinson's disease on, 118
  Pick's disease on, 79
  progressive supranuclear palsy (PSP) on, 110
  subacute sclerosing panencephalitis (SSPE) on, 200, 201
  Wilson's disease on, 131
Electrolyte abnormalities, 232–234
Embolic vascular occlusions, 173
Emotional changes
  cerebral trauma and, 309
  definition of dementia and, 1
  mental status examination of, 23–24
  Pick's disease and, 77–78
Empty-sella syndrome, 351
Encephalitis, and chronic bacterial meningitis, 209–211
Encephalitis subcorticalis chronica progressiva, 161
Encephalopathies
  alcohol-related, 259–260
  arteriosclerotic, 341
  dialysis dementia and, 224
  hepatic, 229
  neurofibrillary tangles in, 66
  pancreatic, 232
  portosystemic, 229–231
  postanoxic, 222
  systemic malignancies and, 235, 236
  uremic, 223–224, 228
  see also Human immunodeficiency virus (HIV) encephalopathy
Endocrine abnormalities, 243–249

dementia of the Alzheimer's type (DAT)
with, 56
depression and, 298
list of principal, 244
malignancies and, 235–236
testing for, 348
Environmental disorientation, and mental
status examination, 29, 36
Epilepsy
dementia with, 321–322
Huntington's disease with, 99
progressive myoclonus, 330–331
Ergot derivatives, 255
Ethical issues, 381–382
Ethosuximide, 253
Evoked response studies
dementia of the Alzheimer's type (DAT)
on, 61
diagnosis with, 360–361, 384
Huntington's disease on, 99
multiple sclerosis and, 317
Parkinson's disease on, 119
Extrapyramidal disorders
amyotrophic lateral sclerosis (ALS)-
parkinsonism-dementia complex with,
139–142
Hallervorden-Spatz syndrome with, 136–
139
Huntington's chorea with, 95–108
idiopathic calcification of the basal
ganglia (ICBG) with, 150–152
Jakob-Creutzfeldt disease with, 190, 191
Parkinson's disease with, 113–128
Pick's disease with, 76, 79
pharmacotherapy and, 368
progressive supranuclear palsy (PSP)
with, 108–113
spinocerebellar degenerations with, 142–
150
subacute sclerosing panencephalitis
(SSPE) with, 201
subcortical dementias with, 9, 95–152
systematic approach to diagnosis of, 12
Wilson's disease with, 128–136
Extrapyramidal type, Jakob-Creutzfeldt
disease, 191
Eye movement disturbances
dementia of the Alzheimer's type (DAT)
and, 56–57
progressive supranuclear palsy (PSP) and,
110
senility and, 339–340

Fabry's disease, 329
Familial amyloid angiopathy, 71
Family
amyotrophic lateral sclerosis (ALS)-
parkinsonism-dementia complex in,
139

caregivers issues and, 380
dementia of the Alzheimer's type (DAT)
inheritance in, 47–48, 57, 64
home care and, 374–376
Jakob-Creutzfeldt disease inheritance in,
189
legal counseling and, 380–381
mental status examination of patient and,
23
multiple sclerosis and, 314
Pick's disease inheritance in, 75
treatment issues and, 385
Family therapy, 373, 380
Finger agnosia, 29, 30
Fisher Test, 283
Folate deficiency, 238, 242–243, 322, 348
Forgetfulness
mental status examination of, 33
senility and, 336–337
Friedreich's syndrome, 143–145
Frontal lobe
degenerations of, 90–92
intracranial neoplasms and, 313
Pick's disease and, 75, 79, 81, 84, 90
senility and changes to, 338, 342
tumors of, 301
Frontopyramidal type, Jakob-Creutzfeldt
disease, 191
Fungal meningitis, 207–208

Gait disturbances
dementia pugilistica with, 310
hydrocephalic dementia with, 279–280
mast syndrome with, 332
senility and, 340
Gamma-aminobutyric acid (GABA)
dementia of the Alzheimer's type (DAT)
and, 70
Huntington's disease and, 99, 103, 104
Gamma globulin, and multiple sclerosis,
316–317
Ganser's syndrome, 305–306, 384
Gaucher's disease, 329
General paresis, 214–216
Gerstmann-Straussler-Scheinker disease
(GSSD), 178, 195, 198–199
early work with, 199
pathological features of, 199
Gerstmann syndrome
Pick's disease and, 89–90
posterior cortical atrophy with, 92
right-to-left disorientation in, 29
Giant cell arteritis, and vascular dementia,
171
Glue sniffing, 256–257
GM_1 gangliosidosis, 328
GM_2 gangliosidosis, 328–329
Gold, 263
Gummas, 216

Hachinski Ischemia Scale, 43–44, 156, 157, 175
Hallervorden-Spatz disease, 136–139
  dementia in, 136–137
  differential diagnosis of, 138
  laboratory evaluation in, 137
  neuropathology of, 137–138
  parkinsonism in, 128
  treatment of, 138–139
Hallucinations
  delirium and, 367
  mania and, 301
  mental status examination and, 36–37
Haloperidol, 251, 252
Halstead-Reitan tests, 41
Head trauma and posttraumatic dementia, 307–308
Health care facility, prevalence of dementia and type of, 5
Helminthic meningitis, 208–209
Hematologic disorders, and vascular dementia, 172–173
Hemisphere function, in mental status examination, 31
Hepatic coma, 229
Hepatic diseases, 229–231, 234
Hepatic encephalopathy, 229
Hepatocerebral degeneration, 231
Hereditary dysphasic dementia, 92
Hereditary spastic ataxia, 144
Herpes encephalitis, 206
Hexamethylamine, 254
Histoplasmosis, 208
Home care, 374–376
Hooper Visual Organization Test, 338
Human immunodeficiency virus (HIV) encephalopathy, 177, 178–180
  dementia with, 180–182
  differential diagnosis of, 180
  early work with, 178
  laboratory features and diagnosis of, 182–184
  neuropathology of, 184–186
  neuropsychological assessment of, 181–182
  pathophysiology of, 186–187
  treatment of, 187–189
Human immunodeficiency virus (HIV) infection
  asymptomatic individuals with, 182
  Centers for Disease Control classification of, 180
  risk factors for, 178, 346
  testing for, 346
Huntington's disease, 95–108
  clinical features of, 98–99
  dementia with, 96–98
  diagnosis of, 12, 104–105

differential diagnosis of, 105–107, 138
  early work with, 114
  inheritance of, 95–96, 104
  juvenile type of, 99
  laboratory evaluation of, 99–101
  neuropathology of, 101–103
  neuropsychological assessment in, 64
  parkinsonism in, 128
  pathophysiology of, 103–104
  treatment of, 107–108
Hyaline inclusion disease, adult-onset neuronal intranuclear, 92
Hydrocephalic dementia, 3, 9, 267–291
  bacterial meningitis with, 207
  cerebral cysts and, 278–279
  cisternography in diagnosis of, 361, 362
  classification of, 269
  diagnostic techniques for, 12, 282–286
  differential diagnosis of, 312
  early work with, 267–268
  EEG studies in, 359
  intelligence and, 268
  mechanism of development of, 268
  nonobstructive communicating, 277–278
  obstructive communicating, 276–277
  obstructive noncommunicating, 274–276
  pathologic states producing, 273–279
  pathology of, 286–288
  pathophysiology of, 269–273
  prognosis in, 290–291
  shunt procedures in, 288–289, 291
  spontaneous arrest of, 273–274
  symptomatology of, 279–282
  treatment of, 288–289, 385
Hyperactivity, in dementia of the Alzheimer's type (DAT), 56
Hyperalgesia, in Pick's disease, 78–79
Hypercalcemia, 233–234, 236, 246–247
Hyperlipidemia, 221
Hypernatremia, 233
Hyperparathyroidism, 246–247
Hypertension
  Binswanger's disease with, 162
  lacunar state with, 159–160
Hyperthyroidism, 244–245
Hypocalcemia, 234, 247
Hypoglycemia, recurrent, 232
Hypomagnesemia, 234
Hyponatremia, 232–233
Hypoparathyroidism
  dementia with, 247
  idiopathic calcification of the basal ganglia (ICBG) with, 151
Hypophonia, 24
Hypothyroidism
  dementia with, 245–246
  lithium carbonate and, 250–251
  parkinsonism with, 127

Hysterical dementia, 294, 304–305, 384

Ideas of reference, 36
Ideational apraxia, 29, 54
Ideomotor apraxia, 54
Idiopathic calcification of the basal ganglia
    (ICBG), 128, 150–152
Illusions, and mental status examination, 36–
    37
Immune system and immunosuppression
    acquired immunodeficiency syndrome
        (AIDS) and, 183
    dementia of the Alzheimer's type (DAT)
        and, 71–72
    human immunodeficiency virus (HIV)
        encephalopathy and, 179, 187
    hydrocephalic dementia and, 276
    kidney transplantation and, 229
    meningitis with, 207, 211
    progressive multifocal leukoencephalo-
        pathy (PML) and, 203
Inappropriate antidiuretic hormone
    syndrome, 232, 233, 249, 256
Incontinence
    dementia of the Alzheimer's type (DAT)
        with, 57
    hydrocephalic dementia and, 282
    long-term care issues and, 367
    mental status examination and, 23
    Pick's disease and, 76, 79
Industrial agents, dementias associated with,
    250, 264
Infantile neuroaxonal dystrophy, 66
Infarctions
    Binswanger's disease with, 161–162
    border-zone, 168
    cortical, 163–168
    CT scans of, 353
    endocrine abnormalities with, 237
    hydrocephalic dementia and, 278
    lacunar state with, 157–160
    mixed cortical and subcortical, 169
    multiple small, 168
    SPECT studies of, 363
    see also Vascular dementias
Inheritance patterns
    amyotrophic lateral sclerosis (ALS)-
        parkinsonism-dementia complex and,
        139
    dementia of the Alzheimer's type (DAT)
        and, 47–48
    Huntington's disease and, 95–96, 104
    multiple sclerosis and, 314–315
    Pick's disease and, 75
Inherited disorders, and dementia, 322–334
Insight of patient, on mental status
    examination, 37–38
Insulinoma, 232

Intellectual impairment
    anemic anoxia and, 221–222
    aphasia differential diagnosis with, 13
    cerebellar and olivopontocerebellar
        degeneration with, 146
    definition of dementia and, 1–2
    dementia of the Alzheimer's type (DAT)
        with, 48, 54–55
    dialysis dementia with, 224
    epilepsy and, 322
    examination of, see Mental status
        examination
    general paresis with, 214
    Hallervorden-Spatz disease with, 136
    hydrocephalic dementia and, 268, 274
    idiopathic calcification of the basal
        ganglia (ICBG) with, 151
    kidney transplantation and, 229
    metabolic disturbances and, 219
    Parkinson's disease with, 116–117, 121–
        122
    Pick's disease with, 88
    posttraumatic dementia and, 308
    prevalence of dementia with, 5
    progressive supranuclear palsy (PSP)
        with, 109
    pseudodementia and, 293
    pulmonary insufficiency and anoxia with,
        220
    schizophrenia and, 302, 303–304
    senility and, 338
    toxic dementias and, 250
    vascular dementia with, 154, 156
    Wilson's disease with, 129
Interferon, 254
Intracranial neoplasms, 312–314
Ischemia Scale (Hachinski), 43–44, 156, 157,
    175
Isotope cisternography, and diagnosis, 361–
    362

Jakob-Creutzfeldt disease, 72, 177, 178, 189–
    191
    clinical variants of, 191
    differential diagnosis of, 197–198
    early work with, 189
    EEG studies in, 190, 192, 193, 358
    frontal lobe degeneration with, 91
    differential diagnosis of, 57, 79, 84
    etiology and transmissability of, 195–197
    laboratory evaluation of, 192–193
    neuropathology of, 193–195
    posterior cortical atrophy with, 92
    stages of, 190–191
    treatment of, 197
Japanese encephalitis, 206
JC virus, 205
Joseph's disease, 148

Judgment
    dementia of the Alzheimer's type (DAT)
        and, 54
    Huntington's disease with, 98
    mental status examination of, 37–38
Juvenile paresis, 215
Juvenile type of Huntington's disease, 99
Juvenile variant of Wilson's disease, 129, 130

Kayser-Fleischer rings, in Wilson's disease,
    130, 135
Kearns-Sayre syndrome, 332
Kidney transplantation, 229
Klüver-Bucy syndrome
    dementia of the Alzheimer's type (DAT)
        with, 55, 88
    herpes encephalitis with, 206
    Pick's disease and, 77, 78, 88, 89
Kuf's disease, 329
Kuru, 198
    clinical characteristics of, 198
    transmission of, 177, 178, 195, 197, 198

Lacunar state, 156, 157–160
    clinical characteristics of, 159–160
    differential diagnosis of, 162–163
    evaluation of, 175
    vessels involved in, 157
Lafora bodies, 330–331
Language disturbances
    definition of dementia and, 1
    dementia of the Alzheimer's type (DAT)
        with, 51–52, 57, 64
    differential diagnosis of dementia
        syndrome with, 13, 14, 16
    Huntington's disease with, 97
    mental status examination of, 24–27, 39
    Pick's disease and, 76, 88–89
    senility and, 337
Lead, 260–261, 348
Learning
    depression and, 297
    mental status examination of, 32, 39
Left hemisphere function, in mental status
    examination, 31
Legal counseling, 380–381
Leigh's disease, 330
Leukoaraiosis, 341
Leukodystrophies, 322–328
Levodopa
    Huntington's disease and, 104–105, 108
    Parkinson's disease and, 122, 123–124
    toxicity with, 255
Lewy bodies, in Parkinson's disease, 121,
    126
Limbic encephalitis, 205, 237–238
Listeria, 211
Lithium carbonate, 250–251, 301
Liver disease

    dementia in metabolic disturbances with,
        229–231
    Wilson's disease and, 130, 132–133
Logoclonia, in dementia of the Alzheimer's
    type (DAT), 52
Long-term care
    behavioral management and, 368–373
    caregivers and, 379–380
    co-occurring medical disorders and, 366–
        368
    day care and, 376–377
    ethical issues and, 381–382
    home care and, 374–376
    legal counseling and, 380–381
    nursing home care and, 377–379
    respite care and, 377
Long-term memory, on mental status
    examination, 32–33
Lung carcinoma
    cerebellar degeneration with, 149
    endocrine abnormalities with, 236
    limbic encephalitis with, 205, 237
Luria tests, 28, 41
Lyme disease, 211
Lymphoproliferative disorders
    dementia of the Alzheimer's type (DAT)
        and, 48, 73
    progressive multifocal leukoencephalo-
        pathy (PML) and, 203

Machado disease, 148
Magnesium abnormalities, 233–234
Magnetic resonance imaging (MRI)
    aging and changes on, 341
    angular gyrus syndrome on, 165
    Binswanger's disease on, 163
    dementia of the Alzheimer's type (DAT)
        on, 62
    diagnosis with, 355–356, 384
    Hallervorden-Spatz disease on, 137
    human immunodeficiency virus (HIV)
        encephalopathy on, 183–184
    hydrocephalic dementia on, 282
    lacunar state on, 160
    multiple sclerosis on, 317
    Parkinson's disease on, 119
    Pick's disease on, 79, 89
    subacute sclerosing panencephalitis
        (SSPE) on, 201
    Wernicke-Korsakoff syndrome on, 241
    Wilson's disease on, 131
Malignancies
    CNS infections associated with, 237–238
    metabolic disturbances and, 235–236
    structural abnormalities produced by,
        236–237
Malingering, 306
Manganese, 262
Mania, 384

Huntington's disease with, 97
pseudodementia with, 294, 301–302
Marchiafava-Bignami disease, 259
Mast syndrome, 332
Measles virus, and subacute sclerosing
    panencephalitis (SSPE), 200, 202
Membranous lipodystrophy, 327
Memory disturbances
    amnesia differential diagnosis with, 14
    aphasia differential diagnosis with, 13
    cerebellar and olivopontocerebellar
        degeneration with, 146
    chronic or recurrent hypoglycemia and,
        232
    classification of dementias and, 9, 10
    confabulation and, 33
    definition of dementia and, 1, 3
    dementia of the Alzheimer's type (DAT)
        with, 48–50, 64
    depression and, 297
    differential diagnosis of dementia
        syndrome with, 14, 17
    forgetfulness and, 33
    Hallervorden-Spatz disease with, 136
    Huntington's disease with, 97–98
    hydrocephalic dementia with, 281
    immediate recall in, 30–31
    learning new material and, 32
    mental status examination of, 30–33, 39
    metabolic conditions and, 217
    multiple sclerosis and, 315
    Parkinson's disease and, 114, 117
    Pick's disease and, 76, 78, 79, 88
    retrieving old learned material and, 32–
        33
    senility and, 336–337
    specialized tests of, 42
    toxic conditions and, 217
    Wernicke-Korsakoff syndrome and, 239,
        240
Meningitis, chronic, 207–212, 215–216
Meningovascular syphilis, 215–216
Mental status changes, 384
    amyotrophic lateral sclerosis (ALS)-
        parkinsonism-dementia complex with,
        139, 141–142
    chronic or recurrent hypoglycemia and,
        232
    chronic renal failure and, 223
    depression and, 300
    dialysis dementia and, 225
    Friedreich's syndrome with, 143
    Ganser's syndrome and, 305
    Gerstmann-Straussler-Scheinker disease
        (GSSD) with, 199
    Hallervorden-Spatz disease with, 136
    human immunodeficiency virus (HIV)
        encephalopathy with, 179–180, 183
    Huntington's disease and, 96

hydrocephalic dementia and, 281
intracranial neoplasms with, 313
limbic encephalitis with, 237
Pick's disease with, 76
portosystemic encephalopathy with, 230
progressive multifocal
    leukoencephalopathy (PML) with,
    203–204
pulmonary insufficiency and anoxia with,
    220
senility and, 338, 344
serum calcium abnormalities with, 233,
    246
subcortical dementias with, 10
subdural hematoma and, 311–312
Mental status examination, 19–44
    body part identification on, 30
    clinical use setting in, 20–37
    dressing difficulties on, 30
    cognitive functions on, 33–35
    finger agnosia on, 30
    general appearance and behavior on, 22–
        23
    hysterical dementia on, 304
    insight and judgment on, 37–38
    language functions on, 25–27
    memory on, 30–33
    metabolic disturbances on, 219
    minimum screening with, 38–40
    mood and affect on, 23–24
    motor aspects of verbal speech on, 25
    motor sequences on, 30–31
    praxis on, 28–29
    psychological testing with, 40–44
    right-left orientation on, 29
    short testing of, 43–44
    speech and language on, 24
    state of awareness on, 20–22
    thought content on, 35–37
    topographic orientation on, 29
    visuospatial functions on, 27–28
Mephenytoin, 253
Mercury, 261–262, 348
Metabolic disturbances, 217, 219–249, 334
    acute confusional states with, 2, 16
    chronic anoxia with, 220–222
    chronic renal failure with, 223–229
    deficiency states and, 238–243
    dementia of the Alzheimer's type (DAT)
        and, 62
    differential diagnosis of dementia
        syndrome with, 16, 17
    electrolyte abnormalities with, 232–234
    Ganser's syndrome and, 305, 306
    hepatic diseases with, 229–231
    laboratory tests in diagnosis of, 347
    list of principal, 218
    malignancies and, 235–237
    pancreatic disorders with, 232

porphyria with, 234–235
state of awareness in, 21
see also specific conditions
Metachromatic leukodystrophy (MLD), 322–
        325
Metals
    dementias associated with, 250, 260–263
    testing for, 348
Methotrexate, 254
N-methyl-D-aspartate (NMDA), in
        Huntington's disease, 103
Methyldopa, 252
Mini-Mental State Examination, 43, 58
Mitochondrial encephalomyopathies, 331–
        332
Mitochondrial myopathy, encephalopathy,
        lactic acidosis, and strokelike episodes
        (MELAS), 332
Mixed dementias
    classification of, 9
    systematic approach to diagnosis of, 11–
        12
Monilia, 208
Mood disturbances
    Hallervorden-Spatz disease with, 136
    Huntington's disease with, 96–97
    mania and, 301
    mental status examination of, 23–24
    metabolic or toxic conditions and, 217
    multiple sclerosis and, 316
    pseudodementia and, 294–302
    senility and, 338–339
    subcortical dementias with, 11
    Wilson's disease with, 129
Motor abnormalities
    apraxia with, 28–29
    dementia pugilistica with, 310–311
    depression and, 300–301
    differential diagnosis of dementia
        syndrome with, 16
    hepatocerebral degeneration with, 231
    Huntington's disease with, 98–99
    hydrocephalic dementia with, 279–281
    idiopathic calcification of the basal
        ganglia (ICBG) with, 150
    mental status examination of, 25, 30–31
    metabolic or toxic conditions and, 217,
        218
    multiple sclerosis with, 316
    senility and, 336, 340
    speech production and, 25
    subcortical dementias with, 10, 11, 25
Motor apraxia, 25, 29
Movement disorders, 384
    Huntington's disease with, 98–99
    Parkinson's disease with, 117–118
    prevalence of dementia with, 5
Multi-infarct dementia, 8, 63
    classification of, 156, 158

depression in, 299
differential diagnosis of, 311
endocrine abnormalities with, 237
etiologies of, 169, 170–171
infarctions producing, 169
terminology regarding, 153–154
Multiple-loop test, 31
Multiple sclerosis, 64, 314–319
    clinical manifestations of, 315–316
    differential diagnosis of, 319
    laboratory evaluation of, 316–317
    pathology and pathogenesis of, 318
    treatment of, 318–319
Musical ability tests, 42
Mutism, 24
    dementia of the Alzheimer's type (DAT)
        with, 52, 62
    dialysis dementia and, 225
    Pick's disease and, 76, 79, 89
Mycobacterial meningitis, 211
Myelin, diseases of, 319, 320
Myocardial infarction, and vascular
        dementia, 173
Myoclonus, 384
    dementia of the Alzheimer's type (DAT)
        with, 57
    dialysis dementia and, 224, 225
    differential diagnosis of syndromes with,
        331, 332
    epilepsy with, 330–331
    Jakob-Creutzfeldt disease with, 190, 191,
        193
    Pick's disease with, 79
    subacute sclerosing panencephalitis
        (SSPE) with, 200, 201
Myoclonus epilepsy with ragged red fibers
        (MERRF), 332
Myotonic dystrophy, 333–334
Myxedema, 245–246

Naming
    dementia of the Alzheimer's type (DAT)
        and, 51, 54
    differential diagnosis of dementia
        syndrome and, 17
    mental status examination of, 26–27
    senility and, 337
National Institute of Neurologic and
        Communicative Disorders and Stroke
        (NINCDS), 8, 58, 386
Neoplasms
    cerebellar degeneration with, 149–150
    intracranial, 312–314
    serum calcium abnormalities with, 233
Neurobrucellosis, 211
Neuritic plaques, in dementia of the
        Alzheimer's type (DAT), 67–68, 71
Neurobrucellosis, 211
Neurofibrillary tangles

dementia of the Alzheimer's type (DAT)
with, 64–67, 69, 71, 386, 387
dementia pugilistica with, 311
differential diagnosis of conditions with,
65–67
progressive supranuclear palsy (PSP)
with, 112
vascular dementias with, 153
Neuroleptic therapy
dementia caused by, 251–252
long-term care issues and, 368, 370
parkinsonian complications of, 126–127
Neuronal alterations
amyotrophic lateral sclerosis (ALS)-
parkinsonism-dementia complex with,
140–141
dementia of the Alzheimer's type (DAT)
with, 64–65
Hallervorden-Spatz disease with, 138
Huntington's disease with, 102–104
Jakob-Creutzfeldt disease with, 193–194
niacin deficiency and, 243
Pick's disease with, 79–80, 82
Neuronal storage diseases, 328–330
Neuropsychological impairment, 384
alcoholic dementia and, 258
amnesia differential diagnosis with, 14
definition of dementia and, 2
dementia and patterns of, 9
Friedreich's syndrome and, 143
industrial agents and pollutants and, 264
multiple sclerosis and, 315
Parkinson's disease and, 116
Pick's disease and, 77
psychological testing of, 40
schizophrenia and, 302–303
vascular dementia with, 156
Neuropsychological testing
dementia assessment with, 42–43
dementia of the Alzheimer's type (DAT)
on, 50, 63–64, 387
depression on, 297
human immunodeficiency virus (HIV)
encephalopathy and, 181–182, 183–
184
hydrocephalic dementia and, 282
multiple sclerosis and, 315
Parkinson's disease on, 117
schizophrenia on, 302–303
specialized areas for, 42
variety of instruments available for, 40–
41
Wilson's disease and, 129
Neurosyphilis, 212–214, 346
Neurotransmitters
aging and senility and, 344
dementia of the Alzheimer's type (DAT)
and, 70
depression and, 298–299

Huntington's disease and, 103
Niacin deficiency, 238, 243
Nickel, 263
Nigro-spino-dentatal degeneration, 148
Nitrogen mustard, 254
Norepinephrine
dementia of the Alzheimer's type (DAT)
and, 70
depression and, 298
Normal-pressure hydrocephalus (NPH), 269,
276–277
air studies in, 356–357
causes of, 277
increased ventricular size in, 272–273
Nuclear medicine investigations, and
diagnosis, 361–364
Nursing homes
long-term management issues and, 377–
379
pharmacotherapy and, 369
wandering and long-term care in, 367–
368

Obsessional ruminative states, 306
Obsessional thoughts, on mental status
examination, 36
Occipital type, Jakob-Creutzfeldt disease,
191
Occupational impairment, and definition of
dementia, 3
Olivopontocerebellar degeneration, 145–150
clinical characteristics of, 146–147
dementia in, 145–146
differential diagnosis of, 147–150
Operant techniques, 373
Oral contraceptives, 255
Organic brain syndrome
definition of dementia and, 2–3
personality changes in, 24
Organochlorine compounds, 264
Orientation, in mental status examination,
29, 31
Oxygen deprivation
anemic anoxia and, 221
chronic cardiac disease and, 221
pulmonary insufficiency and anoxia with,
220, 221

Paget's disease, 351
Palilalia, in dementia of the Alzheimer's
type (DAT), 52
Pancreatic disorders, 232
Pancreatitis, 232
Panencephalopathic type, Jakob-Creutzfeldt
disease, 191
Panhypopituitarism, 248–249
Papova viruses, with progressive multifocal
leukoencephalopathy (PML), 203, 205

Paralysis agitans, 113–114; *see also*
    Parkinson's disease
Paraneoplastic cerebellar degeneration, 149–
    150
Paraneoplastic encephalomyelitis, 205, 238
Paraneoplastic limbic encephalitis, 178
Paraphasia, 25
    dementia of the Alzheimer's type (DAT)
        with, 51, 53
    Pick's disease and, 78
Parasitic meningitis, 208–209
Parkinsonism
    drug-induced, 126–127
    postencephalitic, 124–126
    see also Amyotrophic lateral sclerosis
        (ALS)-parkinsonism-dementia
        complex
Parkinson's disease, 113–128
    clinical characteristics of, 117–118
    dementia with, 114–117
    depression compared with, 295, 296–297
    differential diagnosis of, 112–113, 124–
        128
    laboratory evaluation of, 118–119
    neuropathology of, 119–121
    neuropsychological assessment in, 64
    pathophysiology of, 121–122
    systematic approach to diagnosis of, 12
    treatment of, 122–124, 385
D-penicillamine, in Wilson's disease, 135–
    136
Peripheral neuropathy, 264–265, 384
Pernicious anemia, and vitamin B12
    deficiency, 241
Persecution beliefs, 36
Personality changes, 384
    chronic or recurrent hypoglycemia and,
        232
    classification of dementias and, 10
    definition of dementia and, 2
    dementia of the Alzheimer's type (DAT)
        with, 55
    Hallervorden-Spatz disease with, 136
    Huntington's disease with, 96
    intracranial neoplasms with, 313
    mental status examination and changes
        in, 24
    multiple sclerosis and, 316
    organic brain dysfunction with, 24
    progressive supranuclear palsy (PSP)
        with, 109
    Pick's disease with, 77
    senility and, 338–339
    Wilson's disease with, 129
Phenobarbital, 253
Phenothiazine drugs, 251–252
Phenytoin, 253, 322
Pick bodies, 80, 82–83, 84
Pick's disease, 45, 75–87

age at onset of, 75
biopsy in diagnosis of, 79–80, 349
classification of, 9
clinical characteristics of, 75–79
CT scans in, 79, 354
differential diagnosis of, 3, 87–90, 301
early work with, 75
etiology of, 86
Klüver-Bucy syndrome and, 77
laboratory evaluation of, 79–81
neurofibrillary tangles in, 66
neuropathology of, 81–86
Pick bodies in, 82–83
primary progressive aphasia with, 92
stages of, 75–79
systematic approach to diagnosis of, 11–
    12
treatment of, 86–87
Pituitary adenoma, 247
Pneumoencephalography, 356–357
Polioencephalopathy, 328–330
Pollutants, dementias associated with, 250,
    264
Polycythemia vera, 221
Polydrug abuse, 256
Polysaccharide metabolism, 329–330
Porphyria, 234–235
Portosystemic encephalopathy, 229–231
Positron emission tomography (PET)
    dementia of the Alzheimer's type (DAT)
        on, 59
    depression on, 297–298
    diagnosis with, 363–364, 384
    human immunodeficiency virus (HIV)
        encephalopathy on, 184
    Huntington's disease on, 100–101
    hydrocephalic dementia on, 285
    Pick's disease on, 79
    progressive multifocal leukoencephalo-
        pathy (PML) on, 204
    progressive supranuclear palsy (PSP) on,
        111
    vascular dementia evaluation with, 175
    Wilson's disease on, 131–132
Postanoxic dementia, 222
Postencephalitic dementias, 206
Postencephalitic parkinsonism, 124–126, 138
Posterior cortical atrophy, 92–93
Postmeningitic dementia, 211–212
Posttraumatic dementia, 307–312
    cerebral trauma and, 308–310
    dementia pugilistica and, 310–311
    subdural hematoma and, 311–312
Praxis, mental status examination of, 28–29
Preoccupation, and mental status
    examination, 36
Presenile dementia, 7
Prevalence of dementia, 3–8, 46–47
Primary degenerative dementia (PDD), 386

Primary progressive aphasia, 92
Prion, 178, 195–196, 387
Process approach to tests, 41
Progressive dialysis encephalopathy, 224
Progressive multifocal leukoencephalopathy
    (PML), 178, 183–184, 203–205
    clinical characteristics of, 203–204
    diseases associated with, 203, 204
    etiology and pathology of, 204–205
    treatment of, 205
Progressive myoclonus epilepsy, 330–331
Progressive rubella encephalitis, 178, 202–
    203
Progressive subcortical gliosis, 91
Progressive supranuclear palsy (PSP), 108–
    113
    clinical characteristics of, 109–110
    dementia with, 109
    differential diagnosis of, 112–113
    hydrocephalic dementia and, 278
    laboratory investigations in, 110–111
    neurofibrillary tangles in, 66
    neuropathology of, 111–112
    neuropsychological assessment in, 64
    parkinsonism in, 128
    treatment of, 112
Propranolol hydrochloride, 253
Prosopagnosia, in dementia of the
    Alzheimer's type (DAT), 54
Protozoan meningitis, 208–209
Proverb interpretation, 34–35
Pseudobulbar palsy, 109
Pseudodementias, 293–306
    diagnostic criteria for, 293–294
    frequency of, 294
    Ganser's syndrome and, 305–306
    hysterical dementia and, 304–305
    list of principal disorders, 294
    mood disorders and, 294–302
    schizophrenia and, 302–304
    use of term, 293
Psychiatric disorders, 384
    dementia definition and, 3
    see also Pseudodementias and specific
        disorders
Psychological testing, 40–44
    dementia assessment with, 42–43
    specialized areas for, 42
    variety of instruments available for, 40–
        41
Psychosis and psychotic episodes
    dementia of the Alzheimer's type (DAT)
        with, 55
    differential diagnosis of, 304
    epilepsy and, 322
    Huntington's disease with, 96
    kidney transplantation and, 229
    multiple sclerosis and, 316
Psychotherapy, and long-term care, 372–373

Psychotropic agents, 250–252, 368
Pulmonary insufficiency, and anoxia, 220–
    221

Radiologic examinations, and diagnosis, 351–
    357
Radiotherapy, 253, 254–255
Rating scales for dementia, 43–44
Raven Matrices, 338
Reactive depression, 339
Reaction times, and senility, 336
Reading, mental status examination of, 27
Recall, on mental status examination, 30–31
Remote memory, on mental status
    examination, 32–33
Renal failure, 223–229
    dialysis and dialysis dementia and, 224–
        229
    differential diagnosis of mental status
        changes in, 223
    kidney transplantation and, 229
    testing for, 348
    uremia and, 223–224
    uretorosigmoidostomy and, 229
Respite care, 377
Retrieval problems, on mental status
    examination, 32–33
Right hemisphere function, in mental status
    examination, 31
Right-to-left disorientation, in mental status
    examination, 29
Rigidity, 384
    amyotrophic lateral sclerosis (ALS)-
        parkinsonism-dementia complex with,
        140
    Parkinson's disease with, 118, 121
    progressive supranuclear palsy (PSP)
        with, 109–110
Rubella encephalitis, progressive, 178, 202–
    203
Rush, Benjamin, 2

St. Louis encephalitis, 206
Sarcoidosis, and vascular dementia, 171–172
Scales for dementia, 43–44
Schilder's disease, 325
Schizophrenia, 384
    differential diagnosis of, 304, 323
    Huntington's disease with, 97
    neuropsychological assessment of, 302–
        303
    pseudodementia with, 294, 302–304
Screening, with mental status examination,
    38–40
Secondary memory consolidation, on mental
    status examination, 32
Seizures
    dementia of the Alzheimer's type (DAT)
        with, 57

dementia pugilistica and, 310
differential diagnosis of dementia with, 321
EEG studies in diagnosis of, 359–360
Huntington's disease with, 99
Pick's disease with, 88, 89
Self-perceptions, on mental status examination, 36–37
Senescence, use of term, 335–336
Senile dementia, 219, 343
Senility, 335–344
    causes of, 341–343
    clinical alterations in, 336–340
    differential diagnosis of, 343
    laboratory changes in, 340–341
    treatment of, 343–344
    use of term, 335–336
Sensory disturbances, in multiple sclerosis, 316
Sensory radicular neuropathy, 333
Serotonin
    dementia of the Alzheimer's type (DAT) and, 70
    depression and, 298
Serum, and diagnosis, 346–348
Sexual behavior
    caregivers and, 380
    dementia of the Alzheimer's type (DAT) and, 56
Short-term memory, on mental status examination, 32
Shunts, with hydrocephalic dementia, 288–289, 291, 385
Shy-Drager syndrome, 128
Simian virus 40, 205
Single photon emission computed tomography (SPECT)
    dementia of the Alzheimer's type (DAT) on, 59, 62
    diagnosis with, 362–363, 384
    Huntington's disease on, 101
    hydrocephalic dementia on, 285
    Pick's disease on, 79
Sleep disturbances
    dementia and, 56, 221
    delirium and, 367
Slowness, and senility, 336
Social behavior impairment
    definition of dementia and, 3
    dementia of the Alzheimer's type (DAT) with, 55
    Pick's disease and, 76
Solvents, dementias associated with, 256–257, 264
Speech disturbances
    dementia of the Alzheimer's type (DAT) with, 53, 62
    dialysis dementia and, 224, 225

differential diagnosis of dementia syndrome with, 16
Ganser's syndrome and, 305–306
mental status examination of, 24–25
Parkinson's disease with, 116
subcortical dementias with, 10
Spinocerebellar ataxia, 198; see also Gerstmann-Straussler-Scheinker disease (GSSD)
Spinocerebellar degeneration, 142–150
Spongiform encephalopathy
    Alper's disease with, 200
    Jakob-Creutzfeldt disease with, 194, 196
Straussler disease, 198; see also Gerstmann-Straussler-Scheinker disease (GSSD)
Striatonigral degeneration, autosomal dominant, 148
Subacute necrotizing encephalomyelopathy, 330
Subacute sclerosing panencephalitis (SSPE), 66, 178, 200–202
    clinical features of, 200–201
    etiology and pathology of, 202
    laboratory evaluation of, 201
Subarachnoid hemorrhages, and hydrocephalic dementia, 276–277, 290
Subcortical dementias
    classification of, 9
    clinical features of, 9, 10–11
    differential diagnosis of, 343
    dilapidation in, 10
    Huntington's disease with, 97
    motor disturbances in, 25, 31
    systematic approach to diagnosis of, 11–12
    treatment of, 385
    use of term, 9
Subdural hematoma, 311–312
Suicide and suicide attempts, and Huntington's disease, 96
Superficial hemosiderosis of the CNS, 319–321
Support groups, 380
Supranuclear gaze palsies, 210–211
Sydenham's chorea, 105
Syphilis
    dementia with, 212–214
    meningitis with, 211, 216
    meningovascular, 215–216
Systemic disturbances
    intellectual consequences of, 219
    laboratory tests in diagnosis of, 347
Systemic lupus erythematosus (SLE), and vascular dementia, 169–171, 174

Tardive dyskinesia, in Huntington's disease, 106–107

Temporal arteritis, and vascular dementia, 171
Temporal lobe
    conditions causing degenerations of, 90, 91
    herpes encephalitis and, 206
    intracranial neoplasms and, 313
    Pick's disease and, 75, 79, 81, 82, 84
Tests, see Mental status examination; Neuropsychological testing
Thalamic dementias, 198, 313
Thallium, 263
Thiamine deficiency, 238–240
Thought content, and mental status examination, 35–37
Thrombocytopenia, in Wilson's disease, 130, 131
Thrush, 208
Thyrotoxicosis, 244–245
Tin poisoning, 263
Tissue samples, 349
Toluene, 256
Topographic disorientation, on mental status examination, 29
Torulosis, 207–208
Toxic dementias, 217, 249–264
    acute confusional states with, 2, 16
    differential diagnosis of dementia syndrome with, 16, 17
    Ganser's syndrome and, 305, 306
    laboratory tests in diagnosis of, 347
    list of principal, 250
    prevalence of dementia with, 5
    state of awareness in, 21
    treatment of, 384–385
    see also specific conditions
Trails test, 28, 129
Tranquilizers
    dementia caused by, 251–252, 256
    Huntington's disease treatment with, 107–108
Traumatic brain injury (TBI), 308–310
Tremor, 230, 384
Treponema pallidum, 212, 215
Tricyclic antidepressants, 251
Tuberculous meningitis, 209
Tuberous sclerosis, 66
Tumors, and hydrocephalic dementia, 277
Twin studies, and dementia of the Alzheimer's type (DAT), 48

Unidentified bright objects (UBOs), 356
Unverricht-Lundborg disease, 330
Uremic encephalopathy, 223–224, 228
Uretorosigmoidostomy, 229
Urinalysis, 348
Uveitis, 211

Vascular dementias, 153–176
    characteristics of, 154–156
    cortical infarctions with, 163–168
    depression with, 300
    differential diagnosis of, 154, 156, 165
    etiologies of, 169–173
    evaluation of, 174–175
    Ischemia Scale (Hachinski) in, 43–44, 156, 157, 175
    prevalence of, 8
    systematic approach to diagnosis of, 12
    terminology regarding, 153–154
    treatment of, 175–176
    types of, 156–159
Venereal Disease Research Laboratory (VDRL) test, 213
Ventriculography, 356–357
Viruses
    dementia of the Alzheimer's type (DAT) etiology and, 72–73, 387
    dementias produced by, 178
    Jakob-Creutzfeldt disease and, 195–196
    kuru and, 198
Visuospatial skills
    classification of dementias and, 9
    definition of dementia and, 1
    dementia of the Alzheimer's type (DAT) with, 50–51, 57, 64
    Hallervorden-Spatz disease with, 136
    mental status examination of, 27–28
    Parkinson's disease and, 117
    Pick's disease and, 76, 78, 79, 88
    senility and, 338
    specialized tests of, 42
Vitamin B_{12} deficiency, 240–242, 348
Vitamin deficiency states, 238–243, 348
Von Economo encephalitis, 124–126

Waldenström macroglobulinemia, 221
Wandering, and long-term care issues, 367, 372
Wechsler Adult Intelligence Scale, 14
    dementia of the Alzheimer's type (DAT) on, 50, 64
    Huntington's disease on, 98
    senility and, 337, 338
Wechsler Memory Test, 41, 129
Wernicke-Korsakoff syndrome, 238–240
Western equine encephalitis, 206
Whipple's disease, 209–210
White-matter hyperintensities, 356
Wilson's disease, 128–136, 334
    clinical features of, 130
    dementia with, 129
    early work with, 128–129
    laboratory evaluation of, 130–133
    liver disease in, 130
    pathology of, 133

pathophysiology of, 133–134
testing for, 348
treatment of, 134–136, 385
variants of, 129
Word lists
  dementia of the Alzheimer's type (DAT)
    and, 51

mental status examination with, 32
Writing, mental status examination of, 27

Xanthomatosis, cerebrotendinous, 328
X-ray studies, and diagnosis, 351–352

Zinc transport, in Pick's disease, 86

Friedrich's Ataxia — Alan
                    & Sister

Muscular Charcot Test   Ruth
                        Pushek

Parkinson's Caregivers — "Chrysler
                           wonder"
              YEARS OF
              Healing SXS

Cadmium poisoning after
spray painting
his new airplane
in a hanger that
was not well ventilated
He himself was a
prominent Neurologist

Alzheimer's dx that
Testing & evaluation
with Dr. Danny Watson